THERAPEUTIC APPLICATIONS OF PROSTAGLANDINS

THERAPEUTIC APPLICATIONS OF PROSTAGLANDINS

Edited by
John R Vane
DSc, FRS

Chairman, The William Harvey Research Institute, London

and
John O'Grady
MD, FRCP, FFPM

Medical Director for Europe, Daiichi Pharmaceutical Co. Ltd, London
Visiting Professor of Clinical Pharmacology, University of Vienna, Austria

Edward Arnold
A division of Hodder & Stoughton
LONDON BOSTON MELBOURNE AUCKLAND

1993

© 1993 Edward Arnold

First published in Great Britain 1993

Distributed in the Americas by Little, Brown and Company
34 Beacon Street, Boston, MA 02108

British Library Cataloguing in Publication Data

Vane, J. R.
  Therapeutic Applications of Prostaglandins.
  I. Title   II. O'Grady, John
  615
  ISBN 0-340-56022-3

Whilst the advice and information in this book is believed to be true and
accurate at the date of going to press, neither the author nor the
publisher can accept any legal responsibility or liability for any errors or
omissions that may be made. In particular (but without limiting the
generality of the preceding disclaimer) every effort has been made to
check drug dosages; however, it is still possible that errors have been
missed. Furthermore, dosage schedules are constantly being revised
and new side effects recognised. For these reasons the reader is
strongly urged to consult the manufacturer's printed instructions before
administering any of the drugs recommended in this book.

Typeset in 10/11pt Century Old Style by Rowland
Phototypesetting Limited, Bury St Edmunds, Suffolk.
Printed and bound in Great Britain for Edward Arnold,
a division of Hodder and Stoughton Limited, Mill Road,
Dunton Green, Sevenoaks, Kent TN13 2YA by
Butler and Tanner Limited, Frome and London.

Preface

Prostaglandin research has provided one of the most rapidly growing areas in the biological sciences. It had its beginnings in the detection of their activity in the early 1930s followed by the isolation and determination of the structure of the primary prostaglandins and the discovery that they are biosynthesized from essential fatty acids in almost all animal cells. In 1971 it was shown that the mode of action of aspirin-like drugs was by prevention of the biosynthesis of prostaglandins. This provided both an understanding of the basis for the therapeutic actions of aspirin and also a tool with which to study the physiological and pathological influences of the prostaglandins.

In 1974 the unstable endoperoxide intermediates in the prostaglandin cascade were isolated and identified. This laid the foundation for the discovery of the chemical structure of thromboxane A_2, a very potent but also very short lived substance made by the platelets which acts both as a vasoconstrictor and to induce platelets to come together to form a thrombus.

In 1976 it was established that the blood vessel wall manufactured a further unstable member of the prostaglandin family. This substance was first called PGX and then, when its chemical structure was determined, renamed prostacyclin. Prostacyclin has actions opposite to those of thromboxane A_2, being a vasodilator and powerfully preventing or reversing platelet clumping. The discovery of prostacyclin was followed by an explosion of research into its formation and activity, providing the basis of our understanding of why the healthy blood vessel wall is immune to the thrombosis which occurs when blood comes into contact with most foreign surfaces.

Research directed towards understanding the physiological and pharmacological roles of prostaglandins has been matched in recent years by clinical investigations to determine whether these substances or their chemical analogues have value in the treatment of disease in man. Given the ubiquitous nature of the prostaglandins and their potent and widespread effects on biological systems it is not surprising that the potential clinical indications which have been explored are diverse. They range from the important and established place of prostaglandins in termination of pregnancy and prevention of gastroduodenal ulceration through their life-saving effects in the management of congenital heart disease in the newborn to their actions in the treatment of intractable cardiac failure.

The present volume provides a comprehensive review of the potential therapeutic applications of prostaglandins written by experts in their use. It gives an up-to-date account of those areas where prostaglandins have been established as important therapeutic agents and also of those areas in which active investigation is still under way. To put these clinical perspectives into context the early chapters review the history, biochemical and pharmacological activities of prostaglandins, the opportunities for chemical analogues and mimetics and the ways in which novel delivery methods and formulations may overcome problems of absorption and instability.

We intend this book to provide a basis from which the now established therapeutic uses of the prostaglandins can be even further extended and explored.

John R Vane
John O'Grady
London, 1993

Contents

Contributors

Erik Änggård, MD, PhD
Professor of Pharmacology, The William Harvey Research Institute, St Bartholomew's Hospital Medical College, London EC1M 6BQ, UK

J J F Belch, MB ChB, MD, FRCP
Reader and Consultant Physician, Department of Medicine, University of Dundee, Ninewells Hospital and Medical School, Dundee DD1 9SY, UK

Bernd Buchmann, PhD
Research Associate, Research Laboratories of Schering AG, D-1000 Berlin 65, Germany

Andrew Bush, MD, MRCP
Senior Lecturer in Paediatric Respiratory Medicine, National Heart and Lung Institute, London SW3 2NP, UK

A Yazdani Butt, MRCP
Clinical Fellow, Papworth Hospital, Papworth Everard, Cambridge CB3 8RE, UK

Marc Bygdeman, MD, PhD
Professor of Obstetrics and Gynecology, and Medical Director, Karolinska Hospital, S-104 01 Stockholm, Sweden

A A Calder, MD, FRCP, FRCOG
Professor and Head of Department of Obstetrics and Gynaecology, University of Edinburgh, Edinburgh EH3 9EW, UK; Honorary Consultant Obstetrician and Gynaecologist, Simpson Memorial Maternity Pavilion and Royal Infirmary of Edinburgh

Robert A Coleman, MIBiol, PhD
Senior Research Associate, Department of Cardiovascular and Respiratory Pharmacology, Glaxo Group Research Limited, Ware, Hertfordshire SG12 0DP, UK

Christy L Cooper, PhD
Division of Clinical Research, Wellcome Research Laboratories, Burroughs Wellcome Company, Research Triangle Park, North Carolina 27709, USA

James W Crow, PhD
Associate Director and Project Leader, Division of Clinical Research, Wellcome Research Laboratories, Burroughs Wellcome Company, Research Triangle Park, North Carolina 27709, USA; Adjunct Associate Professor, School of Pharmacy, University of North Carolina at Chapel Hill, North Carolina

Donald M Demke, MD
Clinical Research Manager, Clinical Development Unit I, The Upjohn Company, Kalamazoo, Michigan 49001, USA

Jørn Dyerberg, Md, DmedSc
Chief Physician, Medi-Lab a.s., DK-1304 Copenhagen K, Denmark

M G Elder, MD, FRCS, FRCOG
Professor of Obstetrics and Gynaecology, Institute of Obstetrics and Gynaecology, Royal Postgraduate
   Medical School, London W12 0NN, UK

Rod Flower, PhD, DSc
Professor of Biochemical Pharmacology, The William Harvey Research Institute, St Bartholomew's Hospital
   Medical College, London EC1M 6BQ, UK

A E S Gimson, MB BS, MRCP
The Institute of Liver Studies, King's College School of Medicine and Dentistry, London SE5 9PJ, UK

H Graf
Research Laboratories of Schering AG, D-1000 Berlin 65, Germany

M Greaves, MD, FRCP, MRCPath
Reader in Haematology and Honorary Consultant Physician, Royal Hallamshire Hospital, Sheffield S10 2JF, UK

Richard J Gryglewski, MD, hcDSc
Professor of Pharmacology, Nicolaus Copernicus University School of Medicine, 31 531 Cracow, Poland

Jacqueline G Hanss, BSc
Research Assistant, Department of Clinical Pharmacology, Royal Postgraduate Medical School, London
   W12 0NN, UK

C J Hawkey, DM, FRCP
Professor of Gastroenterology, Division of Gastroenterology, University Hospital, Nottingham NG7 2UH, UK

T W Higenbottam, BSc, MA, MD, FRCP
Consultant Physician and Director of the Respiratory Physiology Department, Papworth Hospital, Papworth
   Everard, Cambridge CB3 8RE, UK

Patrick P A Humphrey, BPharm, PhD, DSc, FRPharmS
Director, Glaxo Institute of Applied Pharmacology, Department of Pharmacology, University of Cambridge,
   Cambridge CB2 1QJ, UK

Ulrich Klar, PhD
Research Associate, Research Laboratories of Schering AG, D-1000 Berlin 65, Germany

Steen Dalby Kristensen, MD, DMSc
University Department of Cardiology, Skejby Hospital, DK-8200 Aarhus N, Denmark

Otto I Linet, MD, PhD
Director, Clinical Development, The Upjohn Company, Kalamazoo, Michigan 49001, USA

Walker A Long, MD
Director, Cardiopulmonary Medicine, Division of Clinical Research, Wellcome Research Laboratories,
   Burroughs Wellcome Company, Research Triangle Park, North Carolina 27709, USA; Research Associate
   Professor and Attending Physician, Department of Pediatrics, University of North Carolina at Chapel Hill,
   Chapel Hill, North Carolina

J F Martin, MD, FRCP
British Heart Foundation Professor of Cardiovascular Science, Department of Medicine, King's College School of Medicine & Dentistry, London SE5 9JP, UK; Honorary Consultant Physician, King's College Hospital, London, and Head of Cardiovascular Research, Wellcome Research Laboratories

Hartmut Rehwinkel, PhD
Research Associate, Research Laboratories of Schering AG, D-1000 Berlin 65, Germany

G M Rubanyi
Research Laboratories of Schering AG, D-1000 Berlin 65, Germany

Elliot A Shinebourne, MD, FRCP
Consultant Paediatric Cardiologist, Royal Brompton National Heart and Lung Hospital, London SW3 2NP, UK

Helmut Sinzinger, MD
Professor of Nuclear Medicine and Atherosclerosis Research, Wilhelm Auerswald Atherosclerosis Research Group, A-1090 Vienna, Austria

G Stock
Research Laboratories of Schering AG, D-1000 Berlin 65, Germany

Graham W Taylor, BA, PhD
Senior Lecturer, Department of Clinical Pharmacology, Royal Postgraduate Medical School, London W12 0NN, UK

Helmut Vorbrüggen, PhD
Deputy Head, Research Laboratories of Schering AG, D-1000 Berlin 65, Germany

J Wallwork, FRCS
Consultant Cardiothoracic Surgeon and Director of Transplant Service, Papworth Hospital, Papworth Everard, Cambridge CB3 8RE, UK

Åke Wennmalm, MD, PhD
Professor of Clinical Physiology, Department of Clinical Physiology, Gothenburg University, Sahlgrensk's Hospital, S-413 45 Gothenburg, Sweden

William S Wheeler, MD
Division of Clinical Research, Wellcome Research Laboratories, Burroughs Wellcome Company, Research Triangle Park, North Carolina 27709, USA

B J R Whittle, PhD, DSc
Head, Department of Pharmacology, Wellcome Research Laboratories, Beckenham, Kent BR3 3BS, UK

1 Essential fatty acids and prostaglandins – an introductory overview

Erik Änggård and Rod Flower

In the 1930s Sir Henry Dale coined the term *autopharmacology* to describe the pharmacological actions of naturally occurring substances which he described as local hormones. At that time most interest was focused on acetylcholine and histamine. Both these simple chemical messengers are derived from amino acids. Many other hormones too are themselves amino acids, or derived from amino acids, or are peptides. Few investigators at that time could have anticipated the emergence of an entirely new group of hormones derived from lipids. At the time, these were regarded as a heterologous collection of 'greasy' substances whose main function was as structural components of tissues. In adipose tissue the neutral lipids represented a useful metabolic store: in the diet 'fat' was a convenient, though not essential, source of nutritional energy. That we now know this view to be naïve, to say the least, is due to a sequence of seminal, though apparently unrelated, findings made in the 1920s and 1930s, namely the discovery of the essential fatty acids and the prostaglandins.

Essential fatty acids

In the 1920s it was recognized that certain lipids were necessary for survival and reproduction in small rodents. The first of these factors was initially designated factor X by Evans and Scott, and later named vitamin E (tocopherol) when the pure compound with vitamin-like activity was isolated in 1936. Another vitamin-like lipid factor was found by George and Mildred Burr to be present in the fatty acid fraction of the diet and was provisionally named vitamin F.[1] Absence of vitamin F led to severe growth retardation, reproductive failure and characteristic dermatological changes such as flaky skin and a scaly tail. After assessing the curative value of many different oils of defined fatty acid composition and individual fatty acids the Burrs were able to show that the active factor was in fact linoleic acid.[2] At the same time they coined the phrase 'essential fatty acid' to denote the importance of the linoleic group of unsaturated fatty acids for the well-being of the organism.

This fundamental discovery of the Burrs initiated an entirely new field of lipid research, and rapid advances were soon made in understanding their role in tissue growth and cell membrane function. In the last 30 years the availability of modern separation techniques and radioactive isotopes has enabled lipid biochemists to map out detailed pathways of essential fatty acid biosynthesis and metabolism.[3,4]

The most abundant *saturated* fatty acids are palmitic (C-16) and stearic acids (C-18). They are mostly derived from dietary intake of lipids but can also be made endogenously from two-carbon fragments derived from intermediary metabolism. These can, if need be, become desaturated to form unsaturated fatty acids belonging to the ω7 series (palmitoleic acid) and ω9 series (oleic acid). In essential fatty acid deficiency this endogenous pathway is activated, presumably to compensate for the failing intake of polyunsaturated fatty acids. The essential fatty acids of the ω3 and ω6 series must be taken through the diet. The interconversions of the polyunsaturated fatty acids of this series are shown in Fig. 1.1.

Today the term 'essential fatty acid' (EFA) embraces the group of unsaturated fatty acids which cannot be made by mammals. Quantitatively arachidonic acid (20:4ω6) is the most abundant of the EFAs in land-dwelling animals (including man) although this depends to a large extent on the diet. Eicosapentaenoic acid (EPA, 20:5ω3) is almost undetectable in most land-dwelling species but is present in much larger amounts in the tissues of marine animals and, therefore, of any species living mainly on a diet of marine animals. Eskimos and other ethnic groups with a diet high in fish, seal and whale meat have much higher levels of EPA and other ω3 fatty acids. It is believed that the lower incidence of heart disease in such ethnic groups is related to the high intake of ω3 EFAs.[5]

Although the Burrs discovered the essential nature of the polyunsaturated fatty acids, it took over 30 years for this finding to be linked to molecular mechanisms regulating cell function. In 1964 Bergström *et al.* and Van Dorp *et al.* independently discovered that 20:3ω6, 20:4ω6 and 20:5ω3 were the obligatory precursors of the prostaglandins, a newly discovered family of lipid hormones.[6,7] The prostaglandins as a separate entity had, however, been established much earlier.

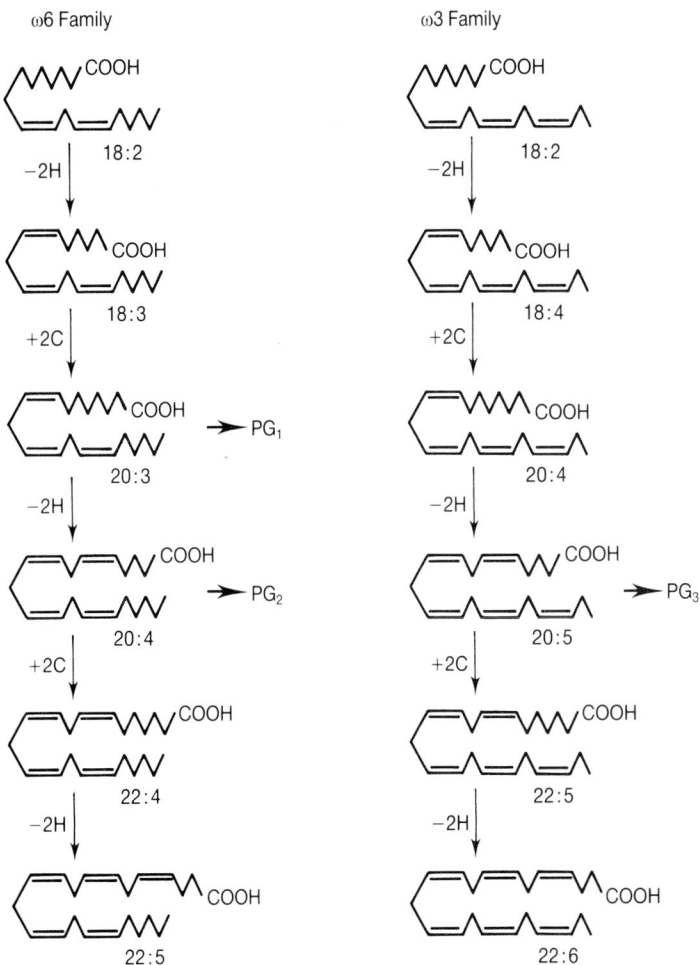

Fig. 1.1 Interconversion of essential fatty acids of the ω6 and ω3 series.

Prostaglandins and related substances

In 1933 and 1934 Goldblatt and von Euler independently described the presence of a vasodepressor and smooth muscle stimulating factor in human seminal fluid.[8,9] Von Euler established that it had acidic lipid properties and was present in the male accessory genital glands and, therefore, proposed the name 'prostaglandin' for the new substance.[9] It is now realized that the main source of prostaglandins in the semen is the vesicular gland rather than the prostate but, by then, the name had become firmly established.

After the Second World War von Euler encouraged a young biochemist, Sune Bergström, to purify prostaglandin and to characterize it further chemically. The first attempt led to a 500 000-fold purification of a sheep vesicular gland extract. The purified factor was a nitrogen-free unsaturated hydroxy-fatty acid with a UV absorption at 280 nm. After a decade of refining chromatographic techniques, Bergström and Sjövall were able to isolate two crystalline prostaglandins, named prostaglandin E_1 and F_1, in 1960.[10,11] The complete structures of these compounds were reported by Bergström et al. in 1963.[12] The chemical structure proved to be a five-membered ring with two side chains of which one carried a carboxyl group. The hypothetical parent acid was named 'prostanoic acid' (Fig. 1.2). In the prostaglandins themselves double bonds are present at carbon 5 (cis) and 13 (trans) and in some compounds also at carbon 17 (cis). Functional groups are typically present at carbons 9, 11 and 15. Thus prostaglandin E_2 (Fig. 1.2) is chemically named 9-keto-11,15-dihydroxy-prosta-5(cis), 13 (trans) dienoic acid.

It was soon recognized that the prostaglandins could conveniently be divided into families denoted by a letter (A–J) after the letters PG. This suffix initially indicated the method by which that particular PG could be isolated or formed. Thus PGE was more soluble in Ether, PGF had higher affinity for phosphate buffer ('Fosfat' in Swedish), PGA was formed by treatment with dilute Acid and PGB by treatment with a Base such as sodium hydroxide. At the time of writing the prostaglandin family ranges from PGA to PGJ. Almost 200 derivatives of prostanoic acid have now been shown to occur naturally and many more synthesized in the pharmaceutical industry. The main structural features of the prostaglandins are shown in Fig. 1.2. The subscript number, as in PGE_1 and PGE_2, indicates the number of double bonds (in this case one and two respectively) in the side chains of the molecule.

Several new developments came in the 1970s. In 1971 Vane[13] and his colleagues[14] discovered that aspirin and virtually all other non-steroidal anti-inflammatory drugs (NSAIDs) inhibited prostaglandin synthesis. This provided not only a biochemical basis for the antipyretic, analgesic and anti-inflammatory reactions of NSAIDs but also a

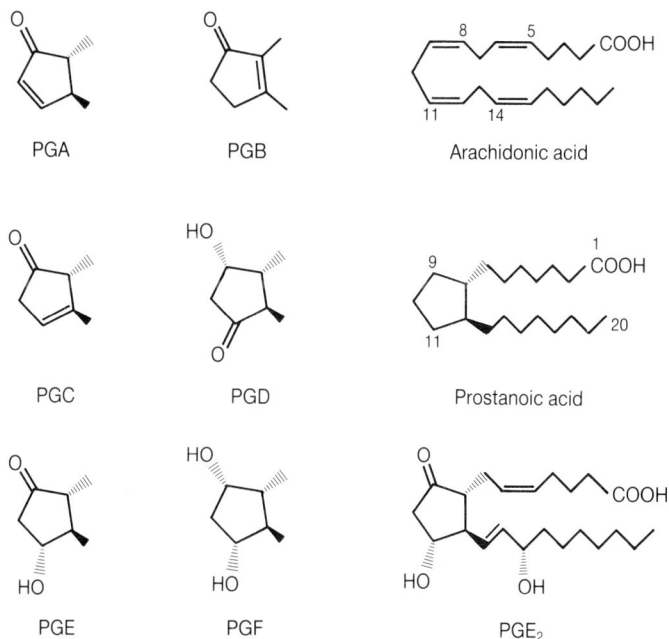

Fig. 1.2 Structures of arachidonic acid, prostanoic acid, PGE_2 and the ring structures of other main prostanoids.

tool to evaluate the role of prostaglandins in patho-physiology. Vane proposed that the therapeutic actions as well as the side effects of the NSAIDs could be explained by the inhibition of prostaglandin biosynthesis.[13] Time has largely borne out this view and this concept has led to the rational design of several anti-inflammatory drugs. More recently, NSAID design has been directed towards inhibition of an inducible form of the PGH synthase.[15] It is hoped that the specific inhibition of this iso-enzyme could lead to therapeutic benefit with less side effects.

Another important development in the early 1970s was the isolation of the cyclic endoperoxide PGH$_2$.[16,17] The presence of this prostaglandin as an intermediate in the prostaglandin biosynthesis had already been postulated by Samuelsson on the basis

of experiments with $^{18}O_2$.[18] Endoperoxides with a hydroperoxy group at position 15 were called PGG whilst those with an alcohol group were called PGH.

Studies by Piper and Vane[19] had indicated the presence of a labile 'rabbit aorta contracting sub-stance' (RCS) released from anaphylactically shocked lung and suggested that it might be identical to the postulated[18] prostaglandin endoperoxide inter-mediate. A 'labile aggregation stimulating sub-stance' (LASS) was also found to be present in platelets in response to thrombotic stimuli.[20] Finally, in 1973 the postulated endoperoxides were isolated by Hamberg and Samuelsson[16] and by Nugteren and Hazelhof,[17] and found to contract vascular and respir-atory smooth muscle and to cause platelet aggrega-tion. The availability of pure PGG$_2$/H$_2$[21] led to a new impetus in prostaglandin research and several new

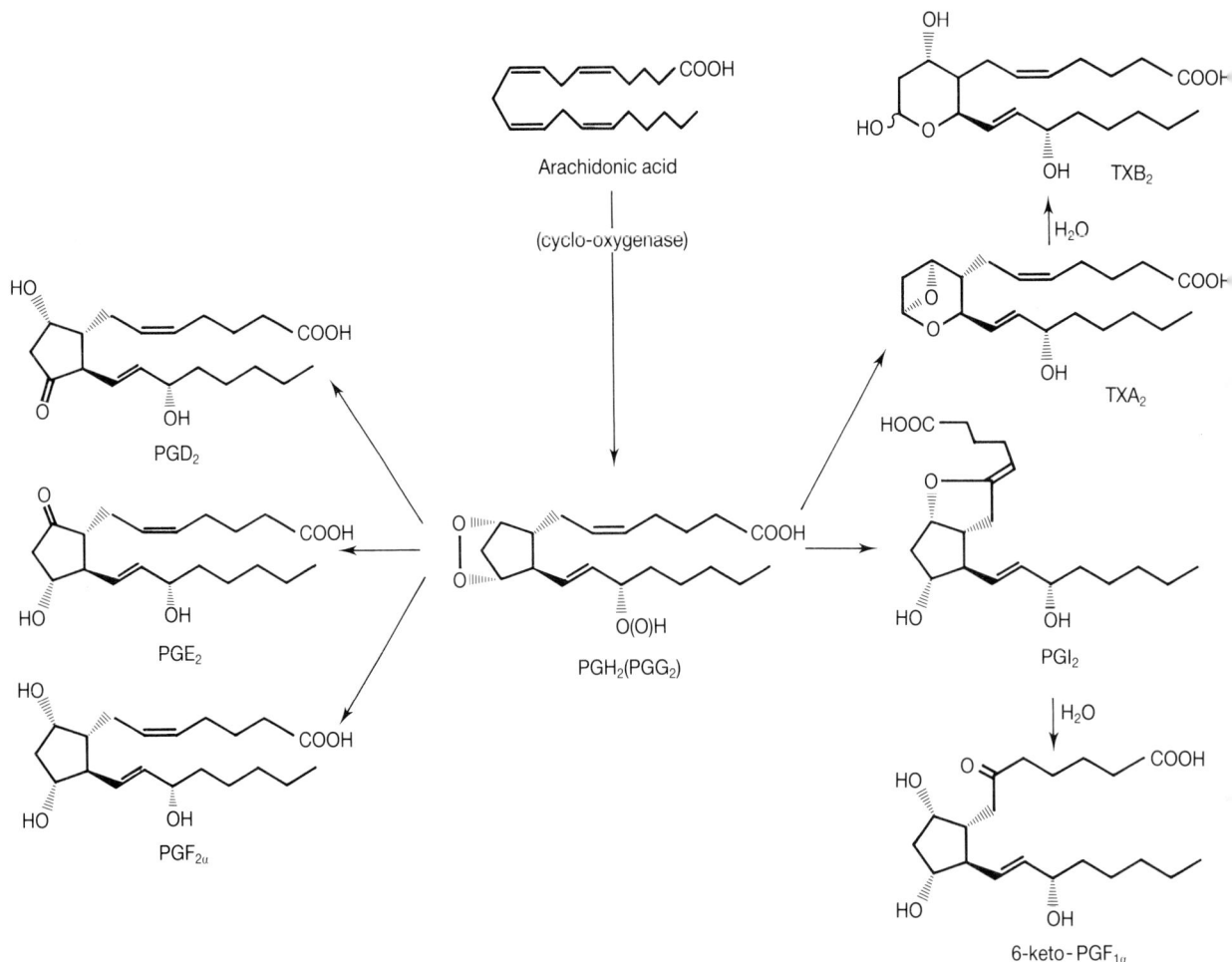

Fig. 1.3   Formation of prostanoids from arachidonic acid through the labile intermediate PGG$_α$.

pathways were discovered. A labile aggregatory vasoconstrictor substance (presumably identical to RCS) was found to be the major endoperoxide metabolite in lung and in platelets.[22] This was found to have a new oxetane ring structure and was subsequently named thromboxane A_2 (TXA$_2$). Its structure is found in Fig. 1.3. In aqueous solution it rapidly decomposes to TXB$_2$.

Another pathway for metabolism of endoperoxides was found by Moncada, Vane and others[23] working with bovine aortic microsomes. They showed the formation of a labile substance provisionally termed 'prostaglandin X' which had vasodilator and anti-aggregatory properties. The structure was quickly

established in collaboration with Upjohn chemists, and the trivial name 'prostacyclin' (PGI$_2$) was adopted.[24] Its structure is shown in Fig. 1.3. Prostacyclin has a half-life of minutes in blood. It degrades to 6-keto-PGF$_{1\alpha}$ (Fig. 1.3) which is now widely used as an index of prostacyclin formation.

A number of additional oxygenation pathways of arachidonic acid have also been described (Fig. 1.4). Perhaps the most important is the 5-lipoxygenase pathway leading to the formation of leukotrienes.[25] This group of substances was earlier described as the slow-reacting substance of anaphylaxis (SRS-A), as they were released from anaphylactically challenged tissue. The leukotrienes (LT) designated

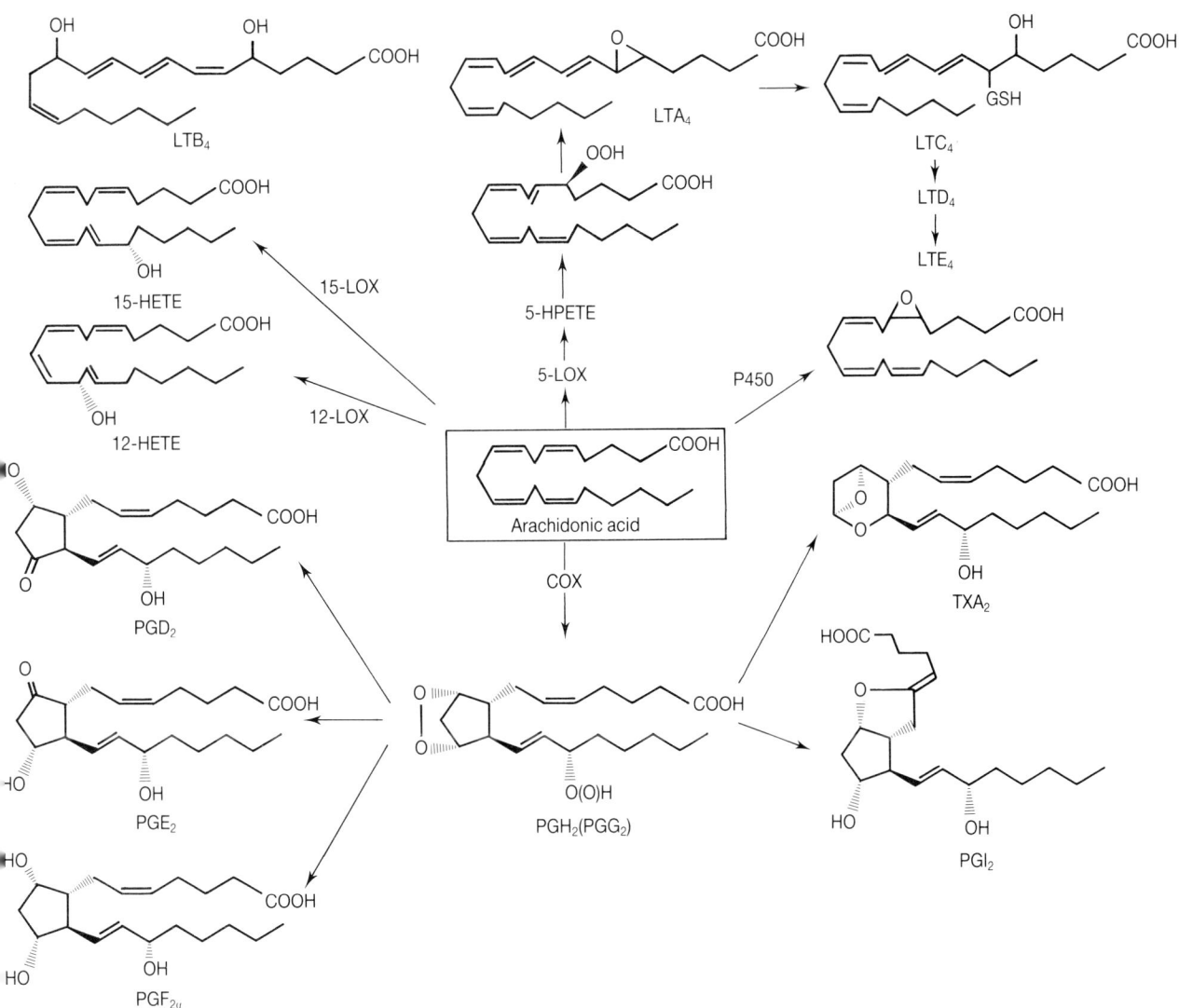

Fig. 1.4 The main pathways in the transformation of arachidonic acid by cellular oxygenases.

LTA_4, LTB_4 mediate neutrophil chemotaxis, and the peptide-containing leukotrienes LTC_4, LTD_4 and LTE_4 cause bronchoconstriction and increased vascular permeability.

Other lipoxygenases attach oxygen at the 12 and 15 positions. The 12-hydroperoxy (12-HPETE) and 12-hydroxy fatty acids (12-HETE) may inhibit neurotransmitter release in platelets and in the brain. The role of the 15-lipoxygenase pathway is at present not clear. An overview of the formation of prostaglandins and related factors from essential fatty acids is indicated in Fig. 1.4.

Arachidonic acid can also be metabolized by cytochrome P450 to epoxides at each of the four double bonds.[26] Some of these (e.g. the 5, 6 epoxide) can be converted by PGH synthase into 5-hydroxy PGs.[27] Finally, lipoxins (LX) have been shown to be formed from 15-HETE in neutrophil suspension.[28] They are trihydroxytetraenoic acids; e.g. 5,6,15-trihydroxyeicosatetraenoic acid (LXA_4). Several positional isomers exist.

The term 'prostaglandins' originally described derivatives of prostanoic acid but the term 'prostanoids' is now used to include also cyclo-oxygenase products, including prostacyclin and thromboxanes. The term 'eicosanoids' encompasses all 20-carbon fatty acids including products from cyclo-oxygenase, lipoxygenases and cytochrome P450-catalysed oxygenation products.

Metabolism of prostanoids

The earliest work on the metabolic transformation of PGs was performed by Änggård and Samuelsson.[29] They showed that both PGE and PGF compounds undergo rapid dehydrogenation at carbon-15 catalysed by 15-hydroxy-prostaglandin dehydrogenase. This enzyme, which occurs in several isoforms, is abundant in lung, liver and kidney.[30] The resulting 15-keto metabolites are much less biologically active as compared to the parent PG, and the initial metabolic transformation, therefore, represents a biological inactivation.[31] Indeed, Ferreira and Vane using the blood-bathed organ technique showed that PGE_2 and $PGF_{2\alpha}$ compounds were inactivated by a single passage across the lung.[32] However, PGA_2 and PGI_2 were less actively removed and could, therefore, survive longer in the circulation.

The second step in the metabolism of the prostaglandins is the saturation of the Δ^{13} double bond. This step, catalysed by a $\Delta^{13,14}$-reductase, can act only on prostaglandins that have first undergone oxidation of the 15-hydroxyl group.[33] The major metabolite in homogenates of lung, kidney and other tissues and also in plasma is the 15-keto,13,14-dihydro prostaglandin metabolite.

In lung homogenates 13,14-dihydro-15-hydroxy metabolites (e.g. dihydro-PGE_1) also occurred as a major metabolite of primary prostaglandins. These compounds do not arise from the direct reduction of the Δ^{13} double bond of the parent PG but from the reduction of the 15-hydroxyl group of the 13,14-dihydro-15-keto metabolites.[33] Dihydro-PGE_1 is almost as biologically active as PGE_1.[31] It is also resistant to inactivation by the lung. Following infusion of PGE_1 in humans, high concentrations of dihydro-PGE_1 have been observed.[34] Therefore, PGE_1 and, by inference, other primary PGs could act through more long lived 13,14-dihydro metabolites.

Although PGI_2 is inactivated by non-enzymatic mechanisms to 6-keto-$PGF_{1\alpha}$ it is also metabolized by the 15-hydroxyprostaglandin dehydrogenase pathway to 6,15-diketo metabolites.[35,36]

The lungs occupy a strategic position between the venous and arterial circulation. They are, therefore, ideally placed to remove hormones such as bradykinin, histamine and the prostaglandins which may leak into the circulation, with deleterious results. In the case of many prostaglandins, a single passage usually results in over 90% destruction. Others may selectively pass across the lungs.[37]

Thus a dual enzyme system catalyses the early steps in the metabolic removal of prostaglandins. However, this is not the final metabolic step. Two more enzymatic processes occur in order to convert the prostanoids into a more polar form suitable for excretion by the kidney. This occurs by shortening the carboxyl side chain through β-oxidation and by introducing another carboxyl group by oxidation of the ω end of the molecule.[38] The enzymes catalysing these reactions are present largely in the liver and kidney. The final end metabolite occurring in the urine is, therefore, a molecule with 16 or 18 carbons and with carboxyl groups on both side chains. The main urinary metabolites (MUM) for the major prostanoids are shown in Figs. 1.5 and 1.6.

Prostaglandin D_2 is a prostaglandin found most abundantly in mast cells,[39] in skin[40] and in the brain.[41,42] It does not follow the established pattern of metabolic degradation, at least not in man. Following the injection of PGD_2 into the circulation a substantial part is recovered as $PGF_{2\alpha}$ metabolites.[43,44] Therefore, at some stage a reduction of the 11-keto group of PGD_2 must take place but it is not clear whether PGD_2 is converted to $PGF_{2\alpha}$-like

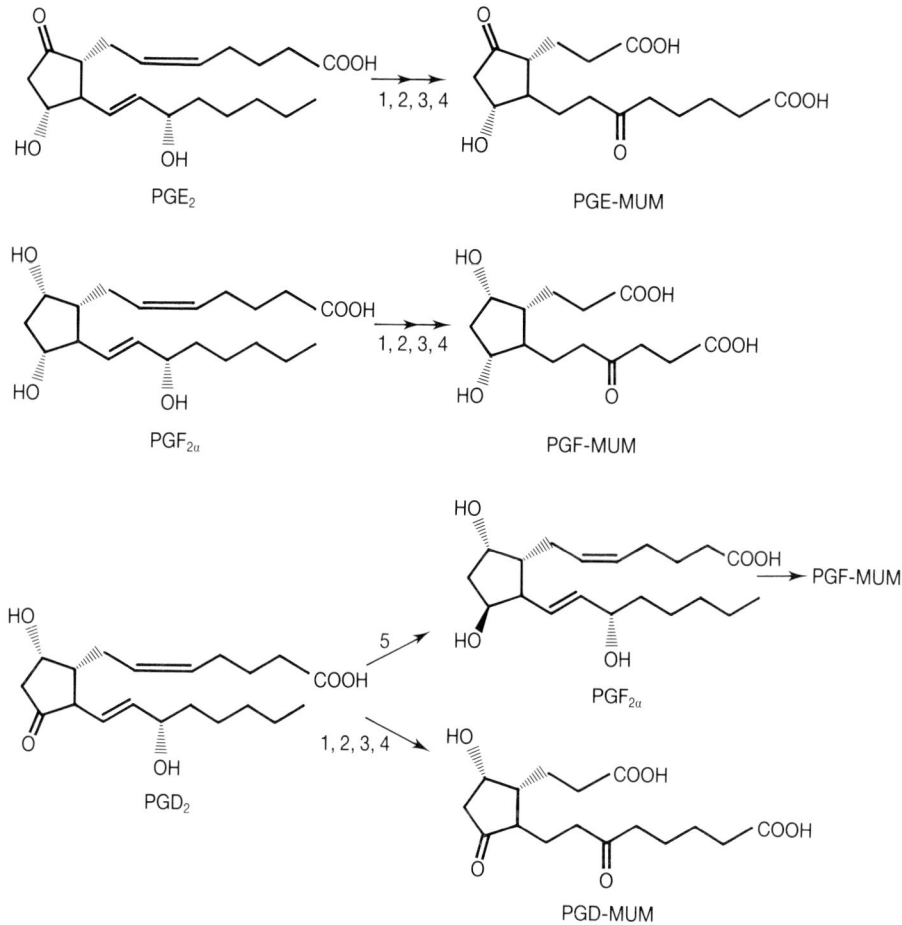

Fig. 1.5 Main metabolic pathways for PGE$_2$, PGF$_{2\alpha}$ and PGD$_2$ in man. Main urinary metabolites indicated by MUM. Enzymatic mechanisms involved are 15-OH-dehydrogenase (1), 13,14-reductase (2), β-oxidation (3) and ω-oxidation (4).

structures before or after metabolism by 15-hydroxyprostaglandin dehydrogenase.

The measurement of urinary prostaglandin metabolites (e.g. PGE-MUM, PGF-MUM, dinor thromboxane B$_2$ and dinor-6-keto-PGF$_{1\alpha}$) can provide only an index of the endogenous production of prostaglandins. Obviously, hormonal factors, diet, disease or drugs can influence the prostaglandin-metabolizing enzymes which in turn can alter the proportion of the metabolite measured.[45-49] For instance, the prostaglandin dehydrogenase is sensitive to hormonal control, as illustrated by the pregnant female of several mammalian species. The prostaglandin-metabolizing activity of the lung and placenta of the pregnant animal is greatly enhanced by up to 20-fold. This is presumably because several prostaglandins, particularly PGF$_{2\alpha}$, have a potent contractile effect on the uterus and it would clearly be disastrous to have high levels of this compound circulating mid-term, as it may cause abortion. There is some evidence that the high levels of prostaglandin dehydrogenase fall immediately before parturition, allowing levels of oxytocic prostaglandins to rise. There are also age-related changes in prostaglandin-metabolizing enzymes in cells. This is especially well studied with respect to neonatal animals. Pathological conditions are also known to influence prostaglandin metabolism. Endotoxin shock is associated with elevated levels of plasma prostaglandin. Whereas undoubtedly this is due to enhanced rate of formation and release it is also clear that the metabolic capacity is reduced.

Medicinal chemists synthesizing prostaglandin analogues for therapeutic purposes have long been mindful of the efficient metabolic degradation of endogenous prostaglandins and have devised ways of creating metabolically more stable analogues.[50] The most obvious ways are to block the dehydrogenation

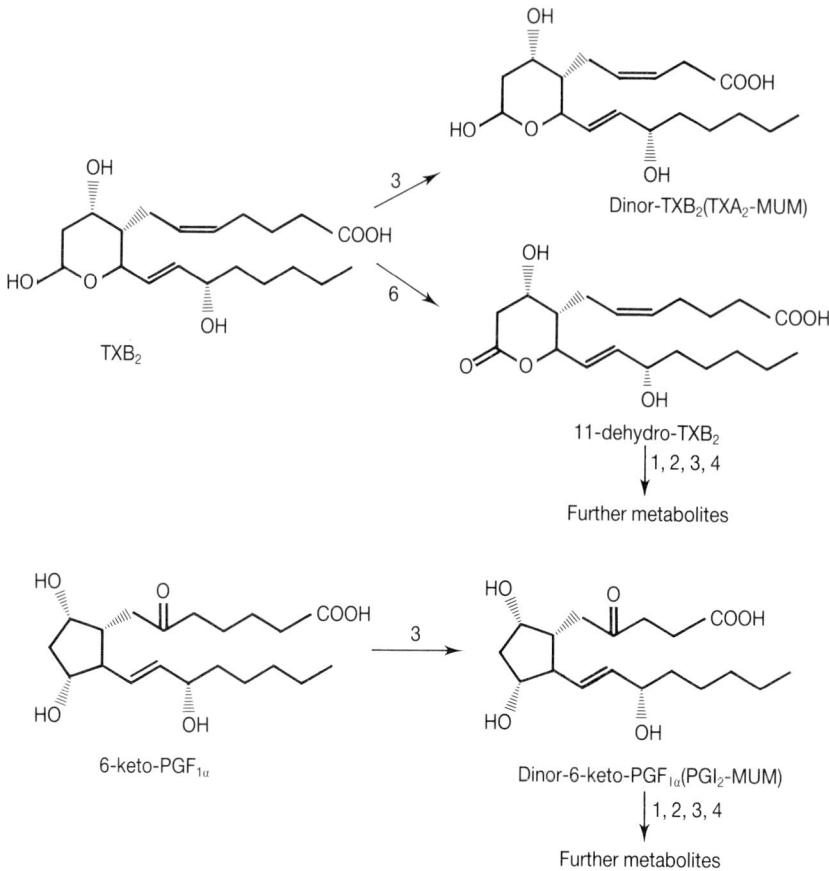

Fig. 1.6   Main metabolic pathways for PGI$_2$ and TXA$_2$. PGI$_2$ is rapidly converted to 6-keto-PGF$_{1\alpha}$ and TXA$_2$ to TXB$_2$, from which the main urinary metabolites are derived. TXB$_2$ is excreted either unchanged or following a single step of β-oxidation (3) to dinor-TXB$_2$. A large part of TXB$_2$ is also dehydrogenated (6) to 11-dehydro-TXB$_2$ which is then further transformed by 15-OH-dehydrogenase (1), 13,14-reductase(2), β-oxidation (3) and ω oxidation (4). A substantial part of 6-keto-PGF$_{1\alpha}$ is excreted as dinor-6-keto-PGF$_{1\alpha}$.

at carbon-15 by substituting the 15 or 16 hydrogen for a methyl group, and to block β-oxidation by substitution at the carboxyl end of the molecule.

Actions of prostanoids

Prostanoids are, with few exceptions, local hormones. The action of prostanoids in any given cell or tissue depends on the interactions of several factors:

1. On the type (20:3ω6, 20:4ω6, 20:5ω3) and availability of precursor in the cellular pool available to the local PGH synthase
2. The activity/turnover rate of the PGH synthase and cofactors
3. The profile of endoperoxide-metabolizing enzymes
4. The profile and density of prostanoid receptors on the local target cells

Because prostanoids have so many diverse actions

(reviewed in reference 59) we can give only an outline of the biological activities displayed by this diverse group of substances. These are presented in Table 1.1.

Cardiovascular actions

Arachidonic acid (20:4,ω6) is a potent vasoactive agent producing vasodilatation in the kidney, gastrointestinal and other vascular beds.[51] Homo-γ-linoleic acid (20:3ω6) is less potent and eicosapentaenoic acid (20:5ω3) is relatively inactive. These effects must be ascribed to the transformation to prostanoids in the body as the effects are abolished by NSAIDs. PGE$_2$, PGD$_2$ and PGI$_2$ are vasodilatory and cause hypotension when injected into the blood stream.[52,53] PGF$_{2\alpha}$ causes vasoconstriction when added to vascular strips *in vitro*. Injected intravenously into rabbits, however, its effects are hypotensive, probably due to a constriction of pulmonary blood vessels.[52,54] PGE$_2$, PGD$_2$ and PGI$_2$ also inhibit platelet aggregation by stimulating the formation of cyclic cAMP.[55]

Table 1.1   Biological actions of prostanoids

Cardiovascular	Increased blood flow/hypotension	PGE_2, PGI_2, PGD_2
	Decreased blood flow	TXA_2, $PGF_{2\alpha}$
	Inhibition of platelet aggregation	PGI_2, PGE_2, PGD_2
	Stimulates platelet aggregation	TXA_2, $PGG_2(H_2)$
Renal	Decreased blood flow	TXA_2, $PGF_{2\alpha}$
	Increased blood flow	PGI_2, PGE_2
	Increased renin release	PGI_2
	Increased H_2O transport	PGE_2
Respiratory	Bronchoconstriction	$PGF_{2\alpha}$, TXA_2
Gastrointestinal	Inhibition of acid secretion	PGE_2
	Cytoprotection	PGE_2
	Increased blood flow	PGI_2
	Increased motility, diarrhoea	PGE_2, $PGF_{2\alpha}$
Brain	Sleep–wake cycle	PGE_2, PGD_2
	Long-term potentiation	20:4
Female reproduction	Uterine motility, parturition	$PGF_{2\alpha}$
	Luteolysis	$PGF_{2\alpha}$
Male reproduction	Fertility?	PGE, 19-OH-PGE_1

Prostanoids endogenously formed in the vascular endothelium, in particular PGI_2, contribute to endothelial thromboresistance. The therapeutic effects of PGE_1 and stable prostacyclin analogues in peripheral vascular disease are probably due to a reversal of the microcirculatory dysfunction by dilatation and enhanced thromboresistance by inhibiting the clumping and sticking of platelets and leucocytes to the vascular wall.[57]

TXA_2 formed by aggregating platelets is a potent vasoconstrictor and mediator of the aggregation response.[22,55] The short half-life of TXA_2 has made studies on its effects difficult and most available data are from studies *in vitro*. The 11,9-epoxymethano analogue of PGH_2 U-46619 is claimed to be a stable TXA_2 mimetic.[56] U-46619 is a potent vasoconstrictor of coronary and renal arteries and increases blood pressure. The most important action of TXA_2 is most likely its proposed proaggregatory effect which is the molecular basis for the use of low dose aspirin and thromboxane synthesis inhibitors in the prevention and treatment of cardiovascular disease. Dosage schedules of aspirin are kept low so as to inhibit platelet thromboxane formation while sparing the formation of endothelial PGI_2.[58]

Renal

One of the earliest effects found for prostaglandins was that PGE_1 blocked the action of the antidiuretic hormone on renal water permeability.[60] This is mediated through activation of the adenylate cyclase in the collecting ducts. Activation of the renal prostanoid system by infusion of arachidonic acid leads to enhanced renal blood flow, particularly in the medulla,[51] and the release of renin, an effect thought to be mediated by PGI_2.[61] Renal failure is associated with enhanced production of TXA_2 having vasoconstrictor action.[62] Long-term intake of NSAIDs can have a deleterious effect on kidney function, particularly in diseases such as congestive heart failure, renal insufficiency and liver cirrhosis. It is thought that this is due to impaired renal synthesis of vasodilating prostanoids rich in PGI_2.[63]

Gastrointestinal

PGE_2 and PGI_2 are present in every part of the gastrointestinal tract, with the higher rates of synthesis in the stomach.[64] PGE_2 and PGI_2 in gastric mucosa are thought to have a role in controlling gastric acid secretions, protecting the mucosal barrier and regulating blood flow and motility.[65] Inhibition of gastric prostanoid production by aspirin and other NSAIDs is, therefore, associated with gastric mucosal erosion and bleeding. PGE_2 analogues as well as PGI_2 have been shown to inhibit gastric acid secretion and prevent gastric side effects of NSAIDs.[66,67] Prostaglandins have, therefore, been proposed to act as 'cytoprotective' agents in the gastric mucosa.[68] Over all, prostaglandins with anti-ulcer effects protect the mucosa by two different mechanisms: inhibition of acid secretion and stimulation of bicarbonate and mucosal secretion. PGE and PGF compounds also lead to increased contractions and motility in the gastrointestinal tract. Intake of $PGF_{2\alpha}$ (e.g. in vaginal pessaries to stimulate uterine contractions) is, therefore, frequently associated with abdominal cramps and diarrhoea.

Brain

The role of the eicosanoids in the brain has been intensively studied but is not well understood. PGE_2 and PGD_2 synthesis is specifically localized and the actions of these prostanoids suggest a role in the sleep–wake cycle.[42] Arachidonic acid and some of its lipoxygenase metabolites are implicated in neurotransmission and 'long-term potentiation', a phenomenon thought to be connected with memory.[69] PGE_2 and PGF_2 are synthesized by decidua and myometrium. The capacity of these tissues to produce prostaglandins rises progressively during pregnancy.

Reproduction

$PGF_{2\alpha}$ and PGE_2 have strong effects on uterine motility. Either the natural prostanoids or analogues are used to induce therapeutic abortion, and, at the end of term, to stimulate cervical ripening and onset of labour.[70] In cattle and horses $PGF_{2\alpha}$ has a luteolytic effect and is used by veterinary surgeons to synchronize oestrus prior to artificial insemination programmes.[71]

The very high levels of PGE_1 compounds and 19-hydroxylated PGE compounds in human seminal fluids are suggestive of a physiological role but as yet are not clarified. A role in ejaculation was suggested early by von Euler but has not been confirmed. A subgroup of sterile men were found to have reduced seminal fluid levels of PGE compounds.

Prostanoid receptors

In recent years a general classification of prostaglandin receptors has emerged.[72] Prostanoid receptors are denoted by 'P' after the letter describing the family of prostanoid. Thus a prostaglandin F receptor is called FP, thromboxane receptor TP and so on. This is shown in Table 1.2.

A range of analogues have been synthesized to interact with specific receptors. Some of the more selective agonists and antagonists are listed in Table 1.2. Others interact less specifically and could also have inhibitory effects on prostanoid biosynthesis. Thus some thromboxane receptor antagonists also inhibit thromboxane synthesis.

The effector pathways of prostanoids are either through the activation of adenylate cyclase or through the inositol phosphate/diacylglycerol pathway. Activation of DP, EP_2 and IP receptors leads to elevation of cAMP.

There appears to be a coupling between cyclic nucleotide effector pathways as activation of adenylate cyclase, e.g. by IP receptors, and activation of guanylate cyclase by nitric oxide (NO) or a NO-donor are synergistic with respect to many effects (e.g. on vascular smooth muscle and on platelets).[73,74]

Prostanoids in disease

Due to the multiplicity of effect observed following application of prostaglandins, many roles for prostanoids and other eicosanoids have been proposed in

Table 1.2 Prostanoid receptors (After TIPS, January 1991[77])

Name	DP	EP_1, EP_2, EP_3	FP	IP	TP
Prostanoid	PGD	PGE	PGF	PGI_2	TXA
Potency order	D>E,F,I,T	E>F,I>D,T	F>D>E>I,T	I>D,E,F>T	T=H>>D,E,F,I
Synthetic-selective agonists	BW-255C ZK-110841	EP_1: 17-phenyl-ω-trinor E_2 EP_2: butaprost EP_3: enoprostil GR-63799 MB-28767	Fluprostene	Cicaprost Iloprost	U-46619 STA_2 I-BOP
Synthetic-selective antagonists	BW-A868C	EP_1: SC-19220 AH 6809	—	—	GR-32191 SQ-29548

disease states. The most compelling evidence has been in diseases of eicosanoid *overproduction*: here it is postulated that the normal defensive and protective roles of the eicosanoids have become exaggerated with deleterious effects. Then it is possible to show elevated levels of the relevant eicosanoids, correlation with symptoms of disease and finally amelioration by treatment with eicosanoid synthesis inhibitors, such as aspirin, NSAIDs and corticosteroids. Some conditions with overproduction of eicosanoids are:

1. Inflammation (PGE_2, LT)
2. Asthma, hayfever ($PGF_{2\alpha}$, TXA_2, LT)
3. Mastocytosis (PGD_2, LT)
4. Hypercalcaemia of cancer (PGE_2, $PGF_{2\alpha}$)
5. Bartter's syndrome ($PGI_{2\alpha}$, PGE_2)
6. Patent ductus arteriosus (PGE_2, PGI_2)
7. Dysmenorrhoea($PGF_{2\alpha}$)
8. Biliary colic/Ureterolithiasis ($PGF_{2\alpha}$, TXA_2)
9. Unstable angina (TXA_2)
10. Transient ischaemic attacks (TXA_2)

In other diseases an *underproduction* of prostaglandins has been postulated. The evidence here is less clear cut. Measurement of eicosanoid levels in blood is fraught with methodological problems, particularly so at lower levels. Accurate measurement of urinary metabolites has been possible in only a few well equipped and experienced laboratories. There is also, as yet, no established method for the enhancement of a failing eicosanoid system, except in frank EFA deficiency. There are, however, some diseases in which it seems likely that a hypofunctioning prostanoid system could be a contributory factor to the pathophysiology.

Atherosclerosis

In endothelial dysfunction arising as a consequence of the oxidative modification of lipoproteins in the vascular wall or in diabetes there is decreased release of PGI_2.[75,76] There is, therefore, the potential for impaired balance between endothelial prostacyclin production and platelet release of TXA_2 as well as mitogens such as platelet-derived growth factor.

Hypertension

Long-term treatment with NSAIDs leads to decreased renal production of prostanoids and sometimes to hypertension. Low-renin hypotension is associated with lower urinary excretion of prostaglandins. As prostanoids are involved in renin release, renal vasodilatation and handling of water a hypofunctioning renal prostanoid system could be an early biochemical lesion in hypertension.

Gastroduodenal ulceration

PGE compounds stimulate mucus and bicarbonate formation as well as inhibiting gastric acid secretion. Pharmacologically induced underproduction of prostanoids by NSAIDs causes erosion and ulceration of the gastric mucosa. It is not known if gastroduodenal ulcers are associated with decreased mucosal PG production. However, stable PGE analogues have a healing effect both in idiopathic and in NSAID-induced ulcers.

The therapeutic strategy for treating a hypofunctioning prostanoid system must be to stimulate the failing prostanoid production by dietary supplement of precursor acids and by the avoidance of NSAIDs in these conditions. In the future it may be possible to use selective IP and EP receptor agonists to enhance a failing endogenous defence system.

Concluding remarks

The fascinating development of eicosanoid biology originates from the seminal discoveries made by Burr and Burr and by von Euler in the 1930s. The main impetus for the modern development came through the isolation of the pure compounds and structural determination of prostaglandins, thromboxanes, leukotrienes and other eicosanoids by Bergström, Sjövall, Samuelsson and Hamberg in Sweden. The link to the essential fatty acids stimulated the interest further. The discovery by Vane that aspirin and related drugs blocked the formation of prostaglandin provided an invaluable tool for elucidating their role in physiology and disease. The role of the eicosanoid system in human biology is becoming increasingly well understood. Modulation of the eicosanoid system by more specifically influencing the production, metabolism and actions of individual eicosanoids is likely to lead to new methods both for prevention and for treatment of many common diseases.

References

1. Burr GO, Burr MM. A new deficiency disease produced by the rigid exclusion of fat from the diet. *J Biol Chem* 1927; **82**: 345–67.

2. Burr GO, Burr MM. On the nature and role of the fatty acids essential in nutrition. *J Biol Chem* 1930; **86**: 587–621.

3. Holman RT. General introduction for polyunsaturated acids. *Prog Chem Fats Other Lipids* 1966; **9**: 3–12.

4. Mead JF, Willis AL. The essential fatty acids: their derivation and role. In: Willis AL (ed), *Handbook of Eicosanoids, Prostaglandins and Related Lipids*, vol 1, part A. Boca Raton FL: CRC Press, 1989: 85–117.

5. Dyerberg J, Bang HO. Haemostatic function and platelet unsaturated fatty acids in eskimos. *Lancet* 1979; **2**: 433–5.

6. Bergström S, Danielsson H, Samuelsson B. The enzymatic formation of prostaglandin E_2 from arachidonic acid. *Biochim Biophys Acta* 1964; **90**: 207–10.

7. Van Dorp DA, Beerthius RK, Nugteren DH, Vonkeman H. The biosynthesis of prostaglandins. *Biochim Biophys Acta* 1964; **90**: 211–17.

8. Goldblatt MW. A depressor substance in seminal fluid. *J Soc Chem Ind (Lond)* 1933; **84**: 208–18.

9. von Euler VS. On the specific vasodilating and plain muscle stimulating substances from accessory genital glands in man and certain animals. *J Physiol (Lond)* 1936; **88**: 213–34.

10. Bergström S, Sjövall J. The isolation of prostaglandin F from sheep prostate glands. *Acta Chem Scand* 1960; **14**: 1693–700.

11. Bergström S, Sjövall J. The isolation of prostaglandin E from sheep prostate glands. *Acta Chem Scand* 1960; **14**: 1701–5.

12. Bergström S, Ryhage R, Samuelsson B, Sjövall J. The structures of prostaglandins E_1, $F_{1\alpha}$ and $F_{1\beta}$. *J Biol Chem* 1963; **238**: 3555–64.

13. Vane JR. Inhibition of prostaglandin biosynthesis as a mechanism of action for aspirin-like drugs. *Nature* 1971; **231**: 232–5.

14. Smith JB, Willis AL. Aspirin selectively inhibits prostaglandin production in human platelets. *Nature* 1971; **231**: 235–7.

15. Xie W, Robertsson DL, Simmons DL. Mitogen-inducible prostaglandin G/H synthase: a new target for non-steroidal anti-inflammatory drugs. *Drug Dev Res* 1992; **25**: 239–65.

16. Hamberg M, Samuelsson B. Detection and isolation of an endoperoxide intermediate in prostaglandin biosynthesis. *Proc Natl Acad Sci USA* 1973; **70**: 899–903.

17. Nugteren DH, Hazelhof E. Isolation and properties of intermediates in prostaglandin biosynthesis. *Biochim Biophys Acta* 1973; **236**: 448–61.

18. Samuelsson B. On the incorporation of oxygen in the conversion of 8,11,14 eicosatrienoic acid to prostaglandin E_1. *J Am Chem Soc* 1965; **87**: 3011–13.

19. Piper PJ, Vane JR. Release of additional factors in anaphylaxis and its antagonism by anti-inflammatory drugs. *Nature* 1969; **223**: 29–35.

20. Willis AL, Vane FM, Kuhn PC, Scott CG, Perkins M. An endoperoxide aggregator (LASS) formed in platelets in response to thrombotic stimuli: purification, identification and unique biological significance. *Prostaglandins* 1974; **8**: 453–507.

21. Hamberg M, Svensson J, Wakabayashi T, Samuelsson B. Isolation and structure of two prostaglandin endoperoxides that cause platelet aggregation. *Proc Natl Acad Sci USA* 1974; **71**: 345–9.

22. Hamberg M, Svensson J, Samuelsson B. Thromboxanes: a new group of biological active compounds derived from prostaglandin endoperoxides. *Proc Natl Acad Sci USA* 1975; **72**: 2994–8.

23. Moncada S, Gryglewski RJ, Bunting S, Vane JR. An enzyme isolated from arteries transforms prostaglandin endoperoxides to an unstable substance that inhibits platelet aggregation. *Nature* 1971; **231**: 663–5.

24. Johnson RA, Morton DR, Kinner JH, *et al*. The chemical structure of prostaglandin X (prostacyclin). *Prostaglandins* 1976; **12**: 915–28.

25. Samuelsson B. The leukotrienes: a new group of biologically active compounds including SRS-A. *Trends Pharmacol Sci* 1980; **1**: 227–30.

26. Chacos N, Folck JR, Wistrom C, Capdevila J. Novel epoxides formed during liver cytochrome P-450 oxidation of arachidonic acid. *Biochem Biophys Res Commun* 1982; **104**: 916–22.

27. Oliw EM. Metabolism of 5(6) oxido-eicosatrienoic acid by ram seminal vesicles. Formation of five stereoisomers of 5-hydroxy prostaglandin I_1. *J Biol Chem* 1989; **259**: 2716–21.

28. Sirhan CN, Hamberg M, Samuelsson B. Lipoxins: a novel series of biologically active compounds formed from arachidonic acid in human leukocytes. *Proc Natl Acad Sci USA* 1984; **81**: 5335–9.

29. Änggård EE, Samuelsson B. Metabolism of prostaglandin E in guinea-pig lung: the structures of two metabolites. *J Biol Chem* 1964; **239**: 4097–102.

30. Änggård EE, Larsson C, Samuelsson B. The distribution of 15-hydroxy prostaglandin dehydrogenase and prostaglandin-13-reductase in tissues of the swine. *Acta Physiol Scand* 1971; **81**: 396–404.

31. Änggård EE. The biological activities of three metabolites of prostaglandin E_1. *Acta Physiol Scand* 1966; **66**: 509–10.

32. Ferreira SH, Vane JR. Prostaglandins: their disappearance from and release into the circulation. *Nature* 1967; **216**: 868–73.

33. Änggård EE, Larsson C. The sequences of the early steps in the metabolism of prostaglandin E_1. *Eur J Pharmacol* 1971; **14**: 66–70.

34. Peskar B, Hesse WH, Rogatti W, *et al*. Formation of 13,14-dihydro-prostaglandin E, during intravenous infusion of prostaglandin E, in patients with peripheral arterial occlusive disease. *Prostaglandins* 1991; **41**: 225–8.

35. Sun FF, Taylor BM. Metabolism of prostacyclin in the rat. *Biochemistry* 1978; **17**: 4096–101.

36. Rosenkranz B, Fischer C, Weimar KE, Frolich JC.

Metabolism of prostacyclin and 6-ketoprostaglandin $F_{1\alpha}$ in man. *J Biol Chem* 1980; **255**: 10194–8.

37. McGiff JC, Terragno NA, Strand JC, Lee JB, Lonigro AJ, Ng KKF. Selective passage of prostaglandins across the lung. *Nature* 1969; **223**: 742–5.

38. Samuelsson B, Granström E, Green K, Hamberg M. Metabolism of prostaglandins. *Ann NY Acad Sci* 1971; **180**: 138–63.

39. Lewis RA, Soter NA, Diamond PT, Austen KF, Oates JA, Roberts LS. Prostaglandin D_2 generation after activation of rat and human mast cells with anti-IgE. *J Immunol* 1982; **129**: 1627–31.

40. Morow JA, Awad JA, Oates JA, Roberts W. Identification of skin as a major site of prostaglandin D_2 release following oral administration of Niacin in humans. *J Invest Dermatol* 1992; **98**: 812–15.

41. Abdel-Halim MS, Hamberg M, Sjöquist E, Änggård E. Identification of prostaglandin D_2 as a major prostaglandin in homogenates of rat brain. *Prostaglandins* 1977; **14**: 633–43.

42. Hayaishi O. Molecular mechanisms of sleep–wake regulation roles of prostaglandins D_2 and E_2. *FASEB J* 1991; **5**: 2575–81.

43. Ellis CK, Smigel MD, Oates JA, Octz O, Sweetman BJ. Metabolism of prostaglandin D_2 in the monkey. *J Biol Chem* 1979; **254**: 4152–63.

44. Barrow SE, Harvey N, Ennis M, Chappell GG, Blair IA, Dollery CT. Measurement of prostaglandin D_2 and identification of metabolites in human plasma during intravenous infusion. *Prostaglandins* 1984; **28**: 743–54.

45. Paulsrud JR, Miller ON. Inhibition of 15-OH prostaglandin dehydrogenase by several diuretic drugs. *Fed Proc* 1974; **33**: 590.

46. Stone KJ, Hart M. Inhibition of renal PGE_2-9-ketoreductase by diuretics. *Prostaglandins* 1976; **12**: 197–207.

47. Tai HH, Hollander CS. Regulation of prostaglandin metabolism activation of 15-OH-PGDH by chlorpromazine and imipramine related drugs. *Biochim Biophys Acta* 1976; **68**: 814–20.

48. Alam NA, Clary P, Russell PT. Depressed placental prostaglandin E_1 metabolism in toxaemia of pregnancy. *Prostaglandins* 1973; **4**: 363–70.

49. Nakano J, Prancan AV. Metabolic degradation of prostaglandin E_1 in the lung and kidney of rats in endotoxic shock. *Proc Soc Exp Biol Med* 1973; **144**: 506–8.

50. Muchowski JM, Willis AL. Synthetic prostanoids in chemistry of the eicosanoids. In: Willis AL (ed), *Handbook of Eicosanoids*, vol II, part B, Boca Raton FL: CRC Press, 1987: 19–153.

51. Änggård E, Larsson C. Stimulation and inhibition of prostaglandin biosynthesis: opposite effects on blood pressure and blood flow distribution. In: Robinson HJ, Vane JR (eds), *Prostaglandin Synthesis Inhibitors*. New York: Raven Press, 1974: 311–16.

52. Weeks JR. Prostaglandins. *Annu Rev Pharmacol* 1972; **12**: 317–36.

53. Dusting GJ, Mullane KM, Moncada S. Prostacyclin and vascular smooth muscle. In: Zanchetti A, Farazi RC (eds), *Handbook of Hypertension*, vol 7: *Pathophysiology of Hypertension – Cardiovascular Aspects*. Amsterdam: Elsevier, 1986: 408–26.

54. Änggård E, Bergström S. Biological effects of an unsaturated trihydroxy acid ($PGF_{2\alpha}$) isolated from normal swine lung. *Acta Physiol Scand* 1963; **58**: 1–12.

55. Moncada S, Vane JR. Pharmacology and endogenous roles of prostaglandin endoperoxides, thromboxane A_2 and prostacyclin. *Pharmacol Rev* 1978; **30**: 293.

56. Bundy GL. The synthesis of prostaglandin endoperoxide analogues. *Tetrahedron Lett* 1975; **24**: 1957–60.

57. De Gaetano G, Bertele V, Cerlesti C. Mechanism of action and clinical use of prostanoids. In: Dormandy JA, Stock G (eds), *Critical Limb Ischaemia*. Berlin: Springer, 1990: 117–37.

58. Ritter JM, Cockcroft JR, Doktor HS, Beecham J, Barrow SE. Differential effect of aspirin on thromboxane and prostaglandin biosynthesis in man. *Br J Clin Pharmacol* 1989; **28**: 573–9.

59. Vane JR, Botting RM. Biological properties of cyclooxygenase products. In: Cunningham F (ed), *The Handbook of Immunopharmacology*, vol 10: *Lipid Mediators*. (In press.)

60. Orloff J, Zusman R. Role of prostaglandin E (PGE) in the modulation of action of vasopressin on water flow in the urinary bladder of the toad and mammalian kidney. *J Membr Biol* 1978; **40**: 297–304.

61. Larsson C, Weber P, Änggård E. Arachidonic acid increases and indomethacin decreases plasma renin activity in the rabbit. *Eur J Pharmacol* 1978; **28**: 391–4.

62. Morrison AR, Nishikawa K, Needleman P. Thromboxane A_2 biosynthesis in the ureter obstructed isolated perfused kidney of the rabbit. *J Pharmacol Exp Ther* 1978; **205**: 1–8.

63. Robert A, Nezamis JE, Phillips JP. Inhibition of gastric secretion by prostaglandin. *Am J Dig Dis* 1967; **12**: 1073–6.

64. Whittle BJR, Salmon JA. Biosynthesis of prostacyclin and prostaglandin E_2 in gastrointestinal tissue. In: Furnberg LA (ed), *Intestinal Secretions*. Welwyn Garden City: Smith Kline French Publications, 1983: 69–73.

65 Whittle BJR. Relationship between the prevention of rat gastric erosion and the inhibition of acid secretion of prostaglandins. *Eur J Pharmacol* 1976; **40**: 233–9.

66. Robert A, Schulz JR, Nezamis JE. Gastric antisecretory and anti-ulcer properties of PGE_2, 15-methyl PGE_2 and 16,16-dimethyl PGE_2. *Gastroenterology* 1976; **70**: 359–70.

67. Whittle BJR, Moncada S, Vane JR. Formation of prostacyclin by the gastric mucosa and its action on gastric function. *Prostaglandins* 1978; **15**: 704–5.

68. Robert A. Antisecretory, anti-ulcer, cytoprotective and diarrhoeagenic properties of prostaglandins. *Adv Prostaglandin Thromboxane Res* 1976; **2**: 507–20.

69. Piomelli D, Greengaro P. Lipoxygenase metabolites of arachidonic acid in neuronal transmembrane signalling. *TIPS* 1990; **11**: 367–73.

70. Bygdeman M, Gottlieb K, Svanborg K, Swahn ML. Role of prostaglandins in human reproduction – recent advances. *Adv Prostaglandin Thromboxane Leukotriene Res* 1987; **17**: 1112–16.

71. Horton EW, Poyser NL. Uterine luteolytic hormone. A physiological role for prostaglandin $F_{2\alpha}$. *Physiol Rev* 1976; **56**: 595–651.

72. Eglen RM, Whiting RL. Classification of prostanoid receptors. In: Willis AL (ed), *Handbook of Eicosanoids*, vol II; Drugs acting via the eicosanoids. Willis AL (ed), CRC Press, 1989: 273–84.

73. Levin RI, Weksler BB, Jaffe EA. The interaction of sodium nitroprusside with human endothelial cells and platelets. Nitroprusside and prostacyclin synergistically inhibit platelet function. *Circulation* 1982; **66**: 1299–307.

74. De Caterina R, Giannessi D, Bernini W, Mazzone A. Organic nitrates: direct antiplatelet effects and synergism with prostacyclin. *Throm Haemost* 1988; **59**: 207–11.

75. Pomerantz KB, Hajjar DP. Eicosanoids in regulation of arterial smooth muscle cell phenotype proliferative capacity and cholesterol metabolism. *Arteriosclerosis* 1989; **9**: 413–29.

76. Fitzgerald G, Catello F, Oates JA. Eicosanoid biosynthesis in human cardiovascular disease. *Hum Pathol* 1987; **18**: 248–52.

77. Watson S, Abbott A. TIPS Receptor Nomenclature. *Trends Pharmacol Sci* 1991; suppl, January.

2 Prostanoid receptors: their function and classification

Robert A Coleman and Patrick PA Humphrey

Prostaglandins, produced from dietary fatty acids, are synthesized *de novo* by a wide variety of cells throughout the body and can subsequently have extensive actions on the same cells and/or on others (see review[1]). It remains to be determined precisely how physiologically important these actions of the prostaglandins are, but they have undoubted pathophysiological importance. This is clearly demonstrated by the obvious therapeutic value of non-steroidal anti-inflammatory drugs (NSAIDs). These drugs are clinically effective because they inhibit the prostaglandin cyclo-oxygenase enzyme, thereby preventing the synthesis of all prostaglandins and the thromboxanes.[2] NSAIDs, like aspirin, thus prevent the algesic and inflammatory actions of prostaglandins of the E series[3,4] and the vasoconstrictor and platelet pro-aggregatory effects of thromboxane A_2.[5,6] However, the fact that the chronic use of NSAIDs causes side effects, such as gastrointestinal ulceration and bleeding, suggests that the prostaglandins do have an important physiological, cytoprotective role in protecting the gastrointestinal mucosa.[7,8]

The multiple pharmacological actions of exogenous prostaglandins have been studied at length, and although it was initially thought that they might act as membrane ionophores, it is now accepted that prostaglandins, like other local hormones, produce their effects by interacting with specific protein receptors in cell membranes (see review[9]). These receptors are termed 'prostanoid' rather than 'prostaglandin' receptors to include those activated by the thromboxanes.[1,10,11]

Prostanoid receptors

The first evidence for the existence of more than a single type of prostanoid receptor came from the work of Pickles, who studied the effects of a range of PGE and PGF analogues on isolated preparations of rabbit jejunum and guinea-pig and human myometrium.[12] The different profiles of agonists he observed led him to the conclusion that there were at least three different types of prostanoid receptor. Further evidence for different prostanoid receptor types was subsequently presented by Andersen and Ramwell, who compared the relative agonist potencies of the naturally occurring A, E and F series prostaglandins.[13] The question of prostanoid receptor subtypes in the lung was addressed by Collier and Gardiner, who compared the relative potencies of a number of synthetic prostanoid agonists.[14] They came to the conclusion that airways contain three different types of prostanoid receptor – one mediating bronchodilatation (ψ-receptors), another bronchoconstriction (χ-receptors) and another cough (ω-receptors). Whilst these three research groups undoubtedly provided clear indications that different types of prostanoid receptors really do exist, it is difficult to draw any comprehensive conclusions from their studies. Thus, Collier and Gardiner, like Pickles, used mainly synthetic agonists with poorly defined pharmacological profiles for their comparisons, whereas Pickles chose preparations that we know contain heterogeneous receptor populations. Andersen and Ramwell compared *in vitro* and *in vivo* data, the latter being of limited value

15

in such quantitative studies owing to the range of processes that can influence agonist potency in the whole animal.[15]

Our own work, which we started with other colleagues at Ware in the early 1980s, was aimed at the development of an overall working classification of prostanoid receptors that was both robust and comprehensive. Our starting point was a systematic, quantitative comparison of the agonist potencies of the natural prostanoids, PGD_2, PGE_2, $PGF_{2\alpha}$, PGI_2, and TXA_2 on isolated tissues. Care was taken to avoid tissue preparations that we believed contained more than one prostanoid receptor type.[10] It soon became apparent that prostanoid receptors could in fact be classified in terms of their relative sensitivities to these five naturally occurring prostanoids.[10] Thus, there appeared to be five types of prostanoid receptor, each characterized by a particularly high agonist potency for one of the five naturally occurring prostanoids. We therefore devised a simple and logical system of nomenclature that is based on this observation. We termed prostanoid receptors P-receptors, this being preceded by a letter indicating the more potent of the natural prostanoids at that particular receptor. We therefore named the five prostanoid receptors DP-, EP-, FP-, IP- and TP-receptors.

Our classification has indeed proved itself useful and is now being widely used. However, in the absence of a range of selective antagonists for the various receptors and their postulated subtypes the initial scheme may be something of an oversimplification. Nevertheless, confirmatory data have been provided from a number of laboratories, and there is now good evidence that three or more subtypes of EP-receptor exist,[16] and these have been termed arbitrarily EP_1, EP_2 and EP_3. The numeric subscript is not intended to suggest any specificity for 1, 2 or 3 series prostanoids. Indeed, we believe that all three subtypes of EP-receptor naturally subserve PGE_2. In addition, it has been suggested that subtypes of TP-receptor also exist, but this is a matter of controversy and has not been convincingly established except between species.[17,18] Hopefully, more good drug tools will be identified soon to provide further insight into the characterization of prostanoid receptors and subtypes. Certainly a greater understanding will come from the use of modern techniques in molecular biology. Indeed, two prostanoid receptors have now been cloned, the TP- and EP_3-receptors.[19,20] Excitingly, the cloned receptors, when transfected into COS cells, exhibited the characteristics predicted from functional studies in whole tissues.

Table 2.1 Current status of prostanoid receptor classification

Prostanoid receptor	Subtype	Selective agonist	Selective antagonist	Radiolabelled ligand	Intracellular transduction mechanism
DP		BW 245C ZK110841	BW A868C	[³H]PGD$_2$	↑ cAMP
EP	EP_1	—	AH6809 SC-19220		IP$_3$/DG
	EP_2	Butaprost AH13205	—	[³H]PGE$_2$	↑ cAMP
	EP_3*	Enprostil GR63799	—		↓ cAMP (IP$_3$/DG?)
FP		Fluprostenol Cloprostenol	—	[³H]PGF$_{2\alpha}$	IP$_3$/DG
IP		Iloprost Cicaprost	—	[³H]iloprost	↑ cAMP
TP*		U-46619	Vapiprost (GR32191) BAYu3405	[³H]U-46619 [³H]SQ 29548	IP$_3$/DG

*Receptor amino acid sequence recently elucidated (TP- and EP$_3$-receptors; see text).
IP$_3$/DG: stimulation of phosphoinositide metabolism.
↑ ↓ cAMP: stimulation or inhibition of adenylyl cyclase.
This scheme is a simplified and updated summary from reference 9. For further details, see text.

Prostanoid receptor classification

The current status of the classification of prostanoid receptors[9] is summarized in Table 2.1. The proposed scheme will be considered here in relation to the essential, and now universally agreed, criteria for receptor characterization (I–V) outlined in Table 2.2 (see review[21]). Thus, before one can be confident of proper characterization of a receptor type, one must have functional data with selective agonists and antagonists (receptor blocking drugs), describing their activity in quantitative terms, with relative efficacies or equipotent concentration ratios for agonists and affinity measures (reciprocal dissociation constants) for antagonists. Ideally too, binding studies should be carried out with a suitable radioligand, to give reliable measures of affinity for agonists as well as antagonists. An understanding of intracellular second messengers (the 'transducing system') linked to a given receptor also gives relevant information about the receptor type and amino acid structure; i.e. is it a G-protein linked and a seven-transmembrane receptor or a ligand-gated ion channel with multiple subunits? Obviously the definitive 'fingerprint' of the receptor will be the full amino acid sequence and receptor topography. However, it would seem unwise to give all receptors with different amino acid sequences different names, since some homologous receptors with small sequence differences may be functionally identical.

Each of the receptor characterization criteria mentioned here and summarized in Table 2.2 will be discussed in relation to each of the known prostanoid receptor types listed in Table 2.1. It should be noted that the receptors were originally classified largely on the basis of data with agonists, but gradually corroborative data have been generated with antagonists as such compounds have become available.

I. Selective prostanoid agonists

Since the mid-1970s, a variety of prostaglandin-like (prostanoid) structures have been synthesized, which display selectivity for prostanoid receptor subtypes. The degree of selectivity obtained for DP-, FP- and TP-receptors is particularly good with, for example, the agonists BW 245C, fluprostenol and U-46619, respectively. However, although EP-receptor selective agonists are available, the situation is complicated by the occurrence of several EP-receptor subtypes, though prostanoids with selectivity for one or more subtypes have been identified.

DP-Receptor agonists

A variety of diverse actions have now been identified for PGD_2, ranging from inhibition of platelet aggregation, vasodilation, modulation of allergen-induced mediator release and an effect on the central nervous system involving the control of sleep. The most

Table 2.2 Criteria for receptor characterization

I.	Selective agonists	Is there a unique rank order of potency of agonists at the receptor being characterized? What are their relative equipotent concentration ratio values? Are there agonists with high selectivity for the receptor compared with their potency at other receptors?
II.	Selective antagonists (receptor blocking drugs)	Are potent and specific antagonists available which can antagonize the actions of agonists by blocking the receptor? Are these antagonists selective for one type or subtype of receptor, as measured by relative dissociation constants?
III.	Ligand binding affinities	Dissociation constants (affinity measures) for ligand (selective agonists and antagonists) from such studies should correlate with data from functional studies. Provides additional data on agonist affinity measures, difficult to obtain from functional studies
IV.	Intracellular transduction mechanisms	Useful information which further defines receptor under investigation, but such data probably do not provide a definite correlate of receptor type or subtype
V.	Molecular structure	Receptor structure and amino acid sequence provide definitive evidence of receptor identity. However, receptors that are structurally different may not be different in terms of their function (i.e. the 'active-site' may be identical)

The criteria for classification (I–V) provide a 'fingerprint' for the basis of identifying distinct receptors. Rigorous classification of receptors in relation to drug action and therapeutics demands proper definition of each for definitive characterization (see reference 21).

thoroughly characterized PGD_2-sensitive system is that which is found on human platelets. A comprehensive review of the biological actions of PGD_2 and mimetics has been produced by Giles and Leff.[22]

PGD_2, like the other natural prostanoids, is only relatively selective for its own receptors, and possesses moderately potent agonist activity at both FP- and TP-receptors.[11,23] For a given degree of platelet inhibition, the PGD_2 metabolite, $9\alpha,11\beta$-PGF_2, appears to possess relatively more TP-receptor agonist activity than PGD_2.[24,25] In contrast, 9-deoxy-Δ^9-PGD_2 (PGJ_2), a dehydration product of PGD_2, is as potent as the parent compound at inhibiting platelet aggregation and producing vasodilatation, but is more specific, possessing less activity on EP- and FP-receptors.[26] Similarly, the 9β derivative of PGD_2 is also relatively more specific than PGD_2 for DP-receptors. In a study conducted by Narumiya and Toda,[27] BW 245C and 9β-PGD_2 were shown, like PGD_2, to potently inhibit human platelet aggregation, and also to relax the rabbit transverse stomach strip. The similarity of the equipotent concentrations of the compounds is indicative of a single subtype of DP-receptor existing in the two systems.

A more recently described DP-receptor agonist which appears to have a similar potency and selectivity to BW 245C, is the 9-chloro analogue of PGE_2, ZK110841.[28] Neither BW 245C nor ZK110841 is obviously closely structurally related to PGD_2, but perhaps the most unexpected compound to display DP-receptor agonist activity is the PGI_2 analogue, RS93520, which possesses some modest IP-receptor agonist activity on human platelets, but is substantially more potent as a DP-receptor agonist.[29] The structures of a range of DP-receptor agonists are shown in Fig. 2.1.

EP-Receptor agonists

Whilst many analogues of PGE_2 have been synthesized, it is important to stress that the biological actions of these agonists are not necessarily all mediated by EP-receptors. For example, 16,16-dimethyl PGE_2, ICI 80205 and Wy17186 all have TP-receptor agonist activity on vascular smooth muscle and blood platelets, whilst PGE_1 has IP-receptor agonist activity.[30,31] Despite this, many analogues of PGE_2 demonstrate selectivity of action within EP-receptors (Table 2.3).

16,16-Dimethyl PGE_2, 9-methylene PGE_2, ICI 80205 and 17-phenyltrinor PGE_2 all demonstrate a moderate degree of EP$_1$-receptor selectivity, but each also has a relatively high agonist potency at EP$_3$-receptors.[31,32] In contrast, AH13205[33] and buta-

Table 2.3 EP-Receptor subtype selectivity for range of EP-receptor agonists

	EP$_1$	*EP$_2$*	*EP$_3$*
PGE_2	+++	+++	+++
PGE_1	++	+++	+++
AY23626	+	+++	+++
Sulprostone	++	—	+++
Iloprost	+++	+	+
17-Phenyl-ω-trinor PGE_2	+++	+	++
9-Methylene PGE_2	+++	+	++
ICI 80205	++++	+	+++
16,16-Dimethyl PGE_2	+++	++	++++
Wy17186	+	+	+++
Butaprost	—	++	—
AH13205	—	++	—
Misoprostol	+	+++	+++
Rioprostil	+	+++	+++
Enprostil	++	+	++++
GR63799	++	+	++++

++++, agonist potency of $\geq$ 10-fold more than PGE_2; +++, agonist potency of a similar order to that of PGE_2; ++, agonist potency of $\geq$ 10-fold less than PGE_2; +, agonist potency of $\geq$ 100-fold less than PGE_2; —, inactive.
Data from references 9, 32, 33 and 36.

prost (TR4979)[34] (Fig. 2.2) are both highly selective agonists at EP$_2$-receptors. Although neither AH13205 nor butaprost is a highly potent agonist at EP$_2$-receptors, both are essentially inactive on preparations containing EP$_1$- and EP$_3$-receptors (see Table 2.4). Wy17186 acts as a moderately potent and selective EP$_3$-receptor agonist, but the usefulness of this compound is limited by its TP-receptor agonist activity. Many EP-receptor agonists are selective for two of the EP-receptor subtypes over the other one, thus sulprostone is a potent EP$_1$- and EP$_3$-receptor agonist, but with dramatically reduced potency at EP$_2$-receptors, whereas AY23626 is a potent EP$_2$- and EP$_3$-receptor agonist, but is weak at EP$_1$-receptors (see Table 2.3). These two compounds have proved invaluable in the characterization of the various subtypes of EP-receptor.[16] The structures of AY23626 and sulprostone are illustrated in Fig. 2.2. In contrast, two other PGE_2 analogues, PGE_1 and 11-deoxy PGE_1, are essentially non-selective, although they are marginally weaker at EP$_1$- than at EP$_2$- and EP$_3$-receptors.

A number of PGE_2 analogues have been synthesized as gastrointestinal cytoprotective agents; for example, misoprostol, rioprostil, enprostil and GR63799[35,36] (Fig. 2.3). All four are potent EP$_3$-receptor agonists, and it is believed that this activity

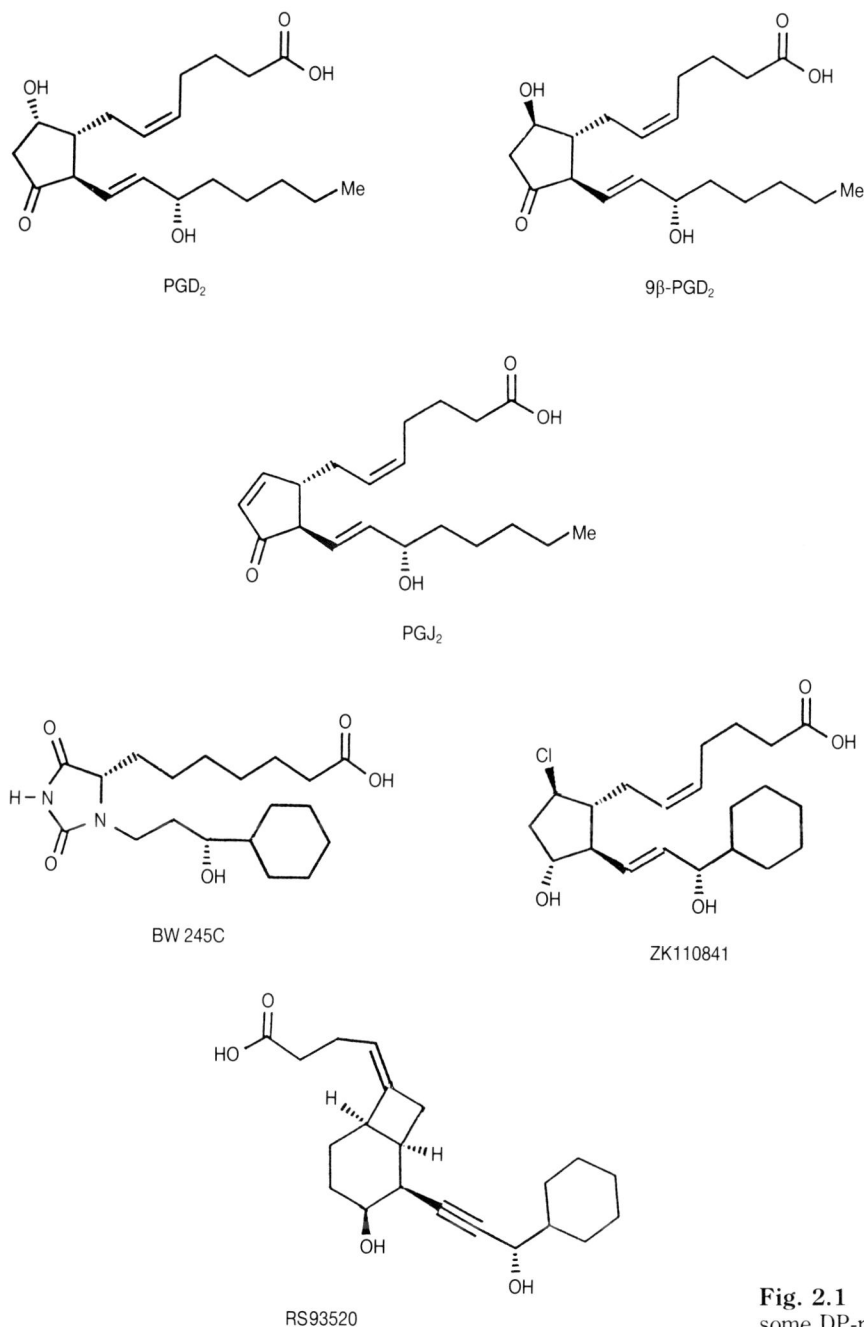

PGD₂

9β-PGD₂

PGJ₂

BW 245C

ZK110841

RS93520

Fig. 2.1 The chemical structures of some DP-receptor agonists.

is responsible for their ability to protect against gastrointestinal damage produced by high doses of NSAIDs. Despite this, their selectivity profiles differ, misoprostol and rioprostil both exhibiting additional potent EP₂-receptor agonist activity, although neither has potent agonist actions at EP₁-receptors.[31,35] In contrast, both enprostil and GR63799 have modest EP₁-receptor agonist activity but both are essentially devoid of activity at EP₂-receptors (see Table 2.3). An agonist need not be a PGE₂ analogue for it to behave as an EP-receptor agonist; a good example of this is the stable PGI₂

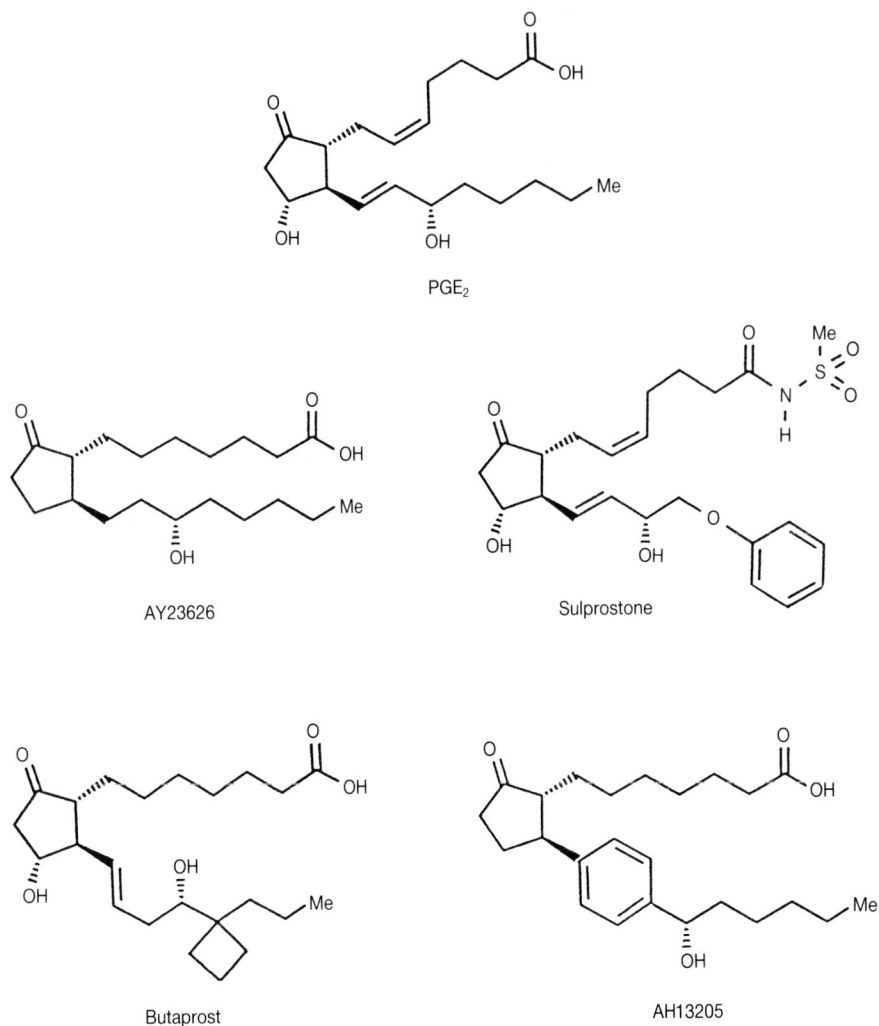

PGE₂

AY23626

Sulprostone

Butaprost

AH13205

Fig. 2.2 The chemical structures of some EP-receptor agonists.

analogue, iloprost (ZK-36374), which is not only a potent IP-receptor agonist on both platelets and vascular smooth muscle but also a potent agonist at EP$_1$-receptors.[37] Interestingly, iloprost has no measurable agonist activity at either EP$_2$- or EP$_3$-receptors.

FP-Receptor agonists

The two 16-phenoxy analogues of PGF$_{2\alpha}$, fluprostenol and cloprostenol[38] (Fig. 2.4) were, like PGF$_{2\alpha}$ itself, potent luteolytic agents in a number of domestic animal species. The fact that PGF$_{2\alpha}$ is far more potent in this action than the other natural prostanoids suggests that FP-receptors are involved. The high potency of fluprostenol and cloprostenol as contractile agents on the FP-receptor-containing prep-

arations, dog and cat iris sphincter muscle, characterize these two compounds as potent FP-receptor agonists.[39] A number of other PGF$_{2\alpha}$ analogues have also been developed as luteolytic agents; for example, prostalene, fenprostalene and tiaprost.[40] Of these compounds, we have evaluated fluprostenol, cloprostenol, prostalene and PGF$_{2\alpha}$, as well as some close analogues, PGF$_{1\alpha}$, PGF$_{2\beta}$ and PGD$_2$, on a range of prostanoid receptor-containing tissues.[30,39] Others have reported data with tiaprost and fenprostalene.[40] These data demonstrate that fluprostenol is the most selective of the FP-receptor agonists, showing not only high potency at FP-receptors but also a quite remarkable degree of selectivity, being essentially inactive at DP-, EP-, IP- and TP-receptors. Whilst other compounds are also

Table 2.4 Distribution of prostanoid receptors in various tissues and cell types

Tissue/Cell type	Response	
	Stimulation*	Inhibition†
Smooth muscle:		
Vascular	TP, (EP$_3$)	DP, EP$_2$, IP
Respiratory	TP, (EP$_1$)	EP$_2$
Gastrointestinal	EP$_1$, EP$_3$, FP, TP	EP$_2$, (DP), (IP)
Uterine	EP$_1$, EP$_3$, FP, TP	(DP), (EP$_2$), (IP)
Ocular	EP$_1$, FP, TP	EP$_2$
Inflammatory cells:		
Monocytes		DP, EP$_2$
Granulocytes		DP, EP$_2$
Lymphocytes		EP$_2$
Neurons:		
Autonomic		EP$_3$, (DP), (IP)
Afferent sensory	EP$_2$, IP	
Myofibroblasts	TP	
Platelets	EP$_3$, TP	IP, (DP)
Adipocytes		EP$_3$
Corpus luteum	FP	
Epithelial cells	EP$_3$	EP$_2$

*Contraction of smooth muscle and myofibroblasts, activation of inflammatory cells to release mediators, depolarization of neurons, aggregation of platelets, luteolysis of the corpus luteum and secretion from epithelial cells.
†Relaxation of smooth muscle, inhibition of mediator release from inflammatory cells, hyperpolarization of neurons, inhibition of aggregation by platelets, lipolysis by adipocytes and secretion by epithelial cells.
Receptor types commonly found in each cell type, or ( ) found only in those from particular species. Data from reference 9.

as potent as fluprostenol at FP-receptors, none is as selective.

IP-Receptor agonists

PGI$_2$ itself has only a relatively low selectivity for IP-receptor agonists, as it also has agonist activity at both EP$_1$- and TP-receptors.[30,31] Although many PGI$_2$ analogues have been synthesized and tested for biological activity, there is little information available regarding their specificity for IP-receptors. The emphasis of the chemical effort in this area appears to have centred on attempts to produce chemically and metabolically stable PGI$_2$ analogues which optimistically might retain the platelet inhibitory effect, but not the vasodilator effect, of the parent compound.

The first stable analogue of PGI$_2$ which was as potent as the parent compound at inhibiting platelet aggregation and relaxing vascular smooth muscle was iloprost.[41] Intriguingly, it is in general more specific than PGI$_2$ itself since, unlike the latter, it lacks any measurable EP$_2$-, EP$_3$- or TP-receptor agonist activity. However, in addition to its potent IP-receptor agonist activity, iloprost also possesses potent, albeit partial, agonist activity at EP$_1$-receptors, thereby mediating contraction of the guinea-pig trachea, rat stomach fundus and bovine iris sphincter muscle.[31]

Further work by the same group yielded cicaprost,[42,43] a compound that is more potent than either PGI$_2$ or iloprost as an inhibitor of platelet aggregation, as a relaxant of bovine coronary artery strip and as a vasodilator. However, in contrast to iloprost, cicaprost has little or no activity on EP$_1$-receptors,[32] and appears to be the most selective IP-receptor agonist yet described.

It is not certain whether all IP-receptors are of the same type, or whether subtypes of IP-receptor exist. Various pharmacological studies have been interpreted to indicate that differences may exist between IP-receptors on platelets from different species, and between IP-receptors on platelets and vascular smooth muscle.[44] However, differences in stimulus–response coupling or receptor density in the biological systems under comparison may well have been responsible for the differences observed. Regardless of the possible existence of IP-receptor subtypes, the distribution of IP-receptors is variable, at least in the vasculature, where in some beds IP-receptors are scarce or absent.[45,46]

Perhaps the most unexpected putative IP-receptor agonist is octimibate, a compound structurally unrelated to prostanoids, yet which displays agonist activity on primate platelets and vascular smooth muscle.[47] Interestingly, unlike iloprost, it is only a weak agonist on platelets from non-primate species, which suggests the existence of species-dependent IP-receptor subtypes. Nevertheless, octimibate demonstrates no selectivity of action between primate platelet and vascular IP-receptors. The structure of octimibate is compared with those of PGI$_2$ and its stable analogues, iloprost and cicaprost in Fig. 2.5.

TP-Receptor agonists

Many studies have been conducted with authentic biosynthetically generated TXA$_2$, but its instability, with a half-life of about 30 seconds in aqueous solution at 37°C and pH 7.4, makes it virtually unusable for quantitative pharmacological studies. Also, bio-

Enprostil

Misoprostol

Rioprostil

GR63799

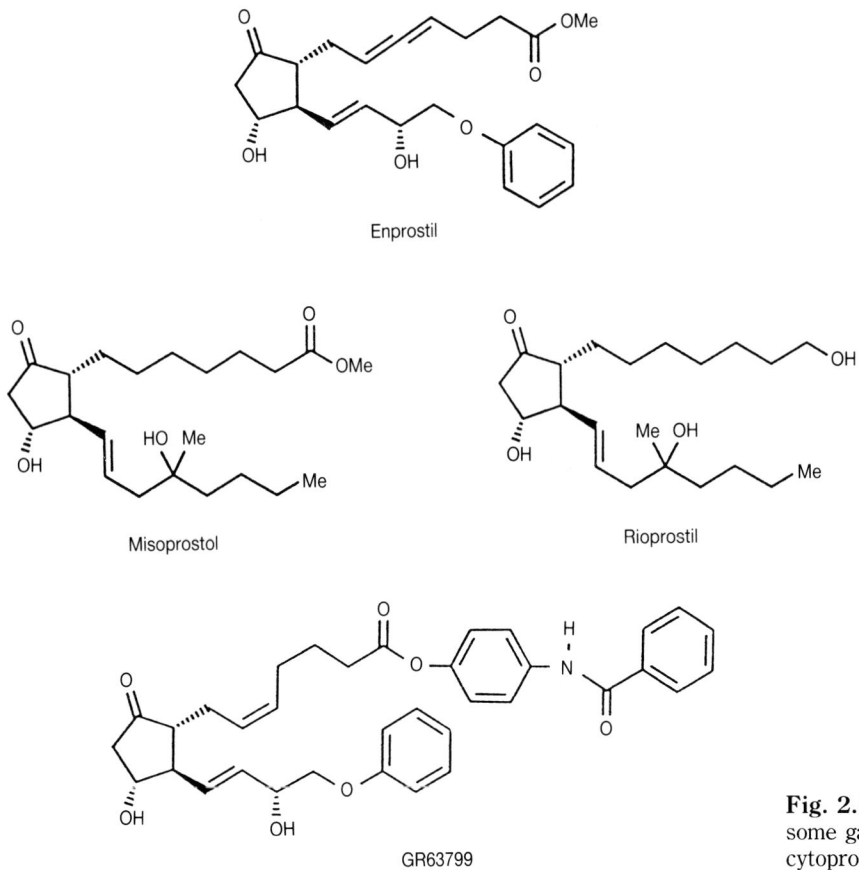

Fig. 2.3   The chemical structures of some gastric antisecretory/cytoprotective prostanoid agonists.

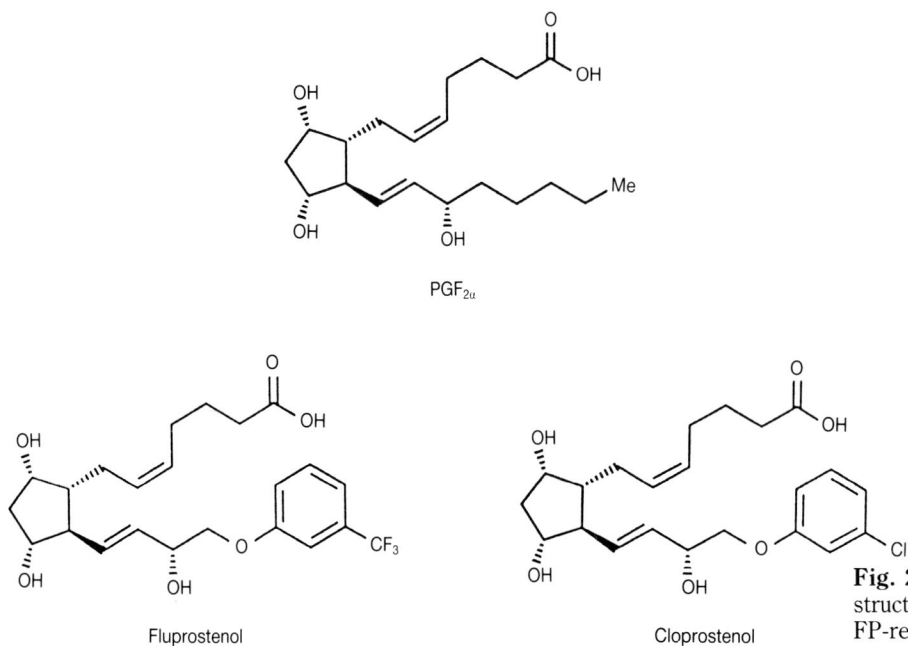

PGF$_{2\alpha}$

Fluprostenol

Cloprostenol

Fig. 2.4   The chemical structures of some FP-receptor agonists.

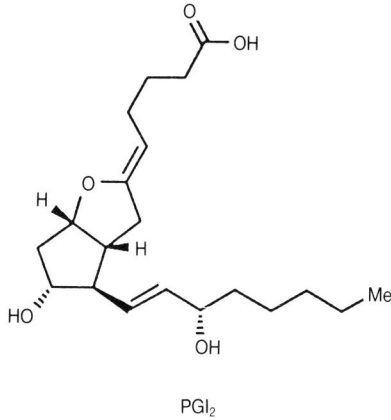

PGI$_2$

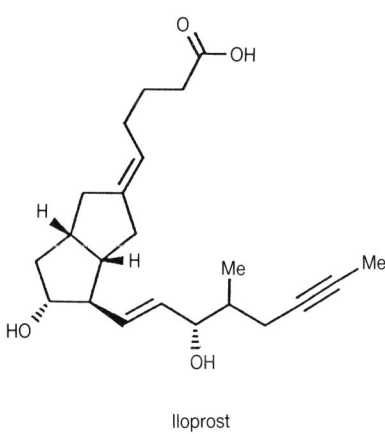

Iloprost

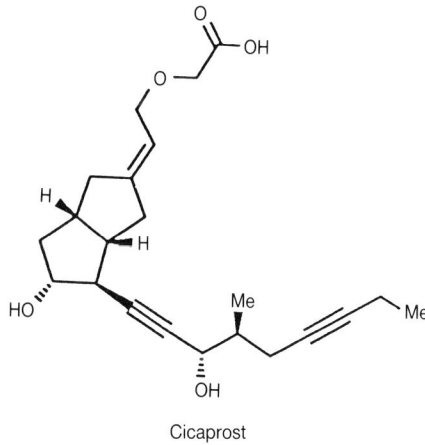

Cicaprost

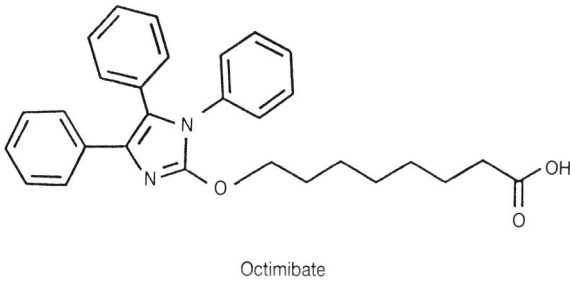

Octimibate

Fig. 2.5 The chemical structures of some IP-receptor agonists.

synthetic TXA$_2$ is invariably contaminated with PGH$_2$, which complicates the interpretation and quantification of the activity of TXA$_2$, as PGH$_2$ has actions in its own right, and may also be converted to other prostaglandins.[48]

Stable analogues of PGH$_2$ have provided the most useful TP-receptor agonists. Of these, U-46619 (11α, 9α-epoxymethano PGH$_2$) and its corresponding 9α, 11α-epoxymethano analogue (U-44069)[49] (Fig. 2.6) re-

main the best characterized, and the former the most widely used TP-receptor agonist. U-46619 closely mimics the contractile actions of TXA$_2$, being a potent and full contractile agonist on a wide range of TP-receptor-containing preparations, but is weak on preparations containing only other prostanoid receptor types.[50] The compound is of similar potency to synthetic TXA$_2$ at causing human platelet aggregation and contraction of vascular smooth muscle re-

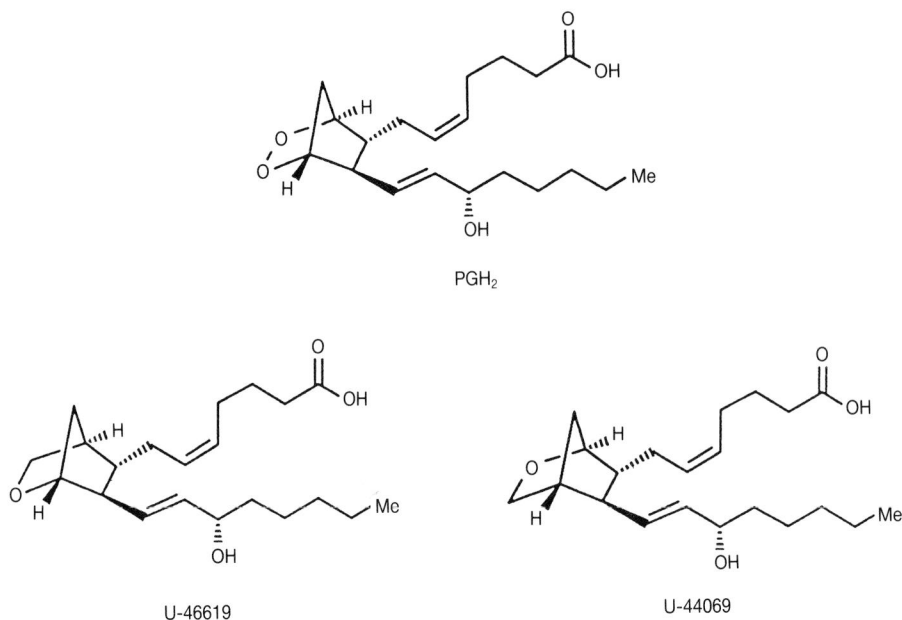

PGH$_2$

U-46619

U-44069

Fig. 2.6 The chemical structures of PGH$_2$ and stable epoxymethano analogues (TP-receptor agonists).

spectively *in vitro*.[51] In anaesthetized animals, U-46619 appears to be equipotent with synthetic TXA$_2$ in causing bronchoconstriction and vasoconstriction. U-44069 possesses a profile of action similar to U-46619, although it is less potent and appears to be a partial agonist on human platelets as well as on various vascular smooth muscle preparations.[52,53]

The fact that U-46619 is an analogue of PGH$_2$ rather than TXA$_2$ has prompted some speculation as to whether, in preparations where PGH$_2$ and TXA$_2$ produce similar effects (e.g. platelets), U-46619 is acting as a PGH$_2$ mimetic via PGH$_2$-sensitive receptors, or as a TXA$_2$ mimetic via TP-receptors. The evidence cited above and that presented by Armstrong *et al.*[54] strongly supports the contention that both U-46619 and PGH$_2$ are TXA$_2$ mimetics, and act at TP-receptors.

Other potent TP-receptor agonists discovered at about the same time as U-46619 are 9,11-azo-PGH$_2$ (U-51093)[55] and PGF$_{2\alpha}$-acetal,[56] 9,11-azo-PGH$_2$ being of similar potency to U-46619 on platelets and vascular smooth muscle. Other similar analogues are 9,11-ethano-PGH$_2$ and its ω-tetranor-16-*p*-fluorophenoxy derivative, EP 011, as well as the more potent 9α,11α-oxa-10a-homo analogues, EP 171 and SQ 26655, and the various thia derivatives of TXA$_2$, including STA$_2$.[57] The structures of EP 011 and EP 171 are shown in Fig. 2.7. The TP-receptor agonist activities of various analogues of PGE$_2$, such as Wy17186, its 15(*S*) epimer (Wy40659) and its

16-methyl analogue, Wy19110, upon human platelets have also been described.[58]

II. Selective prostanoid receptor blocking drugs

Despite considerable efforts by various groups over the years, only a limited number of specific prostanoid receptor blocking drugs have been developed, and, with the exception of TP-receptor blocking drugs, few of these are obviously prostanoid-like in structure. However, despite this, various blocking drugs for some of the receptors have been identified, and they have proved invaluable in the classification of prostanoid receptors.

DP-Receptor blocking drugs

The first compound identified as a DP-receptor blocking drug was the phloretin derivative, N-0164, which antagonized the anti-aggregatory action of PGD$_2$ on human platelets, with tenfold higher concentrations being required to antagonize the effects of PGI$_2$ and PGE$_1$. N-0164 was also shown to antagonize the anti-aggregatory effect of BW 245C, and inhibit PGD$_2$-induced elevation of cAMP in human platelets.[59] However, N-0164 also possesses other actions, and was in fact first identified, like the parent compound, polyphloretin phosphate, as an EP-receptor blocking drug, antagonizing contractions of gastrointestinal smooth muscle induced by PGE$_2$ and

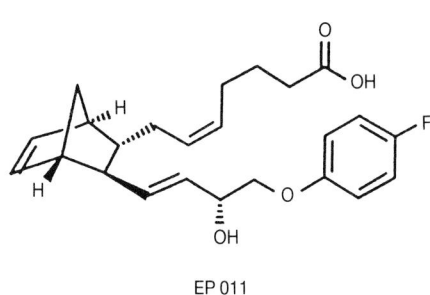

EP 011

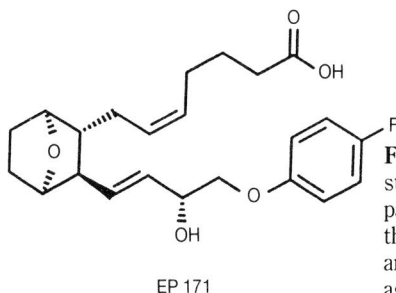

EP 171

Fig. 2.7 The chemical structures of parafluorophenoxy thromboxane A$_2$ analogues (TP-receptor agonists).

PGF$_{2\alpha}$.[60] The compound was also subsequently shown to exhibit thromboxane synthase inhibitory activity, TP-receptor blocking activity and cAMP phosphodiesterase inhibitory activity.

A more specific DP-receptor blocking drug is AH6809, which antagonizes the anti-aggregatory effects of PGD$_2$ and its mimetics BW 245C and 9α, 11β-PGF$_2$ but not those of PGI$_2$ or the adenosine mimetic NECA upon human platelets.[61] Whilst AH6809 has a pA$_2$ of approximately 6.5 at DP-receptors, it also displays a similar potency in blocking EP$_1$-receptors;[62] thus, while the compound can be used experimentally for characterizing DP-receptors, more specific compounds are required.

The most potent and specific DP-receptor blocking drug reported to date is BW A868C, a structural analogue of BW 245C.[63] This compound displays high antagonist potency against the anti-aggregatory effects of PGD$_2$ upon human platelets (pK$_B$ 9.3) but is without effect upon other prostanoid receptors. BW A868C is also active *in vivo*,[64] and should prove to be a major advance in studying the pharmacology of PGD$_2$ and its analogues. The structures of AH6809 and BW A868C are compared in Fig. 2.8.

EP-Receptor blocking drugs
Although there are at least three different subtypes of EP-receptors, to date specific antagonists for only one of them have been described, namely the EP$_1$-receptor subtype. One of the first specific prostanoid antagonists reported was SC-19220[65] (Fig. 2.9), and this has since been identified as a specific EP$_1$-receptor blocking drug, exhibiting pA$_2$ values of 5.2–5.6 in a range of EP$_1$-receptor-containing preparations.[62] Since then, AH6809 has been identified which possesses a similar profile of action. AH6809 is between 10 and 30 times more potent than SC-19220, with pA$_2$ values in the range 6.5–7.0.[62] However, unlike SC-19220, AH6809 also possesses some blocking activity at both DP- and TP-

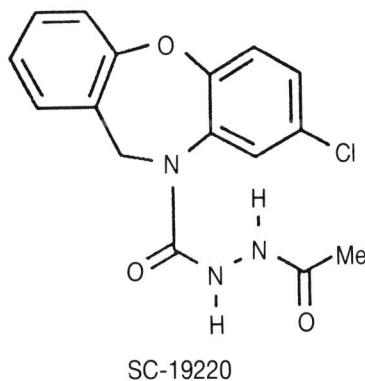

AH6809

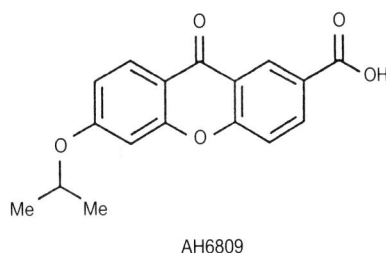

BW A868C

Fig. 2.8 The chemical structures of two DP-receptor blocking drugs.

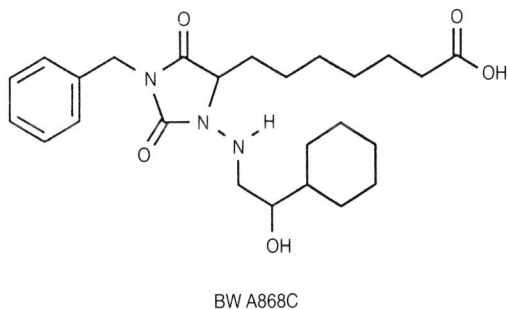

SC-19220

Fig. 2.9 The chemical structure of the dibenzoxazepine EP-receptor blocking drug SC-19220.

receptors. Whilst both compounds have proved valuable in the characterization of prostanoid receptors, both have their limitations. For example, the combination of poor aqueous solubility and low potency of SC-19220 makes its usefulness *in vivo* limited.[39] Furthermore, despite its higher potency and aqueous solubility, AH6809 also has limited usefulness *in vivo*, since it has been found to be extensively protein bound ($\simeq$ 97%).[66]

A number of analogues of SC-19220 have been synthesized, in which the acetyl function has been replaced with *n*-butanolyl, isobutanol and *n*-hexanyl functions. However, although increase in length of this function was associated with higher EP_1-receptor antagonist potency, it was also associated with a reduced specificity of action. Thus, despite its low potency, SC-19220 remains the most useful of this series of compounds.[67] Whilst one further analogue, the *n*-chloropentanoyl derivative, SC-25469,[68] has been reported to exhibit EP_1-receptor blocking activity, there is no published information relating to its potency.

Another compound that displays weak (pK_B=5.7) but specific prostanoid EP_1-receptor blocking activity is the NSAID meclofenamic acid.[69] This compound also exhibits some TP-receptor blocking activity. Meclofenamic acid is particularly effective in the treatment of dysmenorrhoea, but whether this is a reflection of its EP_1-receptor blocking activity is not clear.

Three other prostanoid antagonists which undoubtedly inhibit at least some EP_1-receptor mediated effects include the phloretin derivatives, polyphloretin phosphate (PPP), diphloretin phosphate (DPP) and N-0164 (see review 9). Additionally, there is evidence that these compounds, like AH6809, also possess some antagonist activity against responses mediated by DP- and TP-receptors. Although it is not clear whether any of these three compounds clearly behaves as a competitive receptor blocking drug, their apparent specificity of action, albeit weak, would be expected to make them of some use for the pharmacological characterization of prostanoid receptors. However, they are not generally highly regarded as pharmacological tools, and are now seldom used.

None of the EP-receptor blocking drugs described so far is obviously structurally related to the prostanoids. However, a prostanoid analogue, 13,14-didehydro-20-methylcarbaprostacyclin (FCE-22176)[70] (Fig. 2.10), has been described which may possess EP_1-receptor blocking activity. This compound is a prostanoid antagonist on guinea-pig

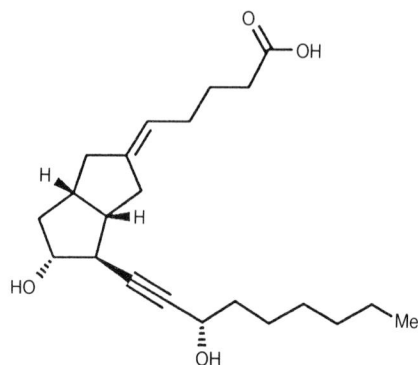

Fig. 2.10   The chemical structure of the putative EP_1-receptor blocking PGI_2 analogue, FCE-22176.

trachea, a preparation containing EP_1-receptors. The claim that this PGI_2 analogue possesses potent EP_1-receptor blocking activity is interesting in the light of the high EP_1-receptor agonist activity observed with another PGI_2 analogue, iloprost.[37]

FP-Receptor blocking drugs

To date, no compounds have been reported that specifically antagonize prostanoid-induced effects mediated by FP-receptors – e.g. luteolysis, contraction of dog and cat isolated iris sphincter or $PGF_{2\alpha}$-induced bronchoconstriction in the dog. Although there are compounds that have been reported to exhibit antagonist activity on preparations that we believe to contain FP-receptors – namely, 13,14-didehydro-20-methyl-$PGF_{2\alpha}$ (K 10136)[71] *N*,*N*-dimethylamino-$PGF_{2\alpha}$ (amino-$PGF_{2\alpha}$) and *N*,*N*-dimethylamido-$PGF_{2\alpha}$ (amido-$PGF_{2\alpha}$)[72] – we have not been able to confirm that any had FP-receptor blocking activity.[9] Rather, all three compounds appear to resemble the parent compound, $PGF_{2\alpha}$, in that they exhibit agonist activity on FP-receptor-containing preparations such as dog and cat iris sphincter but are only weak or inactive on those containing other prostanoid receptor types. None of the three compounds was obviously a partial agonist with respect to $PGF_{2\alpha}$ on any of the FP-receptor-containing preparations, and, of the three compounds, K 10136 was particularly potent, being only about five times less potent than $PGF_{2\alpha}$ itself.

IP-Receptor blocking drugs

The synthesis of PGI_2 analogues has yielded many IP-receptor agonists, but as yet no specific IP-receptor blocking drug has been identified. However, there are compounds that might serve as chemical starting points; for example, (5Z)-6a-carba-PGI$_2$ [(5Z)-carbacyclin].[46] This compound behaved as a full IP-agonist in human platelets, but in rat mesenteric arterial myocytes it displayed partial agonist activity and was able to antagonize adenylyl cyclase activation produced by PGI$_2$, PGE$_1$ and (5E)-carbacyclin. In addition, this compound also antagonized PGI$_2$-induced relaxation of the rabbit isolated mesenteric artery.

TP-Receptor blocking drugs

In contrast to the problems encountered in developing antagonists at receptors for the stable prostaglandins, it appears to be much simpler to identify TP-receptor blocking drugs. For example, compounds of such widely differing chemical structures as the phloretin phosphates, meclofenamic acid and trimethoquinol have been found to possess weak TP-receptor blocking activity. However, the elucidation of the chemical structures of the prostaglandin endoperoxide intermediates and, subsequently, of TXA$_2$ led to the development of not only potent stable mimetics but also antagonists. The first analogues of these naturally occurring prostanoids with antagonist activity were 9,11-azoprosta-5,13-dienoic acid (azo analogue I),[73] 9,11-epoxyiminoprosta-5,13-dienoic acid[74] and pinane thromboxane A$_2$ (PTA$_2$),[75] but all three are in fact partial agonists, exhibiting anatagonist activity on blood platelets and agonist activity on many smooth muscle preparations. The structure of PTA$_2$ is shown in Fig. 2.11.

Further work has resulted in the development of TP-receptor blocking drugs of many different chemical types. A series of 7-oxabicyclo[2.2.1]heptane prostaglandin analogues (e.g. SQ 29548) were developed by the Squibb group,[76] and at the same time we at Glaxo discovered the chemically novel TP-receptor blocking drug AH19437.[77] From AH19437, we developed AH23848[78] and eventually GR32191[18] (vapiprost), both of which have been shown to be potent and long-lasting TP-receptor blocking drugs in humans. Whilst of similar potency to AH23848, GR32191 lacks the partial agonist activity exhibited by the former compound as well as by many other TP-receptor blocking drugs.

Structural refinements to various PGH$_2$ analogues which acted as partial TP-receptor agonists on platelets and vascular smooth muscle led to the discovery by Jones and his colleagues of the specific, albeit relatively weak, TP-receptor blocking drug, EP 045,[79] and subsequently the more potent compound, EP 092.[80]

Independently, a further group, at ICI, developed a series of TP-receptor blocking drugs such as ICI 192605.[81] These were, like the compounds from the Squibb, Glaxo and Edinburgh University groups, highly potent and specifically acting compounds. The chemical structures of GR32191, SQ 29548, EP 092 and ICI 192605 are shown in Fig. 2.12.

Various compounds have been developed which, although they are structurally unrelated to prostaglandins (Fig. 2.13), have been reported to possess potent and specific TP-receptor blocking activity. Among these is the benzylsulfonamido analogue, BM 13505,[82] which has a pA$_2$ of about 7.7 at TP-receptors. There is now evidence, however, that this compound displays weak partial agonist activity on both platelets and vascular smooth muscle. Detailed structure–activity relationships have been reported on indole-2-propanoic acid derived TP-antagonists such as L-655240.[83] This compound is slightly more potent than BM 13505, with a pA$_2$ of at least 8.0. A further TP-receptor blocking drug structurally unrelated to the prostanoids but which shows marked potency is BAYu3405,[84] which is of the order of 10 times more potent than BM 13505. The structures of some of these 'non-prostanoid' TP-receptor blocking drugs are shown in Fig. 2.13.

For many TP-receptor blocking drugs, comprehensive information on the profile of action upon other prostanoid receptor types is lacking. However, GR32191, AH23848, ICI 192605, SQ 29548, EP 092 and BAYu3405 have all been shown to be without effect upon IP- and DP-receptors (human platelets), FP-receptors (dog iris) and EP$_1$-, EP$_2$- and EP$_3$-receptors in concentrations of up to 1–10 μM.[9,18,85]

The availability of potent TP-receptor blocking drugs has led to some studies that have focused on TP-receptor subclassification. The TP-receptors in rabbit aorta appear to be different from those in

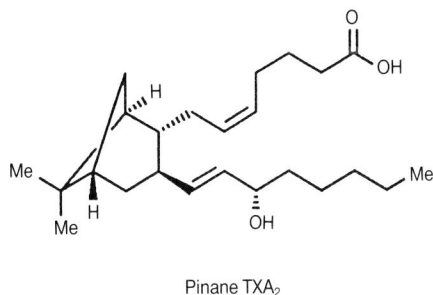

Pinane TXA$_2$

Fig. 2.11 The chemical structure of the partial TP-receptor agonist, pinane TXA$_2$.

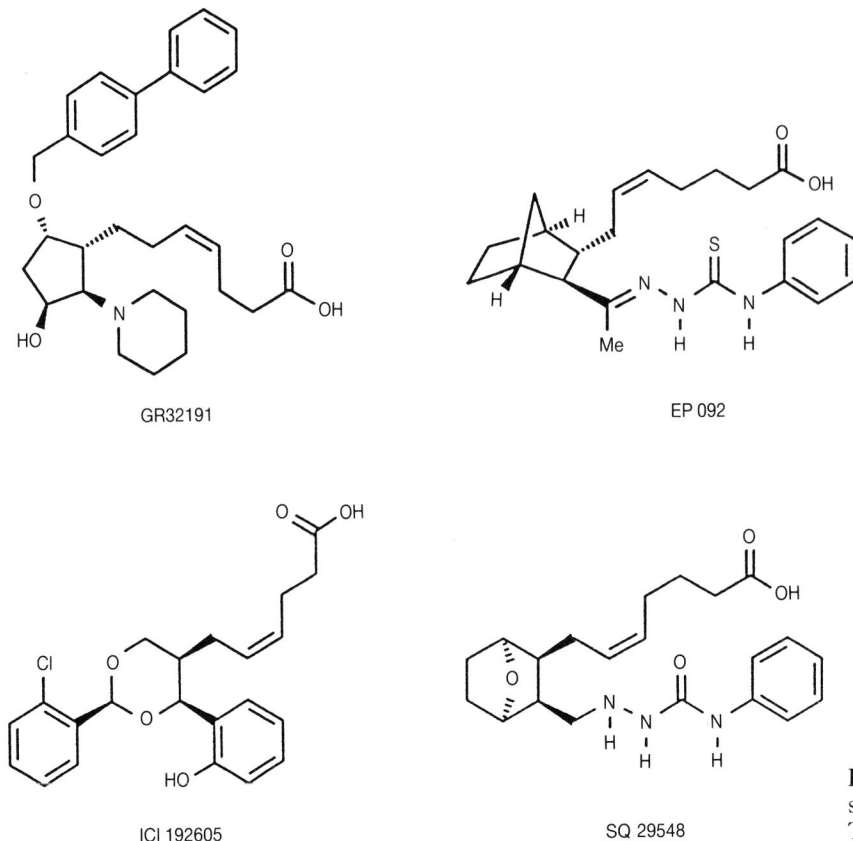

GR32191

EP 092

ICI 192605

SQ 29548

Fig. 2.12   The chemical structures of some prostanoid TP-receptor blocking drugs.

other species, pA_2 values for several compounds being almost one order of magnitude lower than on vascular smooth muscle preparations from other species. Evidence for the existence of a subtype of TP-receptor in the rabbit has been reported by several authors who have examined vascular smooth muscle, airways smooth muscle and platelets.[18] Interestingly, not all blocking drugs differentiate rabbit TP-receptors from those of other species; for example, BM 13177, BM 13505 and BAYu3405 show no such differentiation.[9,85]

Various groups have suggested that there are differences between platelet and vascular TP-receptors both between and within species. However, it is clear that further, more carefully controlled, studies are necessary before a firm conclusion can be drawn regarding the possible existence of subtypes of TP-receptors within a single species.

III. Ligand binding studies

When we first reviewed the literature on prostanoid ligand binding studies some years ago, we were fascinated by the fact that binding sites have been identified that are characterized by a high affinity at each of the natural prostanoids. Thus, at each site, one of the natural prostanoids has a higher affinity than any of the others, an observation entirely consistent with our proposed classification of prostanoid receptors on the basis of functional data.

PGD$_2$-specific binding sites

In the light of pharmacological evidence that distinct receptors exist for PGD$_2$ in platelets from some (e.g. man) but by no means all species, it is interesting that high affinity PGD$_2$-specific binding sites have also been isolated from human platelets.[86] A rank order of binding affinity at these sites is: D$_2$ (1) >I$_2$ (25) >E$_1$ (75) >F$_{2\alpha}$ (100) >E$_2$ (>100) (relative binding affinities, PGD$_2$ = 1). That these binding sites are identical to the DP-receptor characterized

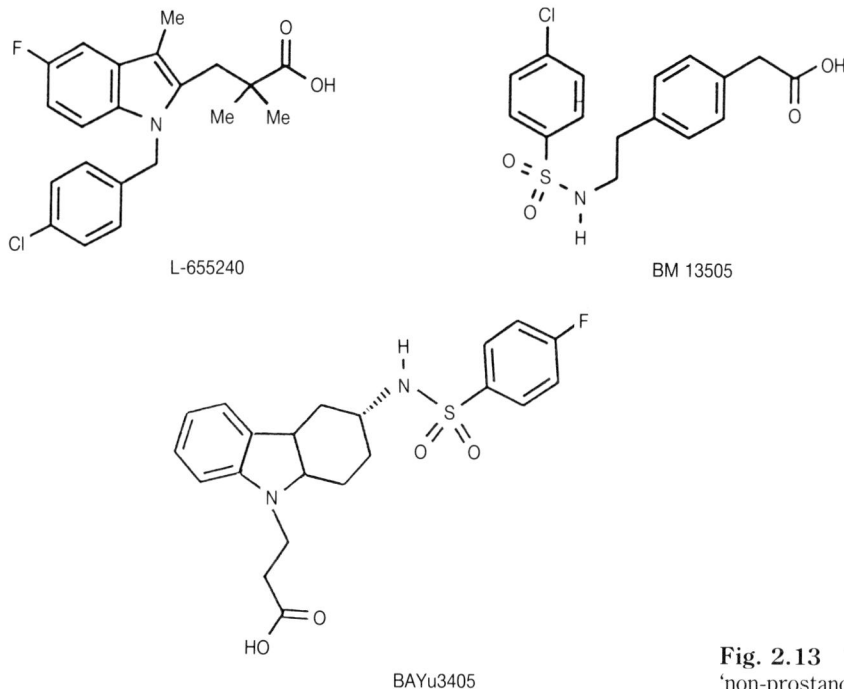

Fig. 2.13 The chemical structures of some 'non-prostanoid' TP-receptor blocking drugs.

in functional studies is given strong support by the finding that the selective DP-receptor agonist BW 245C displaces [³H]PGD$_2$ but not [³H]PGI$_2$ or [³H]iloprost from human and bovine platelets respectively.[87]

PGE-specific binding sites

In studies in which [³H]PGE$_2$ was used as radioligand, high affinity (K_D <10 nM) [³H]PGE$_2$-specific binding sites have been identified in adipocytes, corpus luteum, myometrium, kidney, intestinal epithelium, liver, heart, brain and blood platelets.[9] The presence of these high affinity binding sites has been associated in some tissues with a functional response, usually an effect on adenylyl cyclase, giving some support to the proposition that these binding sites are indeed functional receptors. Furthermore, in a number of studies, rank orders of binding affinities for at least some of the natural prostanoids, as well as the two synthetic PGE analogues sulprostone and AY23626, have been reported.[88,89] Interestingly, the binding affinities of sulprostone and AY23626 relative to PGE$_2$ on rat adipocytes, which are known to contain EP$_3$-receptors, are similar to the relative potencies of these two analogues on a range of preparations containing EP$_3$ but not EP$_1$- or EP$_2$-receptors.[9,90]

PGF-specific binding sites

Most studies on [³H]PGF$_{2\alpha}$-specific binding sites have been conducted on fractions from corpus luteum.[9] PGF$_{2\alpha}$ and a number of structural analogues of PGF$_{2\alpha}$ (e.g. cloprostenol and fluprostenol) are potent luteolytic agents in a range of animal species, being, as far as is known, the most potent of the naturally occurring prostanoids in this respect. A comparison of the relative binding affinities of a range of both natural prostanoids and of fluprostenol and cloprostenol at luteal binding sites with their FP-receptor agonist potencies reveals an excellent correlation.[9] It appears, therefore, that the PGF-specific binding sites in luteal membranes are similar to FP-receptors, and further suggests that, at least in animals, FP-receptors are responsible for prostanoid-induced luteolysis.

PGI-specific binding sites

Studies performed on human and bovine platelets, on homogenates of bovine coronary arteries, on NCB-20 neuronal somatic hybrid cell membranes and on homogenates of guinea-pig lung with [³H]PGI$_2$, [³H]PGE$_1$ and/or [³H]iloprost as the radioligand have provided evidence for PGI-specific binding sites in all of the tissues.[9]

It is interesting that not only are the rank orders

of prostanoid binding similar for all of the PGI_2 binding sites isolated but, omitting only PGD_2, for which distinct receptors exist on platelets, they also reflect the rank order of potency of the prostanoids in inhibiting platelet aggregation. These data are therefore consistent with the specific PGI_2 binding sites in vascular smooth muscle, blood platelets, cultured neuronal cells and guinea-pig lung being identical to functional IP-receptors. Finally, the putative IP-receptor agonist, octimibate, competes for [^{3}H]iloprost binding on primate platelet membranes,[47] providing further evidence that this compound does indeed have affinity for IP-receptors.

TXA_2-specific binding sites

In addition to a range of selective TP-receptor agonists, there exists a wide variety of specific and potent TP-receptor blocking drugs, and it is the latter that are the ideal ligands for binding studies. Not surprisingly, many studies have been carried out on platelet membranes using both labelled agonists and antagonists as ligands, and their binding has been displaced with both unlabelled agonists and antagonists.[9] The earlier ligands used include [^{3}H]-labelled 9,11- and 11,9-epoxymethano-PGH_2 (U-44069 and U-46619, respectively),[91,92] both of which are potent selective TP-receptor agonists, and [^{3}H]13-azaprostanoic acid (13-APA)[93] and [^{125}I]13-aza,16-*p*-hydroxyphenyl-pinane-TXA_2 (PTA-OH),[94] both of which are TP-receptor blocking drugs. The K_D value for PTA-OH determined on platelets from binding studies and the K_B value determined from pharmacological studies are very similar, being 14.5–40 nM and 11 nM respectively. This similarity is consistent with the common identity of binding site and receptor. Similarly, 13-APA has a binding affinity on platelet membranes of 100 nM, which corresponds to the pharmacologically derived pK_B.

Comparisons of the abilities of ranges of agonists and/or antagonists to inhibit ligand binding with their pharmacological activities in platelet aggregation studies revealed impressive correlations. In human washed platelets, binding of [^{3}H]U-44069 was displaced not only by unlabelled U-44069 and its close analogue, U-46619, but also by both PGH_2 and authentic TXA_2.[95] Kattelman *et al.* examined a range of structurally unrelated TP-receptor blocking drugs, SQ 29548, ONO 3708, BM 13177 and 13-APA, on human platelet membranes,[96] and again obtained identical rank orders of binding affinity and TP-receptor antagonist potency using the two techniques. In their study on guinea-pig platelets, Halushka *et al.*[91] displaced [^{125}I] PTA-OH binding

with a range of synthetic TP-receptor agonists and antagonists. Whilst all of the agonists both aggregated platelets and displaced labelled ligand from the platelet binding sites, the rank orders of potency for the two effects were different, whereas, in contrast, there was an excellent correlation with the antagonists. The apparent inconsistency with the agonist data presumably reflects differences in the respective efficacies of the agonists. Interestingly, these authors compared similar data for the antagonists in both guinea-pig and dog platelets, and found correlation within each species but differences between species. This suggests that whilst the binding sites are indeed the same as functional TP-receptors, the TP-receptors in dog and guinea-pig platelets may be different.

More recently, the more potent TP-receptor blocking drugs SQ 29548 and GR32191 (vapiprost) have been tritiated for use as radiolabelled ligands.[97,98] [^{3}H]SQ 29548 is a good specific ligand which has been shown to associate and dissociate rapidly from human platelets, consistent with its being a competitively acting antagonist.[97,98] However, the binding of [^{3}H]GR32191 under similar conditions is characterized by its slow dissociation, which correlates with vapiprost's unique pharmacological profile in platelets where, unlike in smooth muscle, it behaves functionally as a partly insurmountable receptor blocker.[18,98] Hence, although the kinetics of [^{3}H]GR32191's interaction with the human platelet TP-receptor make it less useful than [^{3}H]SQ 29548 as a radioligand for general use, they do seem to explain vapiprost's antagonist profile *in vitro* as well as, in part, its very long duration of action in man.[99]

IV. Intracellular transduction mechanisms

At least four prostanoid receptor types mediate contraction of smooth muscle, i.e. EP_1-, EP_3-, FP- and TP-receptors. Contraction of smooth muscle involves a rise in concentration of free Ca^{2+} in the cytoplasm, and evidently, activity at these receptors may be transduced via changes in the concentration of intracellular Ca^{2+}. Evidence that Ca^{2+} is the second messenger for TP-receptor activation is abundant, but is less so for EP- and FP-receptors. The contraction of smooth muscle by TXA_2 mimetics involves increases in intracellular free Ca^{2+}, of both extracellular and intracellular origin, resulting from the opening of receptor-operated Ca^{2+} channels in the plasma membrane and the mobilization of intracellular Ca^{2+} from the sarcoplasmic reticulum.[100,101]

The latter effect may be triggered by influx of extra-cellular Ca^{2+} and/or involve phosphatidylinositol turnover.[102] Most of the work relating TP-receptor activation to Ca^{2+} mobilization is in human platelets, where TXA_2 mimetics induce platelet aggregation by elevating free intracellular Ca^{2+}, possibly through an influx of extracellular Ca^{2+} and/or by the mobilization of Ca^{2+} from intracellular stores.[102,103] This latter release of Ca^{2+} is thought to be mediated via the hydrolysis of phosphatidylinositol-4,5-diphosphate in the plasma membrane. A good correlation exists between the degree of TP-receptor occupancy with U-44069, phosphatidylinositol hydrolysis and the rise in cytosolic free Ca^{2+}, all of which are antagonized by the TP-receptor blocking drug EP 045.[102]

EP$_1$-receptors mediate contraction in guinea-pig trachea, and Creese and Denborough have reported[104] that this effect is absolutely dependent on extracellular Ca^{2+}. However, there is no clear evidence linking EP$_3$-receptor agonist activity with alterations of intracellular Ca^{2+} levels. EP$_3$-receptors mediate inhibition of neurotransmitter release in guinea-pig vas deferens, an effect that is believed to be associated with a decrease in the intracellular levels of cAMP.[105] This is also the case with prostanoid-induced antilipolytic activity in adipocytes which is mediated by EP$_3$-receptors,[90] and is associated with a decrease in adenylyl cyclase activity.[106,107] These data all suggest that EP$_3$-receptors mediate their effects through inhibition of adenylyl cyclase. However, EP$_3$-receptors can also mediate the contraction of smooth muscle preparations (e.g. chick ileum and rabbit renal artery), an event not usually associated with changes in cAMP. The explanation for this apparent inconsistency is not yet clear, but it is possible that EP$_3$-receptors are coupled to different transducing mechanisms in different tissues.

Prostanoid-induced luteolysis in many species is mediated by FP-receptors, and it is associated with an increase in intracellular Ca^{2+} in the luteal cells.[108] As removal of extracellular Ca^{2+} had no effect on the luteolytic action of PGF$_{2\alpha}$, presumably mobilization of intracellular Ca^{2+} is involved. Indeed, Raymond et al. have shown that PGF$_{2\alpha}$ stimulates phosphatidylinositol turnover in isolated luteal cells, implicating Ca^{2+} as the second messenger.[109]

Three prostanoid receptor types mediate relaxation of smooth muscle, i.e. EP$_2$-, DP- and IP-receptors. Since relaxation of smooth muscle is often associated with intracellular increases in cAMP, it seems likely that activity at EP$_2$-, DP- and IP-receptors is transduced via intracellular cAMP. In-

direct evidence associating EP$_2$-receptors with cAMP is derived from the observation that PGE$_2$-induced relaxation of vascular and airway smooth muscle is accompanied by increases in intracellular cAMP.[104,110] A more direct association between EP$_2$-receptors and cAMP may be found in enterocytes; Hardcastle et al. have reported that PGE$_2$ increases cAMP levels in rat isolated enterocytes, and that dibutyryl cAMP stimulates intestinal secretion.[111] These data indicate that increase in intestinal secretion is mediated by EP$_2$-receptors via increased levels of intracellular cAMP.

Experiments on platelets and on intestinal mucosa have provided further evidence that DP- and IP-receptors are associated with increases in cAMP; inhibition of platelet aggregation is mediated by DP- and IP-receptors, and in both cases there is a good correlation between stimulation of adenylyl cyclase and this inhibition.[112] Taken together with the observation that dibutyryl cAMP inhibits platelet aggregation,[113] these results link DP- and IP-receptor stimulation with adenylyl cyclase stimulation and cAMP elevation. Additional, albeit indirect, evidence relating DP- and IP-receptors with cAMP is the observation of Simon et al. that PGE$_2$, PGI$_2$ and PGD$_2$ are approximately equipotent in stimulating adenylyl cyclase activity in human colonic mucosa,[114,115] indicating that EP-, IP- and DP-receptors may all be involved. Unfortunately, complementary studies on colonic secretion were not carried out.

Paradoxically, low concentrations of PGE$_2$ have been reported to inhibit adenylyl cyclase and antagonize the anti-aggregatory action of PGD$_2$ and PGI$_2$.[116] The importance of adenylyl cyclase inhibition in this platelet aggregatory action is debatable and the receptor types involved as yet uncharacterized, though it appears to be of the EP rather than TP type (see reference 9).

V. Molecular structure of prostanoid receptors

The pharmacology of prostaglandins outlined here is entirely consistent with their actions being mediated by a variety of membranal receptor types. Their associated transduction mechanisms seem to involve either activation of phosphoinositide metabolism or positive or negative effects on adenylyl cyclase. This, together with the relatively slow nature of the responses produced by the prostaglandins, is indicative of a family of receptors that are G-protein linked.[117]

Direct evidence has now been obtained in human

platelets, using antibodies to the C-terminal region of G-protein α-subunits, that a specific G-protein is involved in the aggregatory response to the TP-receptor agonist U-46619.[118] Following purification of the human platelet TP-receptor, a DNA clone encoding this receptor from human placenta has been obtained.[19] As would be expected for a G-protein linked receptor, the placental cDNA encodes a protein of 343 amino acids, which has seven putative α-helical transmembrane domains. When transfected into COS-7 cells, the receptor bound drugs with affinities similar to those of the platelet receptor. Of particular interest, Northern blot analysis of TP-receptor mRNA from various human tissues indicated that the receptor is the same in platelets and in vascular smooth muscle, although those from man and rat appeared to be different.[19]

Excitingly, another prostaglandin receptor has now been cloned by Narumiya's group. This receptor has been isolated from a mouse cDNA library using the sequence of the human TP-receptor employing the polymerase chain reaction and cross-hybridization screening.[20] The functional cDNA clone identified consists of 365 amino acid residues, again with the anticipated seven putative transmembrane hydrophobic domains. The receptor, when transfected into COS cells, displayed the specific [^{3}H]PGE$_2$ binding characteristics of the EP$_3$-receptor subtype. In CHO cells permanently expressing the cDNA, PGE$_2$ and the prostanoid receptor agonist MB28767 decreased forskolin-induced cAMP formation in a concentration-dependent manner. Thus, on the basis of evidence to date, the receptor has the distinct features of the EP$_3$-receptor.

Clearly, more studies are needed, but the early data from molecular biology approaches are entirely consistent with the more extensive pharmacological data. Undoubtedly, the structural information will give us a better understanding of the overall classification of prostaglandin receptors, and will ultimately aid the design of new, potentially valuable medicines which will come from work in this area.

References

1. Johnson M, Carey F, McMillan RM. Alternative pathways of arachidonate metabolism: prostaglandins, thromboxane and leukotrienes. *Essays Biochem* 1983; **19:** 40–141.
2. Vane JR. Inhibition of prostaglandin synthesis as a mechanism of action for aspirin-like drugs. *Nature* 1971; **231:** 232–5.
3. Ferreira SH, Vane JR. New aspects of the mode of action of non-steroidal drugs. *Annu Rev Pharmacol* 1974; **14:** 57–73.
4. Kuehl FA Jr, Egan RW. Prostaglandins, arachidonic acid and inflammation. *Science* 1980; **210:** 978–84.
5. Roth GJ, Majerus PW. The mechanism of the effect of aspirin on human platelets. 1. Acetylation of a particulate fraction protein. *J Clin Invest* 1975; **56:** 624–32.
6. Moncada S, Vane JR. Unstable metabolites of arachidonic acid and their role in haemostasis and thrombosis. *Br Med Bull* 1978; **34:** 129–35.
7. Hart ED. Indomethacin and gastric ulcer. *Br J Med* 1965; **2:** 1000–1.
8. Robert A. Antisecretory, antiulcer, cytoprotective and diarrheogenic properties of prostaglandins. *Adv Prostaglandin Thromboxane Res* 1976; **2:** 507–20.
9. Coleman RA, Kennedy I, Humphrey PPA, Bunce KT, Lumley P. Prostanoids and their receptors. In: Hansch C, Sammes PG, Taylor JB (eds), *Comprehensive Medicinal Chemistry.* Oxford: Pergamon Press, 1990: 643–714.
10. Kennedy I, Coleman RA, Humphrey PPA, Levy GP, Lumley P. Studies on the characterization of prostanoid receptors: a proposed classification. *Prostaglandins* 1982; **24:** 667–89.
11. Coleman RA, Humphrey PPA, Kennedy I, Lumley P. Prostanoid receptors – the development of a working classification. *Trends Pharmacol Sci* 1984; **5:** 303–6.
12. Pickles VR. The myometrial actions of six prostaglandins: consideration of a receptor hypothesis. In: Bergström S, Samuelsson B (eds), *Nobel Symposium,* vol 2: *Prostaglandins.* Stockholm: Almquist & Wicksell, 1967: 79–83.
13. Andersen NH, Ramwell PW. Biological aspects of prostaglandins. *Arch Intern Med* 1974; **133:** 30–50.
14. Gardiner PJ, Collier HOJ. Specific receptors for prostaglandins in airways. *Prostaglandins* 1980; **19:** 819–41.
15. Kenakin TP. *Pharmacologic Analysis of Drug-Receptor Interaction.* New York: Raven Press, 1987.
16. Coleman RA, Kennedy I, Sheldrick RLG. Further evidence for the existence of three subtypes of PGE$_2$-sensitive (EP-) receptors. *Br J Pharmacol* 1987; **91:** 323P.
17. Ogletree ML, Allen GT. Interspecies differences in thromboxane receptors: studies with thromboxane receptor antagonists in rat and guinea-pig smooth muscles. *J Pharmacol Exp Ther* 1992; **260:** 789–94.
18. Lumley P, White BP, Humphrey PPA. GR32191, a highly potent and specific thromboxane A$_2$ receptor blocking drug on platelets and vascular and airways smooth muscle *in vitro. Br J Pharmacol* 1989; **97:** 783–94.
19. Hirata M, Hayashi Y, Ushikubi F, *et al.* Cloning and expression of cDNA for a human thromboxane A$_2$ receptor. *Nature* 1991; **349:** 617–20.

20. Sugimoto Y, Namba T, Honda A, *et al.* Cloning and expression of cDNA for mouse prostaglandin E receptor EP_3 subtype. *J Biol Chem* 1992; **267**: 6463–6.

21. Kenakin TP, Bond RA, Bonner TI. The definition of pharmacological receptors. *Pharmacol Rev* **44**: 351–62.

22. Giles H, Leff P. The biology and pharmacology of PGD_2. *Prostaglandins* 1988; **35**: 277–300.

23. Coleman RA, Sheldrick RLG. Prostanoid-induced contraction of human bronchial smooth muscle is mediated by TP-receptors. *Br J Pharmacol* 1989; **96**: 688–92.

24. Beasley RCW, Featherstone RL, Church MK, *et al.* Effect of thromboxane receptor antagonist on PGD_2 and allergen induced bronchoconstriction. *J Appl Physiol* 1989; **66**: 1685–93.

25. Giles H, Bolofo ML, Lydford SJ, Martin GR. A comparative study of the prostanoid receptor profile of $9\alpha,11\beta$-prostaglandin F_2 and prostaglandin D_2. *Br J Pharmacol* 1991; **104**: 541–9.

26. Bundy GL, Morton DR, Peterson DC, Nishizawa EE, Miller WL. Synthesis and platelet aggregation inhibitory activity of prostaglandin D analogues. *J Med Chem* 1983; **26**: 790–9.

27. Narumiya S, Toda N. Different responsiveness of prostaglandin D_2-sensitive systems to prostaglandin D_2 and its analogues. *Br J Pharmacol* 1985; **85**: 367–75.

28. Thierauch K-H, Stürzebecher C-St, Schillinger E, *et al.* Stable 9β- or 11α-halogen-15-cyclohexyl-prostaglandins with high affinity to the PGD_2 receptor. *Prostaglandins* 1988; **35**: 853–68.

29. Alvarez R, Eglen RM, Chang LFK, *et al.* Stimulation of prostaglandin D_2 receptors on human platelets by analogs of prostacyclin. *Prostaglandins* 1991; **42**: 105–19.

30. Coleman RA. Studies Towards a Classification of Prostanoid Receptors. PhD Thesis. Council for National Academic Awards. 1983.

31. Dong YJ, Jones RL, Wilson NH. Prostaglandin E receptor subtypes in smooth muscle: agonist activities of stable prostacyclin analogues. *Br J Pharmacol* 1986; **87**: 97–107.

32. Lawrence RA, Jones RL, Wilson NH. Characterization of receptors involved in the direct and indirect actions of prostaglandins E and I on the guinea-pig ileum. *Br J Pharmacol* 1992; **105**: 271–8.

33. Nials AT, Coleman RA, Hartley D, Sheldrick RLG. AH13205 – a novel selective prostanoid EP_2 agonist. *Br J Pharmacol* 1991; **102**: 24P.

34. Gardiner PJ. Characterisation of prostanoid relaxant/inhibitory receptors (ψ) using a highly selective agonist, TR4979. *Br J Pharmacol* 1986; **87**: 45–56.

35. Collins PW. Development and therapeutic role of synthetic prostaglandins in peptic ulcer disease. *J Med Chem* 1986; **29**: 437–43.

36. Bunce KT, Clayton NM, Coleman RA, *et al.* GR63799 – a novel prostanoid with selectivity for EP_3-receptors. *Adv Prostaglandin Thromboxane Leukotriene Res* 1990; **21**: 379–82.

37. Sheldrick RLG, Coleman RA, Lumley P. Iloprost – a potent EP_1- and IP-receptor agonist. *Br J Pharmacol* 1988; **94**: 334P.

38. Dukes M, Russell W, Walpole AL. Potent luteolytic agents related to prostaglandin $F_{2\alpha}$. *Nature* 1974; **250**: 330–1.

39. Coleman RA. Methods in prostanoid receptor classification. In: Benedetto C, McDonald-Gibson RG, Nigam S, Slater TF (eds), *Prostaglandins and Related Substances: a Practical Approach*. Oxford: IRL Press, 1987: 267–303.

40. Jackson PS, Jessup R. Secondary pharmacological properties of prostaglandins. *Vet Rec* 1984; **114**: 168.

41. Schrör K, Darius H, Matzky R, Ohlendorf R. The antiplatelet and cardiovascular actions of a new carbacyclin derivative (ZK36374) – equipotent to PGI_2 in vitro. *Naunyn Schmiedeberg's Arch Pharmacol* 1981; **316**: 252–5.

42. Stürzebecher C-St, Haberey M, Muller B, *et al.* Pharmacological profile of ZK96480, a new chemically and metabolically stable prostacyclin analogue with oral availability and high PGI_2 intrinsic activity. In: Schrör K (ed), *Prostaglandins and other Eicosanoids in the Cardiovascular System*. Basel: Karger, 1985: 485–91.

43. Stürzebecher C-St, Haberey M, Muller B, *et al.* Pharmacological profile of a novel carbacyclin derivative with high metabolic stability and oral activity in the rat. *Prostaglandins* 1987; **31**: 95–109.

44. Wilson NH, Armstrong RA, Jones RL. Novel prostaglandin endoperoxide analogues having prostacyclin-like actions on platelets from human and horse but not from rat and rabbit. *Adv Prostaglandin Thromboxane Res* 1987; **17**: 491–5.

45. Lumley P, Humphrey PPA, Kennedy I, Coleman RA. Comparison of the potencies of some prostaglandins as vasodilators in three vascular beds of the anaesthetised dog. *Eur J Pharmacol* 1982; **81**: 421–30.

46. Corsini A, Folco GC, Fumagalli R, Nicosia S, Moe MA, Oliva D. (5Z)-Carbacyclin discriminates between prostacyclin receptors coupled to adenylate cyclase in vascular smooth muscle and platelets. *Br J Pharmacol* 1987; **90**: 255–61.

47. Merritt JE, Brown AM, Bund S, *et al.* Octimibate, a potent non-prostanoid inhibitor of platelet aggregation, acts via the prostacyclin receptor. *Br J Pharmacol* 1991; **102**: 260–6.

48. Bhagwat SS, Hamann PR, Still WC. Synthesis of thromboxane A_2. *J Am Chem Soc* 1985; **107**: 6372–6.

49. Malmsten C. Some biological effects of prostaglandin endoperoxide analogs. *Life Sci* 1976; **18**: 169–76.

50. Coleman RA, Humphrey PPA, Kennedy I, Levy GP,

Lumley P. Comparisons of the actions of U-46619, a stable prostaglandin H_2 analogue, with those of prostaglandin H_2 and thromboxane A_2 on some isolated smooth muscle preparations. *Br J Pharmacol* 1981; **73:** 773–8.

51. Richards IV, Oostveen JA, Griffin RL, Bunting S. Pulmonary pharmacology of synthetic thromboxane A_2. *Adv Prostaglandin Thromboxane Res* 1987; **17:** 1067–72.

52. Jones RL, Wilson NH, Armstrong RA, Dong YJ. Receptors for thromboxane and prostaglandins. *Proc IUPHAR 9th Congr Pharmacol, London* 1984; **2:** 293–301.

53. Jones RL, Peesapati V, Wilson NH. Antagonism of the thromboxane-sensitive contractile systems of the rabbit aorta, dog saphenous vein and guinea-pig trachea. *Br J Pharmacol* 1982; **76:** 423–38.

54. Armstrong RA, Jones RL, Wilson NH. The effect of thromboxane antagonism on aggregation and release in human platelets. *Br J Pharmacol* 1983; **78:** 159P.

55. Corey EJ, Nicolaou KC, Machida Y, Malmsten CL, Samuelsson B. Synthesis and biological properties of a 9,11-azo-prostanoid. *Proc Natl Acad Sci USA* 1975; **72:** 3355–8.

56. Portoghese PS, Larson DL, Abatjoglou AG, Denham EW, Gerrard JM, White JG. A novel prostaglandin endoperoxide mimic, prostaglandin $F_{2\alpha}$ acetal. *J Med Chem* 1977; **20:** 320–1.

57. Wilson NH, Jones RL. Prostaglandin endoperoxide and thromboxane A_2 analogs. *Adv Prostaglandin Thromboxane Res* 1985; **14:** 393–425.

58. MacIntyre DE. Platelet prostaglandin receptors. In: Gordon JL (ed), *Platelets in Biology and Pathology*, vol 2. Amsterdam: Elsevier/North Holland, 1981: 211–46.

59. MacIntyre DE, Gordon JL. Discrimination between platelet prostaglandin receptors with a specific antagonist of bisenoic prostaglandins. *Thromb Res* 1977; **11:** 705–13.

60. Eakins KE, Rajadhyaksha V, Schroer R. Prostaglandin antagonism by sodium *p*-benzyl-4-[1-oxo-2-(4-chlorobenzyl)-3-phenyl propyl] phenyl phosphonate (N-0164). *Br J Pharmacol* 1976; **58:** 333–9.

61. Keery RJ, Lumley P. AH6809, a prostaglandin DP-receptor blocking drug on human platelets. *Br J Pharmacol* 1988; **94:** 745–54.

62. Coleman RA, Humphrey PPA, Kennedy I. Prostanoid receptors in smooth muscle: further evidence for a proposed classification. In: Kalsner S (ed), *Trends in Autonomic Pharmacology*, vol 3. London: Taylor & Francis, 1985: 35–49.

63. Giles H, Leff P, Balofo ML, Kelly MG, Robertson AD. The classification of prostaglandin DP-receptors in platelets and vasculature using BWA868C, a novel selective and potent competitive agonist. *Br J Pharmacol* 1989; **96:** 291–300.

64. Hamid-Bloomfield S, Whittle BJ. Antagonism of PGD_2 vasodepressor responses in the rat *in vivo* by the novel, selective antagonist, BWA868C. *Br J Pharmacol* 1989; **96:** 307–12.

65. Sanner JH. Antagonism of prostaglandin E_2 by 1-acetyl-2-(8-chloro-10,11-dihydrobenz[b,f] [1,4] oxazepine-10-carbonyl) hydrazine (SC-19220). *Arch Int Pharmacodyn Ther* 1969; **180:** 46–56.

66. Coleman RA, Denyer LH, Sheldrick RLG. The influence of protein binding on the potency of the prostanoid EP_1-receptor blocking drug, AH6809. *Br J Pharmacol* 1985; **86:** 203P.

67. Sanner JH, Mueller RA, Schulze RH. Structure–activity relationships of some dibenzoxazepine derivatives as prostaglandin antagonists. *Adv Biosci* 1973; **9:** 139–48.

68. Drower EJ, Stapelfeld A, Mueller RA, Hammond DL. The antinociceptive effects of prostaglandin antagonists in the rat. *Eur J Pharmacol* 1987; **133:** 249–56.

69. Head SA, Louttit JB, Coleman RA. The actions of meclofenamic acid at prostanoid receptors. *Br J Pharmacol Proc Suppl* 1992; **106:** 106P.

70. Fassina G, Froldi G, Caparrotta L. A stable isosterically modified prostacyclin analogue, FCE22176, acting as a competitive antagonist to prostacyclin in guinea-pig trachea and atria. *Eur J Pharmacol* 1985; **113:** 459–60.

71. Ceserani R, Gandolfi C, Longiave D, Mandelli V. A new selective antagonist of prostaglandins: 20-methyl-13,14-didehydro-$PGF_{2\alpha}$. *Prostaglandins Med* 1979; **2:** 455–7.

72. Maddox YT, Ramwell PW, Shiner CS, Corey EJ. Amide and 1-amino derivatives of F prostaglandins as prostaglandin antagonists. *Nature* 1978; **273:** 549–52.

73. Gorman RR, Bundy GL, Peterson DC, Sun FF, Miller OV, Fitzpatrick FA. Inhibition of human platelet thromboxane synthetase by 9,11-azaprosta-5,13-dienoic acid. *Proc Natl Acad Sci USA* 1977; **74:** 4007–11.

74. Fitzpatrick FA, Bundy GL, Gorman RR, Honohan T. 9,11-Epoxyiminoprosta-5,13-dienoic acid is a thromboxane A_2 antagonist in human platelets. *Nature* 1978; **275:** 764–6.

75. Nicolaou KC, Magolda RL, Smith JB, Aharony D, Smith EF, Lefer AM. Synthesis and biological properties of pinane-thromboxane A_2, a selective inhibitor of coronary artery constriction, platelet aggregation and thromboxane formation. *Proc Natl Acad Sci USA* 1979; **76:** 2566–70.

76. Sprague PW, Heikes JE, Harris DN, Greenberg R. Stereo controlled synthesis of 7-oxabicyclo [2,2,1] heptane prostaglandin analogues as TxA_2 antagonists. *Adv Prostaglandin Thromboxane Res* 1980; **6:** 493–6.

77. Coleman RA, Collington EW, Geisow HP, *et al.* AH19437, a specific thromboxane receptor blocking drug. *Br J Pharmacol* 1981; **72:** 524–5P.

78. Brittain RT, Boutal L, Carter MC, *et al.* AH23848:

a thromboxane receptor blocking drug that can clarify the pathophysiologic role of thromboxane A2. *Circulation* 1985; **72**: 1208–18.

79. Jones RL, Wilson NH. Thromboxane receptor antagonism shown by a prostanoid with a bicyclo [2,2,1] heptane ring. *Br J Pharmacol* 1981; **73**: 220–1P.

80. Armstrong RA, Jones RL, Wilson NH. Effect of the thromboxane receptor antagonist EP092 endotoxin shock in the sheep. *Prostaglandins* 1985; **29**: 703–13.

81. Brewster AG, Brown GR, Foubister AJ, Jessup R, Smithers MJ. The synthesis of a novel thromboxane receptor antagonist 4(Z)-6-(2-o-chlorophenyl-4-o-hydroxyphenyl-1,3-dioxan-cis-5-yl) hexenoic acid ICI 192605. *Prostaglandins* 1988; **36**: 173–8.

82. Lefer AM. Daltroban (BM13505) – a highly specific, potent thromboxane receptor antagonist. *Drugs Future* 1988; **13**: 999–1005.

83. Hall RA, Gillard J, Guindon Y, *et al.* Pharmacology of L-655,240 (3-[1-(4-chlorobenzyl)-5-fluoro-3-methyl indol-2-yl] 2,2-dimethylpropanoic acid); a potent selective thromboxane/prostaglandin endoperoxide antagonist. *Eur J Pharmacol* 1987; **135**: 193–201.

84. Rosentreter U, Boeshagen H, Seuter F, Perzborn E, Fiedler VB. Synthesis and absolute configuration of the new thromboxane antagonist 3(R)-3-(4-fluorophenylsulphonamido)-1,2,3,4-tetrahydro-9-carbazole propanoic acid and comparison with its exantiomer. *Arzneimittelforschung* 1989; **39**: 1519–21.

85. McKenniff MG, Norman P, Cuthbert NJ, Gardiner PJ. BAYu3405, a potent and selective thromboxane A2 receptor antagonist on airway smooth muscle *in vitro*. *Br J Pharmacol* 1991; **104**: 585–90.

86. Cooper B, Ahern D. Characterization of the platelet prostaglandin D2 receptor. *J Clin Invest* 1979; **64**: 586–90.

87. Town MH, Casals-Stenzel J, Schillinger E. Pharmacological and cardiovascular properties of a hydantoin derivative, BW245C, with high affinity and selectivity for PGD2 receptors. *Prostaglandins* 1983; **25**: 13–28.

88. Schillinger E, Prior G, Speckenbach A, Wellershof S. Receptor binding in various tissues of PGE2, PGF2α and sulprostone, a novel PGE2-derivative. *Prostaglandins* 1979; **18**: 293–302.

89. Oien HG, Babiarz EM, Soderman DD, Ham EA, Kuehl FA. Evidence for a PGE-receptor in rat kidney. *Prostaglandins* 1979; **17**: 525–42.

90. Strong P, Coleman RA, Humphrey PPA. Prostanoid-induced inhibition of lipolysis in rat isolated adipocytes: probable involvement of EP3 receptors. *Prostaglandins* 1992; **43**: 559–66.

91. Halushka PV, Mais DE, Garvin M. Binding of a thromboxane A2/prostaglandin H2 receptor antagonist to guinea-pig platelets. *Eur J Pharmacol* 1986; **131**: 49–54.

92. Armstrong RA, Jones RL, Wilson NH. Ligand binding to thromboxane receptors on human platelets: correlation with biological activity. *Br J Pharmacol* 1983; **79**: 953–64.

93. Hung SC, Ghali NI, Venton DL, Le Breton GC. Specific binding of the thromboxane A2 antagonist 13-aza-prostanoic acid in human platelet membranes. *Biochim Biophys Acta* 1983; **728**: 171–8.

94. Burch RM, Mais DE, Pepkowitz SH, Halushka PV. Hydrodynamic properties of a thromboxane A2 prostaglandin H2 antagonist binding site solubilized from human platelets. *Biochem Biophys Res Commun* 1985; **132**: 961–8.

95. Kattelman EJ, Venton DL, Le Breton GC. Characterisation of U-46619 binding in unactivated intact human platelets and determination of binding site affinities of four TxA2/PGH2 receptor antagonists (13-APA, BM13177, ONO3708 and SQ29547). *Thromb Res* 1986; **41**: 471–81.

96. Hedberg A, Hall SE, Ogletree ML, Harris DN, Liu EC-K. Characterisation of [5,6-³H] SQ29,548 as a high affinity radioligand binding to thromboxane A2/prostaglandin H2-receptors in human platelets. *J Pharmacol Exp Ther* 1988; **245**: 786–92.

97. Armstrong RA, Lumley P, Humphrey PPA. Characteristics of [³H]-GR32191 binding to the thromboxane (TP-) receptor of human platelets. *Br J Pharmacol Proc Suppl* 1989; **98**: 843P.

98. Armstrong RA, Lumley P, Humphrey PPA. Reduction in the number of thromboxane TP-receptors (Bmax) on human platelets after exposure to GR32191. *Br J Pharmacol Proc Suppl* 1990; **99**: 113P.

99. Loutzenhiser R, Van Breeman C. Mechanism of activation of isolated rabbit aorta by PGH2 analogue U-44069. *Am J Physiol* 1981; **241**: C243–9.

100. Toda N. Mechanism of action of carbacyclic thromboxane A2 and its interaction with prostaglandin I2 and verapamil in isolated arteries. *Circ Res* 1982; **51**: 675–82.

101. Itoh T, Ueno H, Kuriyama H. Calcium induced calcium release mechanism in vascular smooth muscles – assessments based on contractions evoked in intact and saponin-treated skinned muscles. *Experientia* 1985; **41**: 989–96.

102. Pollock WK, Armstrong RA, Brydon LJ, Jones RL, MacIntyre DE. Thromboxane-induced phosphatidate formation in human platelets. Relationship to receptor occupancies and to changes in cytosolic free calcium. *Biochem J* 1984; **219**: 833–42.

103. MacIntyre DE, Shaw AM, Bushfield M, MacMillan LJ, McNicol A, Pollock WK. Endogenous and pharmacological mechanisms for the regulation of human platelet cytosolic free Ca^{2+}. *Nouv Rev Fr Hematol* 1985; **27**: 285–92.

104. Creese BR, Denborough MA. The effects of prostaglandin E2 on contractility and cyclic AMP levels of guinea-pig tracheal smooth muscle. *Clin Exp Pharmacol Physiol* 1981; **8**: 616–17.

105. Gutman Y, Boonjaviroj P, Eckstein L. Mechanism of PGE and alpha adrenergic effects on release of catecholamines. *Adv Biosci* 1979; **18**: 341–5.
106. Losert W, Loge O, Schillinger E, Casals-Stenzel J. On the pharmacology of sulprostone. In: Friebel K, Schneider A, Würfel H (eds), *International Sulprostone Symposium*. Berlin: Schering, 1979: 47–54.
107. Kather H, Zimmer B. Mechanisms of prostaglandin action on human fat cell lipolysïs. *Adv Prostaglandin Thromboxane Leukotriene Res* 1983; **12**: 253–8.
108. Behrman HR, Luborsky JL, Aten RF, *et al.* Luteolytic hormones are calcium-mediated, guanine nucleotide antagonists of gonadotrophin-sensitive adenylate cyclase. *Adv Prostaglandin Thromboxane Leukotriene Res* 1985; **15**: 601–7.
109. Raymond V, Leung PCK, Labric F. Stimulation by prostaglandin $F_{2\alpha}$ of phosphatidic acid phosphatidylinositol turnover in rat luteal cells. *Biochem Biophys Res Commun* 1983; **116**: 39–46.
110. Somova L, Bojkov B. PGE_2 and $PGF_{2\alpha}$, cyclic nucleotides and reactivity of the rat femoral artery. *Acta Physiol Pharmacol Bulg* 1983; **9**: 36–42.
111. Hardcastle J, Hardcastle PT, Redfern JS. Morphine has no direct effect on PGE_2-stimulated cyclic AMP production by rat isolated enterocytes. *J Pharm Pharmacol* 1982; **34**: 68.
112. Alvarez R, Taylor A, Fazzari JJ, Jacobs JR. Regulation of cyclic AMP metabolism in human platelets. Sequential activation of adenylate cyclase and cyclic AMP phosphodiesterase by prostaglandins. *Mol Pharmacol* 1981; **20**: 302–9.
113. Haslam RJ, Davidson MML, Davies T, Lynham JA, McClenaghan MD. Regulation of blood platelet functional by cyclic nucleotides. In: George WJ, Ignaro LJ (eds), *Advances in Cyclic Nucleotide Research*. New York: Raven Press, 1978: 552–3.
114. Simon B, Kather H, Kommerell B. Activation of human colonic mucosal adenylate cyclase by prostaglandins. *Adv Prostaglandin Thromboxane Res* 1980; **8**: 1617–20.
115. Simon B, Kather H. Human colonic adenylate cyclase. Stimulation of enzyme activity by vasoactive intestinal polypeptide and various prostaglandins via distinct receptor sites. *Digestion* 1980; **20**: 62–7.
116. Andersen NH, Eggerman TL, Harker LA, Wilson CH, De B. On the multiplicity of platelet prostaglandin receptors. 1. Evaluation of competitive antagonism by aggregometry. *Prostaglandins* 1980; **19**: 711–34.
117. Strange PG. The structure and mechanism of neurotransmitter receptors. Implications for the structure and function of the central nervous system. *J Biochem* 1988; **249**: 309–18.
118. Shenker A, Goldsmith P, Unson CG, Spiegel AM. The G protein coupled to the thromboxane A_2 receptor in human platelets is a member of the novel G_q family. *J Biol Chem* 1991; **266**: 9309–13.

3 Metabolism and toxicology of the prostaglandins

Jacqueline G Hanss and Graham W Taylor

The metabolism of arachidonic acid via the cyclo-oxygenase pathway generates a family of potent biologically active lipids known as the prostanoids; these include the classic prostaglandins E_2, D_2 and $F_{2\alpha}$, as well as prostacyclin (PGI_2) and thromboxane A_2 (TXA_2) (Fig. 3.1). These compounds possess a wide spectrum of activity, which is often species, sex and tissue dependent. The prostanoids have been implicated in a number of pivotal mechanisms of clinical importance, in homoeostasis as well as in disease. Although the prostanoids have been known for many years, it is only recently that they have found clinical applications.

Levels of prostanoids *in vivo* depend on their rate of synthesis, and this is regulated by phospholipase mobilization of arachidonic acid from phospholipids, its oxygenation in the presence of cyclo-oxygenase and finally through the action of the various synthases. Circulating and tissue prostanoid concentrations are also dependent on their rate of metabolism.

Metabolism

In general, metabolism leads to a reduction or inactivation of the biological effects of the prostanoid, whilst at the same time facilitating renal clearance by increasing the number of polar function groups in the substances. Metabolism can occur in a number of tissues, particularly in the lung, the liver and the kidney.

The metabolism of the prostanoids appears at first sight to be complex, numerous metabolites arising from a few primary bioactive prostaglandins. This picture can be considerably simplified when it is understood that there are only five basic enzymic pathways involved in the metabolism of the prostanoids (Fig. 3.2): dehydrogenation (oxidation) of the 15-hydroxyl function; reduction of the 9-, 11- or 5-oxo function to the corresponding hydroxyl group; reduction of the 13,14 double bond; β-oxidation of the α(C-1 to C-7) side chain; and, finally, cytochrome P450-mediated oxidation of the ω(C-13 to C-20) side chain and the associated oxidations to the aldehyde and acid. These reactions are catalysed by a variety of different enzymes which are not necessarily specific to the prostanoids, and almost certainly play a wider role in metabolic processes than in the control of prostanoid levels alone. A further pathway of biological importance is the non-enzymic hydrolysis that leads to the rapid inactivation of PGI_2 and TXA_2. These reactions are outlined in Fig. 3.2 and are discussed in some detail below.

Hydrolysis

Prostaglandins E_2, D_2 and $F_{2\alpha}$ are stable to hydrolysis (although they can undergo other chemical rearrangements). In contrast, both PGI_2 and TXA_2 are

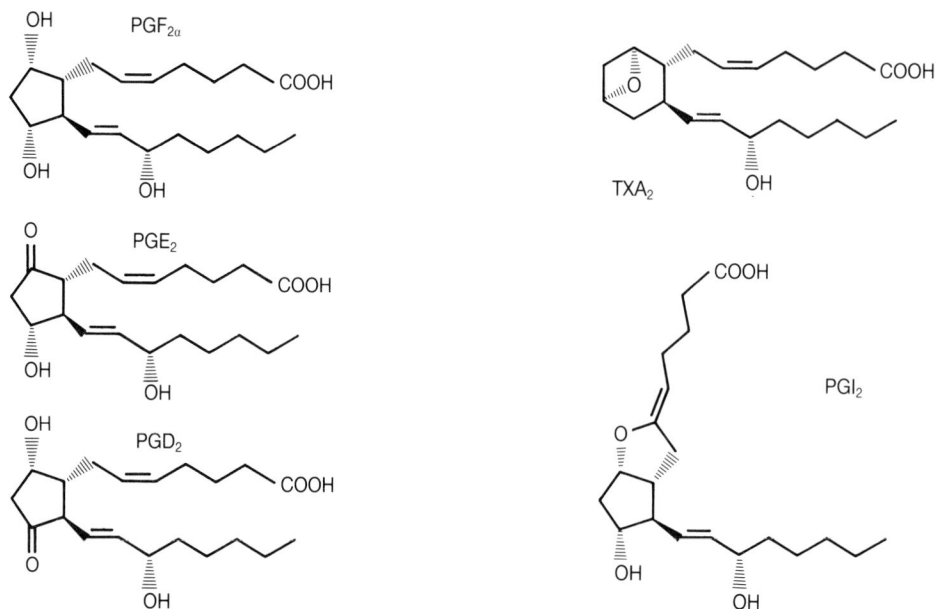

Fig. 3.1 Arachidonic acid is converted to five major prostanoids: PGE_2, PGD_2, $PGF_{2\alpha}$, PGI_2 and TXA_2. Tissue and circulating levels of prostanoids *in vivo* depend on their rate of synthesis and their rate of metabolism.

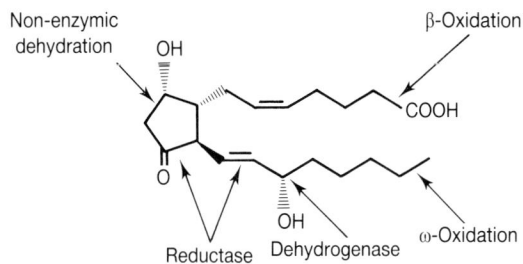

Fig. 3.2 Although the metabolism of the prostanoids appears at first sight to be complex, there are only five major enzymic pathways involved: oxidation of hydroxyl functions to carbonyl groups; reduction of carbonyls back to hydroxyls; reduction of the 13, 14 double bond; β-oxidation; and ω-oxidation. Non-enzymic hydrolysis, dehydration and isomerization reactions are also important.

rapidly hydrolysed in aqueous solution. PGI_2 is hydrolysed by an acid-catalysed mechanism to 6-oxo-$PGF_{1\alpha}$ (Fig. 3.3a). At neutral pH (e.g. in plasma), PGI_2 has a half-life of 2 minutes and can be detected by bioassay on rat aorta using a superfusion cascade.[1,2] It is stable under basic conditions, or in the presence of proteins with basic PGI_2 binding sites such as albumin. TXA_2 is even more labile in solution, with a half-life in plasma of less than 7 seconds, but, again, may be detected by bioassay.[3] TXA_2 has

never been isolated from a biological preparation. It is converted to a stable hydrolysis product, TXB_2 (Fig. 3.3b). Both 6-oxo-$PGF_{1\alpha}$ and TXB_2 may be considered as parent prostanoids which then undergo further metabolism.

Dehydrogenases

The prostaglandin dehydrogenases catalyse the oxidation of hydroxyl functions to the corresponding carbonyl function.

15-Hydroxyprostaglandin dehydrogenase

The initial step in the catabolism of a number of prostanoids is the oxidation of the 15-hydroxy group to the corresponding 15-ketoprostanoid by an NAD^+/$NADP^+$-linked enzyme – 15-hydroxyprostaglandin dehydrogenase (15-PGDH) (Fig. 3.4). These enzymes are cytosolic and fairly widespread in mammalian tissues. There are two families of these enzymes involved in prostanoid metabolism; one group of dehydrogenase uses NAD^+ as a cofactor, and the other group uses $NADP^+$.[4,5] These enzymes are distributed among different tissues, with the $NADP^+$-dependent enzyme found mainly in brain, kidney and red blood cells, and the NAD^+-dependent enzymes in the lung, heart, liver and kidney.[5–7] The 15-PGDH enzymes exhibit a degree of specificity for

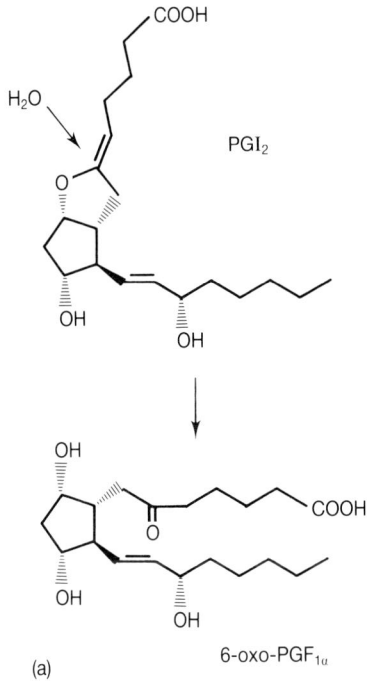

(a)

6-oxo-PGF$_{1a}$

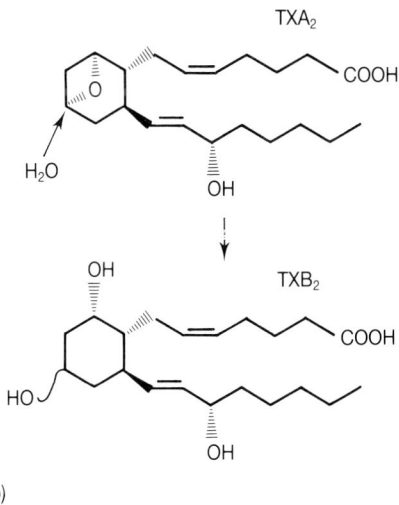

(b)

Fig. 3.3 Both PGI$_2$ and TXA$_2$ are rapidly hydrolysed at neutral pH. PGI$_2$ has a half-life of 2 minutes. TXA$_2$ is even more labile in solution with a half-life in plasma of <7 seconds. (*a*) Hydrolysis of PGI$_2$ to 6-oxo-PGF$_{1a}$. (*b*) Hydrolysis of TXA$_2$ to TXB$_2$.

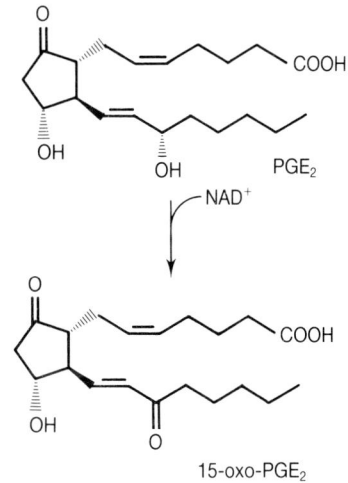

Fig. 3.4 The initial step in the catabolism of a number of prostanoids is the oxidation of the 15-hydroxy group to the corresponding 15-ketoprostanoid by an NAD$^+$/NADP$^+$-linked enzyme – 15 hydroxyprostaglandin dehydrogenase.

to their 15-keto derivatives occurs most rapidly through an NADP$^+$ enzyme.[8] The lung NAD$^+$-dependent PGDH will also oxidize other lipids, including the lipoxygenase product, 15-hydroxyeicosatetraenoic acid (15-HETE) and a number of ω6 hydroxy fatty acids to their corresponding keto derivatives; the enzyme is not specific for the cyclopentane-containing prostaglandins.[9]

PGI$_2$ is a substrate *in vitro* for an NADP$^+$-dependent PGDH enzyme present in kidney and has a similar K_m value to the primary prostaglandins.[10] In contrast, 6-oxo-PGF$_{1a}$ is a much poorer substrate for PDGH and Δ^{13}-reductase.

Inhibitors of 15-PGDH include the substituted phenylazobenzene acetic acid derivatives, Ph CL28A and Ph CK61A[11] which have been shown to increase the output of PGE$_2$ and PGF$_{1a}$ but not that of 6-oxo-PGF$_{1a}$ in rat isolated lung. Sofalcone (a synthetic isoprenyl flavanoid derived from sophoradin) orally administered will also inhibit PGDH, which is present in large amounts in the gastrointestinal tract; this is thought to explain the increase in PGE$_2$ and sofalcone's anti-ulcer properties.[12] Sulphasalazine will also inhibit this pathway.[13]

Other prostaglandin dehydrogenases

9-Hydroxyprostaglandin dehydrogenase (9-PGDH) catalyses an NAD$^+$-dependent oxidation of the 9α-

the various prostaglandins; PGE$_2$, PGF$_{2a}$ and PGB$_2$ are preferentially inactivated by an NAD$^+$-dependent enzyme, whereas the reduction of PGD$_2$ and PGI$_2$

hydroxyl group of PGF$_{2\alpha}$ and its derivatives (15-oxo-13,14-dihydro-PGF$_{2\alpha}$ and 15-keto-PGF$_{2\alpha}$) to the corresponding PGE$_2$ derivatives without affecting other hydroxyl groups in the molecule.[14] This is not thought to be a major pathway of PGF$_{2\alpha}$ metabolism. A similar reduction occurs with 6-oxo-PGF$_{1\alpha}$ (the stable and biologically inactive hydrolysis product of prostacyclin) which is oxidized to the weak anti-aggregatory product 6-oxo-PGE$_1$. An 11-dehydrogenase can convert TXB$_2$ to a long-lived circulating metabolite, 11-dehydro-TXB$_2$.

Reductases

The carbonyl groups present in many prostanoids can be reduced to their corresponding hydroxyl functions by ubiquitous NAD(P)H-dependent reductases.

9-Ketoprostaglandin reductase
There are several 9-ketoprostaglandin reductases that catalyse the conversion of PGE$_2$ to PGF$_{2\alpha}$ (Fig. 3.5a). The reduction is stereospecific and there is no evidence for the formation of the other C-9-hydroxylated enantiomer. These enzymes are found in almost every tissue,[15] and have a wide range of substrate specificity acting as carbonyl reductases at both the 9 and 15 positions of prostaglandins. These enzymes will also reduce carbonyl functions of certain non-prostaglandin compounds although they are not active against cyclohexanone.[16] Interestingly, although these enzymes have such a broad specificity, they will not reduce the 11-keto group of PGD$_2$, which is metabolized by a distinct reductase.

11-Ketoprostaglandin reductase
The 11-carbonyl group in PGD$_2$ is metabolized via a specific 11-ketoreductase to form 9α,11β-PGF$_2$, a compound which has potent biological activity.[17] In contrast to the action of the 9-ketoreductase on PGE$_2$, this enzyme produces the 11β enantiomer of PGD$_2$ (Fig. 3.5b). PGD$_2$ 11-ketoreductase activity is widely distributed in the cytosol fraction of various bovine tissues, especially high in the liver, lung and spleen, and is associated with prostaglandin F synthetase activity.[18] It appears that the reduction of PGH$_2$ to PGF$_{2\alpha}$ and that of PGD$_2$ to 9α,11β-PGF$_2$ occur at different active sites on the same enzyme.[19] It should be noted that formation of these PGF compounds can also occur non-enzymically via auto-oxidation of arachidonate in plasma (see 'Chemical inactivation', later).[20]

15-Ketoprostaglandin Δ^{13}-reductase
Reduction of the Δ^{13,14} double bond by the reductase is the final step in the formation of 13,14-dihydro-15-oxo-PGF$_{2\alpha}$, which is the major circulating metabolite of PGE$_2$ and PGF$_{2\alpha}$ in man (Fig. 3.6). The reaction uses NADPH preferentially and can be inhibited by *p*-chloromercuribenzoic acid.[21]

β-Oxidation

When prostanoids are infused in animals or humans, urinary metabolites consist mainly of dinor and tetranor compounds; the C-1 to C-8 carboxyl side chain is shortened by two or four carbon atoms. This indicates that these arachidonic acid metabolites

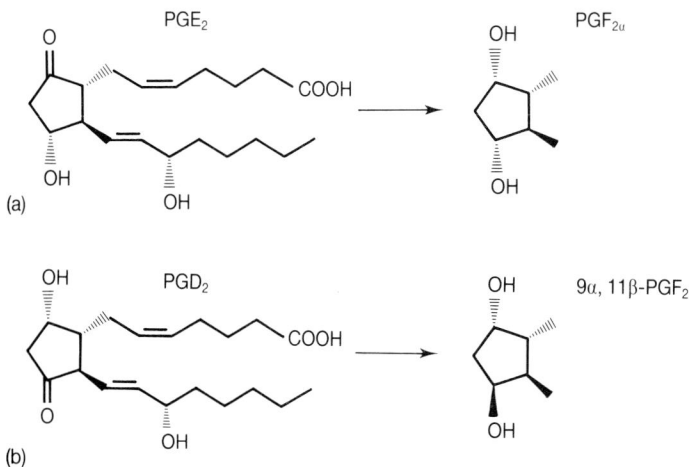

Fig. 3.5   Ubiquitous NAD(P)H-dependent reductases will reduce carbonyl groups present into their corresponding hydroxyl functions. (*a*) There are several 9-ketoprostaglandin reductases which catalyse the conversion of PGE$_2$ to PGF$_{2\alpha}$. (*b*) The 11-carbonyl group in PGD$_2$ is metabolized via a specific 11-ketoreductase to form 9α,11β-PGF$_2$. Note that the stereochemistry of the 11-hydroxyl group differs from that in PGF$_{2\alpha}$.

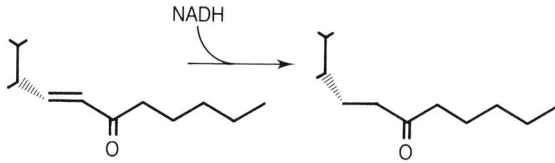

Fig. 3.6 15-Ketoprostaglandin Δ^{13}-reductase catalyses the reduction of the $\Delta^{13,14}$ double bond in many prostanoids. The reaction also uses NADPH.

behave in a manner analogous to long chain fatty acids and can undergo β-oxidation, primarily in the liver. PGE_2 is rapidly metabolized in the liver; it has been suggested that 60% of the rapid PGE_2 inactivation in the hepatocyte system occurred via β-oxidation. Non-β-oxidation accounted for 26% of PGE_2 disappearance.[22] β-Oxidation can occur both in the mitochondria and in peroxisomes; however, the specificities and mode of action of the enzyme complexes involved are markedly different.

Crude mitochondrial fractions from rat or guinea-pig liver will oxidize many saturated and unsaturated fatty acids and medium chain dicarboxylic fatty acids, and also convert a number of prostanoids to their dinor and tetranor metabolites.[23] The substrate specificity of the enzyme complex is broad, although there is a lower capacity to oxidize very long chain fatty acids. This 'β-oxidation spiral' in mitochondria is an FAD^+-, NAD^+- and CoASH-dependent pathway. Two carbons are lost at each cycle, leading eventually to the formation of acetyl CoA (Fig. 3.7). Mitochondria oxidize the major portion of the long chain fatty acids, which, because of their abundance, constitute a major source of metabolic fuel.

The peroxisomal β-oxidation pathway appears to act mainly as a chain-shortening system for fatty acids which in particular can degrade the prostanoids. The peroxisomal fraction of a rat liver homogenate has the highest capacity to β-oxidize prostaglandins with chain shortening of $PGF_{2\alpha}$ and PGE_2 to dinor and tetranor metabolites.[24] The reaction is dependent on NAD^+, CoA, ATP and Mg^{2+} and was stimulated by FAD^+. Incubation of PGE_2 with liver peroxisomes resulted in conversion into several products, one of which was the tetranor PGB_1, the B series prostanoid being formed through non-enzymic dehydration and isomerization of the PGE metabolite (see 'Chemical inactivation', later).[25] The enzymes catalysing β-oxidation in rat liver peroxisomes differ from the corresponding mitochondrial enzymes; they possess a large spectrum of activity and appear to be better equipped to handle polyunsaturated and very long chain fatty acids. In peroxisomes, the first

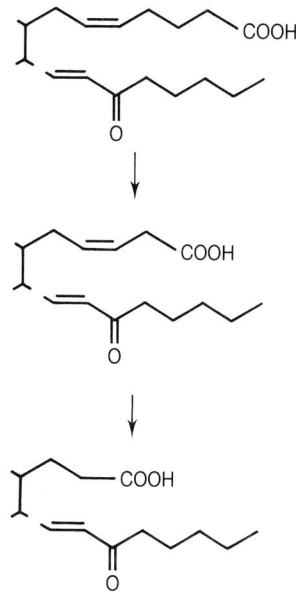

Fig. 3.7 β-Oxidation shortens prostanoids and other fatty acids by two carbon atoms to generate the dinor and tetranor species. The reaction can occur in both mitochondria and peroxisomes.

enzymic step is catalysed by an acyl-CoA oxidase, the second and third steps are catalysed by a bifunctional enzyme and the last step is catalysed by a peroxisomal 3-oxoacyl-CoA thiolase. Interestingly, partial conversion of $PGF_{2\alpha}$ to 2,3-dehydro-$PGF_{2\alpha}$ was observed, indicating that peroxisomal reduction also occurred and suggesting that, in contrast to mitochondrial fatty acid oxidation, the peroxisomal pathway is not tightly coupled.[26] Clofibrate induces peroxisomal proliferation, and it has been demonstrated that hepatocytes from clofibrate-treated rats are able to metabolize PGE_2 more efficiently than control cells,[27] and this has been suggested as a mechanism for modulating the hepatic effects of prostanoids.

The exact physiological role of peroxisomal β-oxidation remains unknown; indeed, the relative importance of peroxisomal and mitochondrial oxidation of the prostanoids has not been defined, although in man, it appears that peroxisomal inactivation of prostanoids is of greater metabolic significance than mitochondrial inactivation. In patients in whom intact peroxisomes are absent (Zellweger syndrome), $PGF_{2\alpha}$ is converted to the ω-oxidized C-20-prostaglandin, 9,11-dihydroxy-15-oxoprost-5-ene-1,20-dioic acid, with little of the tetranor derivative which is the major urinary metabolite in normal subjects.[28] β-Oxidation can be inhibited by the long chain fatty acid, palmitic acid and other inhibitors of oxidative metabolism[29] although it is not clear whether this can have any physiological effects in man.

ω-Oxidation: cytochromes P450

The ω side chain of prostaglandins, like many long chain fatty acids, are hydroxylated by microsomal mono-oxygenases (cytochromes P450) present in liver and kidney, and, to a lesser extent, in the lung (Fig. 3.9). There is a superfamily of these membrane-bound enzymes[30] possessing a wide range of substrate specificities, many of which can be induced by drugs such as phenobarbitone and clofibrate. In man, the main urinary metabolites of many prostanoids are generated through ω-oxidation. Although ω-hydroxy prostaglandins are initially produced, further oxidation to the corresponding carboxylic acid often occurs *in vivo* (Fig. 3.8). Although ω-oxidation generally inactivates the prostanoids, it is possible that these derivatives of some prostaglandins may themselves possess biological activity.

Work on P450-mediated oxidation of prostanoids is complicated by the varied nomenclature used. When the action of a cytochrome P450 on a pro-stanoid is first described, it is then usual to describe the enzyme in terms of its activity: P450$_{ka}$ is a renal enzyme which hydroxylates PGA$_1$,[31] whereas a rabbit enzyme, P450$_{PGω}$, was reported to cause ω-oxidation of a number of prostanoids.[32] In other cases, the enzymes are named after the inducing agents: P450$_{PB-1}$ is a liver enzyme induced by phenobarbitone. It is not always clear from such nomenclature whether these enzymes are similar or markedly different. Recently, a nomenclature for cytochromes P450 was agreed that is based on the gene from which they are transcribed. For example, the inducible benzo(a)pyrene metabolizing enzyme is termed CYP1A1: this defines the enzyme as a cytochrome P450 from family 1, subfamily A, member 1. The new nomenclature for cytochromes P450 and a comparison with the older names can be found in reference 30.

The ω-hydroxylation of fatty acids, leukotrienes and prostaglandins is catalysed by the CYP IVA family. Lauric acid is oxidized preferentially by CYP4A1, although it appears that this is not the major enzyme involved in prostanoid metabolism. In general, the liver possesses the greatest P450 oxidizing capacity;[33] however, both kidney and liver can catalyse ω-oxidation of fatty acids at similar rates.[34]

These enzymes rarely hydroxylate prostanoids only at the ω position, and there are many examples of ω$_{-1}$ and ω$_{-2}$-oxidation; seminal fluid, for example, containing large amounts of 19-hydroxy PGE$_1$ and 19-hydroxy PGE$_2$.[35] There are a number of hepatic cytochromes P450 with different specificities. For example, the specificity of rat liver P450 UT-8 to PGA$_1$ was high whereas P450 UT-2 has moderate PGE ω$_{-2}$-hydroxylation activity. PGA$_1$ undergoes ω-hydroxylation by multiple forms of P450. In the rat liver it has been shown that PGA$_1$ was specifically metabolized by P450 UT-8 with ω-hydroxylation. P450 UT-2 (11B) and PB-1 (11B1) could hydroxylate PGA$_1$ by ω$_{-1}$-hydroxylation, but with low activity.[31,36] Consistent with this report, P450 UT-2 had only slight PGA$_1$ ω$_{-1}$-hydroxylation activity.

Recently, two forms of the P450 causing ω-hydroxylation have been cloned in rabbit kidney. The mRNA for P450 ka-1 was found to be expressed in the liver and kidney whilst the mRNA for P450 ka-2 was expressed in kidney, liver and small intestine. These have ω-hydroxylation toward PGA.[34] A further two have been characterized: P450 kc and P450 kd in this same model.[37] Rabbit pulmonary cytochrome P450p-2 (CYP4A4) has high activity as a prostaglandin ω-hydroxylase.[38] Lung microsomal prostaglandin ω-hydroxylation is mediated by the pregnancy

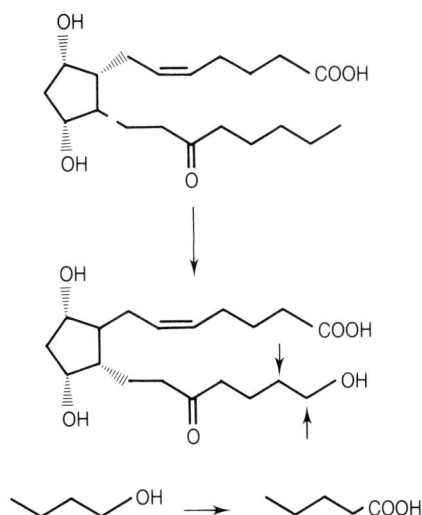

Fig. 3.8 The ω side chain of prostaglandins, like many long chain fatty acids, are hydroxylated by cytochromes P450 to the hydroxy derivatives. There are many examples of ω$_{-1}$- and ω$_{-2}$-oxidation. The hydroxy-prostanoids are often further oxidized *in vivo* by NAD(P)$^+$-dependent cytosolic dehydrogenases (such as ADH) to the carboxylic acid.

inducible P450PG-ω and inhibited by 11-DDYA and 17-ODYA.[39] The ratio between β- and ω-oxidation products in urine can be altered by diet. This ratio (between β- and β+ω-oxidation) was highest for the animals fed fish oil, intermediate after HCO feeding, and lowest for SO administration. The results clearly indicate that various dietary lipids have different effects on the oxidative metabolic pathway of prostanoids.[40,41]

Chemical inactivation

Prostaglandins can also undergo non-enzymic conversion to products that may themselves be metabolized. PGE$_2$ will readily eliminate water under acid conditions to form the $\Delta^{10,11}$ unsaturated product (PGA$_2$). This double bond will rearrange, first, to $\Delta^{11,12}$ (PGC$_2$), which rapidly rearranges to the stable conjugated dienone, PGB$_2$. PGA$_2$ and PGB$_2$ are often found as byproducts in systems in which PGE$_2$ is generated (Fig. 3.9). This is exemplified in a recent study on the metabolism of PGE$_2$ by human fetal membranes: the major metabolite 13,14-dihydro-15-oxo-PGE$_2$ was produced along with PGA$_2$, PGB$_2$ and 13,14-dihydro-15-oxo-PGA$_2$ (Fig. 3.10).[42] PGD$_2$ can also undergo acid-catalysed dehydration, forming PGJ$_2$. Rearrangement and further dehydration can then occur to form Δ^{12}-PGJ$_2$ (Fig. 3.10). 13,14-Dihydro-15-oxo-PGA$_2$ can also undergo further rearrangement, particularly at high pH, to form a bicyclo compound. Recently, Morrow and colleagues noted that a number of PGF compounds were formed in plasma on storage by non-enzymic processes.[20] Not only can this interfere with the

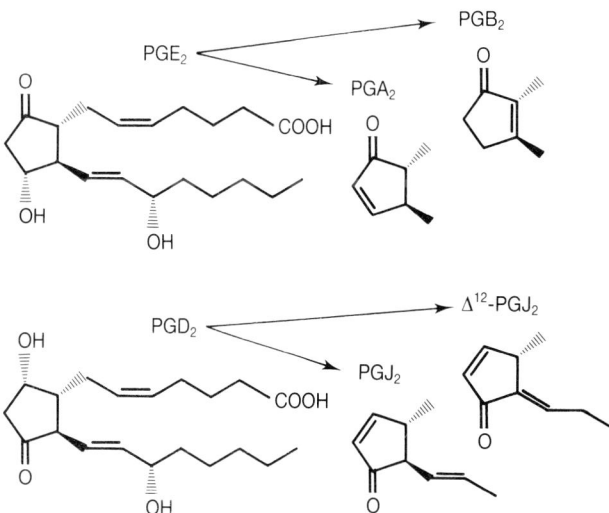

Fig. 3.10 The metabolism of ^{3}H-PGE$_2$ (I) by human fetal membranes leads to the formation of 13,14-dihydro-15-oxo-PGE$_2$ (II) along with PGA$_2$ and PGB$_2$ (II, unresolved) formed through non-enzymic inactivation. 13,14-Dihydro-15-oxo-PGA$_2$ is also produced through metabolism of PGA$_2$ (IV).

quantification of PGF compounds, but it appears that at least one of these compounds, 8-epi-PGF, is a potent renal vasoconstrictor.

Major metabolites in man

If prostanoids are altered in disease, measurement may be used to monitor prostanoid levels and gain an insight into the mechanism and effects of treat-

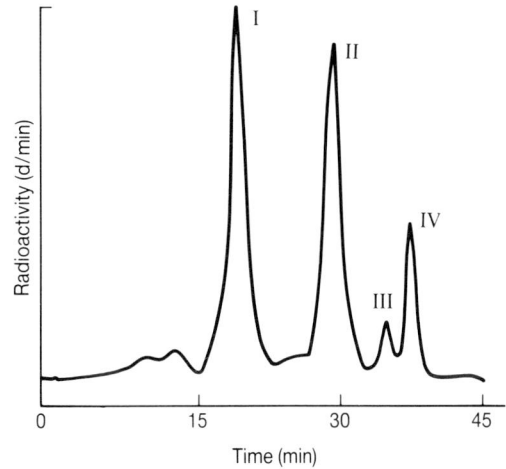

Fig. 3.9 Non-enzymic inactivation of PGE$_2$ leads to the formation of PGA$_2$ and PGB$_2$ by dehydration and isomerization. PGD$_2$ is similarly converted to PGJ$_2$ derivatives.

ment on the disease. Plasma levels of the parent prostanoids are extremely low, as would be expected for local hormones. As the prostaglandins are very rapidly metabolized *in vivo*, attention has been diverted to suitable metabolites. The major metabolites in man of the 2-series prostanoids are summarized below and in Table 3.1.

PGE$_2$ and PGF$_{2\alpha}$ are first modified by 15-PGDH and Δ^{13}-reductase activity, leading to formation of 15-oxo-13,14-dihydro prostaglandins as major circulating metabolites.[43] There is almost complete metabolism of these species during first pass through the lung. Further ω- and β-oxidation leads to chain-shortened tetranor 1,16-dicarboxylic acids (7α-hydroxy-5,11-dioxo-tetranorprosta-1,16-dioic acid and 5α,7α-dihydroxy-11-oxo-tetranorprosta-1,16-dioic acid respectively) as the major urinary metabolites.[44] PGD$_2$ is converted in the circulation to 9α,11β-F$_2$ (9 pg/ml) which is biologically active[45] and then on to 9α,11β-15-oxo-PGF$_2$ and its 13,14 dihydro-15-oxo-derivative which is the major plasma metabolite.[46] The major urinary metabolite is the ω/β-oxidation product, 9α,11β-dihydroxy-15-oxo-2,3,18,19-tetranorprost-5-ene-1,20-dioic acid, which can be used as a marker of PGD$_2$ production *in vivo*, although at least 20 other minor metabolites are also found in urine.[47]

Prostacylin and TXA$_2$ are rapidly hydrolysed in plasma generating low (1–2 pg/ml) circulating levels of 6-oxo-PGF$_{1\alpha}$ and TXB$_2$ respectively. Dinor-6,15-dioxo-13,14-dihydro-PGF$_{1\alpha}$ and its ω-oxidized analogue could also be identified as circulating metabolites.[48] Low levels of circulating 11-dehydro TXB$_2$ are also present,[49] and may offer a way to overcome the problems of *ex vivo* determination of TX levels. The major urinary metabolites are the 2,3-dinor products produced mainly in the liver, and it is generally accepted that these metabolites offer a time-integrated measure of TXA$_2$ and PGI$_2$ turnover in man. Under basal conditions urinary TXB$_2$ and 6-oxo-PGF$_{1\alpha}$ probably arise mainly from the kidney, although this no longer holds under conditions of systemic stimulation.[50]

Toxicology and clinical use

Of the naturally occurring prostanoids, only PGE$_1$, PGE$_2$ (dinoprostone), PGF$_{2\alpha}$ (dinoprost) and PGI$_2$ (epoprostenol) have found clinical applications, although a number of analogues (e.g. enprostil, misoprostol, iloprost) have been developed for clinical use. As many of the biological properties and clinical effects of the prostaglandins are covered elsewhere in this book, we will concentrate here on the generally unwanted effects of prostanoids and their analogues in man.

Clinical pharmacology of the prostanoids

There have been a number of studies investigating the clinical pharmacology of the natural prostaglandins through oral, inhaled or intravenous routes of administration. With the exception of prostacyclin which is rapidly hydrolysed, most prostanoids may be absorbed orally, although this may lead to rapid

Table 3.1 Major metabolites of prostanoids in man

Prostanoid	Plasma	Urine*
PGE$_2$†	13,14-dihydro-15-oxo-PGE$_2$	7α-hydroxy-5,11-dioxo-tetranorprosta-1,16-dioic acid
PGD$_2$†	9α,11β-PGF$_2$ and its 15-oxo-PGF$_2$ and 13,14-dihydro-15-oxo derivatives	9α,11β-dihydroxy-15-oxo-2,3,18,19-tetranorprost-5-ene-1,20-dioic acid
PGF$_{2\alpha}$	13,14-dihydro-15-keto-PGF$_{2\alpha}$	5α,7α-dihydroxy-11-oxo-tetranorprosta-1,16-dioic acid
PGI$_2$/6-oxo-PGF$_{1\alpha}$	6-oxo-PGF$_{1\alpha}$	2,3-dinor 6-oxo PGF$_{1\alpha}$
TXA$_2$/TXB$_2$	TXB$_2$,‡ 11-dehydro-TXB$_2$	2,3-dinor TXB$_2$

*There are numerous urinary metabolites of the endogenous prostanoids. The majority of prostaglandin metabolites are C-18 or C-16 compounds, the result of one or two cycles of β-oxidation.

†Both PGE$_2$ and PGD$_2$ will form chemical dehydration/isomerization products (PGA$_2$, PGB$_2$ and PGJ$_2$).

‡Circulating levels of TXB$_2$ are extremely low (1–2 pg/ml). Reports of raised circulating levels are normally associated with platelet activation on venepuncture.

first-pass metabolism in the liver. Inhaled prostanoids rapidly cross the epithelial barrier and pass into the circulation where they can exert systemic effects. One problem with inhalation is that only a small proportion of the dose (<10%) reaches the second and third generation bronchi with their smooth muscle. A large proportion of the dose is swallowed or (particularly if the particles are charged) bound to the trachea. Most of the pharmacokinetic data on prostanoids has been obtained through infusion studies, and this route, in particular, has increased our awareness of the action and side effects of these compounds.

PGE series

PGE_1 and PGE_2 are vasodilators which cause a small increase in heart rate and decrease blood pressure. PGE_2 is a potent bronchodilator when aerosolized in asthmatics[51] but has only minor pulmonary effects when infused.[52] It causes an increase in the rate and intensity of uterine contractions in pregnant women and can affect gut motility, leading to abdominal cramps. Infusion of PGE_2 (10 µg per minute) has been shown to inhibit acute release of insulin and cause glucose intolerance although some of these effects may be related to the concomitant release of catecholamines.[53] It is rapidly cleared from the circulation, with a half-life of less than 1 minute. PGE_1 (>1 µg/kg per hour), but not PGE_2, causes facial flushing. Infused PGE_1 (1 µg/kg per minute) appears to have a selective effect on the pulmonary vasculature, causing a reduction in the elastic recoil pressure of the lung.[54] It is also rapidly metabolized, but there is now evidence that the biologically active metabolite, 15-oxo-PGE_1, is produced during infusion of PGE_1 and may account for part of its vasodilator activity.

Misoprostol (15-deoxy-16-hydroxy-16-methyl PGE_1) is a PGE_1 analogue which has a longer duration of action and a more selective effect than PGE_1. Misoprostol is extensively metabolized to its biologically active free acid, a de-esterified derivative.[55–57] The major reported side effects of misoprostol for patients taking the recommended dose of 100–200 µg four times daily are diarrhoea and abdominal pain, headache and altered mental status.[58] One report suggests that misoprostol should be administered with caution to patients suffering from urinary stress incontinence as its authors have shown it to induce urinary incontinence.[59]

PGD₂

Unlike the E series prostanoids, PGD_2 is not used clinically. It is a vasodilator and causes intense facial flushing and nasal congestion following infusion at doses where no significant effect on blood pressure or lung function occurred or ADP-induced platelet aggregation was observed, suggesting that PGD_2 is unlikely to be a useful antithrombotic agent.[60]

PGF₂ₐ

$PGF_{2\alpha}$ is rapidly metabolized in the circulation, and thus has a very short biological half-life. $PGF_{2\alpha}$ constricts bronchial, uterine and gastrointestinal smooth muscle, and is a renal vasoconstrictor. Paradoxically, vasodilation occurs following injection into the human brachial artery. Infusion at 240 µg/kg per hour in normal subjects has shown no major cardiovascular effects[61] although it causes significant increase in airway resistance.[62] At doses over 60 µg/kg per hour, $PGF_{2\alpha}$ has been reported to cause stomach cramps and diarrhoea. Its main use is in the induction of labour and as an abortifacient.[63,64]

Prostacyclin

PGI_2 is a potent vasodilator with a threshold for pharmacological effects in man at 120 ng/kg per hour during infusion.[65] It causes a drop in blood pressure and also inhibits platelet aggregation through receptor-mediated mechanisms. These effects are always accompanied by significant side effects which include nausea, emesis, flushing, diaphoresis and restlessness. PGI_2 leads to an increase in renin activity *in vivo*.[66] Its hydrolysis product, 6-oxo-$PGF_{1\alpha}$, is essentially inactive, although there is evidence that it may be metabolized *in vivo* to 6-oxo-PGE_1 which has weak anti-aggregatory properties. The ease of hydrolysis of PGI_2 has led to the development of a number of stable analogues, of which iloprost is perhaps the best known. Iloprost causes a slight increase in heart rate, but little effect on blood pressure. As with PGI_2, infusion of iloprost 2 ng/kg per minute to subjects on peritoneal ambulatory dialysis caused a reversible reduction of platelet PGI_2 sensitivity which was rapidly reversible due to a down-regulation of PGI_2 platelet receptors.[67] Following intravenous infusion, the steady-state plasma levels of iloprost were strictly dose dependent, with a biphasic distribution and half-lives of 3–4 and 30 minutes. After oral administration, absorption of the drug was extremely rapid, achieving a maximum plasma level at ~10 minutes; except for transient side effects (facial flushing and headache), no adverse reactions were observed.[68]

Thromboxane A_2

TXA_2 is a potent aggregator of platelets and can cause bronchoconstriction and renal vasoconstriction *in vivo*. Much of the pharmacoclinical work on this eicosanoid is aimed at preventing its synthesis or antagonizing its action. The stable hydrolysis product, TXB_2, appears to be biologically inactive, with no biological effects following inhalation, ingestion or infusion.[50]

Concluding remarks

We began by noting that the apparently complex metabolic pathway for the prostanoids can be simplified into five major enzymic pathways: two reductions (ketone to hydroxyl and saturation of the 13, 14 double bond) and three oxidations (hydroxyl to ketone, β- and ω-oxidation) together with three chemical reactions (hydrolysis, dehydration and isomerization). Of course, these pathways also lead to the formation of many minor metabolites as well as the major metabolites discussed above. For example, 20 urinary metabolites of TXB_2 have been detected following administration of TXB_2 in man,[49] and a similar number identified following PGD_2 infusions.[47] As in the case of 15-oxo-PGE_1 and 9α,11β-PGF (produced from PGE_1 and PGD_2 respectively), some metabolites will possess biological activity, and this will affect the efficacy of any prostanoid treatment. Thus a knowledge of the metabolism of the prostanoids may be useful in understanding their pharmacological profile *in vivo*.

References

1. Whittiker N, Bunting S, Salmon J, *et al.* The chemical nature of prostaglandin X (prostacyclin). *Prostaglandins* 1976; **12**: 915–28.
2. Vane JR. Adventures and excursions in bioassay: the stepping stones to prostacyclin. *Br J Pharmacol* 1983; **79**: 821–38.
3. Patrono CAD. Biosynthesis and pharmacological modulation of thromboxane in humans. *Circulation* 1990; **81** (suppl I): I12–I15.
4. Watanabe K, Shimizu T, Iguchi S, Wakatsuka H, Hayashi M, Hayaishi O. An NADP-linked prostaglandin D dehydrogenase in swine brain. *J Biol Chem* 1980; **255**: 1779–82.
5. Hansen HS. 15-Hydroxyprostaglandin dehydrogenase. A review. *Prostaglandins* 1976; **12**: 647–79.
6. Lee SC, Levine L. Prostaglandin metabolism II. Identification of two 15-hydroxyprostaglandin dehydrogenase types. *J Biol Chem* 1975; **250**: 548–52.
7. Braithwaite SS, Jarabak J. Studies on a 15-hydroxy-prostaglandin dehydrogenase from human placenta. *J Biol Chem* 1975; **250**: 2315–18.
8. Robinson C, Herbert CA, Bedwell S, Shell DJ, Holgate ST. The metabolism of prostaglandin D_2. Evidence for the sequential conversion by NADPH and NAD^+ dependent pathways. *Biochem Pharmacol* 1989; **38**: 3267–71.
9. Bergholte JM, Soberman RJ, Hayes R, Murphy RC, Okita RT. Oxidation of 15-hydroxyeicosatetraenoic acid and other hydroxy fatty acids by lung prostaglandin dehydrogenase. *Arch Biochem Biophys* 1987; **257**: 444–50.
10. Korff JM, Jarabak J. Isolation and properties of an $NADP^+$ dependent PGI_2 specific 15-hydroxy prostaglandin dehydrogenase from rabbit kidney. In: Lands WE, Smith WL (eds), *Methods in Enzymology*. New York, London: Academic Press, 1982: 153–5.
11. Bakhle YS, Pankhania JJ. Inhibitors of prostaglandin dehydrogenase (Ph CL 28A and Ph CK 61A) increase output of prostaglandins from rat isolated lung. *Br J Pharmacol* 1987; **92**: 189–96.
12. Muramatsu M, Tanaka M, Murakami S, Airhara H. Inhibition of 15-hydroxy prostaglandin dehydrogenase and increase of prostaglandin E_2: effect of sofalcone on rat gastric mucosa. *Life Sci* 1987; **41**: 315–22.
13. Hoult JRS, Bacon KB, Osborne DJ, Robinson C. Organ selective conversion of prostaglandin D_2 to 9α,11β-prostaglandin F_2 and its subsequent metabolism in rat, rabbit and guinea pig. *Biochem Pharmacol* 1988; **37**: 3591 9.
14. Tai HH, Yuan B. Purification and assay of a hydroxy prostaglandin dehydrogenase from rabbit kidney. *Anal Biochem* 1976; **74**: 113–17.
15. Lee SC, Pong SS, Katzen D, Wu KY, Levine L. Distribution of prostaglandin E 9-ketoreductase and types I and II 15-hydroxyprostaglandin dehydrogenase in swine kidney medulla and cortex. *Biochemistry* 1975; **14**: 142–5.
16. Lee SC, Levine L. Purification and regulatory properties of chicken heart prostaglandin E 9-ketoreductase. *J Biol Chem* 1975; **250**: 4549–55.
17. Wendelborn DF, Morrow JD, Roberts LJ. Quantification of 9α,11β-prostaglandin F_2 by stable isotope dilution mass spectrometric assay. *Methods Enzymol* 1990; **187**: 51–62.
18. Urade Y, Watanabe K, Eguchi N, Fujii Y, Hayaishi O. 9α,11β-Prostaglandin F_2 formation in various bovine tissues. *J Biol Chem* 1990; **265**: 12029–35.
19. Watanabe K, Iguchi Y, Iguchi S, Arai Y, Hayaishi O, Roberts LJ II. Stereospecific conversion of prostaglandin D_2 to (5Z, 13E)-(15S)-9α-11β,15-trihydroxy prosta-5-13-dien-1-oic acid (9α,11β-prostaglandin F_2) and of prostaglandin H_2 to prostaglandin $F_{2α}$ by bovine lung prostaglandin F synthase. *Proc Natl Acad Sci USA* 1986; **83**: 1583–7.
20. Morrow JD, Harris TM, Roberts II LJ. Noncyclooxygenase oxidative formation of a series of novel prostaglandins. Analytical ramifications for measure-

ment of eicosanoids. *Anal Biochem* 1990; **184**: 1–10.

21. Hansen HS. Purification and assay of 15-keto-prostaglandin Δ^{13}-reductase from bovine lung. *Methods Enzymol* 1990; **186**: 156–63.

22. Scheper L, Casteels M, Vamecq J, Parmentier G, Van Veldhoven PP, Mannaerts GP. β-Oxidation of the carboxyl side chain of prostaglandin E_2 in rat liver peroxisomes and mitochondria. *J Biol Chem* 1988; **263**: 2724–31.

23. Kolvrae S, Gregersen N. *In vitro* studies on the oxidation of medium chain dicarboxylic acids in rat liver. *Biochim Biophys Acta* 1986; **876**: 515–25.

24. Schepers L, Casteels M, Vamecq J, Parmentier G, Van Veldhoven PP, Mannaerts GP. Beta-oxidation of the carboxyl side chain of prostaglandin E_2 in rat liver peroxisomes and mitochondria. *J Biol Chem* 1988; **263**: 2724–31.

25. Diczfalusy U, Alexson SEH. Peroxisomal chain-shortening of prostaglandin $F_{2\alpha}$. *J Lipid Res* 1988; **29**: 1629–36.

26. Diczfalusy U, Alexson SEH. Identification of metabolites from peroxisomal beta-oxidation of prostaglandins. *J Lipid Res.* 1990; **31**: 307–13.

27. Brass EP, Ruff LJ. Effect of clofibrate treatment on hepatic prostaglandin catabolism and action. *J Pharmacol Exp Ther* 1991; **257**: 1034–8.

28. Diczfalusy U, Kase BF, Alexson SEH, Bjorkhem I. Metabolism of prostaglandin $F_{2\alpha}$ in Zellweger syndrome. *J Clin Invest* 1991; **88**: 978–84.

29. Brass EP, Garrity MJ. Modulation of prostaglandin E_2 catabolism and action by fuel substrates in rat hepatocytes. *Biochim Biophys Acta* 1989; **1010**: 233–6.

30. Nebert DW, Nelson DR, Coon MJ, *et al.* The P450 superfamily: update on new sequences, gene mapping and recommended nomenclature. *DNA Cell Biol* 1991; **10**: 1–14.

31. Tanaka S, Imaoka S, Kusunose E, Kusunose M, Maekawa M, Funae Y. ω- and (ω-1)-hydroxylation of arachidonic acid, lauric acid and prostaglandin A_1 by multiple forms of cytochrome P450 purified from rat hepatic microsomes. *Biochim Biophys Acta* 1990; **1043**: 177–81.

32. Williams DE, Hale SE, Okita RT, Masters BS. A prostaglandin omega-hydroxylase cytochrome P450 (P-P450 PG-omega) purified from lungs of pregnant rabbits. *J Biol Chem* 1984; **259**: 14600–8.

33. Kupfer D, Jansson I, Favreau I, Theoharides AD, Schenkman JB. Regioselective hydroxylation of prostaglandins by constitutive forms of cytochrome P450 from rat liver: formation of a novel metabolite by a female-specific P450. *Arch Biochem Biophys* 1988; **261**: 186–95.

34. Yokotani N, Bernhard R, Sogawa K, *et al.* Two forms of ω-hydroxylase toward prostaglandin A and laurate. *J Biol Chem* 1989; **264**: 21665–9.

35. Taylor PL, Kelly RW. 19-Hydroxylated E prostaglandins as major prostaglandins of human semen. *Nature* 1974; **250**: 665–7.

36. Capdevila JH, Karara A, Waxman DJ, Martin MV, Falck JR, Guenguerich FP. Cytochrome P450 enzyme-specific control of the regio- and enantiofacial selectivity of the microsomal arachidonic acid epoxygenase. *J Biol Chem* 1990; **265**: 10865–71.

37. Yoshimura R, Kusunose E, Yokotani N, Yamamoto S, Kubota I, Kusunose MAD. Purification and characterization of two forms of fatty acid omega-hydroxylase cytochrome P-450 from rabbit kidney cortex microsomes. *J Biochem (Tokyo)* 1990; **108**: 544–81.

38. Powell WS. ω-Oxidation of prostaglandins by lung and liver microsomes. *J Biol Chem* 1978; **253**: 6711–16.

39. Powell WS, Solomon S. Formation of 20-hydroxyprostaglandins by lungs of pregnant rabbits. *J Biol Chem* 1978; **253**: 4609–16.

40. Honstra G, van Houwelingen AC, Kivitis GA, Fischer S, Uedelhoven W. The influence of dietary fish oil on eicosanoid metabolism in man. *Prostaglandins* 1990; **40**: 311–29.

41. Honstra G, vanHouwelingen AC, Kivitis GA, Fischer S, Uedelhoven W. Dietary fish and prostanoid formation in man. *Adv Prostaglandin Thromboxane Leukotriene Res* 1991; **21A**: 225–8.

42. Sullivan MHF, Roseblade CK, Rendell NB, Taylor GW, Elder MG. Metabolism of prostaglandins E_2 and $F_{2\alpha}$ by human fetal membranes. *Biochim Biophys Acta* 1992; **1123**: 342–6.

43. Barrow SE, Cockroft J, Dollery CT, Hickling NE, Ritter JM. Identification of 13,14-dihydro-15-oxo-prostaglandin $F_{2\alpha}$ in the circulation during infusions of bradykinin and prostaglandin E_2 in man. *Br J Pharmacol* 1987; **91**: 245–50.

44. Granstronm E, Samuelsson B. On the metabolism of prostaglandin $F_{2\alpha}$ in female subjects. *J Biol Chem* 1971; **246**: 5254–63.

45. Liston TE, Roberts LJ II. Transformation of prostaglandin D_2 to 9α,11β(15S)-trihydroxyprosta-(5Z,13E)-dien-1-oic acid(α,11β-PGF$_2$): a unique biologically active prostaglandin produced enzymically *in vivo* by humans. *Proc Natl Acad Sci USA* 1985; **82**: 6030–4.

46. Barrow SE, Heavey DJ, Ennis M, Chappell CG, Blair IA, Dollery CT. Measurement of prostaglandin D_2 and identification of metabolites in human plasma during intravenous infusion. *Prostaglandins* 1984; **28**: 743–54.

47. Liston TE, Roberts LJ II. Metabolite fate of radiolabelled prostaglandin D_2 in a normal human male volunteer. *J Biol Chem* 1985; **260**: 13172–80.

48. Rosenkranz B, Fischer C, Frolich JC. Prostacyclin metabolites in human plasma. *Clin Pharmacol Ther* 1981; **29** (3): 420–4.

49. Roberts LJ II, Sweetman BJ, Oates JA. Metabolism of TxB$_2$ in man: identification of 20 urinary metabolites. *Proc Natl Acad Sci USA* 1981; **256**: 8384–93.

50. Taylor IK, Ward PS, O'Shaughnessy K, *et al.* Thromboxane A_2 synthesis in acute asthma and following

antigen challenge. *Am Rev Resp Dis* 1991; **143:** 119–25.

51. Smith AP, Cuthbert MF, Dunlop LS. Effects of inhaled prostaglandins E_1, E_2 and $F_{2\alpha}$ on the airway resistance of healthy and asthmatic man. *Clin Sci Mol Med* 1975; **48:** 421–30.

52. Eklund B, Carlson LA. Central and peripheral circulatory effects and metabolic effects of different prostaglandins given i.v. to man. *Prostaglandins* 1980; **20:** 333–46.

53. Newman WP, Brodows RG. Metabolic effects of prostaglandin E_2 infusion in man: possible adrenergic mediation. *J Clin Endocrinol Metab* 1982; **55:** 496–501.

54. Naeje N, Bracamonte M, Sergijsels R. Influence of parenteral prostaglandin E_1 on lung mechanics in normal man. *Eur J Clin Pharmacol* 1983; **24:** 329–32.

55. Schoenhard G, Opperman J, Kohn FE. Metabolism and pharmacokinetic studies of misoprostol. *Dig Dis Sci* 1985; **30:** 126S–8S.

56. Karim A. Antiulcer prostaglandin misoprostol: single and multiple dose pharmacokinetic profile. *Prostaglandins* 1987; **335:** 40–50.

57. Arns P. Misoprostol. *Am J Med Sci* 1991; **301:** 133–7.

58. Morton MR, Robbins ME. Delirium in an elderly woman possibly associated with administration of misoprostol. *DICP* 1991; **25:** 133–4.

59. Fossaluzza V, DiBenedetto P, Zampa A, DeVita S. Misoprostol-induced urinary incontinence. *J Intern Med* 1991; **230:** 463–4.

60. Heavy DJ, Lumley P, Barrow SE, Murphy MB, Humphrey PP, Dollery CT. Effects of intravenous infusions of prostaglandin D_2 in man. *Prostaglandins* 1984; **28:** 755–67.

61. Karim SM, Somers K, Hillier K. Cardiovascular and other effects of prostaglandin E_2 and F_2 in man. *Cardiovasc Res* 1971; **5:** 255.

62. Fishburne JI, Brenner WE, Braaksma JT, *et al.* Cardiovascular and respiratory responses to intravenous infusion of prostaglandin $F_{2\alpha}$ in the pregnant woman. *Am J Obstet Gynecol* 1972; **114:** 765–72.

63. MacClennen AH, Green RC. Cervical ripening and induction of labour with intravaginal prostaglandin $F_{2\alpha}$. *Lancet* 1979; **1:** 117–19.

64. Karim SM, Sivasamboo R. Termination of second trimester pregnancy with intra-uterine 15(S),15-methyl prostaglandin $F_{2\alpha}$ – a two-dose schedule study. *Prostaglandins* 1975; **9:** 487–94.

65. Lewis PJ, Dollery CT. Clinical pharmacology and potential of prostacyclin. *Br Med Bull* 1983; **39:** 281–4.

66. Patrono C, Pugliese F, Ciabottoni G, *et al.* Evidence for a direct stimulatory effect of prostacyclin on renin release in man. *J Clin Invest* 1982; **69:** 231–9.

67. Modesti PA, Fortini A, Pogessi L, Boddi M, Abbate R, Gensini GF. Acute reversible reduction of PGI_2 platelet receptors after iloprost infusion in man. *Thromb Res* 1987; **48** (6): 663–9.

68. Krause W, Krais T. Pharmacokinetics and pharmacodynamics of the prostacyclin analogue iloprost in man. *Eur J Clin Pharmacol* 1986; **30:** 61–8.

4   Prostaglandins – analogues and mimetics

*Bernd Buchmann, Ulrich Klar, Hartmut Rehwinkel and
Helmut Vorbrüggen*

As described in Chapter 1, the natural prostaglandins PGE_2, $PGF_{2\alpha}$ and PGD_2, prostacyclin (PGI_2) and thromboxane (TXA_2) are formed by specific enzymes from the common biochemical precursor PGH_2, which in turn is derived from arachidonic acid with the enzyme cyclo-oxygenase.

Because of the chemical instability and short biological half-life of the natural prostaglandins and prostacyclin a substantial effort has been made in the last 25 years to synthesize new chemically stable and biologically equipotent analogues, which can be used in medical practice without complicated storage problems and preparations as in the case of the inherently unstable sodium salt of prostacyclin.

In the following text only those prostaglandin or prostacyclin analogues and thromboxane synthase inhibitors or antagonists for which detailed pharmacological data as well as some clinical results have been published or which are of novel types and seem to have therapeutic potential, will be discussed. For these compounds the Chemical Abstracts System Registry numbers [RN], if available, are given with the chemical formulae to facilitate a prompt search in Chemical Abstracts for the most recent information.

Leading references, especially to reviews, will be given. Synthetic pathways are depicted for only a few selected and most promising compounds.

Prostaglandin analogues

The chemistry of prostaglandin analogues has been discussed in detail in two monographs[1,2] and in a review article.[3] The corresponding syntheses as well as patent literature can be easily traced as mentioned above.

Although all PGE_2 analogues stimulate the smooth muscles of the human uterus and intestine, certain compounds such as sulprostone (**1**),[4,5] gemeprost (**2**)[6,7] or meteneprost (**3**)[8,9] (Fig. 4.1) were primarily synthesized as therapeutic agents for cervical dilatation and as abortifacients, whereas other PGE_2 analogues such as misoprostol (**4**)[10] (Fig. 4.2) were developed as cytoprotective and anti-ulcer agents. But all of these compounds can be used to terminate human pregnancies. In particular, successful abortions are almost always achieved when PGE_2 analogues are used in combination with progesterone antagonists such as mifepristone (RU-38486).[11–15]

The introduction of misoprostol (**4**)[10] (for the synthesis see Fig. 4.3) and enprostil (**5**)[16–18] (for the synthesis see Fig. 4.4) as cytoprotective and anti-ulcer agents on the market have made such PGE_2 analogues widely available for a variety of clinical studies.[44–47]

Following the first observations on the cytoprotective as well as antisecretory effects of PGE_2 analogues such as 16,16-dimethyl PGE_2 in the human stomach,[48–51] quite a number of other PGE_2 analogues have been or are being developed primarily

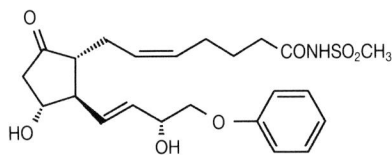

1 ZK-57671; sulprostone[4,5]
[RN 60325-46-4]

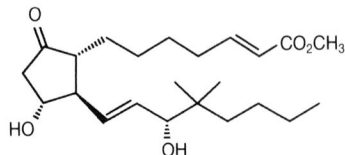

2 ONO-802; gemeprost[6,7]
[RN 64318-79-2]

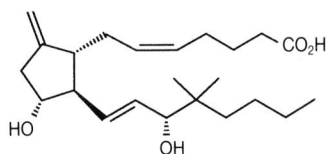

3 U-46785; meteneprost[8,9]
[RN 61263-35-2]

Fig. 4.1   Prostaglandin analogues with pronounced abortifacient activity.

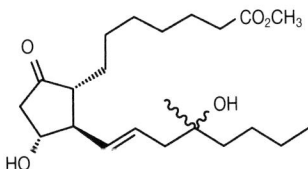

4 SC-29333; misoprostol (rac.)[10]
[RN 59122-46-2]

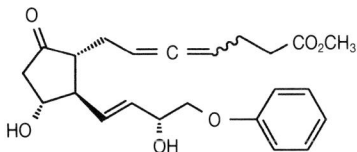

5 RS-84135; enprostil (rac.)[16–18]
[RN 73121-56-9]

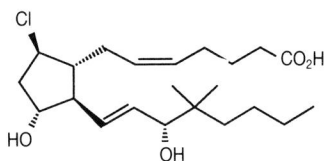

6 ZK-94726; nocloprost[19–21]
[RN 79360-43-3]

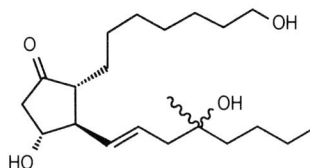

7 ORF-15927; rioprostil (rac.)[22,23]
[RN 77287-05-9]

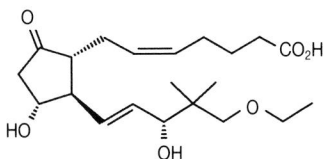

8 HR-260; dimoxaprost (rac.)[24,25]
[RN 90243-98-4]

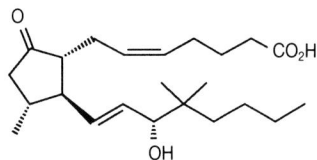

9 Ro-21-6937; trimoprostil[26,27]
[RN 69900-72-7]

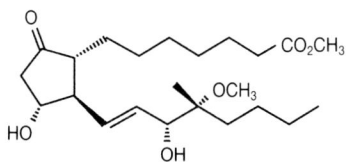

10 MDL-646; mexiprostil[28–30]
[RN 88980-20-5]

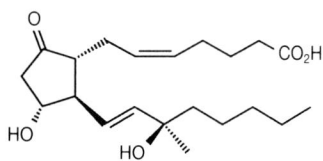

11 U-42842; arbaprostil[31]
[RN 55028-70-1]

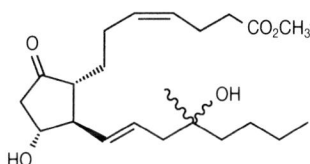

12 SC-34301; enisoprost (rac.)[32,33]
[RN 81026-63-3]

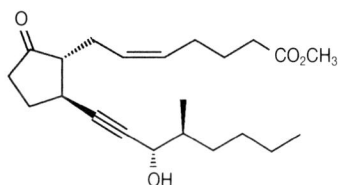

13 FCE-20700[34,35]
[RN 89648-76-0]

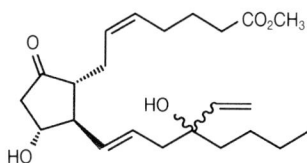

14 CL-115347; viprostol (rac.)[36–38]
[RN 73647-73-1]

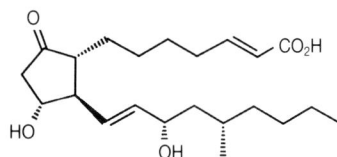

15 ONO-1206; limaprost[39]
[RN 74397-12-9]

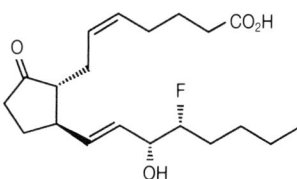

16 Ro-221327[40]
[RN 69900-71-6]

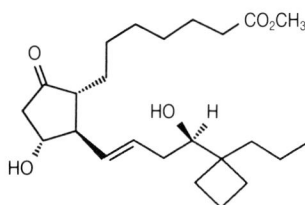

17 Bay-q-4218; butaprost[41]
[RN 69648-38-0]

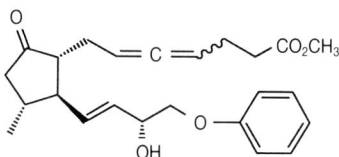

18 RS-18492 (rac.)[42,43]
[RN 103522-44-7]

Fig. 4.2 Prostaglandin analogues with pronounced cytoprotective activity.

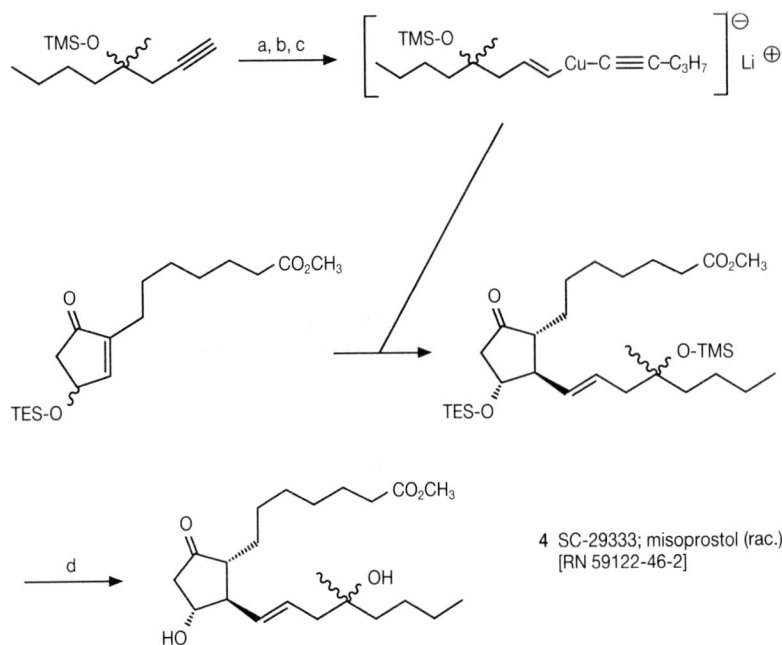

Fig. 4.3   Synthesis of (±)-misoprostol (4). Reagents: a, Bu₃SnH/hv/rt; b, *n*BuLi/THF/ −60°C; c, C₃H₇C≡CCu/HMPT/ Et₂O; d, H₃O⁺.

4 SC-29333; misoprostol (rac.) [RN 59122-46-2]

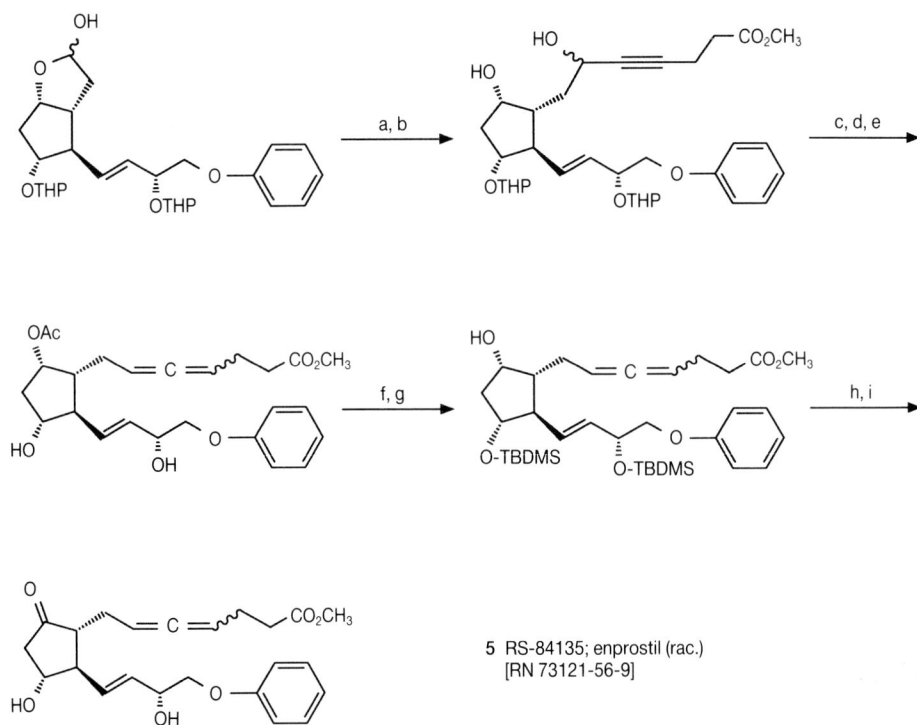

5 RS-84135; enprostil (rac.) [RN 73121-56-9]

Fig. 4.4   Synthesis of (±)-enprostil (5). Reagents: a, Li-C≡C-(CH₂)₂CO₂Li; b, CH₂N₂; c, Ac₂O; d, Me₂CuLi/−70°C; e, AcOH; f, TBDMSCl; g, K₂CO₃/MeOH; h, CrO₃·2Pyr; i, AcOH.

to heal or to prevent the formation of stomach ulcers. In particular, the combination of aspirin or other non-steroidal anti-inflammatory drugs (NSAIDs) with PGE$_2$ analogues has been investigated to prevent the erosion and bleeding of the stomach and intestinal mucosa caused by these NSAIDs.[19,52]

It should be realized, however, that with the exception of nocloprost (6),[19–21] trimoprostil (9),[26,27] FCE-20700 (13)[34,35] and Ro-221327 (16)[40] as well as RS-18492 (18)[42,43] all the other compounds do contain the 9-oxo-11α-hydroxy moiety and are thus, as β-hydroxyketones, chemically unstable especially in the presence of traces of acids or bases. Although addition of buffers or cyclodextrins can stabilize the galenical formulations of these drugs, their inherent instabilities will cause storage problems.

In contrast to misoprostol (4) and the other drugs possessing the β-hydroxyketone moiety, in nocloprost (6) (for the synthesis see Fig. 4.5) the 9-carbonyl group is mimicked by a 9-β-chloroatom, which prevents the elimination of the 11-hydroxy group, thus vastly increasing the chemical stability. Even more importantly nocloprost (6) has the additional advantage that the drug is nearly completely metabolized on oral application during passage of the stomach or intestinal mucosa and liver. Therefore nocloprost (6) on oral administration of therapeutic doses does not cause adverse systemic effects such as uterine contractions or diarrhoea.[53]

In contrast to the above-mentioned uterotropic and cytoprotective PGE$_2$ analogues, viprostol (14)[36–38] (Fig. 4.2) has been primarily characterized as a hypotensive and hair growth promoting agent.

PGD$_2$, which contains a chemically labile β-hydroxyketone moiety, like the above-mentioned PGE$_2$ and most of its analogues, is rapidly degraded to the $\Delta^{9,10}$-ketone or metabolized *in vivo* in particular by the 11-oxoreductase to 11β-PGF$_{2\alpha}$, which is mainly responsible for the pronounced side effects. These problems are avoided in the PGD$_2$ analogues depicted in Fig. 4.6.

Interestingly, introducing a 15-cyclohexyl moiety into the lower side chain of PGD$_2$ and different types of prostanoids amplifies or generates a PGD$_2$ quality.

Following the introduction of the first racemic PGD$_2$ analogue BW-245C (19)[54–56] (Fig. 4.6) and the somewhat related L-644122 (20),[57,58] the potent novel and chemically stable PGD$_2$ agonists ZK-110841 (21a)[59,60] and the chemically and metabolically stable ZK-118182 (21b)[59,61] have been identified and are being investigated for a number of therapeutic applications (e.g. against glaucoma).

Since large amounts of natural PGD$_2$ are formed besides histamine by stimulated mast cells in mastocytosis,[62] PGD$_2$ antagonists like BW-A868C (22)[63,64] are of potential clinical interest in the treatment of this disease.

There is evidence that PGD$_2$ and PGE$_2$ are playing an important role in the sleep–wake cycle[65] so that the potential application of PGD$_2$ and in particular of its stable analogues for sleep induction in human patients is still being discussed. Interestingly, PGD$_2$ analogues diminish the formation of oxygen radicals in leucocytes.[59]

Since 6-oxo-PGE$_1$ possesses biological effects

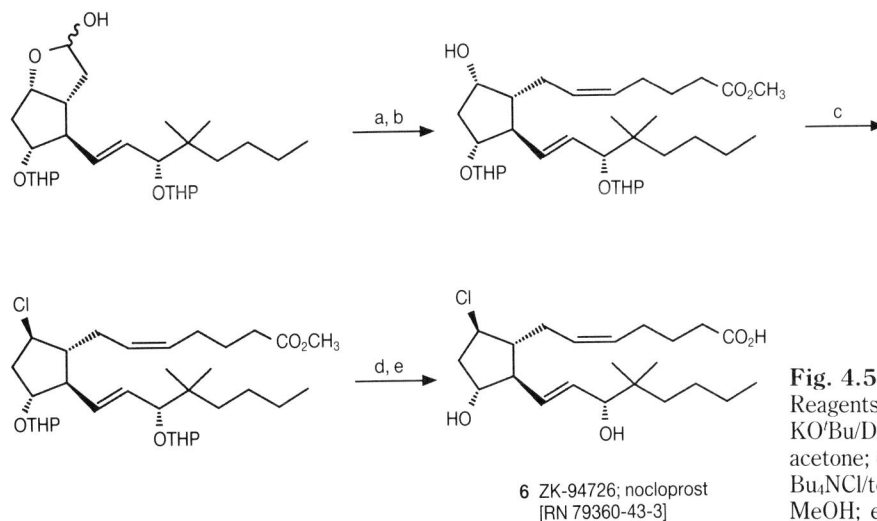

Fig. 4.5 Synthesis of nocloprost (6). Reagents: a, Br$^-$Ph$_3$P$^+$(CH$_2$)$_4$CO$_2$H/ KO^{t}Bu/DMSO/THF; b, K$_2$CO$_3$/CH$_3$I/ acetone; c, CH$_3$SO$_2$Cl/Et$_3$N/toluene then Bu$_4$NCl/toluene; d, amberlyst 15/ MeOH; e, NaOH/MeOH.

6 ZK-94726; nocloprost
[RN 79360-43-3]

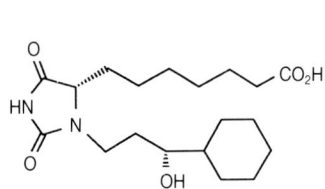

19 BW-245C (rac.)[54–56]
[RN 72814-32-5]

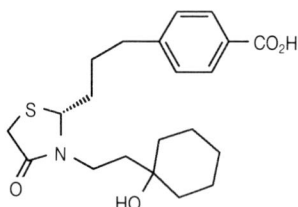

20 L-644122 (rac.)[57,58]
[RN 72313-44-1]

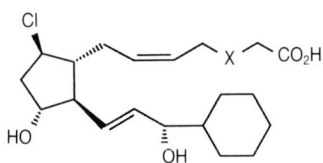

21a (X=CH$_2$): ZK-110841[59,60]
[RN 105595-17-3]
21b (X=O): ZK-118182[59,61]
[RN 120962-76-7]

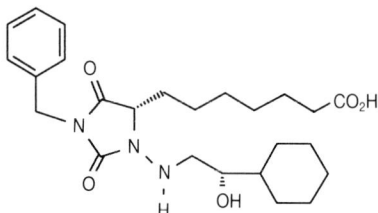

22 BW-A868C (rac.)[63,64]
[RN 118675-50-6]

Fig. 4.6 PGD$_2$ agonists and antagonists.

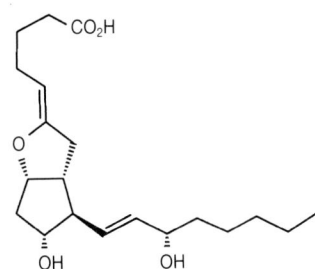

23 Prostacyclin[66]
[RN 35121-78-9]

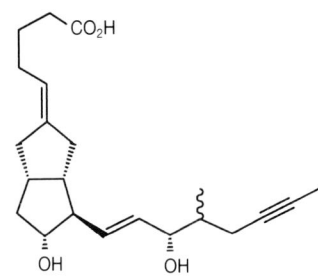

24 ZK-36374; iloprost[72–74]
[RN 78919-13-8]

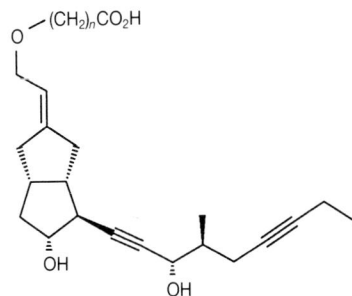

25a (*n*=1): ZK-96480; cicaprost[77,78]
[RN 94079-80-8]

25b (*n*=3): ZK-97959; eptaloprost[79]
[RN 90693-76-8]

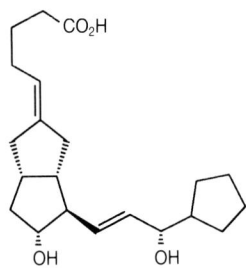

26 OP-41483; ataprost[80–82]
[RN 83997-19-7]

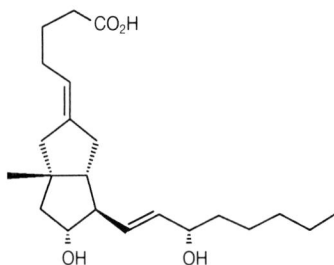

27 U-61431; ciprostene[83–85]
[RN 81845-44-5]

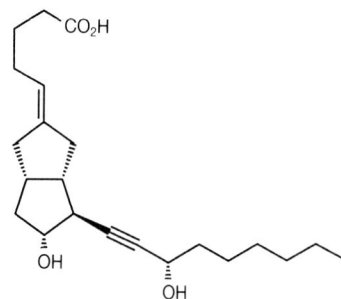

28 FCE-22177/21292[86]
[RN 78542-68-4]

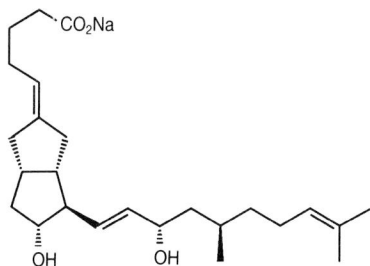

29 R-59274/CS-570[87,88]
[RN 71806-48-9]

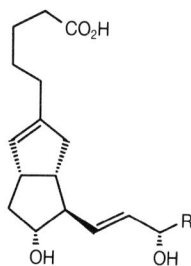

30a (R=C$_5$H$_{11}$): Tei-7165[89,90]
[RN 88911-35-7]
30b (R=c-C$_5$H$_9$): Tei-8107[91]
[RN 116499-12-8]

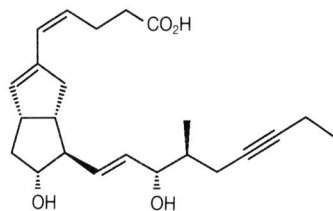

31 KP 10614[92,93]
[RN 130273-99-3]

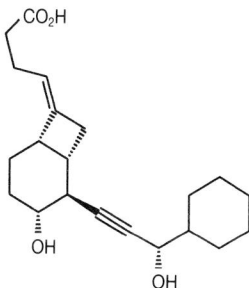

32 RS-93427[94,95]
[RN 105284-21-7]

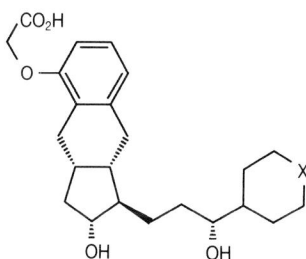

33a (X=CH$_2$): U-68215[96-98]
[RN 99570-57-7]
33b (X=O): U-72382[97]
[RN 101691-66-1]

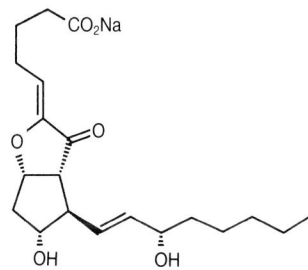

34 CH-5084[99]
[RN 79673-16-8]

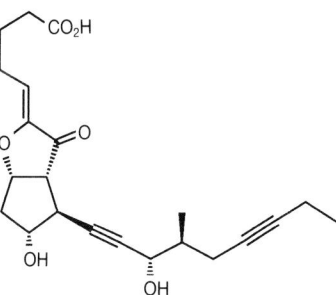

35 ZK-113929[100]
[RN 114409-62-0]

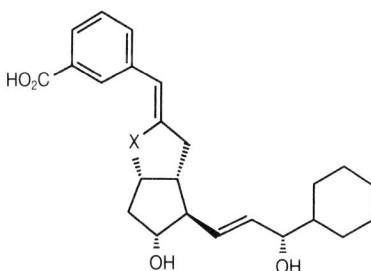

36a (X=CH$_2$): EL-784; naxaprostene[101,102]
[RN 87269-59-8]
36b (X=O): CG-4203; taprostene[103,104]
[RN 108945-35-3]

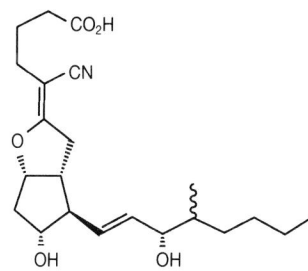

37 ZK-34798; nileprost[105,106]
[RN 71097-83-1]

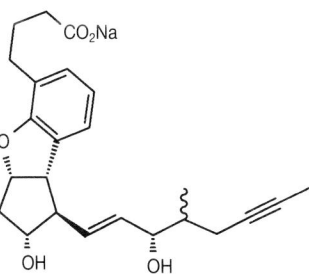

38 TRK-100; beraprost[107-110]
[RN 88475-69-8]

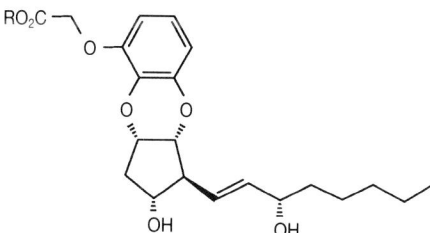

39a (R=H); Shionogi[111]
[RN 120962-70-1]
39b (R=CH$_3$): Shionogi[111]
[RN 120962-54-1]

Fig. 4.7 Compounds with PGI$_2$-mimetic activity.

very similar to those of prostacyclin, its derivatives will be discussed in connection with the prostacyclin analogues.

Prostacyclin analogues

Vane *et al.* discovered in 1976 the natural prostacyclin PGI$_2$ (**23**)[66] (Fig. 4.7), which is formed from the central biosynthetic intermediate PGH$_2$ by the endothelial cells in the vascular wall and which is the most potent natural inhibitor of platelet aggregation and vascular constriction. Due to the inherent chemical instability of the crystalline prostacyclin sodium salt, which strongly limits its application in routine medical practice, an intensive search for chemically and metabolically stable prostacyclin analogues with the same biological profile and potency as **23** was initiated.[67–71]

The first analogue to meet these criteria was the modified carbacyclin analogue iloprost (**24**),[72–74] in which the enolether oxygen of prostacyclin (**23**) is replaced by a methylene group and the lower side chain is further modified in order to enhance the biological potency as well as the metabolic stability. In the last 10 years iloprost has been intensively studied pharmacologically and clinically and has entered clinical practice for the treatment of peripheral arterial occlusive disease (PAOD).[75,76]

Due to the rapid degradation of the upper side chain by β-oxidation, iloprost (**24**) shows only ca. 20% bioavailability on oral application.[112,113] This metabolic pathway is completely blocked by the exchange of the β-methylene group of the upper side chain by an oxygen atom. Further modification of the lower side chain resulted in the biologically even more potent cicaprost (**25a**)[77,78] (for the synthesis see Fig. 4.8) which is metabolically stable and excreted unchanged via urine and faeces.[114] The corresponding prodrug eptaloprost (**25b**)[79] is metabolized *in vivo* by β-oxidation of the upper side chain to cicaprost (**25a**).

In addition to the anticipated biological effects of iloprost (**24**) and cicaprost (**25a**) the recently described antimetastatic properties of cicaprost (**25a**) might be of clinical importance for cancer surgery and the prevention of the spread of cancers.[115–118]

Other carbacyclin analogues such as ataprost (**26**)[80–82] and the less potent ciprostene (**27**),[83–85] FCE-22177 (**28**)[86] and R-59274 (**29**)[87,88] are in various states of clinical development. Shifting the exocyclic double bond into the five-membered ring led to isocarbacyclins like Tei-7165 (**30a**)[89,90] (for

the synthesis see Fig. 4.9), Tei-8107 (**30b**)[91] and KP 10614 (**31**),[92,93] which are equipotent to the corresponding carbacyclins. Some other interesting novel structures are the bicyclo[4.2.0]octane analogue RS-93427 (**32**),[94,95] the tricyclo-analogues U-68215 (**33a**)[96–98] and U-72382 (**33b**),[97] the latter being primarily developed as a cytoprotective and anti-ulcer agent.

Whereas the chemically stable 7-oxoprostacyclins CH-5084 (**34**)[99] and ZK-113929 (**35**)[100] as well as the interphenylene analogues naxaprostene (**36a**)[101,102] and taprostene (**36b**)[103,104] are potent inhibitors of platelet aggregation, the chemically stable 5-cyanoprostacyclin nileprost (**37**) binds to both the PGI$_2$ receptor and the PGE$_2$ receptor and is therefore an excellent therapeutic agent for the treatment of stomach ulcers.[105,106]

The orally active racemic compound beraprost (**38**)[107–110] (for the synthesis see Fig. 4.10) has recently been launched in Japan for the treatment of peripheral arterial occlusive disease (PAOD). In contrast to beraprost (**38**), the corresponding analogue (**39a**)[111] shows only weak platelet aggregation inhibitory properties but its methyl ester (**39b**)[111] is an interesting cytoprotective agent for the treatment of stomach ulcers.

Despite its PGI$_2$-like structure, the aza-analogue piriprost (**40**)[119] is a lipoxygenase inhibitor (Fig. 4.11), while OP-2507 (**41**)[120,121] possesses pronounced cerebrovascular activity.

Modification of the naturally occurring 6-oxo-PGE$_1$[130] led to the 6-oxo-PGE$_1$ analogue ZK-119022 (**42**),[122] containing the lower side chain of cicaprost (**25a**). ZK-119022 (**42**), which shows a biological profile and activity similar to iloprost (**24**) and cicaprost (**25a**), turned out to be a very potent long-acting hypotensive agent on oral application in SHR rats.[131]

Two other modified 6-oxo-PGE$_1$ analogues, however, ornoprostil (**43**)[123,124] and ONO-1082 (**44**)[125] have pronounced cytoprotective properties and might serve as anti-ulcer drugs.

Finally, the rather simple imidazole derivative octimibate (**45**)[126–128] turned out to be a prostacyclin mimetic. Octimibate (**45**) binds to the PGI$_2$/PGE$_1$ receptor of platelets and inhibits ADP-induced aggregation of platelet-rich plasma *in vitro* with an activity of 1/160 of iloprost (**24**).[128]

Potent analogues of octimibate (**45**) such as the pyrazole derivative BMY-42239 (**46**),[129] have recently been described.

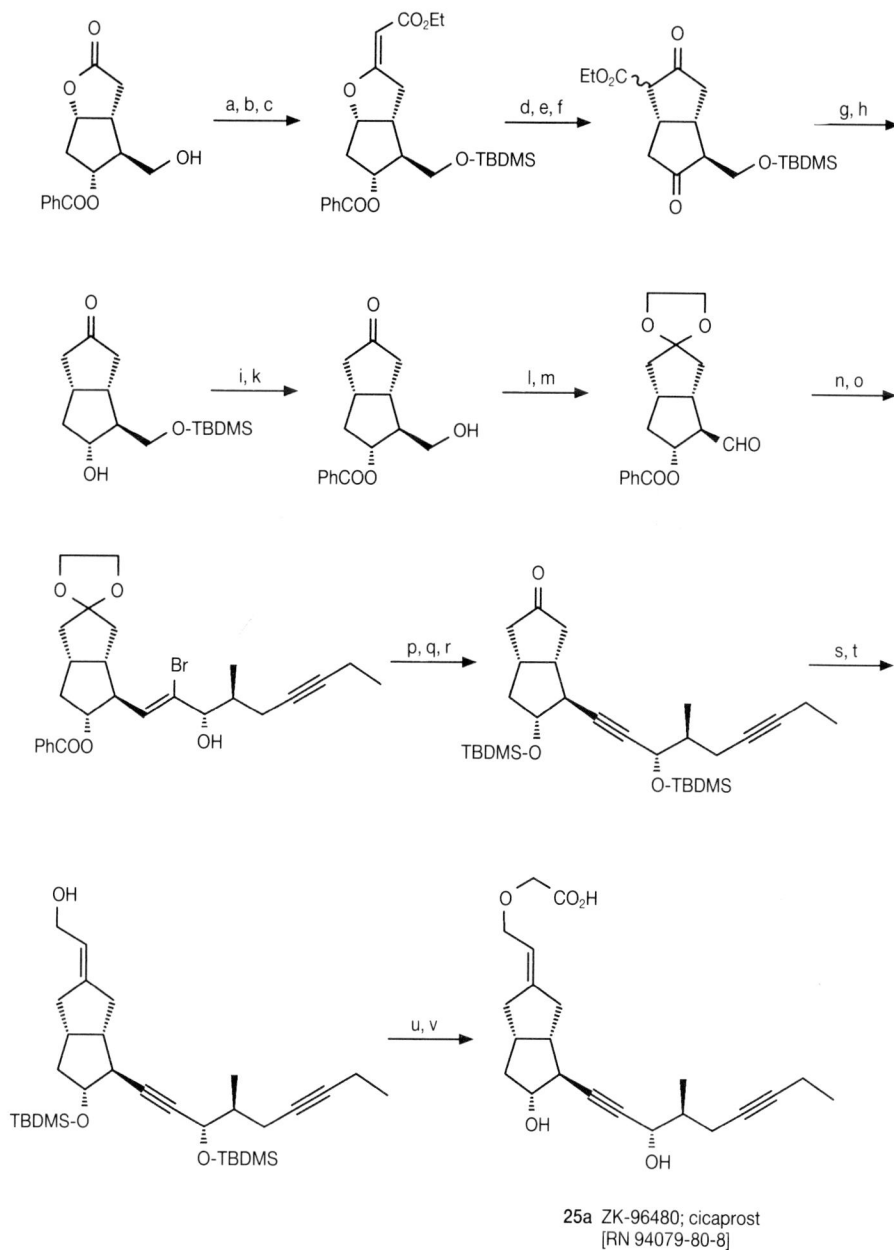

25a ZK-96480; cicaprost
[RN 94079-80-8]

Fig. 4.8 Synthesis of cicaprost (**25a**). Reagents: a, TBDMSCl/DMF/imid.; b, LiCH₂CO₂Et/THF/−70°C; c, PTSA/toluene/25°C; d, K₂CO₃/MeOH/25°C; e, CrO₃·2Pyr; f, DBN/THF/0°C; g, NaBH₄/MeOH; h, 1,4-diazabicyclo[2.2.2]octane/toluene/H₂O/110°C; i, PhCOCl/0°C; k, AcOH/H₂O/THF (65:35:10)/25°C; l, HOCH₂CH₂OH/H⁺; m, CrO₃·2Pyr; n, phosphonate/NaH/NBS/DME/−20°C; o, NaBH₄/MeOH/−40°C; p, 50%aq. NaOH/toluene/cat. Bu₄NHSO₄/25°C; q, HOAc/H₂O; r, TBDMSCl/DMF/imid.; s, (EtO)₂P(O)CH₂CO₂Et/KOᵗBu/THF/0°C; t, DIBAH/toluene/0°C; u, BrCH₂CO₂ᵗBu/50%aq. NaOH/toluene/cat. Bu₄NHSO₄/25°C; v, Bu₄NF/THF/25°C.

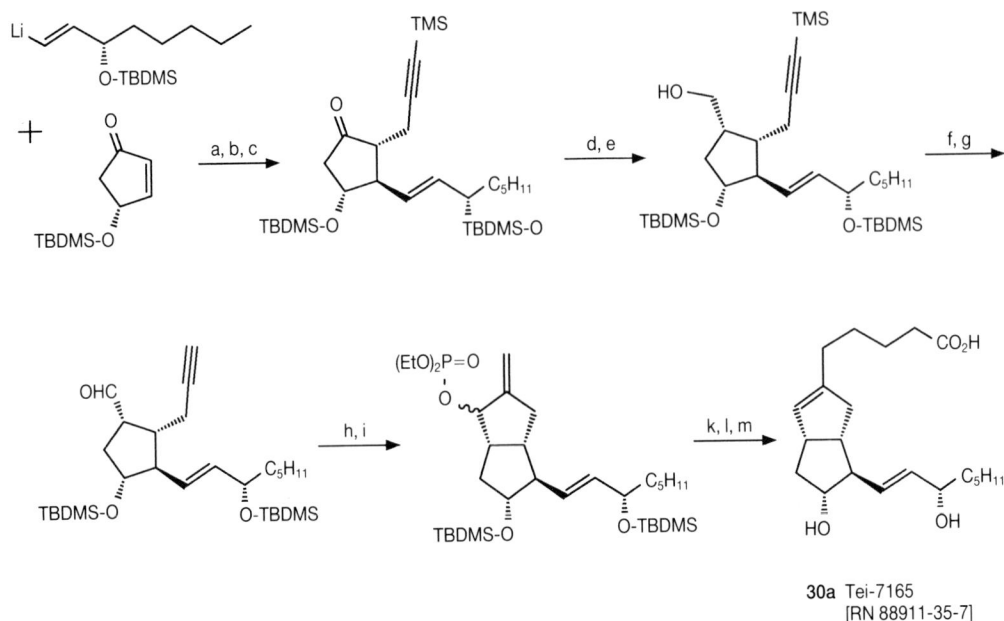

Fig. 4.9 Synthesis of Tei-7165 (**30a**). Reagents: a, Cu-≡-C$_4$H$_9$; b, Ph$_3$SnCl; c, I-CH$_2$-≡-TMS; d, Zn/CH$_2$Br$_2$/TiCl$_4$; e, 9-BBN/H$_2$O$_2$/NaOH; f, NaOCH$_3$; g, Swern oxidation; h, SmI$_2$/*t*-BuOH; i, BuLi/(EtO)$_2$ P(O)Cl/THF; k, IZnCN-CuC$_3$H$_6$CO$_2$CH$_3$; l, Bu$_4$NF; m, LiOH/H$_2$O/THF.

Thromboxane antagonists and synthase inhibitors

Whereas prostacyclin (**23**) raises the cAMP level in platelets and vascular tissue and is thus a potent inhibitor of platelet aggregation and a vasodilator, the extremely labile thromboxane TXA$_2$ (**47a**)[132] (Fig. 4.12), which is formed from the central biosynthetic intermediate PGH$_2$ (**48a**)[135] by thromboxane synthase, counteracts the effects of prostacyclin by inhibiting adenylate cyclase probably via release of bound calcium. TXA$_2$ (**47a**) is a powerful inducer of platelet aggregation and contracts vascular as well as airways smooth muscle. The structure elucidation of the elusive, unstable and biologically potent TXA$_2$ by Samuelsson[147] and its ingenious synthesis years later by Still[148] belong to the outstanding scientific achievements of our time.

Diminishing the effects of TXA$_2$ (**47a**) inhibits the activation of platelets and causes an increase in biological activity of prostacyclin (**23**) or any of its stable analogues. Consequently, thromboxane antagonists and synthase inhibitors have been actively investigated for a number of years and have recently been reviewed in detail.[149–154]

The study of the biological properties and the significance of the very unstable TXA$_2$ (**47a**) only became possible after stable TXA$_2$ mimetics such as the most commonly used U-46619 (**48b**)[136,137] (Fig. 4.12) became available. Unfortunately U-46619 (**48b**) is not a pure TXA$_2$ agonist but has also PGF$_{2\alpha}$-agonistic properties.[156] Other compounds such as EP-171 (**49**),[138–140] I-PTA-OH (**50**)[141,142] or I-BOP (**51b**),[143–145] ZK-131489 (**52**)[146] and 10, 10-difluoro-TXA$_2$ (**47b**)[133,134] are likewise powerful TXA$_2$ mimetics.

Since N-substituted imidazoles are inhibitors of cytochrome P450 and the specific P450 enzyme thromboxane synthase, a number of N-substituted imidazoles such as dazoxiben (**53**),[157–159] dazmegrel (**54**),[160,161] ozagrel (**55**)[162,163] and pirmagrel (**56**)[164,165] have been identified as potent inhibitors of thromboxane synthase (Fig. 4.13). Other potent TXA$_2$-synthase inhibitors such as furegrelate (**57**)[166–168] or OKY-1581 (**58**)[169] incorporate a β-picolyl moiety as pharmacophore.

Because TXA$_2$-synthase inhibitors only block the biosynthesis of TXA$_2$ (**47a**) from PGH$_2$ (**48a**), whereas the formation of the central biosynthetic intermediate PGH$_2$ (**48a**), which also interacts with the TXA$_2$/PGH$_2$ receptor[170–173] on human platelets, is unaffected, these TXA$_2$-synthase inhibitors did not show consistent therapeutic effects in patients.[132]

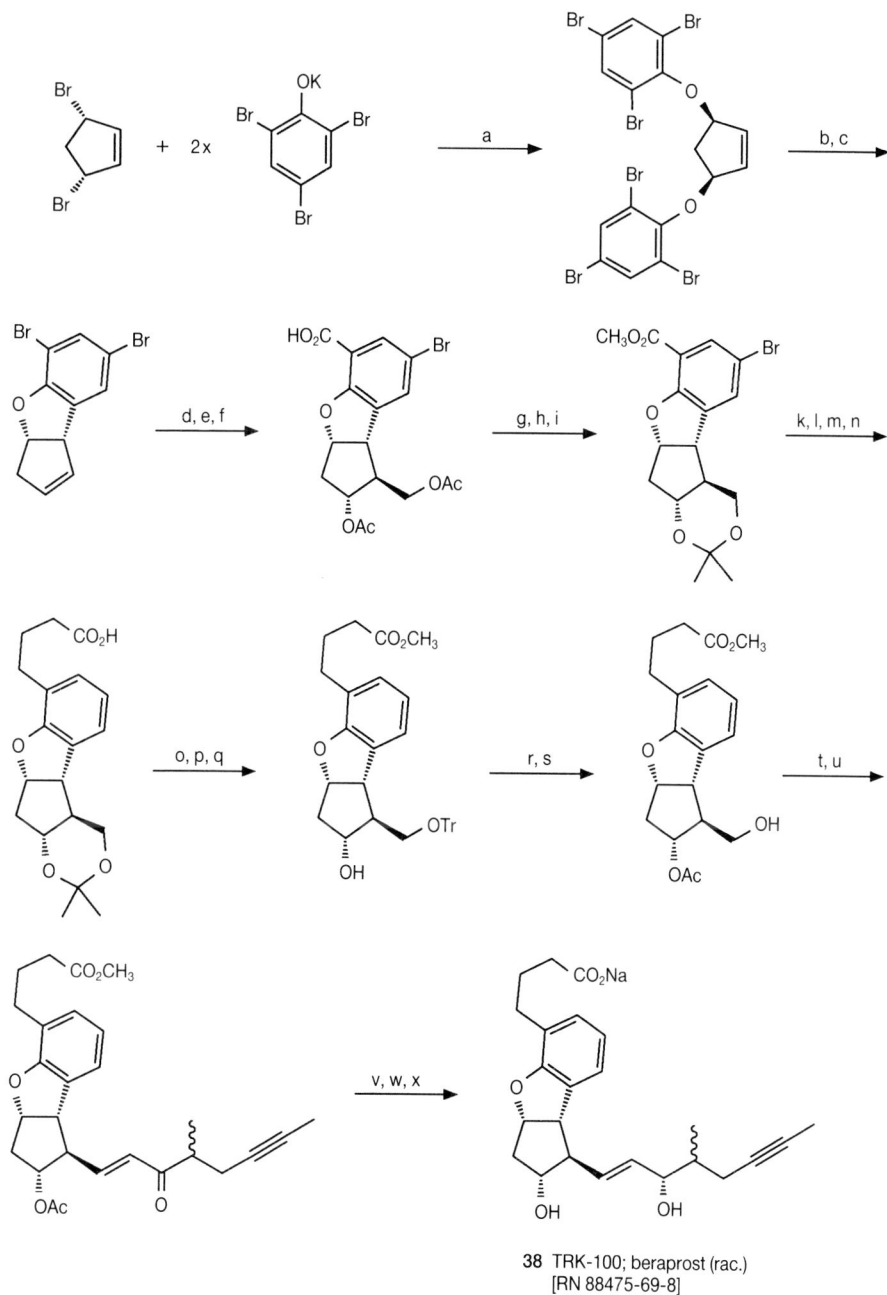

Fig. 4.10 Synthesis of (±)-beraprost (**38**). Reagents: a, 18-crown-6/DME; b, c-C₆H₁₁MgCl; c, CuI; d, c-C₆H₁₁MgCl; e, CO₂; f, (CH₂O)₃/H₂SO₄; g, NaOH; h, CH₂N₂; i, (CH₃)₂C(OCH₃)₂; k, LiAlH₄/THF; l, SOCl₂/Pyr; m, Mg; n, β-propiolactone/CuI; o, CH₂N₂; p, 1 N HCl; q, TrCl/NEt₃; r, Ac₂O/Pyr; s, HCl/MeOH; t, DCC/DMSO; u, phosphonate/NaH/THF; v, NaBH₄/CeCl₃/MeOH; w, NaOMe; x, NaOH.

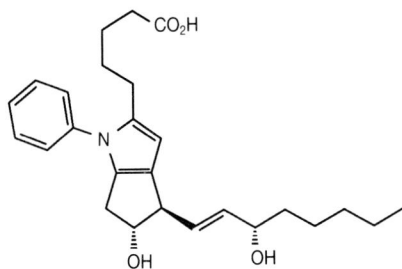

40 U-60257; piriprost[119]
[RN 79672-88-1]

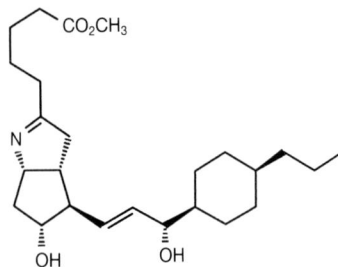

41 OP-2507[120,121]
[RN 101758-79-6]

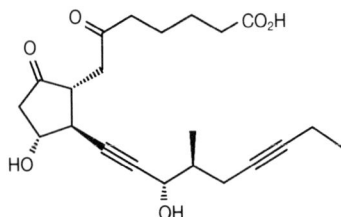

42 ZK-119022[122]
[RN 118610-09-6]

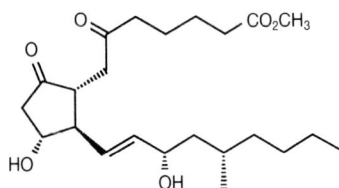

43 OU-1308; ornoprostil[123,124]
[RN 70667-26-4]

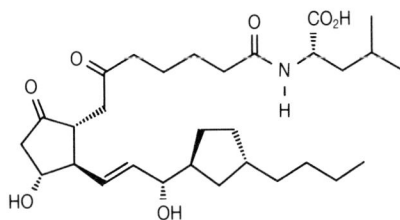

44 ONO-1082[125]
[RN 111111-04-7]

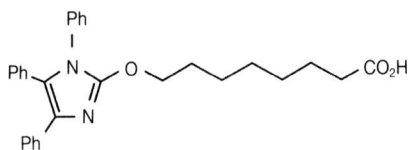

45 Nat-04-152; octimibate[126–128]
[RN 89838-96-0]

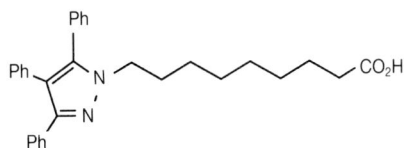

46 BMY-42239[129]
[RN 134701-70-5]

Fig. 4.11   Miscellaneous compounds.

47a R=H: TXA$_2$[132]
[RN 57576-52-0]
47b R=F: 10,10-difluoro-TXA$_2$[133,134]
[RN 121573-36-2]

48a (X=Y=O): PGH$_2$[135]
[RN 127969-05-5]
48b (X=O, Y=CH$_2$): U-46619[136,137]
[RN 56985-40-1]

49 EP-171 (rac.)[138–140]
[RN 122089-44-5]

50 I-PTA-OH[141,142]
[RN 95234-09-6]

51a (X=H): BOP[143–145]
[RN 87983-54-8]
51b (X=I): I-BOP[143–145]
[RN 128719-90-4]

52 ZK-131489[146]
[RN 134642-91-4]

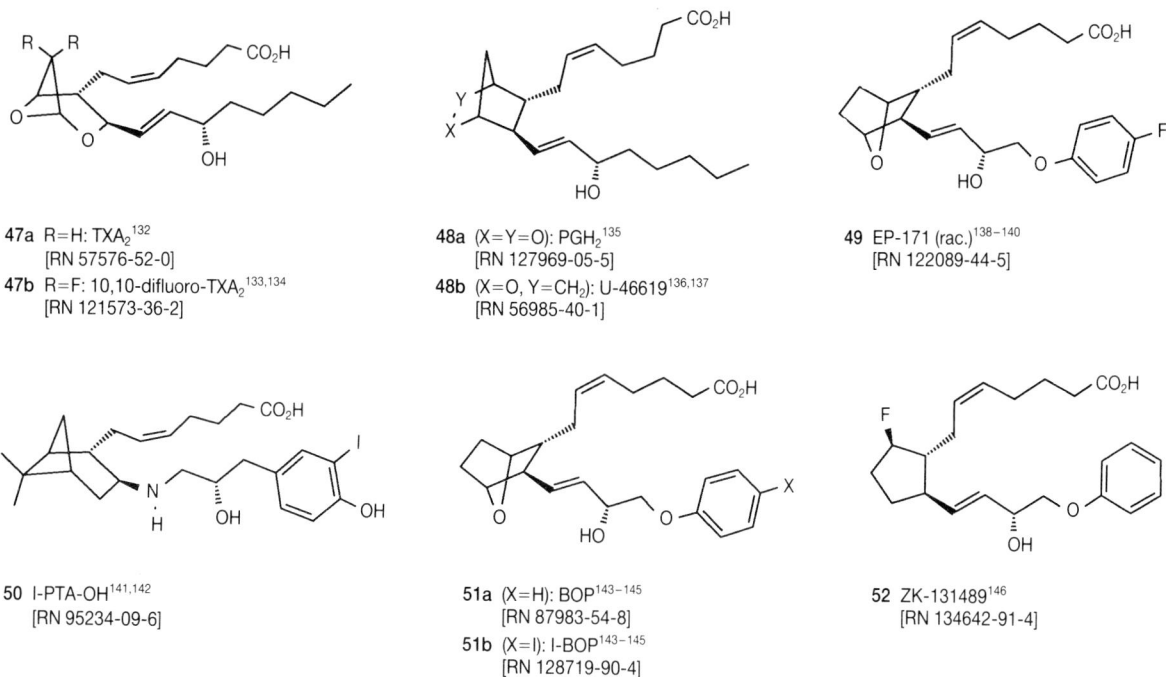

Fig. 4.12 TXA$_2$ agonists.

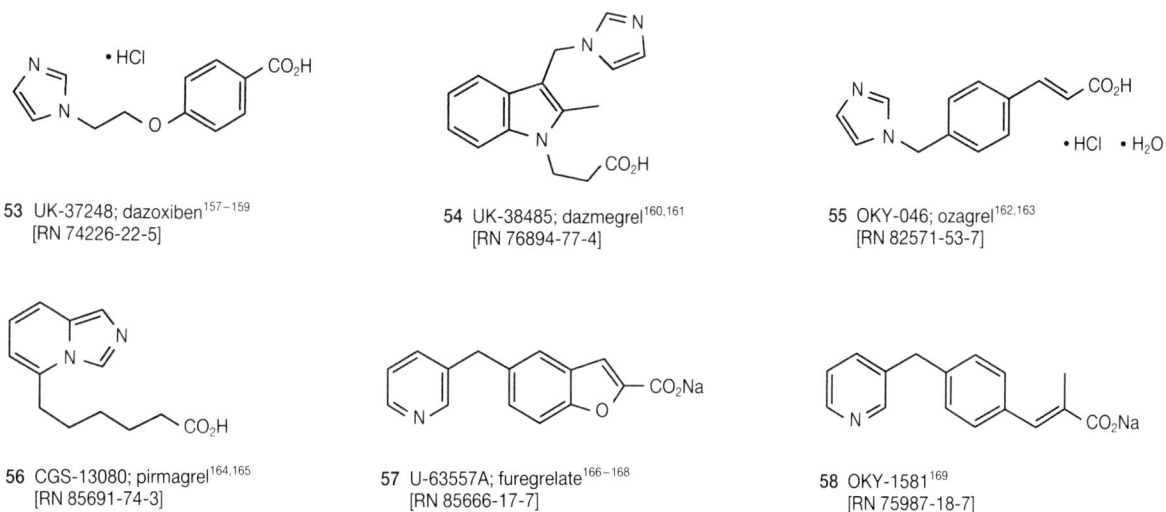

53 UK-37248; dazoxiben[157–159]
[RN 74226-22-5]

54 UK-38485; dazmegrel[160,161]
[RN 76894-77-4]

55 OKY-046; ozagrel[162,163]
[RN 82571-53-7]

56 CGS-13080; pirmagrel[164,165]
[RN 85691-74-3]

57 U-63557A; furegrelate[166–168]
[RN 85666-17-7]

58 OKY-1581[169]
[RN 75987-18-7]

Fig. 4.13 TXA$_2$-synthase inhibitors.

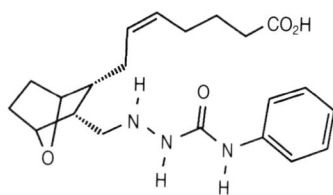

59 SQ-29548[174–176]
[RN 98672-91-4]

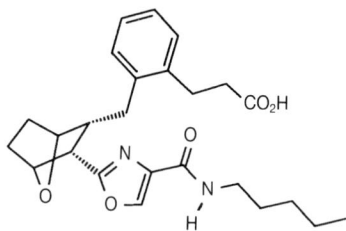

60 BMS-180291[177–179]
[RN 133026-97-8]

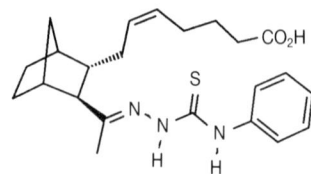

61 EP-092 (rac.)[180,181]
[RN 81806-67-9]

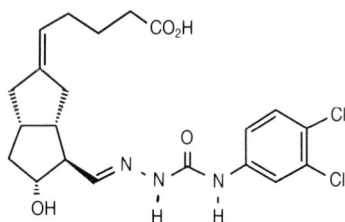

62 ZK-151803[182]

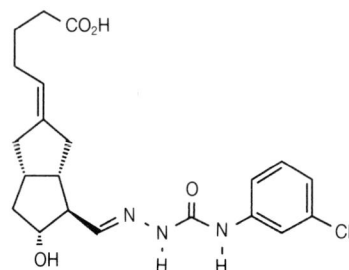

63 ZK-152010[182]

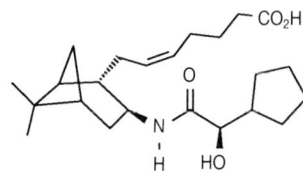

64 ONO-3708[183,184]
[RN 102191-05-9]

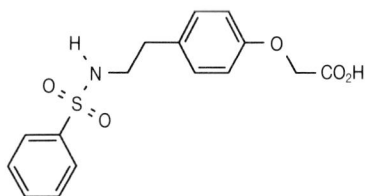

65 BM-13177; sulotroban[185]
[RN 72131-33-0]

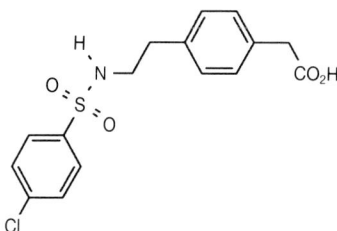

66 BM-13505; daltroban[186]
[RN 79094-20-5]

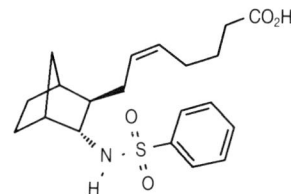

67 S-145 (rac.)[187–190]
[RN 115266-92-7]

In contrast, however, TXA$_2$ antagonists, which block the interaction of both TXA$_2$ (**47a**) and PGH$_2$ (**48a**) with the TXA$_2$/PGH$_2$ receptor, are of much more interest (Fig. 4.14).

One of the first potent and pure TXA$_2$ antagonists without any partial agonistic activity was the analogue SQ-29548 (**59**),[174–176] which in its radiolabelled form became the standard for all subsequent binding studies to the platelet TXA$_2$/PGH$_2$ receptor and other pharmacological studies. Modification of **59** resulted more recently in the synthesis of BMS-180291 (**60**)[177–179] (for the synthesis see Fig. 4.15) which is more potent as well as chemically and metabolically more stable thus having a longer lasting therapeutic effect.

Variation of the semicarbazide moiety in **59** gave rise to EP-092 (**61**),[180,181] ZK-151803 (**62**)[182] and ZK-152010 (**63**)[182] which also possess some additional PGI$_2$-agonistic activity. The α-hydroxyamide ONO-3708 (**64**)[183,184] is also a potent TXA$_2$ antagonist.

Investigations in the field of antidiabetic drugs led to the discovery of the simple ω-carboxysulphonamides sulotroban (**65**)[185] and the much more potent daltroban (**66**).[186] Subsequent efforts by many other groups resulted in more elaborate and biologically more potent ω-carboxysulphonamides such as the racemic S-145 (**67**)[187–190] (for the synthesis see Fig. 4.16), ONO-8809 (**68**)[191,192] and Bay-u-3405 (**69**)[193–198] (for the

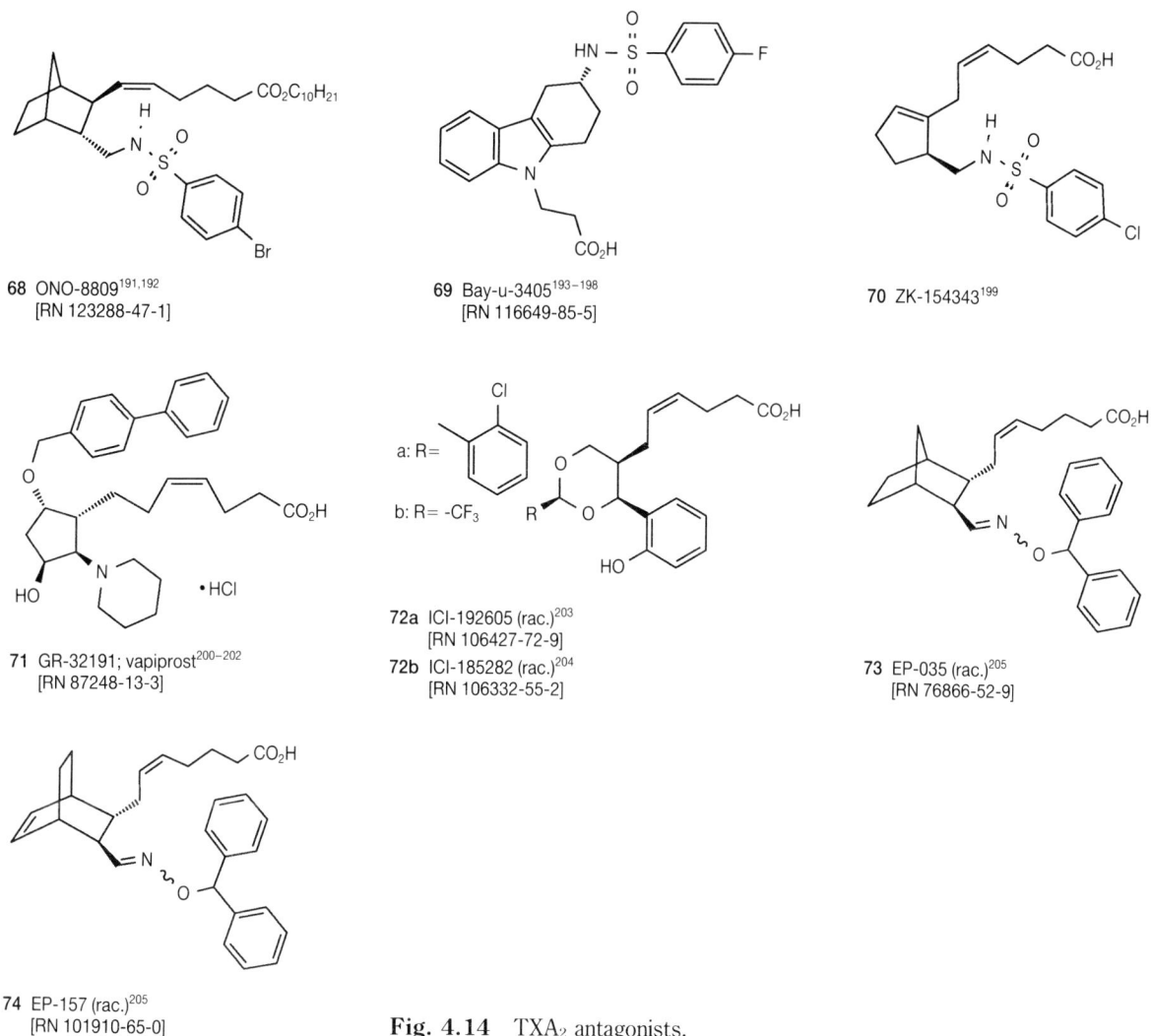

68 ONO-8809[191,192]
[RN 123288-47-1]

69 Bay-u-3405[193–198]
[RN 116649-85-5]

70 ZK-154343[199]

71 GR-32191; vapiprost[200–202]
[RN 87248-13-3]

a: R=

b: R= -CF$_3$

72a ICI-192605 (rac.)[203]
[RN 106427-72-9]

72b ICI-185282 (rac.)[204]
[RN 106332-55-2]

73 EP-035 (rac.)[205]
[RN 76866-52-9]

74 EP-157 (rac.)[205]
[RN 101910-65-0]

Fig. 4.14   TXA$_2$ antagonists.

synthesis see Fig. 4.17) as well as to ZK-154343 (**70**).[199] In all these compounds the ω-carboxy group and the sulphonamide nitrogen are usually separated by about 8–10 atoms to result in biologically active compounds.

The thoroughly investigated long acting vapiprost (**71**)[200–202] and the substituted 1,3-dioxanes such as ICI-192605 (**72a**)[203] and ICI-185282 (**72b**)[204] are also potent TXA$_2$ antagonists.

Unfortunately, all these TXA$_2$ antagonists appear as yet to fail as monotherapy in a number of clinical tests.[206,207] Therefore, compounds with dual activities, such as EP-035 (**73**)[205] or EP-157 (**74**)[205] which inhibit U-46619 (**48b**) as well as ADP, induced platelet aggregation and thus have TXA$_2$-

antagonistic as well as PGI$_2$-agonistic activity, are of particular interest. Since a simultaneous administration of the TXA$_2$ antagonist sulotroban (**65**) with the PGI$_2$-mimetic iloprost (**24**) was shown to possess pronounced synergistic effects,[208] such a combination permits lower doses of a PGI$_2$ agonist and prevents thus or minimizes typical side effects caused by high doses of a PGI$_2$ mimetic.

Combining TXA$_2$-antagonistic with PGI$_2$-agonistic properties within one molecule as indicated in **73** or **74** would furthermore avoid the pharmacokinetic problems inherent with a mixture of the two single entities.

Combinations of a TXA$_2$ antagonist with a TXA$_2$-synthase inhibitor (e.g. daltroban (**66**) and ozagrel

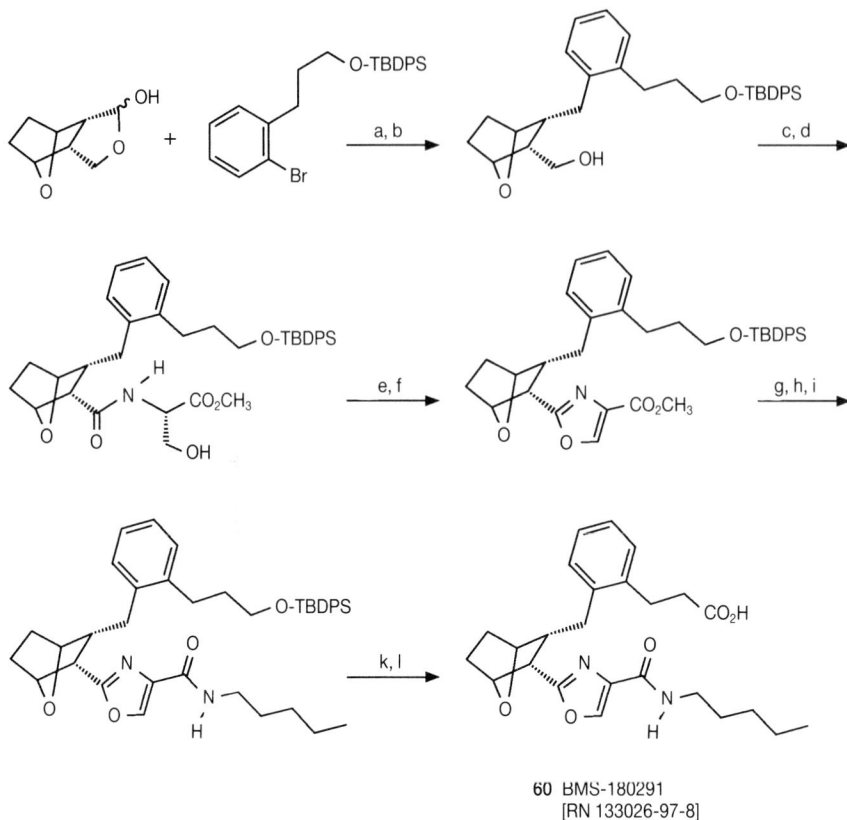

Fig. 4.15 Synthesis of BMS-180291 (**60**). Reagents: a, *t*-BuLi/−100°C; b, moist Pd(OH)$_2$/EtOAc/H$_2$; c, Jones oxidation; d, 1-hydroxybenzotriazole hydrate/L-serine methylester hydrochloride/Et$_3$N/DCC/0°C to rt; e, PPh$_3$/ CCl$_4$/(*i*-Pr)$_2$NEt/CH$_3$CN; f, nickel peroxide/CH$_2$Cl$_2$; g, LiOH/THF/H$_2$O (3:1)/rt; h, oxalyl chloride/benzene; i, *n*-C$_5$H$_{11}$NH$_2$/Et$_3$N/CH$_2$Cl$_2$/0°C; k, 48% aq. HF; l, Jones oxidation.

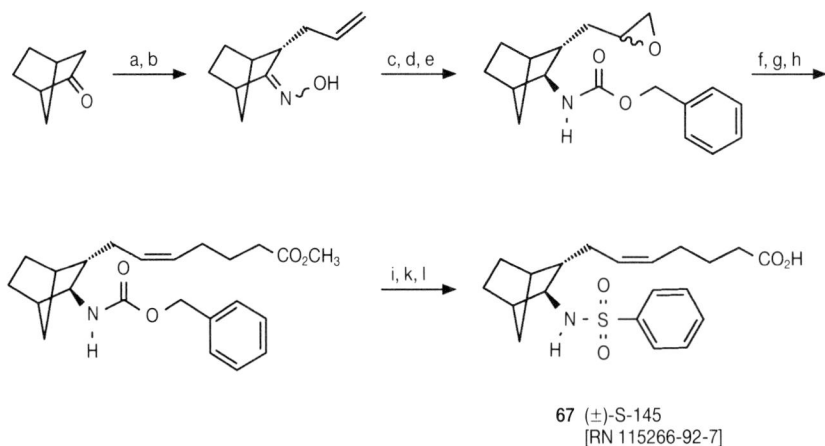

Fig. 4.16 Synthesis of (±)-S-145 (**67**). Reagents: a, allyl bromide/THF/−15°C; b, H$_2$NOH·HCl/KOH/MeOH/0°C; c, LAH/THF/Δ; d, carbobenzoxy chloride/pyridine/CH$_2$Cl$_2$/0°C; e, *m*-CPBA/CH$_2$Cl$_2$/rt; f, HIO$_4$/H$_2$O/dioxane/rt; g, NaH/DMSO/(4-carboxybutyl)triphenylphosphonium bromide/rt; h, CH$_2$N$_2$/ether; i, anisole/TFA/45°C; k, benzenesulphonyl chloride/Et$_3$N/CH$_2$Cl$_2$/rt; l, 1 N KOH, MeOH, rt.

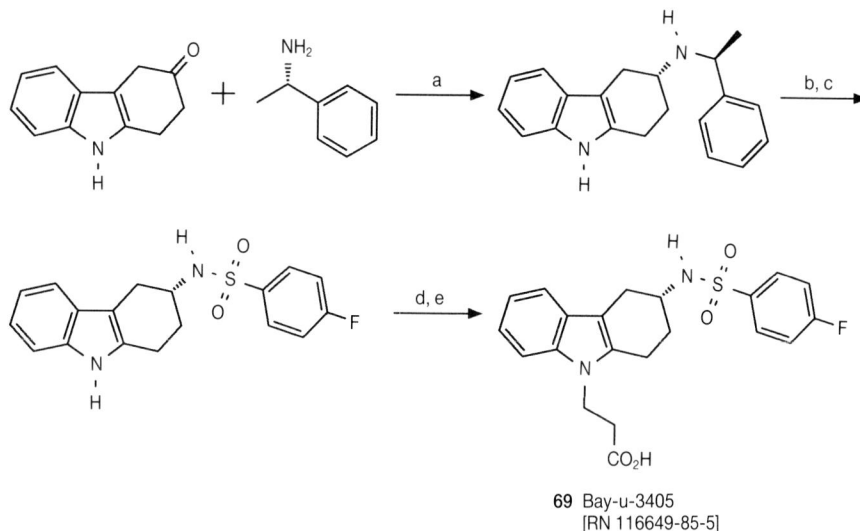

Fig. 4.17 Synthesis of Bay-u-3405 (**69**). Reagents: a, benzene/Δ; Bu₄NBH₄/CH₂Cl₂/−50°C; b, 2 N NaOH/MeOH/ ethyl acetate; HCO₂NH₄/Pd/C (10%)/DMF/Δ; c, 4-fluorobenzenesulphonyl chloride/Et₃N/CH₂Cl₂/rt; d, NaH/ acrylonitrile/DMF/rt; e, 10% KOH/*i*-PrOH/Δ.

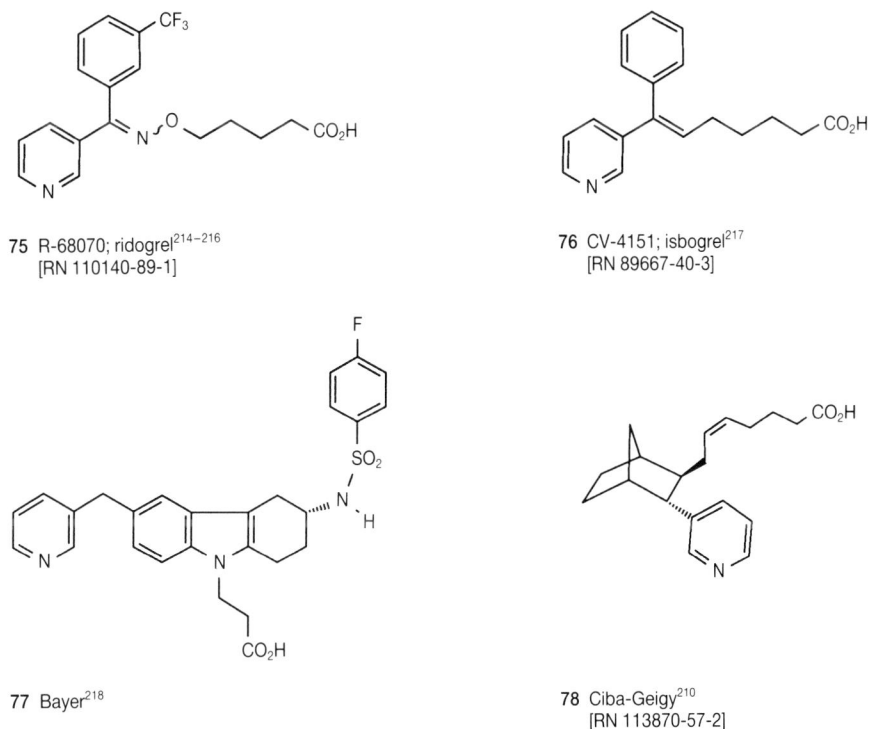

75 R-68070; ridogrel[214–216]
[RN 110140-89-1]

76 CV-4151; isbogrel[217]
[RN 89667-40-3]

77 Bayer[218]

78 Ciba-Geigy[210]
[RN 113870-57-2]

Fig. 4.18 TXA₂-synthase inhibitors with mixed profile.

(55), ICI-185282 (72b) and dazmegrel (54))[209–212] were shown to act synergistically. Therefore, a series of compounds was synthesized with these two properties in one molecule to achieve lower levels of TXA_2 and a more effective blocking of the inter-action of PGH_2 with the TXA_2/PGH_2 receptor. This results in a possible 'redirection'[213] of the endo-peroxide PGH_2 (48a) in platelets towards the syn-thesis of PGI_2 (23) in endothelial cells. Typical for such a combination of TXA_2-antagonistic with TXA_2-synthase inhibiting properties within one molecule are ridogrel (75)[214–216] or isbogrel (76),[217] the Bayer compound 77[218] and the Ciba-Geigy compound 78,[219] which all incorporate the above-mentioned β-picolyl pharmacophore for the additional TXA_2-synthase inhibiting activity (Fig. 4.18).

Finally, other combinations of biological activities have been identified within one molecule, e.g. TXA_2 with serotonin antagonistic activity (L-636499[220]) or TXA_2-synthase and 5-lipoxygenase inhibiting activity in a Takeda compound.[221]

The next years will show which combination of biological activities and in which ratio will be optimal to fight thromboembolic diseases.

References

1. Bindra JS, Bindra R. *Prostaglandin Synthesis*. New York, San Francisco, London: Academic Press, Inc., 1977.
2. Mitra A. *The Synthesis of Prostaglandins*. New York, London, Sydney, Toronto: John Wiley & Sons, 1977.
3. Raduechel B, Vorbrueggen H. Prostaglandin ana-logs. *Adv Prostaglandin Thromboxane Leukotriene Res* 1985; **14**: 263–307.
4. Elger W. Pharmacology of parturition and abortion. *Anim Reprod Sci* 1979; **2**: 133–48.
5. Schmidt Gollwitzer K, Schuessler B, Elger W, Schmidt Gollwitzer M. A new therapeutic for termin-ating intact and disturbed pregnancies: three years of experience with the prostaglandin Esub 2-derivative sulprostone (SHB 286). *Geburtshilfe Frauenheilkd* 1979; **39**: 667–75.
6. Ding JQ, Granberg S, Norstroem A. Clinical effects and cervical tissue changes after treatment with 16,16-dimethyl-trans-Δ^2-PGE1 methyl ester in the first trimester. *Prostaglandins* 1990; **39**: 281–5.
7. Suga H, Konishi Y, Wakatsuka H, Miyake H, Kori S, Hayashi M. Synthesis of 16,16-dimethyl-trans-Δ^2-PGE1 methyl ester (ONO-802). *Prostaglandins* 1978; **15**: 907–12.
8. Eder SE, Chatterjee M, Salvio C. Evaluation of met-eneprost potassium (a PGE2 analogue) for cervical dilation and side effects in nonpregnant women. *Prostaglandins* 1986; **32**: 19–23.
9. Bundy GL, Kimball FA, Robert A, *et al*. Synthesis and biological activity of 9-deoxo-9-methylene and related prostaglandins. *Adv Prostaglandin Throm-boxane Res* 1980; **6**: 355–63.
10. Collins PW. Misoprostol: discovery, development, and clinical applications. *Med Res Rev* 1990; **10**: 149–72.
11. Urquhart DR, Templeton AA, Shinewi F, *et al*. The efficacy and tolerance of mifepristone and prosta-glandin in first trimester termination of pregnancy. UK multicenter trial. *Br J Obstet Gynaecol* 1990; **97**: 480–6.
12. Silvestre L, Dubois C, Renault M, Rezvani Y, Baulieu EE, Ulmann A. Voluntary interruption of pregnancy with mifepristone (RU 486) and a prosta-glandin analog. A large-scale French experience. *N Engl J Med* 1990; **322**: 645–8.
13. Maria B, Stampf F, Goepp A, Dubois C. Termination of early pregnancy through a combination of the anti-progestin and prostaglandin analog. *Eur J Obstet Gynecol Reprod Biol* 1990; **37**: 35–40.
14. Elger W, Beier S, Chwalisz K, *et al*. Studies on the mechanisms of action of progesterone antagonists. *J Steroid Biochem* 1986; **25**: 835–45.
15. Bygdeman M, Swahn ML. Progesterone receptor blockage. Effect on uterine contractility and early pregnancy. *Contraception* 1985; **32**: 45–51.
16. Carpio H, Cooper GF, Edwards JA, *et al*. Synthesis and gastric antisecretory properties of allenic 16-phenoxy-omega-tetranor prostaglandin E analogs. *Prostaglandins* 1987; **33**: 169–80.
17. Roszkowski AP, Garay GL, Baker S, Schuler M, Carter H. Gastric antisecretory and antiulcer properties of enprostil, (±)-11α,15α-dihydroxy-16-phenoxy-17,18,19,20-tetranor-9-oxoprosta-4,5,13(t)-trienoic acid methyl ester. *J Pharmacol Exp Ther* 1986; **239**: 382–9.
18. *Drugs of the Future* 1986; **11**: 986–8.
19. Konturek SJ, Konturek JW, Kwiecien N, *et al*. Gas-tric protection by nocloprost against aspirin damage in humans. *Scand J Gastroenterol* 1991; **26**: 231–6.
20. Konturek SJ, Kwiecien N, Obtulowicz W, Maczka J, Hebzda Z, Oleksy J. Effects of nocloprost on gastric functions in man. *Scand J Gastroenterol* 1991; **26**: 1145–51.
21. *Drugs of the Future* 1986; **11**: 660–2.
22. Kluender H, Corey P. Discovery and synthesis of rioprostil. *Scand J Gastroenterol* 1989; **24** (suppl 164): 1–9.
23. Shriver DA, Katz LB, Rosenthale ME. Gastric anti-secretory and antigastrolesive pharmacology of rio-prostil. *Scand J Gastroenterol* 1989; **24** (suppl 164): 10–20.
24. *Drugs of the Future* 1987; **12**: 1102–3.
25. Bartmann W, Beck G, Jaehne G, Lerch U, Wess G. Synthesis of a biologically active analog of prosta-glandin E2 (racemate and enantiomerically pure com-pounds). *Liebigs Ann Chem* 1987; 321–6.

26. Ishimori A, Kawamura T, Koizumi F. Effect of trimoprostil on gastric secretion in man. *Arzneim-Forsch/Drug Res* 1988; **38** (I): 833–9.
27. UK Trimoprostil study colloborative group. A multicentre comparison of trimoprostil and cimetidine in the treatment of duodenal ulcer. *Scand J Gastroenterol* 1988; **23**: 134–8.
28. Mueller P, Dammann HG, Leucht U, Simon B. An alprostadil analogue and human gastric secretion. *Arzneim-Forsch/Drug Res* 1989; **39** (II): 809–11.
29. Kolb M, van Hijfte L, Ireland RE. A highly convergent synthesis of mexiprostil: 16(R) 16-methoxy 16-methyl PGE₁ methyl ester. *Tetrahedron Lett* 1988; **29**: 6769–72.
30. Guzzi U, Ciabatti R, Padova G, et al. Structure–activity studies of 16-methoxy-16-methyl prostaglandins. *J Med Chem* 1986; **29**: 1826–32.
31. Sugiyama S, Kawabe Y, Kuroiwa M, Goto H, Tsukamoto Y, Ozawa T. Effects of the synthesized prostaglandin E₂-analogue arbaprostil on gastric mucosal lesions in rats. *Arzneim-Forsch/Drug Res* 1989; **39** (II): 1571–3.
32. Dygos JH, Adamek JP, Babiak KA, et al. An efficient synthesis of the antisecretory prostaglandin enisoprost. *J Org Chem* 1991; **56**: 2549–52.
33. Collins PW, Gasiecki AF, Perkins WE, et al. Chemistry and structure–activity relationships of C-17 unsaturated 18-cycloalkyl and cycloalkenyl analogs of enisoprost. Identification of a promising new antiulcer prostaglandin. *J Med Chem* 1990; **33**: 2784–93.
34. *Drugs of the Future* 1985; **10**: 737–9.
35. Arrigoni C, Mizzotti B, Toti D, Faustini F, Ceserani R. Cytoprotective and antisecretory effects of 11-deoxy-13,14-didehydro-16(S)-methyl PGE₂ methylester (FCE 20700). *Prostaglandin Leukot Med* 1984; **15**: 79–89.
36. Olsen EA, DeLong E. Transdermal viprostol in the treatment of male pattern baldness. *J Am Acad Dermatol* 1990; **23** (3 Pt 1): 470–2.
37. Cervoni P, Chan PS. Synthetic stable orally and transdermally long-acting prostaglandin E₂ (PGE₂) congener (viprostol; CL 115,347) and prostacyclin congener (CL 115,999) as antihypertensive agents. *Adv Prostaglandin Thromboxane Leukotriene Res* 1989; **19**: 331–4.
38. Chan PS, Cervoni P, Ronsberg MA, et al. Antihypertensive activity of dl-15-deoxy-16-hydroxy-16(α/β)-vinyl prostaglandin E2 methyl ester (CL 115,347), a new orally and transdermally long-acting antihypertensive agent. *J Pharmacol Exp Ther* 1983; **226**: 726–32.
39. Adaikan PG, Karim SMM. Some pharmacological effects of 17(S) methyl-ω-homo-trans-Δ²-PGE₁ (ONO 1206). *Prostaglandins Med* 1981; **6**: 449–58.
40. Harper SL, Klevans LR, Granger DN. Effects of the antihypertensive prostaglandin analog Ro 22–1327 on regional blood flows in the spontaneously hypertensive rat. *J Cardiovasc Pharmacol* 1987; **9**: 285–90.
41. Gardiner PJ. Characterization of prostanoid relaxant/inhibitory receptors (Ψ) using a highly selective agonist, TR4979. *Br J Pharmacol* 1986; **87**: 45–56.
42. Waterbury LD, Cooper GF, Fried JH. Ocular hypotensive activity of RS-18492, a potent synthetic PGE₂ analog. *Pharmacologist* 1987; **29** (3): 139 (Abs 187).
43. Cooper GF, Fried JH, Waterbury D. 11-Substituted-16-phenoxy- and 16-substituted phenoxyprostatrienoic acid derivatives. *Published European Patent Application*. EP 170258.
44. Lanza FL, Kochman RL, Geis GS, Rack EM, Deysach LG. A double-blind, placebo-controlled, 6-day evaluation of two doses of misoprostol in gastroduodenal mucosal protection against damage from aspirin and effect on bowel habits. *Am J Gastroenterol* 1991; **86**: 1743–8.
45. Ahmed WU, Qureshi H, Alam E, Zuberi SJ. A double-blind study of misoprostol (SC-29333) in the healing of duodenal ulcer. *J Gastroenterol Hepatol* 1991; **6**: 179–80.
46. Morgan AG, Pacsoo C, Taylor P, McAdam WA. A comparison between enprostil and ranitidine in the management of gastric ulceration. *Aliment Pharmacol Ther (Oxford)* 1990; **4**: 635–41.
47. Lanza FL, Robinson MG, Isenberg JI, Basuk PM, Karlin DA. Effect of enprostil on the gastroduodenal mucosa of healthy volunteers. *Aliment Pharmacol Ther (Oxford)* 1990; **4**: 601–13.
48. Bays DE, Finch H. Inhibitors of gastric acid secretion. *Nat Prod Rep* 1990; 409–45.
49. Katz LB, Genna TBS, George H, Greeley Jr GH, Shriver DA. Antisecretory and antigastrin effects of rioprostil in gastric fistula dogs. *Dig Dis Sci* 1987; **32**: 1268–74.
50. *Drugs of the Future* 1983; **8**: 450–2.
51. *Drugs of the Future* 1981; **6**: 317–18.
52. Dixon JS, Page MC. Interactions between nonsteroidal anti-inflammatory drugs and H₂-receptor antagonists or prostaglandin analogs. *Rheumatol Int* 1991; **11**: 13–18.
53. Taeuber U, Brudny-Kloeppel M, Jakobs U, Madetzki C, Mahler M. Pharmacokinetics of nocloprost in human volunteers in dose dependency. *Eur J Clin Pharmacol* in press.
54. Barraclough P, Jackson WP, Harris CJ. Imidazolidin-2-one prostaglandin analogues. *Arch Pharm* 1991; **324**: 473–7.
55. Al-Sinawi LAH, Mekki QA, Hassan S, et al. Effects of hydantoin prostaglandin analogue, BW245C, during oral dosing in man. *Prostaglandins* 1985; **29**: 99–111.
56. Brockwell MA, Caldwell AG, Whittaker N. Heterocyclic prostaglandin analogues. Part 3. The relationship of configuration to biological activity for some

hydantoin prostaglandin analogues. *J Chem Soc Perkin Trans 1* 1981; 706–11.

57. *Drugs of the Future* 1986; **11**: 372–4.
58. Ritter JM, Ludgin JR, Scharschmidt LA, Smith RD, Dunn MJ. Effects of a stable prostaglandin analog, L-644,122, in healthy and hypertensive men. *Eur J Clin Pharmacol* 1985; **28**: 685–8.
59. Schulz BG, Beckmann R, Mueller B, *et al.* Cardio- and hemodynamic profile of selective PGD$_2$-analogues. *Adv Prostaglandin Thromboxane Leukotriene Res* 1991; **21B**: 591–4.
60. Thierauch KH, Stuerzebecher CS, Schillinger E *et al.* Stable 9β- or 11α-halogen-15-cyclohexyl-prostaglandins with high affinity to the PGD$_2$-receptor. *Prostaglandins* 1988; **35**: 855–68.
61. Buchmann B, Skuballa W, Vorbrueggen H. Synthesis of a chemically and metabolically stable and biologically potent PGD$_2$-analogue. *Tetrahedron Lett* 1990; **31**: 3425–8.
62. Roberts LJ, Sweetman BJ. Metabolic fate of endogenously synthesized prostaglandin D$_2$ in a human female with mastocytosis. *Prostaglandins* 1985; **30**: 383–400.
63. Giles H, Leff P, Bolofo ML, Kelly MG, Robertson AD. The classification of prostaglandin DP-receptors in platelets and vasculature using BW A868C, a novel, selective and potent competitive antagonist. *Br J Pharmacol* 1989; **96**: 291–300.
64. Trist DG, Collins BA, Wood J, Kelly MG, Robertson AD. The antagonism by BW A868C of PGD2 and BW 245C activation of human platelet adenylate cyclase. *Br J Pharmacol* 1989; **96**: 301–6.
65. Hayaishi O. Molecular mechanisms of sleep–wake regulation: roles of prostaglandins D$_2$ and E$_2$. *FASEB J* 1991; **5**: 2575–81.
66. Moncada S, Gryglewski RJ, Bunting S, Vane JR. An enzyme isolated from arteries transforms prostaglandin endoperoxides to an unstable substance that inhibits platelet aggregation. *Nature* 1976; **263**: 663–5.
67. Whittle BJR, Moncada S. Platelet actions of stable carbocyclic analogs of prostacyclin. *Circulation* 1985; **72**: 1219–25.
68. Aristoff PA. Synthesis of prostacyclin analogs. *Adv Prostaglandin Thromboxane Leukotriene Res* 1985; **14**: 309–92.
69. Nickolson RC, Town MH, Vorbrueggen H. Prostacyclin-analogs. *Med Res Rev* 1985; **5**: 1–53.
70. Aristoff PA, Harrison AW, Aiken JW, Gorman RR, Pike JE. Synthesis and structure–activity relationship of novel stable prostacyclin analogs. *Adv Prostaglandin Thromboxane Leukotriene Res* 1983; **11**: 267–74.
71. Bartmann W, Beck G, Knolle J, Rupp RH, Schoelkens BA, Weithmann U. Synthesis of stable prostacyclin analogs. *Adv Prostaglandin Thromboxane Leukotriene Res* 1983; **11**: 287–92.
72. Stock G. Iloprost: a stable analog of prostacyclin. In:
Rubanyi GM, Vanhoutte PM (eds). *Endothelium-derived Relaxing Factors: 1st International Symposium on Endothelium-derived Vasoactive Factors, Philadelphia 1989.* Basel, München, Paris: Karger Verlag, 1990: 260–4.
73. Gryglewski RJ, Stock G. *Prostacyclin and its Stable Analogue Iloprost.* Berlin, Heidelberg, New York, London, Paris, Tokyo: Springer Verlag, 1987.
74. Skuballa W, Vorbrueggen H. Ein neuer Weg zu 6a-Carbacyclinen – Synthese eines stabilen, biologisch potenten Prostacyclin-Analogons. *Angew Chem* 1981; **93**: 1080–1. *Angew Chem Int Ed Engl* 1981; **20**: 1046–8.
75. Balzer K, Bechara G, Bisler H, *et al.* Reduction of ischaemic rest pain in advanced peripheral arterial occlusive disease. A double blind placebo controlled trial with iloprost. *Int Angiol* 1991; **10**: 229–32.
76. Ylitalo P, Kaukinen S, Reinikainen P, Salenius JP, Vapaatalo H. A randomized, double-blind, crossover comparison of iloprost with dextran in patients with peripheral arterial occlusive disease. *Int J Clin Pharmacol Ther Toxicol* 1990; **28**: 197–204.
77. *Drugs of the Future* 1986; **11**: 913–17.
78. Skuballa W, Schillinger E, Stuerzebecher CS, Vorbrueggen H. Synthesis of a new chemically and metabolically stable prostacyclin analogue with high and long-lasting oral activity. *J Med Chem* 1986; **29**: 313–15.
79. Skuballa W, Raduechel B, Vorbrueggen H, *et al.* Carbacyclincs and their use as medicaments. *Published German Patent Application.* DE 3226550.
80. Sodeoka M, Ogawa Y, Kirio Y, Shibasaki M. Stereocontrolled synthesis of exocyclic olefins using arene tricarbonyl chromium complex-catalyzed hydrogenation. I. Efficient synthesis of carbacyclin and its analogs. *Chem Pharm Bull* 1991; **39**: 309–22.
81. Fujitani B, Wakitani K. Studies on antiplatelet effects of OP-41483, a prostaglandin I2 analog, in experimental animals. I. Effect on platelet function and thrombosis. *Jpn J Pharmacol* 1990; **52**: 123–30.
82. Fujitani B, Wakitani K. Studies on antiplatelet effects of OP-41483, a prostaglandin I2 analog, in experimental animals. II. Mechanism of its antiplatelet effect. *Jpn J Pharmacol* 1990; **53**: 25–33.
83. Linet OI, Luderer JR, Froeschke M, Welch S, Metzler CM, Eckert SM. Ciprostene in patients with peripheral vascular disease (PVD). An Open-Label, tolerance trial. *Prostaglandins Leukot Essent Fatty Acids* 1988; **34**: 9–14.
84. O'Grady J, Hedges A, Whittle BJR, *et al.* A chemically stable analog, 9β-methylcarbacyclin, with similar effects to epoprostenol (prostacyclin, PGI2) in man. *Br J Clin Pharmacol* 1984; **18**: 921–33.
85. Aristoff PA, Johnson PD, Harrison AW. Synthesis of 9-substituted carbacyclin analogs. *J Org Chem* 1983; **48**: 5341–8.
86. Morley J, Page CP, Paul W, Mongelli N, Ceserani

R, Gandolfi C. A comparative study of PGI2 and two analogs (FCE 21292 and FCE 21258) *in vitro* and *in vivo*. *Prostaglandins Leukot Med* 1983; **11**: 391–9.

87. *Drugs of the Future* 1986; **11**: 918–21.
88. Morita A, Kamoshita K, Ito T, Naito Y, Akiyama K, Kobayashi S. Beneficial effects of sodium salt of 17(R)-methyl-20-isopropylidenecarbacyclin on experimentally-induced ischemic hind limb lesions and blood viscosity. *Arzneim-Forsch/Drug Res* 1986; **36**: 680–3.
89. Tanaka T, Bannai K, Hazato A, Koga M, Kurozumi S, Kato Y. Short synthesis of isocarbacyclin by regioselective S_N2' alkylation of bicyclic allylic esters with zinc-copper reagents. *Tetrahedron* 1991; **47**: 1861–76.
90. Bannai K, Tanaka T, Okamura N, *et al.* Syntheses of isocarbacyclin by highly regioselective alkylation of allylic alcohols. *Tetrahedron* 1990; **46**: 6689–704.
91. Ohtsu A, Fujii K, Kurozumi S. Induction of angiogenic response by chemically stable prostacyclin analogs. *Prostaglandins Leukot Essent Fatty Acids* 1988; **33**: 35–9.
92. Kanayama T, Kimura Y, Iseki K, Hayashi Y, Tamao Y, Mizogami S. Antithrombotic effects of KP-10614, a novel and stable prostacyclin (PGI2) analog. *J Pharmacol Exp Ther* 1990; **255**: 1210–17.
93. Iseki K, Kanayama T, Hayasi Y, Shibasaki M. Synthesis of a new chemically stable prostacyclin analog with high and long-lasting activity. *Chem Pharm Bull* 1990; **38**: 1769–71.
94. Wallach MB. The antihypertensive properties of a synthetic prostanoid: RS-93427. *Prostaglandins Leukot Essent Fatty Acids* 1989; **36**: 35–41.
95. Kluge AF, Kertesz DJ, O'Yang C, Wu HY. Potent prostacyclin analogues based on the bicyclo-[4.2.0]octane ring system. *J Org Chem* 1987; **52**: 2860–8.
96. Shea-Donohue T, Kandasamy A, Dubois A. Effects of a prostacyclin analog, U-68,215, on gastric acid secretion, gastric emptying and systemic blood pressure in primates. *J Pharmacol Exp Ther* 1992; **260**: 1023–7.
97. Alexander DL, Lin CH. The synthesis of benzidene prostacyclin analogs as potential antiulcer agents. *Prostaglandins* 1986; **32**: 647–53.
98. Aristoff PA, Johnson PD, Harrison AW. Total synthesis of a novel antiulcer agent via a modification of the intramolecular Wadsworth–Emmons–Wittig reaction. *J Am Chem Soc* 1985; **107**: 7967–74.
99. Kovacs G, Simonidesz V, Toemoeskoezi I, *et al.* A new stable prostacyclin mimic, 7-oxo-PGI2. *J Med Chem* 1982; **25**: 105–7.
100. Vorbrueggen H, Stuerzebecher CS, Maas M. 7-Oxo prostacyclin derivatives and process for their manufacture. *Published International Patent Application.* WO 87/05900.
101. *Drugs of the Future* 1990; **15**: 233–6.
102. Flohé L, Boehlke H, Frankus E, *et al.* Designing prostacyclin analogs. *Arzneim-Forsch/Drug Res* 1983; **33**: 1240–8.
103. Michel G, Seipp U. *In vitro* studies with the stabilized epoprostenol analog taprostene. Effect on platelets and erythrocytes. *Arzneim-1 Forsch/Drug Res* 1990; **40**: 817–22.
104. Michel G, Seipp U. *In vivo* studies with the stabilized epoprostenol analog taprostene. Effects on platelet functions and blood clotting. *Arzneim-Forsch/Drug Res* 1990; **40**: 932–8.
105. *Drugs of the Future* 1989; **14**: 913–14.
106. Darius H, Thomsen T, Schroer K. Cardiovascular actions *in vitro* and cardioprotective effects *in vivo* of nileprost, a mixed type PGI_2/PGE_2 agonist. *J Cardiovasc Pharmacol* 1987; **10**: 144–52.
107. Murata T, Sakaya S, Hoshino T, Umetsu T, Hirano T, Nishio S. General pharmacology of beraprost sodium, 1st communication: effect on the central nervous system. *Arzneim-Forsch/Drug Res* 1989; **39** (II): 860–6.
108. Murata T, Murai T, Kanai T, *et al.* General pharmacology of beraprost sodium, 2nd communication: effect on the autonomic cardiovascular and gastrointestinal systems, and other effects. *Arzneim-Forsch/Drug Res* 1989; **39** (II): 867–76.
109. Nishio S, Matsuura H, Kanai N, *et al.* The *in vitro* and *in vivo* antiplatelet effects of TRK-100, a stable prostacyclin analog, in several species. *Jpn J Pharmacol* 1988; **47**: 1–10.
110. *Drugs of the Future* 1986; **11**: 956–8.
111. Mori S, Takechi S. Synthesis of benzodioxane prostacyclin analogue. *Heterocycles* 1990; **31**: 1189–99.
112. Hildebrand M, Pfeffer M, Mahler M, Staks T, Windt-Hanke F, Schuett A. Oral iloprost in healthy volunteers. *Eicosanoids* 1991; **4**: 149–54.
113. Hildebrand M, McDonald FM, Windt-Hanke F. Characterization of oral sustained release preparations of iloprost in a pig model by plasma level monitoring. *Prostaglandins* 1991; **41**: 473–86.
114. Hildebrand M, Staks T, Schuett A, Matthes H. Pharmacokinetics of ^{3}H-cicaprost in healthy volunteers. *Prostaglandins* 1989; **37**: 259–73.
115. Schirner M, Schneider MR. Cicaprost inhibits metastases of animal tumors. *Prostaglandins* 1991; **42**: 451–61.
116. Schneider MR, Schillinger E, Schirner M, Skuballa W, Stuerzebecher S, Witt W. Effects of prostacyclin analogues in *in vivo* tumor models. *Adv Prostaglandin Thromboxane Leukotriene Res* 1991; **21B**: 901–8.
117. Giraldi T, Rapozzi V, Perissin L, Zorzet S. Antimetastatic action of stable prostacyclin analogs in mice. *Adv Prostaglandin Thromboxane Leukotriene Res* 1991; **21B**: 913–16.
118. Costantini V, Giampietri A, Allegrucci M, Agnelli G, Nenci GG, Fioretti MC. Mechanisms of the antimetastatic activity of stable prostacyclin analogues: modulation of host immunocompetence. *Adv Prosta-*

glandin Thromboxane Leukotriene Res 1991; **21B:** 917–20.

119. Smith HW, Bach MK, Harrison AW, Johnson HG, Major NJ, Wasserman MA. The synthesis of 6,9-N-phenylimino-$\Delta^{6,8}$-prostaglandin I1. A novel inhibitor of leukotriene C and D synthesis. *Prostaglandins* 1982; **24:** 543–6.

120. *Drugs of the Future* 1989; **14:** 525–8.

121. Iguchi S, Miyata Y, Okuyama S, Miyake H, Okegawa T. Synthesis of 15-cis-(4-n-propylcyclohexyl)-16,17, 18,19,20-pentanor-9-deoxy-6,9α-nitriloprostaglandin F1 methyl ester (OP-2507), a novel anticerebral ischemic agent. *Chem Pharm Bull* 1988; **36:** 1128–34.

122. Klar U, Pletsch A, Skuballa W, Vorbrueggen H. Synthesis of potent 6-oxo and 9-fluoro-PGE₁-derivatives and their biological properties. *Bioorg Med Chem Lett* 1992; **2:** 445–8.

123. Kobayashi K, Arakawa T, Higuchi K, Nakamura H. Gastric cytoprotection by ornoprostil, a PGE₁ analogue, in human subjects. *J Clin Gastroenterol* 1991; **13** (suppl I): S32–6.

124. *Drugs of the Future* 1987; **12:** 1023–4.

125. Wakatsuka H, Okegawa T, Arai Y. Process for the preparation of 6-keto-prostaglandin E1 derivatives as cytoprotective agents. *Published European Patent Application*. EP 232126.

126. Merrit JE, Brown AM, Bund S, *et al*. Primate vascular responses to octimibate, a non-prostanoid agonist at the prostacyclin receptor. *Br J Pharmacol* 1991; **102:** 260–6.

127. Seiler S, Brassard CL, Arnold AJ, Meanwell NA, Fleming JS, Keely Jr SL. Octimibate inhibition of platelet aggregation: stimulation of adenylate cyclase through prostacyclin receptor activation. *Pharmacol Exp Ther* 1990; **255:** 1021–6.

128. Merritt JE, Hallam TJ, Brown AM, *et al*. Octimibate, a potent non-prostanoid inhibitor of platelet aggregation, acts via the prostacyclin receptor. *Br J Pharmacol* 1991; **102:** 251–9.

129. Meanwell NA, Rosenfeld MJ, Wright JJK. Structure–activity relationships associated with 3,4,5-triphenyl-1H-pyrazole-1-nonanoic acid, a nonprostanoid prostacyclin mimetic. *J Med Chem* 1992; **35:** 389–97.

130. Hoult JRS, Moore PK. 6-Keto-prostaglandin E₁: a naturally occurring stable prostacyclin-like mediator of high potency. *Trends Pharmacol Sci* 1986; **7:** 197–200.

131. Unpublished results.

132. Cross PE, Dickinson RP. The story of thromboxane A₂. *Chem Br* 1991; 911–14.

133. Morinelli TA, Okwu AK, Mais DE, *et al*. Difluorothromboxane A₂ and stereoisomers: stable derivatives of thromboxane A₂ with differential effects on platelets and blood vessels. *Proc Natl Acad Sci USA* 1989; **86:** 5600–4.

134. Fried J, John V, Szwedo Jr MJ, *et al*. Synthesis of 10,10-difluorothromboxane A₂, a potent and chemically stable thromboxane agonist. *J Am Chem Soc* 1989; **111:** 4510–11.

135. Coleman RA, Humphrey PPA, Kennedy I, Levy GP, Lumley P. Comparison of the actions of U-46619, a prostaglandin H₂-analogue, with those of prostaglandin H₂ and thromboxane A₂ on some isolated smooth muscle preparations. *Br J Pharmacol* 1981; **73:** 773–8.

136. *Drugs of the Future* 1980; **5:** 453–8.

137. Bundy GL. Synthesis of prostaglandin endoperoxide analogs. *Tetrahedron Lett* 1975; 1957–60.

138. Tymkewycz PM, Jones RL, Wilson NH, Marr CG. Heterogeneity of thromboxane A2 (TP-) receptors: evidence from antagonist but not agonist potency measurements. *Br J Pharmacol* 1991; **102:** 607–14.

139. Jones RL, Wilson NH, Lawrence RA. EP 171: a high affinity thromboxane A2-mimetic, the actions of which are slowly reversed by receptor blockade. *Br J Pharmacol* 1989; **96:** 875–87.

140. Wilson NH, Jones RL, Marr CG, Muir G. Synthesis of oxabicyclo[2.2.1]heptane prostanoids having thromboxane-like activity at sub-nanomolar concentrations. *Eur J Med Chem* 1988; **23:** 359–64.

141. Halushka PV, Mais DE, Garvin M. Binding of a thromboxane A₂/prostaglandin H₂ receptor antagonist to guinea pig platelets. *Eur J Pharmacol* 1986; **131:** 49–54.

142. Mais D, Knapp D, Halushka P, Ballard K, Hamanaka N. Synthesis of thromboxane receptor antagonists with the potential to radiolabel with iodine-125. *Tetrahedron Lett* 1984; **25:** 4207–10.

143. Masuda A, Mais DE, Oatis Jr JE, Halushka PV. Platelet and vascular thromboxane A₂/prostaglandin H₂ receptors. Evidence for different subclasses in the rat. *Biochem Pharmacol* 1991; **42:** 537–44.

144. Mais DE, Saussy Jr DL, Magee DE, Williams CM. Binding of a radioiodinated agonist to thromboxane A₂/prostaglandin H₂ (TxA₂/PGH₂) receptors in guinea pig lung membranes. *Adv Prostaglandin Thromboxane Leukotriene Res* 1991; **21A:** 347–50.

145. Morinelli TA, Mais DE, Oatis Jr JE, Crumbley AJ-III, Halushka PV. Characterization of thromboxane A₂/prostaglandin H₂ receptors in human vascular smooth muscle cells. *Life Sci* 1990; **46:** 1765–72.

146. Klar U, Rehwinkel H, Vorbrueggen H, Thierauch KH, Stuerzebecher CS. 9-Fluor-prostaglandin-Derivate, Verfahren zu ihrer Herstellung und ihre pharmazeutische Verwendung. *Published German Patent Application*. DE 3923797.

147. Hamberg M, Svensson J, Samuelsson B. Thromboxanes: a new group of biologically active compounds derived from prostaglandin endoperoxides. *Proc Natl Acad Sci USA* 1975; **72:** 2994–8.

148. Bhagwat SS, Hamann PR, Still WC. Synthesis of thromboxane A₂. *J Am Chem Soc* 1985; **107:** 6372–6.

149. Hall SE. Thromboxane A$_2$ receptor antagonists. *Med Res Rev* 1991; **11**: 503–79.

150. Gresele P, Deckmyn H, Nenci GG, Vermylen J. Thromboxane synthase inhibitors, thromboxane receptor antagonists and dual blockers in thrombotic disorders. *Trends Pharmacol Sci* 1991; **12**: 158–63.

151. Schroer K. Thromboxane antagonism in blood platelets – pathophysiology, pharmacology, and possible clinical relevance. *Wien Klin Wochenschr* 1991; **103**: 543–53.

152. Patrono C. Thromboxane synthesis inhibitors and receptor antagonists. *Thromb Res* 1990; **suppl 11**: 15–23.

153. Collington EW, Finch H. Thromboxane synthase inhibitors and receptor antagonists. *Annu Rep Med Chem* 1990; **25**: 99–108.

154. Halushka PV. Pharmacology of thromboxane A$_2$ receptor antagonists. *Z Kardiol* 1989; **89** (suppl 3): 42–7.

155. Wilson NH, Jones RL. Prostaglandin endoperoxide and thromboxane A$_2$ analogs. *Adv Prostaglandin Thromboxane Leukotriene Res* 1985; **14**: 393–425.

156. Unpublished results.

157. Martinez GR, Hirschfeld DR, Maloney PJ, Yang DS, Rosenkranz RP, Walker KAM. ((1H-Imidazol-1-yl)methyl)- and ((3-pyridinyl)methyl)pyrroles as thromboxane synthetase inhibitors. *J Med Chem* 1989; **32**: 890–7.

158. Cross PE, Dickinson RP, Parry MJ, Randall MJ. Selective thromboxane synthetase inhibitors. 1. 1-((Aryloxy)alkyl)-1H-imidazoles. *J Med Chem* 1985; **28**: 1427–32.

159. Tyler HM. Dazoxiben: a pharmacological tool or clinical candidate? *Br J Clin Pharmacol* 1983; **15**: 13S–16S.

160. *Drugs of the Future* 1991; **16**: 1047.

161. Rebec MV, Skrinska VA. Pharmacology of UK-38485 (dazmegrel), a specific inhibitor of thromboxane A$_2$ synthetase. *Prostaglandins Leukot Essent Fatty Acids* 1989; **38**: 207–12.

162. Hiraku S, Taniguchi K, Wakitani K, *et al.* Pharmacological studies on the TxA$_2$ synthetase inhibitor; (E)-3-[p-(1H-imidazol-1-ylmethyl)phenyl]-2-propenoic acid (OKY-046). *Jpn J Pharmacol* 1986; **41**: 393–401.

163. Iizuka K, Akahane K, Momose D, *et al.* Highly selective inhibitors of thromboxane synthetase. 1. Imidazole derivatives. *J Med Chem* 1981; **24**: 1139–48.

164. Ford NF, Browne LJ, Campbell T, *et al.* Imidazo(1,5-a)pyridines: a new class of thromboxane A$_2$ synthetase inhibitors. *J Med Chem* 1985; **28**: 164–70.

165. MacNab MW, Foltz EL, Graves BS, *et al.* The effects of a new thromboxane synthetase inhibitor, CGS-13080, in man. *J Clin Pharmacol* 1984; **24**: 76–83.

166. Mohrland JS, Vanderlugt JT, Lakings DB. Multiple dose trial of the thromboxane synthase inhibitor furegrelate in normal subjects. *Eur J Clin Pharmacol* 1990; **38**: 485–8.

167. Johnson RA, Nidy EG, Aiken JW, Crittenden NJ, Gorman RR. Thromboxane A$_2$ synthase inhibitors (5-(3-pyridylmethyl)benzofuran-2-carboxylic acids. *J Med Chem* 1986; **29**: 1461–8.

168. Gorman RR, Johnson RA, Spilman CH, Aiken JW. Inhibition of platelet thromboxane A$_2$ synthase activity by sodium 5-(3'-pyridinylmethyl)benzofuran-2-carboxylate. *Prostaglandins* 1983; **26**: 325–42.

169. *Drugs of the Future* 1985; **10**: 526–7.

170. Furci L, Fitzgerald DJ, Fitzgerald GA. Heterogeneity of prostaglandin H$_2$/thromboxane A$_2$ receptors: distinct subtypes mediate vascular smooth muscle contraction and platelet aggregation. *J Pharmacol Exp Ther* 1991; **258**: 74–81.

171. Tymekewycz PM, Jones RL, Wilson NH, Marr CG. Heterogeneity of thromboxane A$_2$ (TP-)receptors: evidence from antagonist but not agonist potency measurements. *Br J Pharmacol* 1991; **102**: 607–14.

172. Morinelli TA, Halushka PV. Thromboxane-A$_2$/prostaglandin-H$_2$ receptors. *Trends Cardiovasc Med* 1991; **1**: 157–61.

173. Halushka PV, Mais DE, Mayeux PR, Morinelli TA. Thromboxane, prostaglandin and leukotriene receptors. *Annu Rev Pharmacol Toxicol* 1989; **10**: 213–39.

174. Nakane M, Reid JA, Han WC, *et al.* 7-Oxabicyclo[2.2.1]heptylcarboxylic acids as thromboxane A$_2$ antagonists: Aza-ω-chain analogs. *J Med Chem* 1990; **33**: 2465–76.

175. Harris DN, Hall SE, Hedberg A, Ogletree ML. 7-Oxabicycloheptane analogs: modulators of the arachidonate cascade. *Drugs of the Future* 1988; **13**: 153–69.

176. Lefer AM, Darius H. SQ-29548: a highly potent and specific thromboxane A$_2$ receptor antagonist. *Drugs of the Future* 1987; **12**: 367–73.

177. Misra RN, Brown BR, Sher PM, *et al.* Interphenylene 7-oxabicycloheptane TXA$_2$ antagonists. BMS 180,291A: a new clinical candidate. *201st ACS National Meeting Atlanta, Georgia,* 1991; Abst. Medi 160.

178. Misra RN. Preparation of 2-(carbamoylazolyl)-7-oxabicyclo[2.2.1]heptanes as antithrombotics and vasorelaxants. *Published European Patent Application.* EP 391652.

179. Sher PM, Stein PD, Floyd D, Hall SE. Preparation of 7-oxabicycloheptyl-substituted azolecarboxamide prostaglandin analogs useful in the treatment of thrombotic and vasospastic disease. *Published European Patent Application.* EP 374952.

180. Garland RB, Miyano M, Pireh D, Clare M, Finnegan PM, Swenton L. Studies in the synthesis of the thromboxane receptor antagonist EP 092 and its enantiomers. *J Org Chem* 1990; **55**: 5854–61.

181. Booth RFG, Honey AC, Lad N, Tuffin DP, Wade PJ. Inhibitory effect of a selective thromboxane A$_2$ receptor antagonist, EP 092, on platelet aggregation in whole blood *ex vivo* and *in vivo*. *Br J Pharmacol* 1989; **96**: 395–405.

182. Klar U, Rehwinkel H, Vorbrueggen H, Thierauch KH, Verhallen P. Bicyclo[3.3.0]octan-Derivate, Verfahren zu ihrer Herstellung und ihre pharmazeutische Verwendung. *Published German Patent Application*. DE 4010355.

183. Nagai H, Tsuji F, Inagaki N, *et al.* The effect of ONO-3708, a novel TXA$_2$ receptor antagonist, on U-46619-induced contraction of guinea pig and human tracheal strips *in vitro* and on bronchoconstriction in guinea pigs *in vivo*. *Prostaglandins* 1991; **41**: 375–82.

184. *Drugs of the Future* 1987; **12**: 446–9.

185. *Drugs of the Future* 1991; **16**: 1065–6.

186. Lefer AM. Daltroban (BM 13.505) – a highly specific, potent thromboxane receptor antagonist. *Drugs of the Future* 1988; **13**: 999–1005.

187. Ohtani M, Matsuura T, Watanabe F, Narisada M. Enantioselective synthesis of S-1452, an orally potent thromboxane A$_2$ receptor antagonist. *J Org Chem* 1991; **56**: 2122–7.

188. Ezumi K, Yamakawa M, Narisada M. Computer-aided molecular modeling of a thromboxane receptor antagonist S-145 and its related compounds. *J Med Chem* 1990; **33**: 1117–22.

189. Seno K, Hagishita S. Thromboxane A$_2$ receptor antagonists. II. Synthesis and pharmacological activity of 6,6-dimethyl-bicyclo[3.1.1]heptane derivatives with the benzenesulfonylamino group. *Chem Pharm Bull* 1989; **37**: 948–54.

190. Narisada M, Ohtani M, Watanabe F, *et al.* Synthesis and *in vitro* activity of various derivatives of a novel thromboxane receptor antagonist, (±)-(5Z)-7-(3-endo((phenylsulfonyl)amino)bicyclo[2.2.1]hept-2-exo-yl)heptenoic acid. *J Med Chem* 1988; **31**: 1847–54.

191. Wakitani K, Matsumoto R, Imawaka H, *et al.* Anti-thrombotic effect of ONO-8809, a novel TxA$_2$/PG endoperoxide receptor antagonist. *Adv Prostaglandin Thromboxane Leukotriene Res* 1991; **21B**: 599–602.

192. Hamanaka N, Seko T, Miyazaki T, Naka M. The synthesis of potent thromboxane A$_2$/prostaglandin endoperoxide receptor antagonist. *Tetrahedron Lett* 1989; **30**: 2399–402.

193. McKenniff MG, Norman P, Cuthbert NJ, Gardiner PJ. BAY u3405, a potent and selective thromboxane A$_2$ receptor antagonist on airway smooth muscle in vitro. *Br J Pharmacol* 1991; **104**: 585–90.

194. Norel X, Labat C, Gardiner PJ, Brink C. Inhibitory effects of BAY u3405 on prostanoid-induced contractions in human isolated bronchial and pulmonary arterial muscle preparations. *Br J Pharmacol* 1991; **104**: 591–5.

195. Francis HP, Greenham SJ, Patel UP, Thompson AM, Gardiner PJ. BAY u3405 an antagonist of thromboxane A$_2$- and prostaglandin D$_2$-induced bronchoconstriction in the guinea-pig. *Br J Pharmacol* 1991; **104**: 596–602.

196. *Drugs of the Future* 1991; **16**: 701–5.

197. Rosentreter U, Boeshagen H, Seuter F, Perzborn E, Fiedler VB. Synthesis and absolute configuration of the new thromboxane antagonist (3R)-3-(4-fluorophenylsulfonamido)-1,2,3,4-tetrahydro-9-carbazolepropanoic acid and comparison with its enantiomer. *Arzneim-Forsch/Drug Res* 1989; **39** (II): 1519–21.

198. Seuter F, Perzborn E, Rosentreter U, Boeshagen H, Fiedler VB. Inhibition of platelet aggregation *in vitro* and *ex vivo* by the new thromboxane antagonist (3R)-3-(4-fluorophenylsulfonamido)-1,2,3,4-tetrahydro-9-carbazolepropanoic acid. *Arzneim-Forsch/Drug Res* 1989; **39** (II): 1525–7.

199. Klar U, Rehwinkel H, Vorbrueggen H, Thierauch KH, Verhallen P. Cyclopentenderivate, Verfahren zu ihrer Herstellung und ihre pharmazeutische Verwendung. *Published German Patent Application*. DE 4024345.

200. Thomas M, Keery RJ, Charter MK, Scully NL, Chilton JE, Lumley P. The pharmacodynamics and pharmacokinetics of a novel thromboxane receptor blocking drug vapiprost (GR 32191) after single intravenous doses in healthy subjects. *Br J Clin Pharmacol* 1991; **32**: 181 6.

201. Ritter JM, Benjamin N, Doktor HS, *et al.* Effects of a selective thromboxane receptor antagonist (GR32191B) and of glyceryl trinitrate on bleeding time in man. *Br J Clin Pharmacol* 1990; **29**: 431–6.

202. *Drugs of the Future* 1990; **15**: 1087–92.

203. Brown GR, Foubister AJ, Hudson JA. Improved synthetic routes to the novel thromboxane receptor antagonist ICI-192605: activity of synthetic 1,3-dioxane intermediates. *J Pharm Pharmacol* 1990; **42**: 53–5.

204. Lee S. Kilograms of thromboxane antagonists. *Chem Ind* 1987; **7**: 223–7.

205. Armstrong RA, Jones RL, MacDermot J, Wilson NH. Prostaglandin endoperoxide analogs which are both thromboxane receptor antagonists and prostacyclin mimetics. *Br J Pharmacol* 1986; **87**: 543–51.

206. *Scrip* 1991; **1659**: 10.

207. Fiddler GI, Lumley P. Preliminary clinical studies with thromboxane synthase inhibitors and thromboxane receptor blockers. *Circulation* 1990; **81** (suppl I): I-69–78.

208. Stuerzebecher S, Witt W. The PGI$_2$-analogue iloprost and the TXA$_2$-receptor antagonist sulotroban synergistically inhibit TXA$_2$-dependent platelet activation. *Prostaglandins* 1988; **36**: 751–60.

209. Deckmyn H, Gresele P, Van Houtte E, Nenci GG, Vermylen J. Synergism of a thromboxane (Tx) syn-

thase inhibitor (TSI) and a Tx receptor antagonist (TRA) in reducing platelet activation. *Thromb Haemost* 1985; **54**: 114 (Abs 0677).

210. Gresele P, Van Houtte E, Arnout J, Deckmyn H, Vermylen J. Thromboxane synthase inhibition combined with thromboxane receptor blockade: a step forward in antithrombotic strategy? *Thromb Haemost* 1984; **52**: 364.

211. Kanzik I, Zengil H, Ipek N, Çakici I, Abacioglu N, Doertlemez H. Synergism between UK 38 485 and ICI 185 282 against digoxin-induced arrhythmias in guinea-pigs. *Arch Int Pharmacodyn Ther* 1991; **312**: 55–65.

212. Zengil H, Ipek N, Cakici I, Abacioglu N, Kanzik I, Doertlemez H. Synergism between UK 38 485, a thromboxane synthetase inhibitor, and ICI 185 282, a thromboxane receptor antagonist, against digoxin induced arrhythmias. *Eur J Pharmacol* 1990; **183**: 1779 (Abs P.th.132).

213. Gresele P, Deckmyn H, Nenci GG, Vermylen J. Thromboxane synthase inhibitors, thromboxane receptor antagonists and dual blockers in thrombotic disorders. *Trends Pharmacol Sci* 1991; **12**: 158–63.

214. Collen D, Masuda M, Rong Lu H, *et al.* Effect of ridogrel, a combined thromboxane A_2 synthase inhibitor/prostaglandin endoperoxide receptor antagonist, on the lysis of platelet-rich coronary arterial thrombi with recombinant tissue-type plasminogen activator in a canine model. *Fibrinolysis* 1992; **6**: 7–15.

215. De Clerck F, Beetens J, de Chaffoy de Courcelles D, Freyne E, Janssen PAJ. R 68 070: thromboxane A_2 synthetase inhibition and thromboxane A_2/prosta-

glandin endoperoxide receptor blockade combined in one molecule – I. Biochemical profile *in vitro*. *Thromb Haemost* 1989; **61**: 35–42.

216. De Clerck F, Beetens J, Van de Water A, Vercammen E, Janssen PAJ. R 68 070: thromboxane A_2 synthetase inhibition and thromboxane A_2/prostaglandin endoperoxide receptor blockade combined in one molecule – II. Pharmacological effects *in vivo* and *ex vivo*. *Thromb Haemost* 1989; **61**: 43–9.

217. Watts IS, Wharton KA, White BP, Lumley P. Thromboxane (Tx) A_2 receptor blockade and TxA_2 synthase inhibition alone and in combination: comparison of anti-aggregatory efficacy in human platelets. *Br J Pharmacol* 1991; **102**: 497–505.

218. Mueller UE, Niewoehner U, Perzborn E, Bischoff E, Dellweg H-G. Heterocyclisch substituierte Cycloalkano[b]-indolsulfonamide. *Published European Patent Application.* EP 0473024.

219. Bhagwat SS, Gude C, Cohen DS, Lee W, Furness P, Clarke FH. Thromboxane receptor antagonism combined with thromboxane synthase inhibition. 1. (±)-(3-pyridinylbicycloheptyl)alkanoic acids. *J Med Chem* 1991; **34**: 1790–7.

220. Siegfried ME, Bush LR. Dual antagonism by L 636,499 of serotonin and thromboxane A_2 induced aggregation of canine platelets. *Thromb Res* 1990; **60**: 343–53.

221. Ohkawa S, Terao S, Terashita Z-I, Shibouta Y, Nishikawa K. Dual inhibitors of thromboxane A_2 synthase and 5-lipoxygenase with scavenging activity of active oxygen species. Synthesis of a novel series of (3-pyridylmethyl)benzoquinone derivatives. *J Med Chem* 1991; **34**: 267–76.

5 Dietary manipulation of prostaglandin synthesis in man – n-3 polyunsaturated fatty acids and their potential role in the prevention and treatment of cardiovascular disease

Steen Dalby Kristensen and Jørn Dyerberg

Circulating platelets and monocytes and their interaction with the arterial endothelium play key roles in the pathogenesis of cardiovascular disease.[1] Platelets are involved in atherogenesis in that they adhere to the arterial wall where the endothelial cells are damaged or perturbed and release platelet derived growth factor(s) that cause migration and proliferation of the vascular smooth muscle cells.[1] In experimental studies, where animals have been fed high doses of cholesterol, monocytes have been shown to adhere to the vessel wall and to migrate into the subendothelium, where the cells take up lipid-laden material and are converted into foam cells.[1-5] Foam cells are the hallmark of the fatty streak.

The platelet–vessel wall interaction is of particular importance for the formation of the coronary arterial thrombus that causes the acute coronary syndromes of unstable angina pectoris, acute myocardial infarction and sudden cardiac death (for review, see references 6, 7). Evidence from autopsy studies indicate that the primary event in these syndromes is rupture or fissuring of a coronary atherosclerotic plaque.[8-10] However, there is also evidence that the reactivity of the circulating platelets is increased.[7] Breaking of the endothelial barrier leads to adhesion of platelets and the release of proaggregatory and vasoactive substances, such as thromboxane A_2 (TXA_2), ADP and serotonin from the activated platelets. This causes aggregation of the platelets and formation of a platelet thrombus. Finally, activation of the coagulation cascade causes the formation of the coronary platelet-fibrin thrombus.

The diene prostaglandins derived from the n-6 polyunsaturated fatty acid (PUFA) arachidonic acid (20:4), TXA_2 and prostacyclin (PGI_2), are key regulators of the platelet–vessel wall interaction. TXA_2 is mainly formed by platelets and has platelet proaggregatory and vasoconstrictory properties.[11] On the other hand, prostacyclin, mainly formed by the endothelial cells, causes vasodilatation and inhibits platelet aggregation.[12] Aspirin inhibits the cyclooxygenase enzyme[13] and abolishes the formation of both TXA_2 and prostacyclin. The clinical importance of TXA_2 has been emphasized by controlled trials showing that aspirin is beneficial in unstable angina pectoris[14-16] and in acute myocardial infarction.[17,18] Another eicosanoid derived from arachidonic acid, leukotriene (LT) B_4 is a strong chemoattractant for monocytes.[19]

In the present review the evidence that benificial modulation of eicosanoid formation can be obtained after dietary supplementation with n-3 PUFAs present in fatty fish and fish oil is discussed. We will also focus on the experimental studies investigating the effect of n-3 PUFAs on atherogenesis and on trials where n-3 PUFAs have been evaluated in patients with ischaemic heart disease.

Pro- and anti-aggregatory prostaglandins in Greenland Eskimos

The low incidence of acute myocardial infarction[20,21] and clinical observations of frequent episodes of nose bleeding and haemoptysis[22] in native Greenland Eskimos initiated studies of their dietary habits and platelet function. The Eskimo diet is mainly based on marine products like whale, seal and fish, and it was found that Eskimo food contained a very high amount of n-3 PUFAs (eicosapentaenoic acid (20:5), docosapentaenoic acid (22:5) and docosahexaenoic acid (22:6)) and a low amount of n-6 PUFAs, particularly linoleic acid (18:2), compared to a typical Danish diet.[23,24] In Eskimo plasma the content of eicosapentaenoic acid (20:5) was found to be high and the content of arachidonic acid (20:4) was low compared to values obtained in age- and sex-matched Danes.[25] Also the composition of the platelet phospholipids of the Eskimos showed a large increase in the content of n-3 fatty acids compared to Danes.[26] These changes in platelet fatty acid composition were paralleled by changes in platelet function. The Eskimos had a lower platelet count, a longer bleeding time and an impaired platelet aggregation in response to ADP compared to an age- and sex-matched Danish control group.[26] The difference in bleeding time could be abolished by aspirin.[26,27] In Danes aspirin caused a prolongation of the bleeding time, whereas the bleeding time was shortened in Eskimos taking aspirin.[26,27]

The hypothesis was generated that the platelet–vessel wall interaction was favourably shifted towards an antithrombotic state in the Eskimos due

to the formation of triene prostaglandins from eicosapentaenoic acid.[28] *In vitro* studies indicated that the TXA_3 produced from exogenous eicosapentaenoic acid was inactive or less proaggregatory than TXA_2.[29] In platelets eicosapentaenoic acid was found to be a competitive inhibitor of TXA_2 synthesis.[30] In human vasculature exogenous eicosapentaenoic acid was shown to be metabolized to PGI_3,[31,32] which has similar antiaggregatory properties as PGI_2.[33] Although some experimental studies performed on endothelial cell culture suggest that eicosapentaenoic acid may inhibit the conversion of arachidonic acid to prostacyclin, this is not true for perfused human vasculature,[32,34] On the contrary, in a model where intact human umbilical veins were continuously perfused with physiological concentrations of fatty acids, eicosapentaenoic acid was found to enhance the amount of PGI-like material produced from arachidonic acid.[32]

In studies on healthy humans fed a fish diet Fischer and Weber have measured urinary prostaglandin metabolites by gas chromatography–mass spectometry. Their results clearly indicate that TXA_3[35] and PGI_3[36] are formed in man. In a recent elegant study De Caterina *et al.* supplemented patients undergoing coronary bypass surgery with n-3 PUFAs.[37] They showed that prostacyclin production from saphenous vein, aortic or atrial tissue was increased in patients receiving n-3 PUFAs compared to matched control patients. Finally, the hypothesis, that the balance between pro- and antiaggregatory prostaglandins is favourably shifted in Greenland Eskimos, was confirmed in a study where urinary metabolites were measured.[38] Considerable formation of bioactive PGI_3 was shown in the Eskimos, whereas metabolites of this compound were barely detectable in Danish controls. The level of PGI_2 metabolites were also significantly higher in Eskimos than in Danes, whereas the excretion of $TXA_{2,3}$ metabolites were lower in the Eskimos.

Other epidemiological studies on fish consumption and cardiovascular disease

The observation of a low mortality from ischaemic heart disease in Greenland Eskimos mentioned above has inspired others to study the relation between fish consumption and incidence of cardiovascular discasc in diffcrcnt populations.

Studies from Japan have shown that in people

living on an island where the dietary intake of fish was high, the incidence of ischaemic heart disease was lower than in a Japanese population where the dietary fish intake was low (reviewed by Hirai *et al.*[39]). Furthermore, the Japanese that lived on the fishing island had higher serum levels of eicosapentaenoic acid and an impaired platelet aggregability compared to the control group.[39]

In Holland, Kromhout and co-workers[40] studied the dietary intake of fish and the mortality of ischaemic heart disease during 20 years in a cohort of 892 middle-aged men. They reported an inverse correlation between fish consumption and mortality from ischaemic heart disease, even though the intake of fish in this population was low. On the other hand, Simonson and Nordøy[41] reported that Norwegians living in a coastal area with a high intake of fish had a higher incidence of ischaemic heart disease than a control goup of Norwegians with a lower intake of fish. However, interpretation is hampered by the finding that the content of n-3 PUFA in the platelet membranes did not differ between the two groups.

Finally, in the large American MRFIT study dietary fish intake in the Usual Care Group consisting of more than 6000 men aged 35–57 years has been recorded and the group has now been followed for more than 10 years. The daily intake of n-3 PUFAs has recently been reported to be inversely related to total mortality and mortality from ischaemic heart disease.[42] Overall the epidemiological evidence available supports the hypothesis that dietary fish intake offers protection against ischaemic heart disease.

Dietary fish or fish oil supplementation and the platelet–vessel wall interaction

Several investigations have been undertaken in order to elucidate whether dietary supplementation with fatty fish or fish oil with a high content of n-3 PUFAs can beneficially alter the platelet–vessel wall interaction in healthy persons or in patients with vascular disease or cardiovascular risk factors. The amount of n-3 PUFAs provided, the duration of the supplementation and other factors vary considerably from study to study. However, in the following sections we have tried briefly to review the effect of n-3 PUFA supplementations on human platelet function and primary haemostasis.

Platelet count

A 10–20% decrease in platelet count after supplementation with n-3 PUFAs has been reported.[43–47] In a long-term study the decrease in platelet count seemed to be temporary in that normalization of the platelet count occurred during continued supplementation.[48] In most of the studies no significant change in platelet count during n-3 PUFA supplementation could be demonstrated.[37,49–56]

Bleeding time

The cutaneous bleeding time provides an overall estimate of the platelet–vessel wall interaction. The bleeding time has been shown to be shortened in the acute phase of a myocardial infarction.[57,58] In several studies on healthy volunteers[43–45,50,51,59–61] and in patients with coronary atherosclerosis,[37,48] peripheral atherosclerosis[62] or hyperlipidaemia[63] supplementation with n-3 PUFAs has been shown to prolong the bleeding time. This prolongation of the bleeding time has recently been shown to be dose-dependent, however, even at the high dose (9 g n-3 PUFAs per day) only reaching a modest degree of prolongation.[64] In open studies on patients with hyperlipidaemia[65,66] or diabetes mellitus[56] and in a single study on 60 healthy volunteers[55] no change in the bleeding time could be demonstrated.

Measurement of the bleeding time is obviously somewhat subjective. This calls for controlled studies in order to obtain blinding of the investigator performing the bleeding time measurement. Such studies have been conducted using encapsulated fish oil and identical capsules containing vegetable oil as placebo. In a cross-over study in healthy males a small (15%), but statistically significant increase in the bleeding time after supplementation with n-3 PUFAs was reported.[52] In other double-blind studies no effect of n-3 PUFA supplementation on the bleeding time could be demonstrated in healthy volunteers,[67] in patients with angina pectoris[54] or in patients with hyperlipidaemia.[68,69]

Platelet volume

The mean platelet volume is increased in acute myocardial infarction.[70–73] *In vitro* studies indicate that large platelets are more reactive haemostatically than small ones[74] and that large platelets produce more thromboxane B_2 (TXB_2) in response to stimulation with collagen or thrombin.[75] Mean platelet volume has been shown to be inversely correlated to the bleeding time in patients with ischaemic heart disease[76] and the platelet volume seems to be an independent risk factor for an acute myocardial infarction.[77] Accordingly, a decrease in mean platelet volume may be favourable. However, n-3 PUFA supplementation does not seem to cause alterations in mean platelet volume neither in healthy volunteers[52] nor in patients with hypertension[53] or ischaemic heart disease.[54,77]

Platelet aggregation

Induction of platelet aggregation by various agonists has been investigated in numerous studies. In most of these studies ADP- or collagen-induced platelet aggregation has been found to be inhibited after intake of n-3 PUFAs.[37,43,45-47,49,51,65,67,78-88] Only a few studies have found inhibition of thrombin-[60] and adrenaline-induced[37,54,83] aggregation. Platelet aggregation in response to arachidonic acid has been reported to be unaffected[35,37,49,62,67,89] or inhibited[61,82] after n-3 PUFA supplementation.

Serum thromboxane B$_2$ (TXB$_2$)

The stable TXA$_2$ metabolite, TXB$_2$, measured by radioimmunoassay, has been found to be decreased in serum[37,45,47,62,69,90,91] or in plasma after stimulation of platelets[45,49,67,79,81,83,85,86,92,93] in subjects supplemented with n-3 PUFAs.

Platelet release products

Platelet factor 4 and β-thromboglobulin are stable platelet proteins that are present in the platelet α-granules. These proteins are released from activated platelets and elevated plasma levels of these proteins have been claimed to reflect an increased *in vivo* platelet reactivity. A decrease in platelet factor 4[44] and β-thromboglobulin[44,62] has been reported in patients with atherosclerosis after supplementation with n-3 PUFAs. In other studies no such changes have been demonstrated.[54,55,68,69,87]

Prostacyclin/thromboxane urinary metabolites

The measurement of urinary metabolites of prostacyclin and TXA$_2$ by gas chromatography–mass spectrometry avoids the artefacts caused by artificial activation of platelets during blood sampling and is now widely accepted as the best method for assessing *in vivo* production of these prostaglandins.[94] Urinary TXA$_2$ metabolites have been shown to be elevated in patients with unstable angina pectoris and acute myocardial infarction.[95,96] Further improvement of the technique has made it possible to quantify metabolites of both PGI$_2$ and PGI$_3$. Healthy humans on a mackerel diet have an increased output of both PGI$_2$ and PGI$_3$ metabolites in the urine.[36] Healthy humans supplemented with fish oil had a decreased output of TXA$_{2,3}$ metabolites, unaltered PGI$_2$ metabolites and increased excretion of PGI$_3$ metabolites.[46] Knapp *et al.*[62] reported that a fish oil supplementation (10 g n-3 PUFAs daily) decreased the amount of urinary TXA$_{2,3}$ metabolites in both healthy controls and patients with peripheral atherosclerosis. They also found that urinary PGI$_3$ metabolites increased in both groups while PGI$_2$ metabolites were unchanged in the controls, but decreased from elevated to almost normal levels in the patients with atherosclerosis.

Other tests on platelet function

Platelet adhesion has been reported to decrease after supplementation with fish oil in healthy controls[43,83] and in patients with ischaemic heart disease.[37] In another group of patients with ischaemic heart disease supplementation with n-3 PUFAs prolonged platelet survival.[44] In a similar group of patients we found that intraplatelet cyclic AMP was elevated after 12 weeks' supplementation with fish oil, reflecting an inhibition of platelet reactivity that may be caused by an increased production of PGI$_2$ and/or PGI$_3$.[54]

Comments

In summary, the studies reviewed above indicate that the favourable shift in the prostacyclin/thromboxane balance found in Greenland Eskimos also can be induced in healthy volunteers or patients with vascular disease after dietary supplementation with fish and fish oil concentrates. It is also possible to obtain an inhibition of platelet function after intake of n-3 PUFAs, probably in a dose-dependent fashion.[48,62,64,91] However, intake of very low doses of n-3 PUFAs has also been reported to inhibit platelet aggregation.[93,97] Docosahexaenoic acid (22:6, n-3) has been shown to be a competitive inhibitor of prostaglandin biosynthesis[98] and to reduce platelet reactivity independent of its conversion to eicosapentaenoic acid.[99] Docosahexaenoic acid may thus significantly contribute to the potential antithrombotic properties of n-3 PUFAs. The stimulation of prostacyclin synthesis induced by n-3 supplementation as opposed to the inhibition caused by aspirin may be advantageous in terms of prevention of atherosclerosis and thrombosis.

The study by Knapp *et al.*[62] indicates that even with a very high daily intake of fish oil, it is not possible to cause an inhibition of thromboxane synthesis of the same order of magnitude as can be obtained after intake of low dose aspirin. In healthy volunteers on a fish diet, low dose aspirin was found to potentiate the inhibition of ADP-induced platelet aggregation.[100] Also dietary fish[51] or fish oil supplementation[101] have been reported to act synergistically with aspirin in prolonging the bleeding time. Therefore n-3 PUFA may have other important effects on the platelet–vessel wall interaction than the mentioned effects on thromboxane and prostacyclin.

Combination of n-3 PUFA supplementation and low dose aspirin may be promising and needs further evaluation.

Dietary fish and fish oil supplementation – effect on monocyte function

As stated previously, recent experimental studies indicate that circulating monocytes infiltrating the arterial wall may play a key role in early atherogenesis.[1–5]

An important mediator of monocyte chemotaxis is leukotriene B_4 (LTB_4) derived from arachidonic acid. Eicosapentaenoic acid (20:5, n-3) in leucocytes have been shown to be metabolized to leukotriene B_5 (LTB_5) which is a less active chemoattractant than LTB_4[102] (for review see reference 103). Also, supplementation of n-3 PUFA to healthy volunteers inhibits the synthesis of interleukin-1 and tumour necrosis factor in monocytes.[104] Interestingly, monocyte chemotaxis has recently been shown to be inhibited in healthy volunteers after fish oil supplementation.[105]

Although further studies on the role of white cells in human atherosclerosis are needed, the above-mentioned anti-inflammatory effects of n-3 PUFA may well turn out to be very important in the prevention of atherosclerosis.

Other effects of n-3 PUFA

The effect of n-3 PUFA supplementation on plasma lipids has been evaluated in numerous studies (for review, see reference 106). It has consistently been reported that plasma triglycerides decrease after intake of n-3 PUFA both in healthy volunteers and in patients with cardiovascular disease. This is due to a lowering of VLDL and IDL particles in the blood. The effect of n-3 PUFA on plasma levels of other lipids and lipoproteins is less clear.[106]

Although some reports have indicated that n-3 PUFA supplementation may increase plasma levels of the natural inhibitor of the coagulation system, antithrombin III,[52] and decrease plasma levels of the cardiovascular risk factor, fibrinogen,[64,107] others have found no consistent effect of n-3 PUFA on the coagulation system (reviewed by Hornstra[108]). Also the reports on the effect of n-3 PUFA on fibrinolysis have been conflicting. Most studies have now shown that plasma levels of plasminogen activator inhibitor may increase after supplementation with n-3 PUFA (reviewed by Schmidt[109]).

Recently, experiments in swine have indicated that dietary fish oil may enhance the synthesis of endothelial-dependent relaxing factor.[110–112] This factor has been shown to be nitric oxide[113] which also is a strong inhibitor of the platelet–vessel wall interaction.[114]

n-3 PUFA and experimental atherosclerosis and coronary thrombosis

In experimental studies, fish oil supplementation has been shown to prevent atherosclerosis in pigs and monkeys on a high cholesterol diet,[115,116] whereas fish oil supplementation in the hypercholesterolaemic rabbit has been reported either to enhance[117] or to be without effect on fatty streak formation.[118] n-3 PUFA supplementation has been shown to decrease the amount of intimal hyperplasia formed in venous bypass grafts implanted in dogs.[119–121] When endothelial damage and coronary artery thrombus formation is induced in animals by electrical stimulation intraluminally, the size of the developing infarct can be reduced if the animals have been pretreated with fish oil.[122]

n-3 PUFA supplementation in patients with cardiovascular disease

In an open study Saynor *et al.* reported that patients with chronic stable angina pectoris treated with fish oil supplementation experienced a decrease in their number of anginal attacks.[48] In a controlled study on 36 patients with stable angina using vegetable oil as placebo we were unable to confirm this finding.[54] Other investigators have reported that n-3 PUFA supplementation does not reduce the amount of exercise-induced myocardial ischaemia in patients with chronic stable angina pectoris.[123,124]

Recently, large controlled studies on the effect of dietary supplementation with n-3 PUFA on the frequency of restenosis after percutaneous transluminal coronary angioplasty have been initiated. In these studies n-3 PUFA or placebo was given in combination with low dose aspirins and other drugs such as nitrates and calcium blockers. In one of the studies n-3 PUFA supplementation reduced the incidence of restenosis,[125] whereas other groups have been unable to confirm this.[126,127]

Two controlled studies have revealed that n-3 PUFA supplementation reduces blood pressure in patients with mild hypertension.[128,129]

Finally, a large trial on the effect of dietary fish in the secondary prevention of acute myocardial infarction was conducted by Burr and co-workers.[130] This brilliant study convincingly shows that a moderate dietary intake of fish or fish oil after first myocardial infarction reduces mortality and morbidity from ischaemic heart disease.

Conclusion

Dietary supplementation with n-3 PUFA alters beneficially the balance between thromboxane and prostacyclin. n-3 PUFA may also inhibit the platelet–vessel wall interaction through other mechanisms. n-3 PUFAs have important anti-inflammatory effects, at least in part due to changes in leukotriene metabolism, and this may be of potential interest in the prevention of atherogenesis. Other potential beneficial effects of n-3 PUFA include alterations in lipids, reduction of blood pressure and stimulation of synthesis of endothelial-derived relaxing factor. Dietary fish intake has recently been shown to decrease mortality in men after a first myocardial infarct.

Regular dietary fish intake can be recommended for the public in general and for patients with cardiovascular disease in particular.

References

1. Ross R. The pathogenesis of atherosclerosis – an update. *N Engl J Med* 1986; **314**: 488–550.
2. Faggiotto A, Ross R, Harker L. Studies on hypercholesterolaemia in the non-human primate. I. Changes that lead to fatty streak formation. *Arteriosclerosis* 1984; **4**: 323–40.
3. Faggiotto A, Ross R. Studies on hypercholesterolaemia in the non-human primate. II. Fatty streak conversion to fibrous plaque. *Arteriosclerosis* 1984; **4**: 341–56.
4. Rosenfeld ME, Tsukada T, Gown AM, Ross R. Fatty streak initiation in Watanabe heritable hyperlipemic and comparably hypercholesterolemic fat-fed rabbits. *Arteriosclerosis* 1987; **7**: 9–23.
5. Tsukada T, Rosenfeld ME, Ross R, Gown AM. Immunocytochemical analysis of cellular components in atherosclerotic lesions. *Arteriosclerosis* 1986; **6**: 601–13.
6. Fuster V, Badimon L, Badimon J, Adams PC, Turitto V, Chesebro JH. Drugs interfering with platelet functions: mechanisms and clinical relevance. In: Verstraete M, Vermylen J, Lijnen R, Arnout J (eds), *Thrombosis and Haemostasis*. Leuven: University Press, 1987: 349–418.
7. Kristensen SD, Martin JF. Platelet heterogeneity and coronary artery thrombosis. *Platelets* 1991; **2**: 11–17.
8. Falk E. Plaque rupture with pre-existing stenosis precipitating coronary thrombosis. Characteristics of coronary atherosclerotic plaques underlying fatal occlusive thrombi. *Br Heart J* 1983; **50**: 127–34.
9. Falk E. Unstable angina with fatal outcome, dynamic coronary thrombosis leading to infarction and/or sudden cardiac death. Autopsy evidence of recurrent mural thrombosis with peripheral embolization culminating in total vascular occlusion. *Circulation* 1985; **71**: 699–708.
10. Davies MJ, Thomas AC, Knapman PA, Hangartner JR. Intramyocardial platelet aggregation in patients with unstable angina pectoris suffering sudden cardiac death. *Circulation* 1986; **73**: 418–27.
11. Hamberg M, Svensson J, Samuelsson B. Thromboxanes: a new group of biologically active compounds derived from prostaglandin endoperoxide. *Proc Natl Acad Sci USA* 1975; **72**: 2994–8.
12. Moncada S, Gryglewski RJ, Bunting S, Vane JR. An enzyme from arteries transforms prostaglandin endoperoxides to an unstable substance that inhibits platelet aggregation. *Nature* 1976; **263**: 663–5.
13. Roth GJ, Majerus PW. The mechanism of the effect

of aspirin on human platelets. I. Acetylation of a particulate fraction protein. *J Clin Invest* 1975; **56**: 624–32.

14. Lewis HD, Davis JW, Archibald DG, *et al.* Protective effects of aspirin against acute myocardial infarction and death in men with unstable angina. Results of a Veterans Administration Cooperative Study. *N Engl J Med* 1983; **309**: 396–403.

15. Cairns JA, Gent M, Singer J, *et al.* Aspirin, sulfinpyrazone or both in unstable angina. *N Engl J Med* 1985; **313**: 1369–75.

16. Theroux P, Quimet H, MaCans J, *et al.* Aspirin, heparin or both to treat acute unstable angina. *N Engl J Med* 1988; **319**: 1105–11.

17. ISIS-2 collaborative groups. Randomised trial of intravenous streptokinase, oral aspirin, both or neither among 17187 cases of suspected myocardial infarction: ISIS-2. *Lancet* 1988; **2**: 349–60.

18. Husted SE, Nielsen HK, Krusell LR, Færgeman O. Acetylsalicylic acid 100 mg and 1000 mg daily in acute myocardial infarction suspects: a placebo controlled trial. *J Intern Med* 1989; **226**: 303–10.

19. Lee TH, Austen KF. Arachidonic acid metabolism by the 5-lipoxygenase pathway, and the effects of alternative dietary fatty acids. *Adv Immunol* 1986; **39**: 145–75.

20. Kromann N, Green A. Epidemiological studies in the Upernavik, Greenland. *Acta Med Scand* 1980; **208**: 401–6.

21. Bjerregaard P, Dyerberg J. Mortality from ischaemic heart disease and cerebrovascular disease in Greenland. *Int J Epidemiol* 1988; **17**: 514–19.

22. Bang HO, Dyerberg J. The bleeding tendency in Greenland Eskimos. *Dan Med Bull* 1980; **27**: 202–5.

23. Bang HO, Dyerberg J, Hjørne N. The composition of food consumed by Greenland Eskimos. *Acta Med Scand* 1976; **200**: 69–73.

24. Bang HO, Dyerberg J, Sinclair HM. The composition of the Eskimo food in north-west Greenland. *Am J Clin Nutr* 1980; **33**: 2657–61.

25. Dyerberg J, Bang HO, Hjørne N. Fatty acid composition of the plasma in Greenland Eskimos. *Am J Clin Nutr* 1975; **28**: 958–66.

26. Dyerberg J, Bang HO. Haemostatic function and platelet polyunsaturated fatty acids in Eskimos. *Lancet* 1979; **2**: 433–5.

27. Jørgensen KA, Nielsen AH, Dyerberg J. Hemostatic factors and renin in Greenland Eskimos on a high eicosapentaenoic acid intake. *Acta Med Scand* 1986; **219**: 473–9.

28. Dyerberg J, Bang HO, Stoffersen E, Moncada S, Vane JR. Eicosapentaenoic acid and prevention of thrombosis and atherosclerosis? *Lancet* 1978; **2**: 117–19.

29. Gryglewski RJ, Salmon JA, Utatuba FB, Weatherly BC, Moncada S, Vane JR. Effects of all-cis 5,8,11,14,17-eicosapentaenoic acid and PGH$_3$ on

platelet aggregation. *Prostaglandins* 1979; **18**: 453–78.

30. Culp BR, Titus BG, Lands WEM. Inhibition of prostaglandin biosynthesis by eicosapentaenoic acid. *Prostaglandins Med* 1979; **3**: 269–78.

31. Dyerberg J, Jørgensen KA, Arnfred T. Human umbilical blood vessel converts all cis-5,8,11,14,17-eicosapentaenoic acid to prostaglandin I$_3$. *Prostaglandins* 1981; **22**: 857–62.

32. Kristensen SD, Arnfred T, Dyerberg J. Eicosapentaenoic acid potentiates the production of prostacyclin-like material in the arachidonic acid perfused human umbilical vein. *Thromb Res* 1984; **36**: 305–14.

33. Needleman P, Raz A, Minkes MK, Ferrendelli JA, Sprecher H. Triene prostaglandins: prostacyclin and thromboxane biosynthesis and unique biological properties. *Proc Natl Acad Sci USA* 1979; **76**: 944–8.

34. Dyerberg J, Jørgensen KA. The effect of arachidonic and eicosapentaenoic acid on the synthesis of prostacyclin-like material in human umbilical vasculature. *Artery* 1980; **8**: 12–17.

35. Fischer S, Weber PC. Thromboxane A$_3$ (TxA$_3$) is formed in human platelets after dietary eicosapentaenoic acid. *Biochem Biophys Res Commun* 1983; **116**: 1091–9.

36. Fischer S, Weber PC. Prostaglandin I$_3$ is formed *in vivo* in man after dietary eicosapentaenoic acid. *Nature* 1984; **307**: 165–8.

37. De Caterina R, Gianness D, Mazzone A, *et al.* Vascular prostacyclin is increased in patients ingesting ω-3 polyunsaturated fatty acids before coronary artery bypass graft surgery. *Circulation* 1990; **82**: 428–38.

38. Fischer S, Weber PC, Dyerberg J. The prostacyclin/thromboxane balance is favourably shifted in Greenland Eskimos. *Prostaglandins* 1986; **32**: 235–41.

39. Hirai A, Terano T, Tamura Y, Yoshida S. Eicosapentaenoic acid and adult diseases in Japan: epidemiological and clinical aspects. *J Intern Med* 1989; **225** (suppl 1): 69–75.

40. Kromhout D, Bosschieter EB, De Lezenne Coulander C. The inverse relation between fish consumption and 20-year mortality from coronary heart disease. *N Engl J Med* 1985; **312**: 1205–9.

41. Simonsen T, Nordøy A. Ischemic heart disease, serum lipids and platelet in Norwegian populations with traditionally low or high fish consumption. *J Intern Med* 1989; **225** (suppl 1): 83–9.

42. Dolecek TA, Grandits G. Dietary polyunsaturated fatty acids and mortality in the Multiple Risk Factor Intervention Trial (MRFIT). In: Simopoulos AP, Kifer RR, Martin RE, Barlow SM (eds), *Health Effects of n-3 Polyunsaturated Fatty Acids in Seafood.* World Rev. Nutr. Diet. Basel: Karger; 1991; **66**: 205–16.

43. Goodnight SH, Harris WS, Connor VE. The effects of dietary ω-3 fatty acids on platelet composition and

function in man: a prospective, controlled study. *Blood* 1981; **58**: 880–5.

44. Hay CRM, Durber AP, Saynor R. Effect of fish oil on platelet kinetics in patients with ischaemic heart disease. *Lancet* 1982; **2**: 1269–72.

45. Lorenz R, Spengler U, Fischer S, Duhm J, Weber PC. Platelet function, thromboxane formation and blood pressure control during supplementation of the western diet with cod liver oil. *Circulation* 1983; **67**: 504–11.

46. von Schacky C, Fischer S, Weber PC. Long-term effects of dietary marine ω-3 fatty acids upon plasma and cellular lipids, platelet function and eicosanoid formation in humans. *J Clin Invest* 1985; **76**: 1626–31.

47. Houwelingen ACV, Hennissen AAHM, Verbeek-Schippers F, Simonsen T, Kestle ADM, Hornstra G. Effect of moderate fish intake on platelet aggregation in human platelet-rich plasma. *Thromb Haemost* 1988; **59**: 505–13.

48. Saynor R, Verel D, Gillott T. The long-term effect of dietary supplementation with fish lipid concentrate on serum lipids, bleeding time, platelets and angina. *Atherosclerosis* 1984; **50**: 3–10.

49. Siess W, Roth P, Scherer B, Kurzmann I, Boehlig B, Weber PC. Platelet-membrane fatty acids, platelet aggregation and thromboxane formation during a mackerel diet. *Lancet* 1980; **2**: 441–4.

50. Sanders TAB, Vickers M, Haines AP. Effects on blood lipids and haemostasis of a supplement of cod-liver oil, rich in eicosapentaenoic and docosahexaenoic acids, in healthy young men. *Clin Sci* 1981; **61**: 317–24.

51. Thorngren M, Gustafson A. Effects of 11-week increase in dietary eicosapentaenoic acid on bleeding time, lipids and platelet aggregation. *Lancet* 1981; **2**: 1190–3.

52. Mortensen JZ, Schmidt EB, Nielsen AH, Dyerberg J. The effect of n-6 n-3 polyunsaturated fatty acids on hemostasis, blood lipids and blood pressure. *Thromb Haemost* 1983; **50**: 543–6.

53. Norris PG, Jones CJH, Weston MJ. Effects of dietary supplementation with fish oil on systolic blood pressure in mild essential hypertension. *BMJ* 1986; **293**: 104–5.

54. Kristensen SD, Schmidt EB, Andersen HR, Dyerberg J. Fish oil in angina pectoris. *Atherosclerosis* 1987; **64**: 13–19.

55. Rogers S, James KS, Butland BK, Etherington MD, O'Brien JR, Jones JG. Effects of fish oil supplement on serum lipids, blood pressure, bleeding time, haemostatic and rheological variables. *Atherosclerosis* 1987; **63**: 137–43.

56. Schmidt EB, Sørensen PJ, Pedersen JO, *et al.* The effect of n-3 polyunsaturated fatty acids on lipids, haemostasis, neutrophil and monocyte chemotaxis in insulin-dependent diabetes mellitus. *J Intern Med* 1989; **225** (suppl 1): 201–6.

57. Milner PC, Martin JF. Shortened bleeding time in myocardial infarction and its relation to platelet mass. *BMJ* 1985; **290**: 1767–70.

58. Kristensen SD, Bath PMW, Martin JF. Differences in bleeding time, aspirin sensitivity and adrenaline between acute myocardial infarction and unstable angina. *Cardiovasc Res* 1990; **24**: 19–23.

59. von Lossonczy R, Ruiter A, Bronsgeest-Schoute HC, van Gent CM, Hermus RJJ. The effect of a fish diet on serum lipids in healthy human subjects. *Am J Clin Nutr* 1978; **31**: 1340–6.

60. Ahmed AA, Holub BJ. Alterations and recovery of bleeding time, platelet aggregation and fatty acid composition of individual phospholipids in platelets of human subjects receiving a supplement of cod-liver oil. *Lipids* 1984; **19**: 617–24.

61. Atkinson PM, Wheeler MC, Mendelsohn D, Pienaar N, Chetty N. Effects of a 4-week freshwater fish (trout) diet on platelet aggregation, platelet fatty acids, serum lipids and coagulation factors. *Am J Hematol* 1987; **24**: 143–9.

62. Knapp HR, Reilly AGI, Alessandrini P, FitzGerald GA. *In vivo* indexes of platelet and vascular function during fish oil administration in patients with atherosclerosis. *N Engl J Med* 1986; **314**: 937–42.

63. Schmidt EB, Ernst E, Varming K, Pedersen JO, Dyerberg J. The effect of n-3 fatty acids on lipids and haemostasis in patients with type IIa and type IV hyperlipidaemia. *Thromb Haemost* 1989; **62**: 797–801.

64. Schmidt EB, Varming K, Ernst E, Madsen P, Dyerberg J. Dose-response studies on the effect of n-3 polyunsaturated fatty acids on lipids and haemostasis. *Thromb Haemost* 1990; **63**: 1–5.

65. Brox JH, Killie JE, Østerud B, Holme S, Nordøy A. Effects of cod-liver oil on platelets and coagulation in familiar hypercholesterolemia (type IIa). *Acta Med Scand* 1983; **213**: 137–44.

66. Simons LA, Hickie JB, Balasubramaniam S. On the effect of dietary n-3 fatty acids (Maxepa) on plasma lipids and lipoproteins in patients with hyperlipidaemia. *Atherosclerosis* 1985; **54**: 75–88.

67. Brox JH, Killie JE, Gunnes S, Nordøy A. The effect of cod liver oil and corn oil on platelets and vessel wall in man. *Thromb Haemost* 1981; **46**: 604–11.

68. Boberg M, Vessby B, Selinus I. Effects of dietary supplementation with n-6 and n-3 long-chain polyunsaturated fatty acids in serum lipoproteins and platelet function in hypertriglyceridaemic patients. *Acta Med Scand* 1986; **220**: 153–60.

69. Demke DM, Peters GR, Linet OI, Metzler CM, Klott KA. Effects of a fish oil concentrate in patients with hypercholesterolaemia. *Atherosclerosis* 1988; **70**: 73–80.

70. Martin JF, Plumb J, Kilbey RS, Kishk YT. Changes in volume and density of platelets in myocardial infarction. *BMJ* 1983; **287**: 456–9.

71. Cameron HA, Philips R, Ibbotson RM, Carson PHM.

Platelet size in myocardial infarction. *BMJ* 1983; **287:** 449–51.

72. Kishk YT, Trowbridge EA, Martin JF. Platelet volume subpopulations in acute myocardial infarction: an investigation of their homogeneity for smoking, infarct size and site. *Clin Sci* 1985; **68:** 419–25.

73. Trowbridge EA, Martin JF. The platelet volume distribution: a signature of the prethrombotic state in coronary heart disease? *Thromb Haemost* 1987; **58:** 714–17.

74. Thompson C, Eaton KA, Princiotta SM, Kushkin CA, Valeri CR. Size dependent platelet subpopulations: relationship of platelet volume to ultrastructure, enzymatic activity and function. *Br J Haematol* 1982; **50:** 509–19.

75. Jakubowski JA, Thompson CB, Vaillancourt R, Valeri CR, Deykin D. Arachidonic acid metabolism by platelets of differing size. *Br J Haematol* 1983; **53:** 503–11.

76. Kristensen SD, Milner PC, Martin JF. Bleeding time and platelet volume in acute myocardial infarction – a 2 year follow up study. *Thromb Haemost* 1986; **59:** 353–6.

77. Martin JF, Bath PMW, Burr ML. Influence of platelet size on outcome after myocardial infarction. *Lancet* 1991; **338:** 1409–11.

78. Hirai A, Hamazaki T, Terano T, *et al.* Eicosapentaenoic acid and platelet function in Japanese. *Lancet* 1980; **2:** 1132–3.

79. Hirai A, Terano T, Hamazaki T, *et al.* The effect of oral administration of fish oil concentrate on the release and the metabolism of (^{14}C)arachidonic acid and (^{14}C)eicosapentaenoic acid by human platelets. *Thromb Res* 1982; **28:** 285–98.

80. Sanders TAB, Roshanai F. The influence of different types of ω-3 polyunsaturated fatty acids in blood lipids and platelet function in healthy volunteers. *Clin Sci* 1983; **64:** 91–9.

81. Sanders TAB, Hochland MC. A comparison of the influence on plasma lipids and platelet function of supplements of ω-3 and ω-6 polyunsaturated fatty acids. *Br J Nutr* 1983; **50:** 521–9.

82. Miller ME, Anagnostou AA, Ley B, Marchall P, Steiner M. Effect of fish oil concentrates on hemorrheological and hemostatic aspects of diabetes mellitus: a preliminary study. *Thromb Res* 1987; **47:** 201–14.

83. Terano T, Hirai A, Hamazaki T, *et al.* Effect of oral administration of highly purified eicosapentaenoic acid on platelet function, blood viscosity and red cell deformability in healthy human subjects. *Atherosclerosis* 1983; **46:** 321–31.

84. Nagakawa Y, Orimo H, Harasawa M, Morita I, Yashiro K, Murota S. Effect of eicosapentaenoic acid on the platelet aggregation and composition of fatty acid in man. *Atherosclerosis* 1985; **47:** 71–5.

85. Lands WEM, Culp BR, Hirai A, Gorman R. Relation-

ship of thromboxane generation to the aggregation of platelet from humans: effect of eicosapentaenoic acid. *Prostaglandins* 1985; **30:** 819–25.

86. Bradlow BA, Chetty N, van der Westhuyzen J, Mendelsohn D, Gibson JE. The effects of a mixed fish diet on platelet function, fatty acids and serum lipids. *Thromb Res* 1983; **29:** 561–8.

87. Tilvis RS, Rasi V, Viinikka L, Ylikorkala O, Miettinen TA. Effects of purified fish oil on platelet lipids and function in diabetic women. *Clin Chim Acta* 1987; **164:** 315–22.

88. von Shacky C, Weber PC. Metabolism and effects on platelet function of the purified eicosapentaenoic and docosahexaenoic acid in humans. *J Clin Invest* 1985; **76:** 2446–50.

89. Galloway JH, Cartwright IJ, Woodcock BE, Greaves M, Russell RGG, Preston FE. Effects of dietary fish oil supplementation on the fatty acid composition of the human platelet membrane: demonstration of selectivity in the incorporation of eicosapentaenoic acid into membrane phospholipid pools. *Clin Sci* 1985; **68:** 449–54.

90. Beitz J, Schimke E, Liebaug U, *et al.* Influence of a cod liver oil diet in healthy and insulin-dependent diabetic volunteers on fatty acid pattern, inhibition of prostacyclin formation by low density lipoprotein (LDL) and platelet thromboxane. *Klin Wochenschr* 1986; **64:** 793–9.

91. Singer P, Berger I, Luck K, Taube C, Naumann E, Godicke W. Long-term effect of mackerel diet on blood pressure, serum lipids and thromboxane formation in patients with mild essential hypertension. *Atherosclerosis* 1986; **62:** 259–65.

92. Haines AP, Sanders TAB, Imeson JD, *et al.* Effects of a fish oil supplement on platelet function, haemostatic variables and albuminuria in insulin-dependent diabetics. *Thromb Res* 1986; **43:** 643–55.

93. Velardo B, Lagarde M, Guichardant M, *et al.* Decrease of platelet activity after intake of small amounts of eicosapentaenoic acids in diabetics. *Thromb Haemost* 1982; **48:** 344.

94. Fitzgerald GA, Pedersen AK, Patrono C. Analysis of prostacyclin and thromboxane biosynthesis in cardiovascular disease. *Circulation* 1983; **67:** 1174–7.

95. FitzGerald DJ, Roy L, Catella F, FitzGerald GA. Platelet activation in unstable coronary disease. *N Engl J Med* 1986; **315:** 983–9.

96. Henriksson P, Wennmalm Å, Edhag O, Vesterquist O, Green K. *In vivo* production of prostacyclin and thromboxane in patients with acute myocardial infarction. *Br Heart J* 1986; **55:** 543–8.

97. Driss F, Vericel E, Lagarde M, Dechavanne M, Darcet P. Inhibition of platelet aggregation and thromboxane synthesis after intake of small amount of eicosapentaenoic acid. *Thromb Res* 1984; **36:** 389–96.

98. Corey EJ, Shih C, Cashman JR. Docosahexaenoic acid is a strong inhibitor of prostaglandin but not

leukotriene biosynthesis. *Proc Natl Acad Sci USA* 1983; **80**: 3581–4.

99. von Schacky C, Weber PC. Metabolism and effects on platelet function of the purified eicosapentaenoic and docosahexaenoic acids in humans. *J Clin Invest* 1985; **76**: 2446–50.

100. Thorngren M, Gustafson A, Wohlfahrt G. Effects of acetylsalicylic acid on platelet aggregation before and during increase in dietary eicosapentaenoic acid. *Haemostasis* 1983; **13**: 244–7.

101. Harris WS, Silveira S, Dujovne CA. The combined effect of n-3 fatty acids and aspirin on hemostatic parameters in man. *Thromb Res* 1990; **57**: 517–26.

102. Lee TH, Hoover RL, Williams JD, *et al.* Effects of dietary enrichment with eicosapentaenoic acid and docosahexaenoic acid on *in vivo* neutrophil and monocyte leukotriene generation and neutrophil function. *N Engl J Med* 1985; **312**: 1217–24.

103. Schmidt EB, Dyerberg J. n-3 fatty acids and leucocytes. *J Intern Med* 1989; **225** (suppl 1): 151–8.

104. Endres S, Ghorbani R, Kelley VE, *et al.* The effect of dietary supplementation with n-3 polyunsaturated fatty acids on the synthesis of interleukin-1 and tumor necrosis factor by mononuclear cells. *N Engl J Med* 1989; **320**: 265–71.

105. Schmidt EB, Pedersen JO, Varming K, *et al.* n-3 fatty acids and leucocyte chemotaxis. Effects in hyperlipidemia and dose-response studies in healthy men. *Arteriosclerosis Thromb* 1991; **11**: 429–35.

106. Dyerberg J, Schmidt EB. n-3 fatty acids and cardiovascular disease – observations generated by studies in Greenland Eskimos. *Wien Klin Wochenschr* 1989; **101**: 277–82.

107. Høstmark AT, Bjerkedal T, Kierulf Y, Flaten H, Ulshagen K. Fish oil and fibrinogen. *BMJ* 1988; **297**: 180–1.

108. Hornstra G. The effect of n-3 fatty acids on coagulation. In: De Caterina R, Kristensen SD, Schmidt EB (eds), *Fish Oil and Vascular Disease*. Berlin: Springer Verlag, 1992; 65–72.

109. Schmidt EB. n-3 fatty acids and fibrinolysis. In: De Caterina R, Kristensen SD, Schmidt EB (eds), *Fish Oil and Vascular Disease*. Berlin: Springer-Verlag, 1992; 73–8.

110. Shimokawa H, Lam JYT, Chesebro JH, Bowie EJW, Vanhoutte PM. Effects of dietary supplementation with cod-liver oil on endothelium-dependent responses in porcine coronary arteries. *Circulation* 1987; **76**: 898–905.

111. Shimokawa H, Vanhoutte PM. Dietary cod-liver oil improves endothelium dependent responses in hypercholesterolemic and atherosclerotic porcine coronary arteries. *Circulation* 1988; **78**: 1421–30.

112. Komori K, Shimokawa H, Vanhoutte PM. Endothelium-dependent relaxation in response to aggregating platelets in porcine femoral veins and its modulation by diet. *Circulation* 1989; **80**: 401–9.

113. Palmer RMJ, Ferrige AG, Moncada J. Release of nitric oxide accounts for the biological activity of endothelium-derived relaxing factor. *Nature* 1987; **327**: 524–6.

114. Radomski MW, Palmer RMJ, Moncada S. Endogenous nitric oxide inhibits human platelet adhesion to vascular endothelium. *Lancet* 1987; **2**: 1057–8.

115. Weiner BH, Ockene IS, Levine PH, *et al.* Inhibition of atherosclerosis by cod-liver oil in a hyperlipidemic swine model. *N Engl J Med* 1986; **315**: 841–6.

116. Davies HR, Bridenstine RT, Vesselinovitch D, Wissler RW. Fish oil inhibits development of atherosclerosis in rhesus monkeys. *Arteriosclerosis* 1987; **7**: 441–9.

117. Thiery J, Seidel D. Fish oil feeding results in an enhancement of cholesterol-induced atherosclerosis in rabbits. *Atherosclerosis* 1987; **63**: 53–6.

118. Kristensen SD, Roberts KM, Lawry J, Martin JF. The effect of fish oil on atherogenesis and thrombopoiesis in rabbits on high cholesterol diet. *Artery* 1988; **15**: 250–8.

119. Landymore RW, Kinley CE, Cooper JH, MacAulay M, Sheridan B, Cameron C. Cod-liver oil in the prevention of intimal hyperplasia in autogenous vein grafts used for arterial by-pass. *J Thorac Cardiovasc Surg* 1985; **89**: 351–7.

120. Cahill PD, Sarris GE, Cooper AD, *et al.* Inhibition of vein graft intimal thickening by eicosapentaenoic acid: reduced thromboxane production without change in lipoprotein levels or low-density lipoprotein receptor density. *J Vasc Surg* 1988; **7**: 108–17.

121. Casali RE, Hale JA, Lenarz L, Faas F, Morris MD. Improved graft patency associated with altered platelet function induced by marine fatty acids in dogs. *J Surg Res* 1986; **40**: 6–12.

122. Culp BR, Lands WEM, Lucchesi, Pitt R, Romson J. The effect of dietary supplementation of fish oil on experimental myocardial infarction. *Prostaglandins* 1980; **20**: 1021–31.

123. Verheught FWA, Schouten JA, Eeltinte JC, Roos JP. Omega-3 polyunsaturated fatty acids in the treatment of angina pectoris: effect on objective signs of exercise-induced myocardial ischaemia. *Curr Ther Res* 1986; **39**: 208–13.

124. Mehta JL, Lopez LM, Lawson D, Vargovich TJ, Williams LL. Dietary supplementation with omega-3 polyunsaturated fatty acids in patients with stable coronary heart disease. *Am J Med* 1988; **84**: 45–52.

125. Dehmer GJ, Popma JJ, van den Berg EK, *et al.* Reduction in the rate of early restenosis after coronary angioplasty by a diet supplemented with n-3 fatty acids. *N Engl J Med* 1988; **319**: 733–9.

126. Reis GJ, Sipperley ME, McCabe CH, *et al.* Randomised trial of fish oil for prevention of restenosis after coronary angioplasty. *Lancet* 1989; **2**: 177–81.

127. Grigg LE, Kay TW, Valentine PA, *et al.* Determinants of restenosis and lack of effect of dietary supplementation with eicosapentaenoic acid on the

incidence of coronary artery restenosis after angioplasty. *J Am Coll Cardiol* 1989; **13:** 665–72.

128. Knapp HR, FitzGerald GA. The antihypertensive effects of fish oil: a controlled study of polyunsaturated fatty acid supplements in essential hypertension. *N Engl J Med* 1989; **320:** 1037–43.

129. Bønaa KH, Bjerve KS, Straume B, Gram IT, Thelle D. Effect of eicosapentaenoic and docosahexaenoic acids on blood pressure in hypertension. *N Engl J Med* 1990; **322:** 795–801.

130. Burr ML, Lancet ML, Gilbert JF, *et al.* Effects of changes in fat, fish and fibre intakes on death and myocardial reinfarction: Diet and Reinfarction Trail (DART). *Lancet* 1989; **2:** 757–61.

6 Prostaglandins for termination of pregnancy

Marc Bygdeman

Natural prostaglandins such as $PGF_{2\alpha}$ and PGE_2, administered either extra- or intra-amniotically, have been used on a routine basis for termination of second trimester pregnancy in many countries for more than 15 years. More recently, analogues with a more specific effect on the myometrium, a longer duration of action and suitable for intramuscular, vaginal and oral administration have become available. The latest development in non-surgical methods to terminate pregnancy is that of antiprogestins, which enhance the sensitivity of the myometrium to prostaglandin. In this chapter, clinical experience of the established procedures is summarized. For more detailed information, readers are referred to review articles on the subject. The emphasis will be on more recent development in this area.

Mode of action

It is generally accepted that prostaglandins play an important role in the regulation of uterine contractility during pregnancy. $PGF_{2\alpha}$ has been regarded as the intrinsic stimulator of uterine contractility. Evidence for this concept arises from several different observations. Exogenous prostaglandins are able to stimulate uterine contractility during all stages of pregnancy. Increased production of $PGF_{2\alpha}$ and PGE_2 in the different uterine tissues has been demonstrated during labour together with an increased concentration in amniotic fluid, plasma and urine. Furthermore, inhibitors of prostaglandin synthesis can interrupt premature labour.[1]

The use of PGE and PGF compounds for termination of pregnancy depends on their stimulatory effect on uterine contractility and softening effect on the uterine cervix. Prostaglandins are unique in that they are equally effective in stimulating the myometrium in all stages of pregnancy. The threshold dose of a single intravenous injection at mid-pregnancy is about 20 µg of PGE_1 and PGE_2, 100–200 µg of $PGF_{2\alpha}$ and approximately 500 µg of $PGF_{1\alpha}$. The five- to tenfold difference in potency between $PGF_{2\alpha}$ and PGE_2 is independent of route of administration.

PGE_2 and $PGF_{2\alpha}$ are very rapidly metabolized. The half-life of these compounds in the circulation is less than a minute. A more prolonged duration of action can be obtained following extra- or intra-amniotic administration. The half-life of $PGF_{2\alpha}$ in amniotic fluid is between 13 and 20 hours.[2]

A number of prostaglandin analogues have been developed which are not substrates for the initial step of enzymatic degradation by 15-dehydrogenase. In general, these compounds are more potent than the corresponding parent compounds. The duration of action is prolonged and the action more specific on uterine than other smooth muscles. The analogues, which currently are in routine clinical use, are 16,16-dimethyl-trans-Δ^2-PGE_1 methyl ester (gemeprost; Cervagem, May & Baker, Dagenham, UK), 16-phenoxy-17,18,19,20-tetranor PGE_2 methylsulphonylamide (sulprostone; Nalador, Schering AG, Berlin, Germany), and 15(S)-15-methyl $PGF_{2\alpha}$ (carboprost; Prostin, Upjohn, Kalamazoo, Michigan, USA). Gemeprost is administered vaginally, sulprostone intramuscularly, and carboprost intramuscularly or intra-amniotically. To illustrate the difference between an analogue and a parent compound, 15-methyl $PGF_{2\alpha}$ can serve as an example. Following an intravenous injection, 15-methyl $PGF_{2\alpha}$ is approximately 10 times more potent than $PGF_{2\alpha}$. If administered as an intravenous infusion, 5 µg of 15-methyl $PGF_{2\alpha}$ is approximately equally effective as 75 µg $PGF_{2\alpha}$ in stimulating uterine contractility. The greater difference in potency following continuous intravenous infusion compared with that following single intravenous injections is likely to be due to the slow metabolic degradation of the analogue.[3] Following intra-amniotic administration, 2.5 mg 15-methyl $PGF_{2\alpha}$ is even more effective than 50 mg $PGF_{2\alpha}$ in terminating second trimester pregnancy, and the need for repeated or additional treatment is reduced as a result of increased potency and slower metabolic degradation.[4] The half-life of 15-methyl $PGF_{2\alpha}$ in amniotic fluid is 27–31 hours, or approximately double that of $PGF_{2\alpha}$.[5]

Csapo has suggested that the pregnant uterus is an intrinsically active organ which is suppressed by progesterone, especially in early and mid-pregnancy. If this is true, withdrawal of progesterone influence will result in uterine contractions. Recent studies have shown this to be the case. In early pregnancy, treatment with RU 486, a steroid which competes with progesterone at the receptor level, results in uterine contractility. The time from initiation of antiprogestin treatment to increased uterine activity is between 24 and 36 hours. Of clinical importance is the fact that withdrawal of progesterone influence also results in increased sensitivity of the myometrium to prostaglandin.[6,7]

The human cervix contains mainly collagen. The muscle content is 29% in the upper part and decreases to 6% in the lower part of the cervix. It is, however, doubtful if the smooth muscle content is of any physiological importance. Degradation of the collagen and an increase in some dermatan sulphate proteoglycans can at least partly explain the pregnancy-associated softening of the connective tissue. Prostaglandins are most probably involved in cervical ripening occurring during pregnancy. Prostaglandins are synthesized in the human cervix and prostaglandin receptors have been demonstrated; cervical ripening can be induced pharmacologically by treatment with prostaglandin and prostaglandin biosynthesis inhibitors can delay cervical ripening.[8]

Clinical use

A number of prostaglandins and prostaglandin analogues have been used for termination of pregnancy. The present review will concentrate on those compounds which have been introduced on the market or substantially tested.

First trimester pregnancy

It was demonstrated some 20 years ago that $PGF_{2\alpha}$ and PGE_2 administered intravenously could terminate early pregnancy. The high incidence of side effects could be limited if $PGF_{2\alpha}$ was administered into the uterine cavity. However, the drawbacks of such invasive procedures are the requirement of medical skill and the risk of introducing infection in the uterine cavity. With the introduction of prostaglandin analogues the situation improved. Both repeated vaginal administration of gemeprost and meteneprost (9-deoxo-16,16-dimethyl-9-methylene PGE_2; 9-methylene PGE_2) and intramuscular injections of sulprostone have been shown to be highly effective in terminating early pregnancy of up to 49 days of amenorrhoea. The success rate (complete abortion) ranged from 90% to 100% in a number of studies.[9] Approximately 50% of the patients had gastrointestinal side effects and about 30% experienced marked uterine pain. In spite of these fairly good results, prostaglandin therapy has in practice not replaced vacuum aspiration for termination of early pregnancy.[9]

The situation changed with the development of an antiprogestin. RU 486 alone is, however, not sufficiently effective. Several dose schedules have been tested but the frequency of complete abortion seldom exceeds 70% irrespective of the dose of the drug and the duration of treatment. However, a success rate of up to 85% has been achieved with a single 600-mg dose of RU 486 if the treatment is restricted to the first 10 days following the missed menstrual period.[10]

As mentioned previously, treatment with an antiprogestin will release the myometrium from the inhibitory effect of progesterone and induce uterine contractions, but, more important, it will also increase the sensitivity of the myometrium to prostaglandin. Treatment with RU 486 in combination with a small dose of prostaglandin was therefore evaluated. In the first clinical study, 25 mg of RU 486 twice daily was combined with 0.25 mg sulprostone injected intramuscularly. The frequency of complete abortion was 94%.[6] That the combination of RU 486 and a low dose of a prostaglandin analogue (either 0.25 mg sulprostone or 0.5–1.0 mg gemeprost administered vaginally) is a highly effective method of medical abortion during early pregnancy has been shown in a number of clinical studies,[10] and the process has been introduced on the market for routine use in France and the UK. Data from large clinical studies are now available. Recently, 73 French medical centres participated in a large-scale study covering 2115 pregnant women with up to 7 weeks' amenorrhoea seeking voluntary termination of pregnancy. The study compared the effect of a single 600-mg dose of RU 486 followed 36–48 hours later by either an intramuscular injection of sulprostone (mainly 0.25 mg) or vaginal administration of gemeprost (1.0 mg). The overall efficacy rate (complete abortion) was 96%. The failures included persisting pregnancy (1%), incomplete expulsion (2.1%) and a need for haemostatic curettage (0.9%).[11]

Following treatment with RU 486 in combination with prostaglandin analogues, almost all patients will start to bleed irrespective of the outcome of the therapy. The duration of bleeding is between 1 and 2 weeks although, in a few patients, occasional spottings continue until the first menstrual period. The amount of blood loss corresponds to a heavy menstrual period. The mean blood loss has been measured to 81 ml.[12] Most of the side effects are related to prostaglandin therapy. Silvestre *et al.*[11] reported at 15.3% and 7.5% frequency of vomiting and diarrhoea, respectively. With 0.25 mg sulprostone, 14.9% of the women required analgesia. In the UK multicentre study,[13] in which 600 mg of RU 486 was combined with 1.0 mg gemeprost, the results were similar. It is important to note, however, that in this study pregnancies up to the ninth week were included. The ideal dose of RU 486 and prostaglandin remains to be established. On-going studies indicate that the dose of both compounds may be reduced significantly.

Large randomized studies comparing vacuum aspiration and RU 486 in combination with prostaglandin have not yet been performed. The data available indicate that the medical method is as effective as vacuum aspiration.[14] The advantages of vacuum aspiration are shorter duration of bleeding and fewer/less gastrointestinal side effects. However, the medical method avoids the risks associated with surgical intervention; moreover, both treatment of heavy bleeding (0.9%) and the frequency of temperature elevation (0.3%) compare favourably with vacuum aspiration.[11]

Recent studies indicate that treatment with RU

Table 6.1 Termination of early pregnancy by 600 mg RU 486 followed by either gemeprost or sulprostone[11]

Outcome	Percentage of patients
Complete abortion	96.0
Incomplete abortion	2.1
Continuation of pregnancy	1.0
Haemostatic procedure required	0.9
Infection (fever)	0.3

Table 6.2 Termination of early pregnancy: a comparison between vacuum aspiration, prostaglandin and an antiprogestin[14]

Treatment	Dose	Outcome: complete abortion (%)
Vacuum aspiration	—	96
RU 486	150 mg daily for 4 days	60
Gemeprost	1.0 mg every 3rd hour up to 5 times	97
RU 486 + Gemeprost	150 mg daily for 4 days 1.0 mg on day 3	95

486 may also be combined with oral administration of prostaglandin analogues. Two prostaglandin analogues have been shown effective: 9-methylene PGE_2 and the PGE_1 analogue misoprostol (15(S)-15-methyl $PGF_{2\alpha}$ methyl ester) (Cytotec, G.D. Searle & Co., Chicago, USA).[15–17] Misoprostol is widely used to treat peptic ulcer. Oral administration is obviously a convenient route of administration and, according to the limited experience so far available, it seems that a combination of RU 486 and misoprostol is associated with a lower frequency of side effects than if other prostaglandin analogues are used.

In the late first trimester of pregnancy the mechanical dilatation of the cervical canal prior to evacuation can be difficult. In a multicentre study performed by the World Health Organization (WHO) it was demonstrated that vaginal administration of 1.0 mg 15-methyl $PGF_{2\alpha}$ was significantly more effective than a placebo in dilating the cervical canal. The prostaglandin treatment also resulted in a reduced frequency of both operative and postoperative complications.[18] Today, the prostaglandins used most world wide are sulprostone 0.5 mg intramuscularly and gemeprost 1.0 mg vaginally. To allow the termination to be performed on an outpatient basis, the prostaglandins are administered 3–4 hours prior to vacuum aspiration. Both compounds are equally effective and the frequency of gastrointestinal side effects is lower than if PGF analogues are used.[19] Generally, the rate of complications associated with vacuum aspiration rises with increasing gestational age. In a recent study, which comprised 1000 vacuum aspirations, late first and early second trimester patients were pretreated with prostaglandin. The overall result was a total complication rate of about 5% and the frequency was the same in all weeks of pregnancy from the 8th to the 14th week, illustrating that, with prostaglandin treatment, vacuum aspiration may be used safely even in the first weeks of the second trimester.[20]

Second trimester pregnancy

Intrauterine administration of PGE_2 and $PGF_{2\alpha}$ has for many years had an established place in the termination of second trimester pregnancy. For extra-amniotic instillation, prostaglandins are administered via a transcervical catheter by repeated instillations or continuous drip. With $PGF_{2\alpha}$, following an initial test dose of 250 µg, a common dose is 750–1000 µg every second hour up to 36 hours. The corresponding doses for PGE_2 are 50 µg followed by 200 µg. These dose schedules are expected to achieve a success rate of 80–90% within a mean induction-to-abortion time of 20–24 hours. Instead of repeated instillations, a continuous infusion of PGE_2 has been practised by several authors. A common dose is a continuous drip of 100 µg per hour or stepwise increased until uterine contractions are sufficient.[21]

Intra-amniotic administration of prostaglandins is mainly restricted to pregnancy in the 16th week and onwards. Based on multicentre studies performed by the WHO and others, the general consensus indicates that optimal dosage schedules for intra-amniotic administration of $PGF_{2\alpha}$ include either 25 mg repeated after 6 hours or 40–50 mg as a single dose. Single doses of 5–25 mg PGE_2 are equally effective but have been used much less.[4,21]

The analogue 15-methyl $PGF_{2\alpha}$ is also often used for intra-amniotic administration. The optimal dose seems to be 2.5 mg. A single dose of 2.5 mg 15-methyl $PGF_{2\alpha}$ was randomly compared with either 40 mg or 50 mg $PGF_{2\alpha}$. Abortion was successfully induced by 15-methyl $PGF_{2\alpha}$ in approximately 95% of cases, which was significantly better than $PGF_{2\alpha}$

(81% with 40 mg and 88% with 50 mg). The mean induction-to-abortion interval (18–20 hours) was similar with both compounds, and gastrointestinal side effects were within clinically acceptable limits. Injury to the cervix is a risk to be considered with both compounds. In a WHO study the incidence of such injury was 2.5% and occurred mainly in primigravidae patients.[22]

The invasive nature of intrauterine administration of prostaglandins is, however, a drawback and incorrect administration, especially following intra-amniotic instillation where high doses of prostaglandins are used, may cause serious complications. From this point of view, intramuscular or vaginal administration of prostaglandin analogues is preferable. The compounds in current use are carboprost and sulprostone for intramuscular, and gemeprost for vaginal, administration. Carboprost was the first analogue to be investigated on a large scale for termination of second trimester pregnancy. In a multicentre trial performed by the WHO Prostaglandin Task Force, carboprost 0.2 mg i.m. followed by 0.3 mg every 3 hours for a total of 30 hours resulted in a success rate of about 85%. The incidence of vomiting and diarrhoea was high, however, and it was concluded that intramuscular carboprost is of limited value as a primary method for abortion but may be used to finalize the abortion process when the first method has failed.[23] The experience with sulprostone is more favourable: if 0.5 mg sulprostone was administered every 4 hours, the rate of abortion was equally high but the occurrence of gastrointestinal side effects substantially lower.[24]

Treatment with both carboprost and sulprostone has been combined with pretreatment of the cervix with one laminaria tent. In a study performed by the WHO Prostaglandin Task Force, either sulprostone 0.5 mg 4-hourly or carboprost 0.25 mg 2-hourly following 12 hours' pretreatment with one laminaria tent was given to 529 patients in the 13th to 22nd week of pregnancy.[25] In the patients given sulprostone, 95.6% aborted within 24 hours of prostaglandin treatment. The corresponding figure for carboprost was 94.5%. The frequency of gastrointestinal side effects was significantly more common following treatment with the F- rather than the E-analogue. Almost half of the patients did not experience any side effects with the E-analogue. The difference between the two compounds was most marked with regard to the frequency of diarrhoea: only 6% of the patients treated with the E-analogues experienced this type of side effect, compared with 64% in those treated with the F-analogue. It was

Table 6.3 Termination of second trimester pregnancy with prostaglandin (PG) analogues administered vaginally or intramuscularly

Treatment	Route of administration	Dose	Frequency of abortion within 24 h of PG therapy (%)	Reference
Gemeprost	Vaginal	1.0 mg every 3 h	82	26
Laminaria tent + sulprostone	Intracervical Intramuscular	— 0.5 mg every 4 h	95.6	25
RU 486 + gemeprost	Oral Vaginal	600 mg 1.0 mg every 3 h	94	27
RU 486 + 9-methylene PGE_2	Oral Vaginal	200 mg 5 mg every 4 h	100	30

concluded in this study that pretreatment with laminaria followed by either carboprost or sulprostone is a highly effective method to terminate second trimester pregnancy. It is a non-invasive procedure which does not require the medical expertise needed for extra- or intra-amniotic instillation of prostaglandin. The simplicity of the therapy may result in a decreased risk for serious complications. An additional advantage is that the procedure is equally applicable during both early and late second trimester pregnancy. The frequency of gastrointestinal side effects following sulprostone is only slightly higher than that observed following intra-amniotic administration of hypertonic saline.

The vaginal route is as convenient as the intramuscular one. The possibility of using gemeprost for termination of second trimester pregnancy has also been evaluated. Gemeprost 1.0 mg was administered vaginally every 3 hours five times to 113 women in the 12th to 16th week of pregnancy. If abortion did not occur within 24 hours, a further course of five pessaries was described: 82% of the patients aborted within 24 hours and an additional 14% during the second 24-hour period, giving an overall success rate of 96%. Vomiting and diarrhoea occurred in 14% and 20% of the patients, respectively.[26] In a more recent study, pregnancies up to the 18th week were included. In this study 80% of the patients aborted within 24 hours and an additional 14% during the next 24-hour period.[27] Vaginal administration of gemeprost has also been randomly compared with extra-amniotic administration of PGE_2. For gemeprost, the dosage was 1.0 mg every 3 hours five times and for PGE_2 100 μg per hour as a continuous infusion. The frequency of abortion within 24 hours was similar for both treatment schedules, or 77% and 79%, respectively. There was no difference in the mean induction-to-abortion time and with both methods gastrointestinal side effects were equally rare. However, the women treated with gemeprost experienced significantly less uterine pain. It was concluded that gemeprost is an effective alternative to extra-amniotic administration of PGE_2 for the termination of pregnancy in the early second trimester and that the treatment is highly acceptable to patients and staff alike.[28]

Pretreatment with RU 486 seems to be beneficial also in second trimester abortions as judged from a few recent studies. If 200 mg was administered 24 hours prior to extra-amniotic infusion of PGE_2, both induction-to-abortion interval and total dose of PGE_2 were significantly reduced in comparison to pretreatment with placebo.[29] In another study, patients were randomly allocated to receive either 600 mg RU 486 or placebo prior to vaginal administration of 1.0 mg gemeprost 3-hourly five times. In the RU 486 pretreated group, 94% of the patients aborted within 24 hours, compared to 80% in the placebo group. The median interval between administration of prostaglandin and abortion was significantly shorter in the RU 486 group (6.8 hours) than in the placebo group (15.8 hours). The women pretreated with RU 486 also required significantly fewer gemeprost pessaries to induce abortion and reported significantly less pain than the women who received the placebo.[27] In a third study, pretreatment with intracervical PGE_2 gel was compared with 200 mg RU 486 followed by vaginal administration of 5.0 mg 9-methylene PGE_2 every fourth hour for up to 24 hours in patients up to the 23rd week of pregnancy. All patients in the RU 486 pretreated group aborted within 24 hours ($n=23$), whereas, following intracervical PGE_2 administration, 3 patients out of 21 needed additional treatment. The interval from the start of vaginal prostaglandin administration to abortion was shorter, the total dose of 9-methylene PGE_2 lower, and the subjectively estimated degree of pain as described on a six-point analogue scale was significantly less in patients pretreated with RU 486 than in those pretreated with intracervical PGE_2 gel.[30]

Conclusions

Extra- or intra-amniotic administration of $PGF_{2\alpha}$ and, to some extent, PGE_2 has been used for termination of second trimester pregnancy for more than 15 years. The clinical value of these procedures is well established. The use of PGE analogues administered by non-invasive routes seems to offer a number of advantages. Both vaginal and intramuscular administration of these analogues appear to be as effective as intrauterine administration of classic prostaglandins, and gastrointestinal side effects and uterine pain are not increased. The treatment requires minimal interference from skilled medical personnel and the simplicity of the therapy will most likely result in a decreased risk of serious complications. Recent data indicate that the ideal method to terminate second trimester pregnancy will be treatment with antiprogestin followed by vaginal administration of a PGE analogue.

During late first and early second trimester pregnancies, treatment with PGE analogues prior to vacuum aspiration will facilitate the surgical procedure and reduce both the operative and the postoperative rate of complications.

Prostaglandins are highly effective in terminating very early first trimester pregnancy but the frequency of gastrointestinal side effects and uterine pain has limited the clinical usefulness of the procedure. However, if vaginal or intramuscular or possibly oral administration of PGE analogues is combined with pretreatment with antiprogestin, the dose of prostaglandin can be significantly reduced. The combined treatment has already been accepted as a non-surgical alternative to vacuum aspiration for termination of early pregnancy.

References

1. Mitchell MD. Regulation of eicosanoid biosynthesis during pregnancy and parturition. In: Hillier K (ed), *Eicosanoids and Reproduction*. Lancaster: MTP Press, 1987: 108–27.
2. Gréen K, Bygdeman M, Wiqvist N. Kinetic and metabolic studies of prostaglandin $F_{2\alpha}$ administered amniotically for induction of abortion. *Life Sci* 1974; **14**: 2285–97.
3. Toppozada M, Beguin F, Bygdeman M, Wiqvist N. Response of the midpregnant human uterus to systemic administration of 15(S)-15-methyl prostaglandin $F_{2\alpha}$. *Prostaglandins* 1972; **2**: 239–49.
4. Bygdeman M. The use of prostaglandins and their analogues for abortion. *Clin Obstet Gynecol* 1984; **11**: 573–84.
5. Gréen K, Granström E, Bygdeman M, Wiqvist N. Kinetic and metabolic studies of 15-methyl $PGF_{2\alpha}$ administered intra-amniotically for induction of abortion. *Prostaglandins* 1976; **11**: 699–711.
6. Bygdeman M, Swahn ML. Progesterone receptor blockage. Effect on uterine contractility in early pregnancy. *Contraception* 1985; **32**: 45–51.
7. Swahn ML, Bygdeman M. The effect of the antigestin RU 486 on uterine contractility and sensitivity to prostaglandin and oxytocin. *Br J Obstet Gynaecol* 1988; **95**: 126–39.
8. Uldbjerg N, Ulmsten U, Ekman G. The physiological role of eicosanoids in controlling the form and function of the cervix. In: Hillier K (ed), *Eicosanoids and Reproduction*. Lancaster: MTP Press, 1987: 163–83.
9. Swahn ML, Bygdeman M. Medical methods to terminate early pregnancy. In: Bygdeman M (ed), *Baillière's Clinical Obstetrics and Gynaecology, Medical Induction of Abortion*. London: Baillière Tindall, 1990: 293–306.
10. Van Look PFA, Bygdeman M. Antiprogestational steroids: a new dimension in human fertility regulation. In: Milligan SR (ed), *Oxford Reviews of Reproductive Biology*. Oxford: Oxford University Press, 1989: 1–60.
11. Silvestre L, Dubois C, Renault M, Rezvani, Baulieu EE, Ulmann A. Voluntary interpretation of pregnancy with mifepristone (RU 486) and a prostaglandin analogue. *N Engl J Med* 1990; **322**: 645–9.
12. Cameron IT, Michie AF, Baird DT. Therapeutic abortion in early pregnancy with antiprogestin RU-486 alone or in combination with a prostaglandin analogue (gemeprost). *Contraception* 1986; **34**: 459–68.
13. UK Multicentre Trial. The efficacy and tolerance of mifepristone and prostaglandin in first trimester termination of pregnancy. *Br J Obstet Gynaecol* 1990; **97**: 480–6.
14. Cameron IT, Baird DT. Early pregnancy termination: a comparison between vacuum aspiration and medical abortion using prostaglandin (16,16-dimethyl-trans-Δ^2-PGE_2 methyl ester) or the antiprogestagen RU-486. *Br J Obstet Gynaecol* 1988; **95**: 271–6.
15. Swahn ML, Gottlieb C, Gréen K, Bygdeman M. Oral administration of RU 486 and 9-methylene PGE_2 for

oral termination of pregnancy. *Contraception* 1990; **41:** 461–73.

16. Auberry M, Baulieu EE. Activité contragestive de l'association au RU 486 d'une prostaglandine active par vioe orale *C R Hebdom Acad Sci* 1991; **312:** 539–45.

17. Norman JE, Thong KJ, Baird DT. Uterine contractility and induction of abortion in early pregnancy by misoprostol and mifepristone. *Lancet* 1991; **338:** 1233–6.

18. WHO Prostaglandin Task Force. Vaginal administration of 15-methyl $PGF_{2\alpha}$ methyl ester for preoperative cervical dilatation. *Contraception* 1981; **23:** 251–7.

19. WHO Prostaglandin Task Force. Randomized comparison of different prostaglandin analogues and laminaria tent for preoperative cervical dilatation. *Contraception* 1986; **34:** 237–51.

20. Fried G, Östlund E, Ullberg C, Bygdeman M. Somatic complications and contraceptive techniques following legal abortion. *Acta Obstet Gynecol Scand* 1989; **68:** 515–21.

21. Toppozada M, Ismail AAA. Intrauterine drugs in abortion. In: Bygdeman M (ed), *Baillière's Clinical Obstetrics and Gynaecology. Medical Induction of Abortion.* London: Baillière Tindall, 1989: 327–49.

22. WHO Prostaglandin Task Force. Comparison of single intra-amniotic injection of 15-methyl prostaglandin $F_{2\alpha}$ and prostaglandin $F_{2\alpha}$ for termination of second trimester pregnancy. An international multicentre study. *Am J Obstet Gynecol* 1977; **129:** 601–6.

23. WHO Prostaglandin Task Force. Intramuscular administration of 15-methyl prostaglandin $F_{2\alpha}$ for induction of abortion in weeks 10 to 20 of pregnancy. *Am J Obstet Gynecol* 1977; **129:** 593–600.

24. WHO Prostaglandin Task Force. Termination of second trimester pregnancy by intramuscular injection of 16-phenoxy-ω-17,18,19,20-tetranor PGE_2 methyl sulfonylamide. *Int J Gynaecol Obstet* 1982; **20:** 383–6.

25. WHO Prostaglandin Task Force. Termination of second trimester pregnancy with laminaria and intramuscular 15-methyl $PGF_{2\alpha}$ or 16-phenoxy-ω-17, 18,19,20-tetranor PGC_2 methyl sulfonylamide. A randomized multicenter study. *Int J Gynaecol Obstet* 1988; **26:** 129–35.

26. Cameron IT, Michie AF, Baird DT. Prostaglandin-induced pregnancy termination: further studies using gemeprost (16,16-dimethyl-trans-Δ^2 PGE_1 methyl ester) vaginal pessaries in the early second trimester. *Prostaglandins* 1987; **34:** 111–17.

27. Rodger MW, Baird DT. Pretreatment with mifepristone (RU 486) reduces interval between prostaglandin administration and expulsion in second trimester abortion. *Br J Obstet Gynaecol* 1990; **97:** 41–5.

28. Cameron IT, Baird DT. The use of 16,16-dimethyl-trans-Δ^2 prostaglandin E_1 methyl ester (gemeprost) vaginal pessaries for the termination of pregnancy in the early second trimester. A comparison with extra-amniotic prostaglandin E_2. *Br J Obstet Gynaecol* 1984; **91:** 1136–40.

29. Urquhart DR, Templeton AA. Mifepristone (RU 486) and second trimester pregnancy. *Lancet* 1987; **2:** 1405.

30. Gottlieb C, Bygdeman M. The use of antiprogestin (RU 486) for termination of second trimester pregnancy. *Acta Obstet Gynecol Scand* 1991; **70:** 199–203.

7 Prostaglandins for cervical ripening and labour induction

AA Calder and MG Elder

The human uterus is responsible for containing the fetus and its supporting structures during its development and then for their rapid expulsion during parturition. In fulfilling these two contrasting functions, its two principal component parts, the uterine corpus and the uterine cervix, are both required to perform directly opposing activities. Thus the corpus must convert from a state of quiescence to one of dynamic contractility, while the cervix converts from a rigidly closed 'gatekeeper' to a readily opening passageway. Successful pregnancy and parturition require the cervix and corpus to interact in a synchronized fashion. Pregnancy must be maintained until the fetus has reached the appropriate stage of development and organ maturity for birth, and it is increasingly apparent that organ maturation is linked to the processes that trigger the onset of labour. It is also now beyond dispute that prostaglandins play an essential part in these role reversals of both uterine components and in the progressive processes of parturition.[1] Furthermore, these properties of prostaglandins are now widely exploited in clinical practice for cervical ripening and induction of labour.

Cervical physiology

In contrast to the mainly muscular uterine corpus, the cervix is predominantly composed of connective tissue in which collagen is the most important structural element. In the non-pregnant and early pregnant state collagen fibrils are bound together in dense bundles which provide the cervix with its characteristic rigidity.[2] There are other formed elements within the cervix, including elastic fibres and smooth muscle cells, but these are much less abundant.

The ground substance that surrounds the formed elements within the cervix is composed of large molecules in which a variety of glycosaminoglycans (GAGs) are incorporated into proteoglycan complexes. The principal cervical GAGs are chondroitin sulphate and its epimer, dermatan sulphate.[3,4] The proteoglycan complexes consist of a hyaluronic acid chain which links to core proteins with GAG side chains. These protein cores and associated GAGs are in intimate contact with collagen molecules and this relationship is considered to be vital for the appropriate alignment of the collagen fibrils and their consequent mechanical strength.[5-7] The greater the chain length and charge density of the GAGs, the greater is their binding affinity to collagen. Individual GAGs vary considerably in this regard, such that those containing iduronic acid (e.g. dermatan sulphate) will bind most strongly and confer tissue stability in contrast to those containing glucuronic acid which have the opposite effect.[8]

The water content of the cervix increases during pregnancy and this is probably the result of qualitative changes in the GAGs making the ground substance generally more hydrophilic.[9] This increase in tissue hydration may be an important factor in the modification of collagen during the process of cervical ripening. The absolute collagen concentration within the tissue appears to be reduced during this process and this may represent either removal of collagen from the tissue or, alternatively, a relative increase in water and GAG content. Cervical fibroblasts appear to orchestrate the changes within cervical tissue and are known to be responsible for synthesis of both collagen and GAGs as well as being a potential source of those lytic enzymes, including collagenase, that are responsible for degradation of these molecules. A further source of lytic enzymes are white cells, such as neutrophils which are known to produce elastase.[10] This may be important in view of the concept that cervical ripening has much in common with an inflammatory process; indeed, an inflammatory infiltrate has been observed in association with the process of cervical ripening in several experimental circumstances.

As a general observation, the rigidity of connective tissue is related to the age of the collagen and the degree of cross-linking between collagen fibrils; thus older collagen with a lot of cross-linking tends to be tougher than younger collagen. In addition, there may be qualitative changes in the type of collagen expressed within cervical tissue, although this has yet to be examined in great detail. Danforth and his colleagues[11] have, however, demonstrated clear differences between the tightly bound collagen of the non-pregnant and early pregnant cervix in which the ground substance is relatively sparse compared to the situation at term where there is increased ground substance and widely scattered and dissociated collagen fibrils. The overall reduction of collagen has been demonstrated both biochemically[11-13] and histologically using stains specific for polymerized collagen.[9] This latter technique appears to demonstrate a greater reduction in collagen and may reflect the fact that in the ripe cervix at term collagen remains within the cervix but in a non-polymerized state rather than as intact fibres which take up the specific stain.

The processes of collagen breakdown are not fully understood but appear to be under the control of collagenase and elastase, perhaps acting in concert. Uldbjerg and his colleagues[4] have shown a clear relationship between increasing activity of leucocyte elastase and collagenase and decreasing collagen content in the cervix as pregnancy progresses. Thus, as pregnancy proceeds and moves towards parturition, there may be a state of dynamic remodelling of collagen with mature collagen being replaced by newer collagen which has fewer cross-links and is more readily broken down at the time of parturition. Furthermore, Ekman and her

colleagues[14] have demonstrated a relationship between the clinical degree of cervical ripeness at term and the collagen concentration of the tissue.

Cervical ripening is a phenomenon that is recognized to proceed quietly during that part of late pregnancy which is best described as pre-labour, i.e. those 4–5 weeks that precede the clinical onset of labour. Rajabi and his colleagues[15] have demonstrated that a further and very dramatic increase in collagenase activity accompanies the onset of labour proper.

Biological control of cervical ripening

The physiological processes that culminate in parturition have preoccupied scientific investigators throughout the globe. The complex endocrine changes (which have often been described as a cascade) appear to have their origins within the fetus, rather than within the mother. These have been extensively reviewed[16-18] and will not be described in detail here. Suffice it to say that this cascade of changes appears to culminate in the activation of both myometrial contractility and cervical ripening in a co-ordinated and synchronized manner. The prostaglandins probably represent the ultimate link that translates the fetal, and to a lesser extent maternal, messages into the fundamental changes at tissue level. The three prostaglandins that appear to be the most important players in these processes are prostaglandin E_2 (PGE$_2$), prostaglandin $F_{2\alpha}$ (PGF$_{2\alpha}$) and prostacyclin (PGI$_2$). These prostanoids are all produced within uterine tissues. The role of prostacyclin is less clear than the roles of the other two prostanoids and although it may, in future, be shown to participate in the control of myometrial and cervical function, this has not yet been precisely clarified. In view of this uncertainty and because prostacyclin has not been explored to any extent as an agent for influencing the course of labour, it will not be further discussed here.

The principal source of PGE$_2$ in pregnancy is the amniotic membrane. PGF$_{2\alpha}$, on the other hand, is principally produced within the decidua. Between the amnion and the decidua lies the chorion and this contains high concentrations and activity of prostaglandin dehydrogenase (PGDH) which inactivates both these prostanoids.

Prostaglandins clearly play a role in the control of cervical ripening and it is known that both PGE$_2$ and PGI$_2$ (and, to a lesser extent, PGF$_{2\alpha}$) are produced within cervical tissue, a production that increases markedly at term and with the onset of parturition.[19]

Clinical and experimental studies have demonstrated that the prostaglandins (especially PGE_2) are capable of producing cervical softening, effacement and dilatation[20] and it seems highly probable that this represents a biological phenomenon. This assumption is reinforced by the observation that inhibitors of prostaglandins are associated not only with a delay in parturition, but also with a failure of cervical ripening.[21]

Proceeding on the assumption that PGE_2 represents the principal link between the factors that trigger parturition and the changes within cervical tissue that facilitate it, it is appropriate to consider the origin and activation of the prostaglandin E_2 which brings this about. There are two separate and perhaps complementary mechanisms. Since prostaglandin E_2 can be produced within the cervical tissue itself and appears to be produced therein in association with parturition,[19] it is an attractive concept to consider that such PGE_2 is activated by endocrine changes that influence the cervix. The principal candidates for such endocrine changes are progesterone, as an inhibitor thereof, and oestrogens and possibly also relaxin, as promoters of the process. Progesterone is a potent anti-inflammatory agent[22] and might inhibit cervical ripening *in vivo* by preventing neutrophil influx and activation.[23] Furthermore, progesterone is known to inhibit collagenase activity in uterine tissues.[24] Further support for an important role for progesterone in inhibiting cervical ripening comes from the observation that antiprogestins promote cervical softening in early pregnancy[25,26] and at least in animal observations this agent produces an influx of neutrophils to cervical tissues.[27]

The extent to which prostaglandins might participate in these processes is not yet clear, although the antiprogestins are known to stimulate prostaglandin synthesis and reduce its catabolism *in vitro*.[28,29] It is tempting to assume that progesterone might exert the opposite effects.

Oestrogens, on the other hand, especially oestradiol, have been shown to provoke cervical ripening in clinical studies[30,31] and this effect may be mediated by prostaglandin synthesis since oestradiol has been shown to stimulate prostaglandin production within uterine tissues.[32] Furthermore, Fitzpatrick and Dobson, using the sheep as a model, demonstrated oestradiol-induced cervical softening which was associated with increased cervical prostaglandin production.[33]

The third candidate as an endocrine influence on the cervix is relaxin, which, on the basis of both experimental[34] and clinical[35] studies, appears to promote cervical ripening. If indeed relaxin is important within this mechanism, this may be independent of the role of prostaglandins, although it seems more likely that an interactive process may pertain. This, however, remains a matter of speculation until subjected to deeper scrutiny.

The foregoing discussion relates, therefore, to the concept that cervical ripening might follow activation of PGE_2 within cervical tissue as a result of changes in the relative concentrations of those circulating hormones to which that tissue is exposed.

A second mechanism may, however, be worth postulating. The most potent and abundant source of PGE_2 within the uterus is the amniotic membrane. The biological reason for this particular source of prostaglandin synthesis remains unclear. It is now known that its synthesis can be provoked by a number of physiological and pathological influences (see later) but the influence that synthesis might exert on uterine tissues remains unclear. The purpose of amniotic PGE_2 may be largely concerned with interactive processes with the fetus rather than with the uterus, and such a view is supported by recognition of the potent capacity of the chorion to catabolize prostaglandins. It thus appears that the amnion with its enormous potential for PGE_2 production is surrounded by a protective envelope of chorion which prevents direct access of that PGE_2 to the uterine tissues. It may be, however, that that defence against PGE_2 is either withdrawn or overwhelmed in association with parturition. Nakla *et al.*[36] have shown that amniotic prostaglandins are capable of crossing the chorion and escaping the metabolic defences in late pregnancy.

In the light of the above observations it may be worth considering a local effect of amniotic PGE_2 being directed not generally at the cervical tissue as a whole but rather specifically and locally at a critical focus of tissue at the internal cervical os. This, after all, is the only part of the cervix with which the fetal membranes are in intimate contact, and the process of cervical effacement which is an essential component of cervical ripening might well be explained on this basis. A local softening influence at the internal cervical os would explain the progressive 'taking up' phenomenon of cervical effacement whereby the cervix becomes progressively shorter. As the internal os softens it might thus be moulded laterally around the intact forewaters, thereby bringing up the next portion of cervical tissue to the influence of amniotic prostaglandins. Whilst this concept is at best speculative, it accords with the commonplace clinical observation that absence of the fetal membranes adjacent to the cervix, as a result of either their spontaneous or artificial rupture, appears to hinder the process of cervical effacement.[37]

Smooth muscle biochemistry

Much of our knowledge of smooth muscle contraction comes from the study of non-uterine and other smooth muscles with respect to electrophysiological and pharmacological responses. There is increasing evidence that the elements and regulation of the contractile processes are common to all types of smooth muscle.

Myometrium is composed of muscle cells within connective tissue. Contractile forces generated by individual muscle cells are summated and co-ordinated. This is done through intercellular communication by means of areas in the cell membrane, called gap junctions, that facilitate ion and small molecule transfer. These important intercellular contacts are crucial to the conduction of electrophysiological stimuli and, so, synchronization of myometrial contractions. The modulation of gap junction synthesis by various hormones or other agents is critical to the onset and maintenance of labour: a certain number of these are required for labour to commence.[38] Increasing oestrogen receptor content is related to an increased number of gap junctions[39] while progesterone may inhibit synthesis of gap junction protein.[40] The effect of uterine stretching together with oestrogen administration is to increase gap junctions.[41]

Contraction of the myometrial cell takes place when the actin and myosin filaments slide over each other, thereby shortening the overall length of the filament. This action is caused by the formation of cross-bridges between actin and myosin filaments using energy derived from ATP hydrolysis. It can take place only when the activating enzyme myosin light chain kinase has been phosphorylated.

Calcium ions play an important role in smooth muscle contractions. Normally the intracellular concentration of calcium ions is considerably less than in the extracellular environment. Elevation of cytosolic free calcium leads to contractions. This can come about by calcium moving into the cell or being liberated in the free form from intracellular stores. Nuclear calcium concentrations are maintained independently of cytosolic concentrations, which is important for the maintenance of nuclear function.[42] Low resting calcium ion concentrations in cytosol are

maintained by calcium transport ATPase.[43] Calcium channels are either opened (activated) or closed (deactivated). Receptor-operated channels are opened in response to ligands such as neurotransmitters or hormones that bind to specific receptors associated with the channel. G proteins regulate calcium channels by coupling the channels and receptors directly.

Regulation of myometrial contractions

Calcium influx into the cell is detected by a protein, calmodulin, which binds calcium with high affinity. Myosin light chain kinase is a calmodulin-dependent enzyme which has a high affinity for the calmodulin/calcium ion complex. It catalyses the phosphorylation of myosin required for the contraction of smooth muscle. Cyclic AMP is important in the regulation of myometrial contractility, possibly by increasing calcium ion uptake into the sarcoplasmic reticulum and so decreasing free intracellular calcium ion concentration. The activities of adenyl cyclase and phosphodiesterase enzymes, which either increase cyclic AMP synthesis or degrade it respectively, are therefore important in regulating myometrial contractions. β-adrenergic agents inhibit myometrial activity by increasing adenyl cyclase.

Progesterone leads to quiescent myometrium. This is due to a combination of reduced cell-to-cell communication because of fewer gap junctions and an inhibitory effect on prostaglandin synthesis. A potent antiprogestin, RU 486, causes uterine contractions at all gestations.

Prostaglandins

Eicosanoids are produced by all uterine and intrauterine tissues. PGE_2 and $PGF_{2\alpha}$ are thought to be the most important prostaglandins involved in uterine contractions. Other cyclo-oxygenase products such as prostacyclin (PGI_2) can cause myometrial relaxation[44] but this effect is not its primary role. Lipoxygenase and epoxygenase products have also been shown to cause myometrial contractions *in vitro*[45] but again these are not thought to be their primary function. Prostaglandins are thought to cause myometrial contractions by the increased passage of calcium ions across gap junctions and by increasing the numbers of gap junctions. They also lead to the release of calcium from the intracellular stores in the sarcoplasmic reticulum.[46]

The synthesis of prostaglandins by intrauterine tissues and factors controlling these are therefore of great importance in initiating labour. Prostaglandins are synthesized by amnion, decidua and myometrium, and are largely metabolized in the chorion which contains large amounts of prostaglandin dehydrogenase.[47] Prostaglandins are local mediators which are produced close to their site of action and so it is logical that their production in the decidua adjacent to the myometrium would be important. As discussed earlier, production of prostaglandins by amnion and their passage across the chorion with its high concentration of prostaglandin dehydrogenase seem to be a less likely source of the increased prostaglandin levels needed to initiate myometrial contractions. However, it may be that increased prostaglandin synthesis from both tissues is important.

The initial step in the formation of prostaglandins is the release of arachidonic acid from its esterified form in cell membrane phospholipids, principally phosphatidylethanolamine and phosphatidylinositol. This requires phospholipases A_2 and C.[48] Phospholipase A_2 is inhibited by lipocortins.[49] The synthesis of lipocortins is stimulated by progesterone.[50]

Prostaglandin production from fetal membranes requires the availability of free calcium which is thought to act through the stimulation of phospholipase A_2 and C.[51] *In vitro* studies have shown that, by increasing intracellular calcium concentration, prostaglandin production by these cells is increased and, conversely, blocking calcium entry into cells reduces prostaglandin production.

Another factor that may influence or regulate prostaglandin production is an as yet uncharacterized substance called the endogenous inhibitor of prostaglandin synthesis (EIPS).[52,53] It is thought that this is a protein of molecular weight of approximately 60 kDa but this has not yet been characterized. Other factors present in fetal urine[54] and amniotic fluid,[55] which may or may not be growth factors, have been shown to stimulate prostaglandin synthesis in tissue culture. Protein kinase is of importance in relation to prostaglandin generation.[56] Steroid hormones such as oestrogen and progesterone produced locally within the fetal membranes may also modulate prostaglandin production by these tissues. An increase in oestrogen locally within the tissues could have a stimulatory effect on prostaglandin production, as has been shown in the case of PGE_2 by decidual cell preparations. Thus, whilst there is no obvious change in oestrogen : progesterone ratios in the circulation prior to labour there may well be significant changes in their ratio at a tissue level.[57]

The tissue source of prostaglandin production

from intrauterine tissues responsible for labour and the factors regulating it are not clear despite several years of research. Amnion cells in culture produce PGE_2 while the decidual cells produce both PGE_2 and $PGF_{2\alpha}$. The amnion consists of a uniform cell population but the decidua consists of stromal cells and bone-marrow-derived cells – largely macrophages. Both cell types produce increased amounts of PGE_2 in response to cytokines IL-1 and IL-6.[58] Ascending infection that is overt or a covert mild chronic inflammatory response will increase cytokine production from macrophages in the decidua, activation of cyclo-oxygenase enzyme in stromal cells and thence increased production of PGE_2 and $PGF_{2\alpha}$. This may be one of the mechanisms initiating preterm labour. The production of an endogenous prostaglandin synthase inhibitor (EIPS) by the decidua and its suppression may be important factors in the cascade of biochemical events leading to myometrial contractions.

Whatever controls the local increase in prostaglandin production by intrauterine tissues in term or preterm labour, there is little doubt that these compounds are central to the onset of myometrial contractions through the biochemical mechanisms that have been described.

Clinical application of prostaglandins

It follows from what we have already considered that prostaglandins should be good candidates for clinical use in cervical ripening and induction of labour. Ever since it became recognized that the condition of the cervix is the main determinant of successful induction of labour,[60] prostaglandins have been strong contenders for the optimum method. In assessing their efficacy, one of the problems has been the large number of small studies using different doses, formulations, routes of administration, intervals between doses, etc. Despite these deficiencies, analysis of the literature leads to the conclusions that prostaglandins are effective and that the incidence of side effects is higher with the use of $PGF_{2\alpha}$ than with PGE_2. The latter preparation is therefore always used when it is available. Comparison of intravenous oxytocin with PGE_2, administered by a variety of routes, shows that when the latter is used the uterus does less work because of increased cervical compliance and this leads to a reduction in caesarean section and operative delivery rate. There is no difference in the incidence of low Apgar scores of babies born of women whose labour has been induced with either prostaglandins or intravenous oxytocin. The large number of studies precludes comprehensive analysis in this chapter and the reader is referred to a review that covers the literature thoroughly.[59]

The use of prostaglandins for cervical ripening prior to induction of labour

The clinical objective of delivering a baby before it would emerge from the mother in the natural course of events may be desirable if it can be seen to benefit the baby, the mother or both. In some circumstances it is necessary to accept that benefiting one may compromise the other. For instance, the safe delivery of a jeopardized fetus may well entail subjecting the mother to caesarean section or other types of operative procedures, whilst in rare circumstances delivery may be imperative if the mother faces life-threatening complications and this may subject the neonate to the hazards of prematurity.

Direct resort to delivery by caesarean section is sometimes the choice but, most often, if delivery is indicated the obstetrician will wish to accomplish this by induction of labour. It is convenient for the purposes of this chapter to regard cervical ripening and induction of labour as separate clinical procedures but they should of course be considered simply as separate components of the same procedure. Thus the mother who requires delivery and whose cervix is already ripe will require simple induction of labour, whereas if the cervix has not ripened spontaneously a different clinical approach will be required which entails cervical ripening followed by labour induction.

In former times, failure to recognize the need for cervical ripening prior to induction of uterine contractility led to protracted labours and an unacceptably high rate of complications for both mother and offspring.[60] The higher the degree of cervical ripeness that can be attained before the introduction of uterine contractility, the easier will the labour be for both the mother and her baby. The past 20 years have witnessed a learning process during which the ways prostaglandins can be exploited for these clinical objectives have been refined and improved. Much of this learning process has concerned the search for the most appropriate agent, the most effective route of administration and the best vehicle in which to administer it.

Development

The intravenous use of PGE_2 and $PGF_{2\alpha}$ in the late 1960s for induction of labour fell rapidly into disrepute because of side effects such as diarrhoea,

vomiting, local erythema and uterine hypertonus. Extra-amniotic instillation of 300–500 µg of PGE_2 in tylose gel was used in conjunction with amniotomy in a few centres in order to avoid gastrointestinal side effects and to deliver the prostaglandins close to their site of action in the hope that this would have the maximum effect on the cervix.[61] This method did not gain widespread popularity because of the possible risks of rupturing the membranes and the fact that it was perceived as being somewhat invasive.

Oral PGE_2 became the next available therapy developed by the pharmaceutical industry as distinct from being made in the hospital pharmacy. This was initially in solution and then in tablet form used in conjunction with amniotomy.[62] The dose was 0.5 mg hourly, increasing to 1 mg and 1.5 mg hourly depending on the onset of contractions and progress. The dose-related side effects were vomiting and diarrhoea, and as a consequence the method was not particularly successful in those who required more than 1 mg per hour, i.e. primigravid patients.[63] For multigravid patients requiring induction of labour or for patients requiring augmentation of a labour that had started spontaneously, the use of oral tablets can be quite effective.[63]

To eliminate the problem of gastrointestinal side effects, the concept of administering prostaglandins vaginally was developed. PGE_2 was the selected prostaglandin in the UK and in other European countries because of its effect on cervical ripening which is an essential part of the process of labour and which is described later in this chapter. These effects are not seen with the use of $PGF_{2\alpha}$. Despite this, $PGF_{2\alpha}$ was the product developed in some countries such as Australia and South Africa because PGE_2 was not licensed there.

Vaginal PGE_2 can be administered from a number of vehicles. Initially, oral tablets inserted into the vagina were moderately effective, with no gastrointestinal side effects.[64] This prompted the development of a vaginal tablet containing 3 mg of PGE_2 in a lactose/starch tablet base. Concurrent with this development was the use in many hospitals in the UK of Witepsol-based pessaries containing varying amounts of PGE_2 solution which were made up in the hospital pharmacy. Absorption of PGE_2 from the tablet was much slower than from wax pessaries.[65,66] This is because the tablet has to absorb water before disintegration and release of PGE_2. The wax pessaries, however, melt at body temperature and so dissolution of the pessary is rapid and complete and blood levels of PGE_2 as measured by its metabolites rise more quickly. There were a number of cases of hypertonus reported following the use of pharmacy-made pessaries.

The use of 3 mg intravaginal tablets has been shown to be quite effective and to be safe.[67] However, to improve efficacy in terms of inducing labour within a shorter time, delivery systems with a more rapid but controlled release of PGE_2 were required. Gels for delivery intravaginally or within the cervical canal were developed and found to be successful.

The current range of prostaglandin products available for cervical ripening and induction of labour and in widespread use in Europe (and hopefully in an increasing number of other countries) are therefore intravaginal tablets or gel, intracervical gel for those patients with particularly unfavourable cervices at the time of induction, and oral tablets. The use of these will be described in more detail.

Cervical ripening

Interference with the normal course of pregnancy by attempting to induce labour requires to be justified by clinical indications; whilst that is true for all patients, it is doubly true if the cervix is unripe. This is because in such circumstances attempts to provoke labour are much more likely to lead to an unsatisfactory outcome with increased complications for the mother and her baby. On the other hand, if the indication for delivery is compelling, the prostaglandins, especially PGE_2, are highly effective in ripening the cervix prior to the onset of labour and thereby in reducing these complications.

Before prostaglandins were available for this purpose, a variety of techniques were used to try to ripen the cervix, such as mechanical stimulation using balloons and bougies or tents of laminaria. It is interesting to reflect that such benefit as these techniques produced may well have been the result of their provoking the release of endogenous prostaglandins within the maternal tissues. Others favoured the use of drug therapy, such as intravenous infusion of oxytocin over long periods although this was generally fairly fruitless.[68] Local administration of oestrogens[30] and relaxin[35] have theoretical justification and have been shown to produce clinical improvement in the ripeness of the cervix but they have been much less effective in this regard than PGE_2. More recently the antiprogestogen, mifepristone, has been studied and appears to show high promise in this regard although more extensive evidence is required.[69]

Whilst potent synthetic prostaglandin analogues have been exploited with great success for cervical softening in early pregnancy (see Chapter 6) and whilst it is almost certain that they would be very satisfactory for cervical ripening at term, they have not been used for this purpose, partly because naturally occurring prostaglandins are effective and partly because of the cost and difficulty of the fetal toxicology studies that would be required before they could be applied in a viable pregnancy. Of the natural prostaglandins, PGE_2 and $PGF_{2\alpha}$ have both been studied extensively and it is clear that PGE_2 is the more effective for cervical ripening. This is hardly surprising in view of an increasing body of evidence that suggests that PGE_2 may be the dominant prostaglandin during pre-labour, cervical ripening and in early labour whereas $PGF_{2\alpha}$ becomes dominant once labour becomes established.[70,71] In addition to its greater efficacy, PGE_2 also surpasses $PGF_{2\alpha}$ in causing fewer side effects.

The same observation applies in regard to labour induction when the cervix is already ripe. This may seem paradoxical in the light of the foregoing suggestion that $PGF_{2\alpha}$ may be biologically more important in such circumstances but this has recently been at least partially explained[72] by the finding that vaginal administration of PGE_2 leads to a rapid rise in circulating PGE_2 metabolites in the maternal blood several hours before the onset of uterine contractility, a phase of the process that appears to be associated with the appearance of PGF metabolites in the mother's circulation. Thus it would seem that exogenous PGE_2 provokes release of endogenous $PGF_{2\alpha}$ to accomplish its myometrial stimulant effect.

Route of administration

For the purpose of cervical ripening, local administration in the genital tract is unquestionably superior to other routes. There are three choices of local route: vaginal, endocervical and extra-amniotic. That rank order represents an increasing level of both invasiveness and effectiveness. Whilst extra-amniotic administration of PGE_2 in gel via a Foley catheter probably represents the most effective method of cervical ripening,[73] it is much the most invasive and consequently less agreeable for the mother. Vaginal administration is the most acceptable for the mother but, because of the decreased efficacy, a larger dose of prostaglandin is required.[74] The compromise of endocervical administration[75] represents a half-way house in terms of both efficacy and invasiveness, which has much to commend it. The choice of route should take account of the degree of cervical ripeness and other clinical features of the individual case. For most purposes, vaginal therapy will prove adequate whilst the more invasive routes may be reserved for the most unripe cases or for those who show a poor response to vaginal PGE_2.

Vehicle

A variety of vehicles have been explored for all the above routes of administration, including saline solution, lactic-acid-based tablets, wax-based pessaries, water-soluble gels, cross-linked starch polymers and sophisticated hydrogel polymers designed for slow release of the prostaglandin. The gels have found the widest favour and have been applied with success by all three local routes of administration. They appear to allow rapid absorption of the PGE_2. This might be considered a disadvantage, but clinical experience and laboratory studies have shown that, so long as the dose is limited to 2 mg PGE_2 intravaginally or 0.5 mg PGE_2 by the other two routes, this rapid absorption does not constitute a risk to mother or fetus.[76]

The hydrogel polymer approach has much to commend it and may in future prove especially suited to the endocervical route. Technical problems have been encountered, however, with vaginal use of such devices, largely because the *in vivo* release profile does not correspond to the *in vitro* pattern. Devices loaded with larger doses of PGE_2 have been associated with a higher incidence of complications, probably because of more rapid release than intended in certain physical conditions within the vagina, such as variations in moisture and acidity.

Administration of PGE_2 to ripen the cervix may of course be followed by the onset of uterine contractility, and if this happens in parallel with cervical ripening it will generally lead to a satisfactory induction of labour. For the majority of mothers, however, local administration of PGE_2 when the cervix is unripe will simply lead to a gradual improvement in the state of the cervix such that a further procedure (usually the following day) will then result in successful induction of labour. It is becoming increasingly accepted that the best choice for that further procedure is further prostaglandin therapy rather than the more traditional amniotomy and intravenous oxytocin infusion.[77]

Induction of labour when the cervix is already ripe

If the cervix is found to be already ripened, labour can be successfully induced by a wide variety of techniques. Even the fondly remembered 'OBE', which consisted of an assault on the mother's gastrointestinal system with castor oil, a hot bath and a soap and water enema, commonly met with some success if the cervix was very ripe. It has, however, been superseded by more humane and 'user-friendly' procedures. The most widely adopted of these has been amniotomy followed by intravenous titration of oxytocin. It is against the undoubted success of this technique that the prostaglandins must be measured. In general, comparison of intravenous oxytocin with the use of PGE_2 by a variety of routes shows similar results in terms of obstetric outcome as measured by the length of labour, the rates of operative delivery including caesarean section and the wellbeing of the fetus both during labour and after delivery. Where the prostaglandins score more highly is with lower rates of neonatal jaundice and postpartum haemorrhage and in the acceptance of the techniques by the mothers. Intravenous oxytocin, while undoubtedly effective, is unpopular with mothers who feel that it represents control of the labour by the midwife or obstetrician rather than by the mother herself. In contrast, prostaglandin-induced labours are often considered more akin to spontaneous labour.[78]

The large number of studies of varying size and design that have been published in the medical literature precludes a comprehensive analysis in this chapter. The reader is referred to the Oxford Database of Perinatal Trials where this extensive literature has been thoroughly analysed.

Oral PGE_2 tablets for induction or augmentation of labour

Study of the absorption of PGE_2 oral tablets given in a dose of 0.5 mg hourly shows that peak plasma levels of PGE_2 metabolite are reached by 45 minutes. Further doses produced uniform increases in circulating metabolite levels.[79] When oral PGE_2 tablets are used in conjunction with amniotomy and no contractions occur, increasing the dose to 1 mg and then 1.5 mg hourly is appropriate. However, the increased incidence of diarrhoea and vomiting with 1.5 mg oral PGE_2 hourly is significant (25%). The method therefore is not appropriate for women other than those with very favourable cervices and in conjunction with amniotomy[63] or as an augmentation of labour of spontaneous onset with or without ruptured membranes.[80]

Vaginal tablets

Release of PGE_2 from vaginal tablets is slower than from tylose gel or Witepsol pessaries and so the induction process is slower in the former group. Indications for the use of PGE_2 vaginal tablets are the same as for amniotomy and intravenous oxytocin, namely a fetal or maternal reason to terminate the pregnancy. However, the method may not initiate labour quickly. This needs to be considered when deciding on the management, and patients need to be warned of it. The dose regimen is one vaginal tablet containing 3 mg dinoprostone (PGE_2) inserted into the posterior fornix of the vagina. This can be repeated after 6 hours up to a maximum of four doses. Monitoring of uterine activity and fetal heart rate by cardiotocography is essential for 30–60 minutes after the insertion of each vaginal tablet to prevent the potentially harmful effects to the fetus of uterine hypertonus, which occurs rarely. A very small number of patients will not go into labour and will require amniotomy and intravenous oxytocin but it is virtually certain that the use of the vaginal PGE_2 tablets will have softened and effaced the cervix somewhat. The numbers requiring supplementary intravenous oxytocin will depend on how favourable the cervix is at the start of the treatment. If the Bishop score is 4 or more the percentage of patients requiring intravenous oxytocin to augment labour after only a single 3 mg vaginal tablet is low (approximately 10%). Oxytocin should not be used within 4–6 hours of the last dose of prostaglandin, to prevent a synergistic effect leading to hypertonus.

Gastrointestinal side effects with the use of PGE_2 vaginal tablets are very rare, and other side effects such as headache and flushing also are rare. On the other hand, there are significant benefits in that the amount of blood loss at delivery and incidence of neonatal jaundice are reduced by the use of prostaglandins compared with oxytocin. Finally, and very importantly, patients using PGE_2 vaginal tablets prefer the much more gradual onset of contractions and the mobility that they have during labour when compared with the use of amniotomy and intravenous oxytocin.[77] To improve the success rate by means of a more rapid and consistent release rate of PGE_2 from the vehicle, gel preparations have been developed.

Vaginal gel

This contains 1 mg or 2 mg of dinoprostone (PGE_2) in 2.5 ml of triacetin gel. The use of this preparation is gradually superseding the use of vaginal tablets. The product is packaged in a syringe ready for use, and its application into the posterior fornix of the vagina is simple. In primigravid patients with an unfavourable cervix (Bishop score <4) the initial dose should be 2 mg and in all other patients 1 mg. After 6 hours, a second dose may be necessary and in both groups of patients it should be 1 mg if uterine activity is present but labour has not been established or 2 mg if there is no uterine activity detectable. The gel must not be inserted intracervically. The patient should lie in bed for 30–60 minutes after insertion of gel, and uterine activity and fetal heart rate should be monitored by cardiotocography as in the case of vaginal tablets. The trials of this preparation have shown its efficacy and a comparative trial between gel and tablet preparations in primigravid patients with unfavourable cervices shows that the gel preparation is the more effective.[81]

Intracervical gel

This preparation contains 0.5 mg dinoprostone in triacetin gel. It was developed as a method of combining both cervical ripening and then induction of labour by inserting the PGE_2 gel into the cervical canal. It is not widely used in the UK because it is perceived as invasive. It is not always easy to get the gel into the cervical canal and there is often leakage into the vagina, as 2.5 ml of gel will not necessarily fit into the cervical canal if it is rigid and narrow. Finally, there may be leakage or direct injection of the PGE_2 gel into the extra-amniotic space, with the possible risks of uterine hypertonus. Studies carried out in Holland comparing the use of vaginal and endocervical gel have shown that there is no difference in the outcome between vaginal and cervical gels.[82] Given that the use of vaginal gel preparations pose fewer potential problems in administration, these should be preferred.

Special situations

Prostaglandins used for induction of labour after previous caesarean section

Prostaglandin preparations have been used quite frequently for inducing labour in women who have already had a caesarean section despite advice to the contrary in the data sheets. Of obstetric units in the UK, 67% will use prostaglandins for inducing labour in at least some cases after caesarean section. An analysis of their use after caesarean section in

Oxford showed that 74% of women induced with PGE$_2$ gel delivered vaginally. This is the same percentage as those who delivered vaginally after spontaneous onset of labour. The incidence of uterine rupture, which is the main anxiety in these cases, was the same as in spontaneous labour following caesarean section and was very small, namely 0.2%.[83] Interim analysis of data from a prospective randomized study comparing PGE$_2$ with intravenous oxytocin, both used with amniotomy for induction of labour after caesarean section, suggests that PGE$_2$ is more efficacious and reduces the chance of repeat caesarean section. However, the study needs to be enlarged before firm conclusions can be drawn.[83]

Use of PGE$_2$ with ruptured membranes

Oral tablets are an efficacious alternative to the use of intravenous oxytocin for the initiation or augmentation of labour in cases of ruptured membranes.[84] The use of vaginal prostaglandin preparations is stated to be contraindicated in cases of ruptured membranes in the data sheets. The reasons are theoretical. For example, there might be a leakage of the dinoprostone into the extra- and intra-amniotic spaces, giving uncontrolled release or loss of dinoprostone respectively. Another theoretical reason is that infection might be introduced by the insertion of the vaginal prostaglandin preparation. Data published on the use of prostaglandins in this situation suggest that it is effective and causes no problems. The use of prostaglandin vaginal tablets or gel in cases of ruptured membranes for the initiation or augmentation of labour is increasing and can be recommended.

Maternal preference

Uterine pain reflects uterine activity in labour. Measuring uterine activity during labour using an intra-uterine transducer has shown that women induced with vaginal PGE$_2$ gel had a longer pre-established phase of labour and a shorter established phase than those induced by amniotomy and intravenous oxytocin. Total uterine activity was lower in the PGE$_2$-gel treated group, reflecting the increased cervical compliance induced by the prostaglandins. Uterine activity during the 4 hours prior to delivery was the same for both groups.[85] This study illustrates the gradual onset of PGE$_2$-induced labour which is similar to normal labour and is in sharp contrast to the rapid onset of strong labour-like contractions working against a resistant cervix induced by intravenous oxytocin. It is this benefit that patients like. Secondly, the mother's ability to be mobile during the early part of her labour is physiologically and psychologically advantageous.[77]

Conclusions

In view of their crucial biological role in the control of parturition, prostaglandins are a logical choice for the clinical objective of labour induction. PGE$_2$ vaginal and cervical gel preparations are effective in inducing labour, particularly in those women with an unfavourable cervix. They do so with very few side effects. The time to the onset of labour is variable. Their use reduces the incidence of caesarean section, analgesic requirements and blood loss at delivery. They do not adversely affect the neonate. They are as safe as any other form of induction of labour after caesarean section and they can be used in cases of ruptured membranes, either orally or vaginally. Uterine hypertonus is an occasional and unpredictable side effect which necessitates vigilance by means of monitoring after the administration of each dose of PGE$_2$. Oral PGE$_2$ tablets are not now generally used for induction of labour because of their incidence of gastrointestinal side effects. They are, however, useful for augmentation of labour. Gel preparations administered vaginally are the best preparations available at present. Attempts to produce a slow sustained-release PGE$_2$ from a polymer base have not yet attained sufficient reliability for clinical purposes but represent a potentially useful future development.

References

1. Amy JJ, Calder AA, Kelly RW. Prostaglandins and human reproduction. In: Macdonald RR (ed), *Scientific Basis of Obstetrics and Gynaecology*, 3rd edn. Edinburgh: Churchill Livingstone, 1985: 255–303.
2. Danforth DN, Buckingham JC, Roddick JW. Connective tissue changes incident to cervical effacement. *Am J Obstet Gynecol* 1960; **86:** 939–45.
3. von Maillot K, Zimmermann BK, Mohanaradhkrishan V, *et al.* Changes in the glycosaminoglycan distribution pattern in the human uterine cervix during pregnancy and labor. *Am J Obstet Gynecol* 1979; **135:** 503–6.
4. Uldbjerg N, Ulmsten V, Ekman G. The ripening of the human uterine cervix related to changes in collagen, glycosaminoglycans and collagenolytic activity. *Am J Obstet Gynecol* 1983; **147:** 662–6.
5. Lindahl U, Hook M. Glycosaminoglycans and their

binding to biological macromolecules. *Annu Rev Biochem* 1978; **47**: 385.

6. Golichowski A. Cervical stromal interstitial polysaccharide metabolism in pregnancy. In: Naftolin F, Stubblefield PG (eds), *Dilatation of the Uterine Cervix: connective tissue biology and clinical management.* New York: Raven Press, 1980: 99–112.

7. Scott JE, Orford CR. Dermatan sulphate rich proteoglycan associates with rat tail tendon collagen at the d band in the gap region. *Biochem J* 1981; **197**: 213.

8. Obrink B. A study of the interactions between monomeric tropocollagen and glycosaminoglycans. *Eur J Biochem* 1973; **33**: 387–400.

9. Junqueira LCU, Zugaib M, Montes GS, *et al.* Morphologic and histochemical evidence for the occurrence of collagenolysis and for the role of neutrophilic polymorphonuclear leukocytes during cervical dilatation. *Am J Obstet Gynecol* 1980; **138**: 273–81.

10. Uldbjerg N, Ulmsten V, Ekman G. The ripening of the human uterine cervix in terms of connective tissue biochemistry. *Clin Obstet Gynecol* 1983; **26**: 14–26.

11. Danforth DN, Veis A, Breen M, *et al.* The effect of pregnancy and labor on the human cervix: changes in collagen, glycoproteins and glycosaminoglycans. *Am J Obstet Gynecol* 1974; **120**: 641–9.

12. Granstrom L, Ekman G, Ulmsten U, *et al.* Changes in the connective tissue of corpus and cervix uteri during ripening and labour in term pregnancy. *Br J Obstet Gynaecol* 1989; **96**: 1198–202.

13. Uldbjerg N, Ekman G, Malmstrom A, *et al.* Biochemical and morphological changes of human cervix after local application of prostaglandin E_2 in pregnancy. *Lancet* 1981; **1**: 267–8.

14. Ekman G, Malmstrom A, Uldbjerg N. Cervical collagen: an important regulator of cervical function in term labour. *Obstet Gynecol* 1986; **67**: 633–6.

15. Rajabi MR, Dean DD, Beydoon SN, *et al.* Elevated tissue levels of collagenase during dilatation of uterine cervix in human parturition. *Am J Obstet Gynecol* 1988; **159**: 971–6.

16. Calder AA, Greer IA. Physiology of labour. In: Philipp E, Setchell M, Ginsberg J (eds), *Scientific Foundations of Obstetrics and Gynaecology*, 4th edn. Oxford: Butterworth-Heinemann, 1991: 239–53.

17. Turnbull A. The endocrine control of labour. In: Turnbull A, Chamberlain G (eds), *Obstetrics*. Edinburgh: Churchill Livingstone, 1989: 189–204.

18. Challis JRG, Riley SC, Yang K. Endocrinology of labour. *Fetal Med Rev* 1991; **3**: 47–66.

19. Ellwood DA, Mitchell MD, Anderson ABM. The *in vitro* production of prostanoids by the human cervix during pregnancy: preliminary observations. *Br J Obstet Gynecol* 1980; **87**: 210–14.

20. Calder AA. Pharmacological management of the unripe cervix in the human. In: Naftolin F, Stubblefield PG (eds), *Dilatation of the Uterine Cervix*. New York: Raven Press, 1980: 317–33.

21. Lewis RB, Schulman JD. Influence of acetylsalicylic acid, an inhibitor of prostaglandin synthesis, on duration of human gestation and labour. *Lancet* 1973; **2**: 1159.

22. Sitteri PK, Febres F, Clemens LE, *et al.* Progesterone and maintenance of pregnancy: is progesterone nature's immunosuppressant? *Ann NY Acad Sci* 1977; **286**: 384–97.

23. Jeffrey JJ, Koob TJ. Endocrine control of collagen degradation in the uterus. In: Naftolin F, Stubblefield PG (eds), *Dilatation of the Uterine Cervix*. New York: Raven Press, 1980: 135–45.

24. Jeffrey JJ, Coffey RJ, Eizen AZ. Studies of uterine collagenase in tissue culture. II. Effect of steroid hormones on enzyme production. *Biochim Biophys Acta* 1971; **252**: 143.

25. Gupta JK, Johnston N. Effect of mifepristone on dilatation of the pregnant and non-pregnant cervix. *Lancet* 1990; **1**: 1238–40.

26. Radestad A, Bygdeman M, Green K. Induced cervical ripening with mifepristone (RU486) and bioconversion of arachidonic acid in human pregnant uterine cervix in the first trimester. *Contraception* 1990; **41**: 283–92.

27. Chwalisz R. Cervical ripening and induction of labour with progesterone antagonists. *XI European Congress of Perinatal Medicine – Rome, 1988*. Rome: CIC Edizioni Internaziolini, 1988: 60.

28. Kelly RW, Bukman A. Antiprogestagenic inhibition of uterine prostaglandin inactivation: a permissive mechanism for uterine stimulation. *J Steroid Biochem Mol Biol* 1990; **37**: 97–101.

29. Kelly RW, Healy DL, Cameron IT, *et al.* The stimulation of prostaglandin production by two antiprogesterone steroids in human endometrial cells. *J Clin Endocrinol Metab* 1986; **62**: 1116–23.

30. Gordon AJ, Calder AA. Oestradiol applied locally to ripen the unfavourable cervix. *Lancet* 1977; **2**: 1319–21.

31. Allen J, Uldbjerg N, Petersen LK, *et al.* Intracervical 17-β-oestradiol before induction of second trimester abortion with a prostaglandin E_2 analogue. *Eur J Obstet Gynecol Reprod Biol* 1989; **32**: 123–7.

32. Liggins GC, Forster CS, Grieves SA, Forster CS, Knox BS. Parturition in the sheep. In: Knight J, O'Connor M (eds), *The Fetus and Birth*. Amsterdam: Elsevier/Excerpta Medica/North Holland, 1977: 5–25.

33. Fitzpatrick RJ, Dobson H. Softening of the ovine cervix at parturition. In: Ellwood DA, Anderson ABM (eds), *The Cervix in Pregnancy and Labour: clinical and biochemical investigations*. Edinburgh: Churchill Livingstone, 1981: 40–56.

34. von Maillot K, Weiss M, Nagelschmidt M, *et al.* Relaxin and cervical dilatation during parturition. *Arch Gynakol* 1977; **223**: 323–31.

35. MacLennan AH. Cervical ripening and the induction of labour by vaginal prostaglandin $F_{2\alpha}$ and relaxin. In: Ellwood DA, Anderson ABM (eds), *The Cervix in Pregnancy and Labour: clinical and biochemical inves-*

tigations. Edinburgh: Churchill Livingstone, 1981: 187–96.

36. Nakla S, Skinner K, Mitchell BF, Challis JRG. Changes in prostaglandin transfer across human fetal membranes obtained after spontaneous labour. *Am J Obstet Gynecol* 1986; **155**: 1337–41.

37. Calder AA. The human cervix in pregnancy: a clinical perspective. In: Ellwood DA, Anderson ABM (eds), *The Cervix in Pregnancy and Labour: clinical and biochemical investigations*. Edinburgh: Churchill Livingstone, 1981: 317–33.

38. Garfield RE, Puri CP, Csapo AI. Endocrine structural and functional changes in the uterus during premature labor. *Am J Obstet Gynecol* 1982; **142**: 21–7.

39. Saito Y, Sakamoto H, MacLusky NJ, Naftolin F. Gap junctions and myometrial steroid hormone receptors in pregnant and postpartum rats: a possible cellular basis for the progesterone withdrawal hypothesis. *Am J Obstet Gynecol* 1985; **151**: 805–12.

40. Garfield RE, Gasc JM, Baulieu EE. Effects of antiprogesterone RU486 on preterm birth in the rat. *Am J Obstet Gynecol* 1987; **157**: 1281–5.

41. Wathes DC, Porter DG. Effect of uterine distension and oestrogen treatment on gap junction formation in the myometrium of the rat. *J Reprod Fertil* 1982; **65**: 497–505.

42. Williams DA, Becker PL, Fay FS. Regional changes in calcium underlying contraction of smooth muscle cells. *Science* 1987; **235**: 1644–8.

43. Wuytack F, Raeymaekers L, Casteels R. The Ca^{2+} transport ATPases in smooth muscle. *Experientia* 1985; **41**: 900–5.

44. Lumsden MA, Baird DT. The effect of intrauterine administration of prostacyclin on the contractility of the non-pregnant uterus *in vivo*. *Prostaglandins* 1986; **31**: 1011–22.

45. Bennett PR, Elder MG, Myatt L. The effects of lipoxygenase metabolites of arachidonic acid on human myometrial contractility. *Prostaglandins* 1987; **33**: 837–44.

46. Huszar G, Walsh MP. Biochemistry of the myometrium and cervix. In: Wynn RM, Jollie WP (eds), *Biology of the Uterus* (2nd edn). New York: Plenum Medical, 1989: 355–402.

47. Cheung PY, Walton JC, Tai HH, Riley SC, Challis JR. Immunocytochemical distribution and localization of 15-hydroxyprostaglandin dehydrogenase in human fetal membranes, decidua and placenta. *Am J Obstet Gynecol* 1990; **163**: 1445–9.

48. Bleasdale JE, Johnston JM. Prostaglandins and human parturition: regulation of arachidonic acid mobilisation. *Rev Perinatal Med* 1984; **5**: 151–91.

49. Flower R. Lipocortin. *Biochem Soc Trans* 1989; **17**: 276–8.

50. Croxtall JD, Pollard JW, Carey F, Forder RA, White JO. Colony stimulating factor-1 stimulates Ishikawa cell proliferation and lipocortin II synthesis. *J Ster Biochem Mol Biol* 1993; in press.

51. Okazaki T, Okita JR, MacDonald PC, Johnston JM. Substrate specificity of phospholipase A_2 in human fetal membranes. *Am J Obstet Gynecol* 1978; **130**: 432–8.

52. Manzai M, Liggins GC. Inhibitory effects of dispersed human amnion cells on production of prostaglandin E and F by endometrial cells. *Prostaglandins* 1984; **28**: 297–307.

53. Ishihara O, Kinoshita K, Satoh K, Mizuno M, Shimuzu T. An inhibitor of prostaglandin biosynthesis from human decidua: partial purification and properties. *Prostaglandins, Leukot Essent Fatty Acids* 1990; **40**: 223–6.

54. Strickland DM, Saeed SA, Casey ML, Mitchell MD. Stimulation of prostaglandin biosynthesis by urine of the human fetus may serve as a trigger for parturition. *Science* 1983; **20**: 521–2.

55. Mitchell MD, MacDonald PC, Casey ML. Stimulation of prostaglandin E_2 synthesis in human amnion cells maintained in monolayered culture by a substance(s) in amniotic fluid. *Prostaglandins, Leukot Med* 1984; **15**: 399–407.

56. Kniss DA, Mershon J, Su H-C, *et al*. Evidence of a role for protein kinase C in epidermal growth factor-induced prostaglandin E_2 synthesis in amnion cells. *Am J Obstet Gynecol* 1990; **163**: 1883–90.

57. Romero R, Scoccia B, Mazor M, Wu YK, Benveniste R. Evidence for a local change in the progesterone/estrogen ratio in human parturition at term. *Am J Obstet Gynecol* 1988; **159**: 657–60.

58. Khan H, Ishihara O, Sullivan MHF, Elder MG. A comparison of two decidual cell populations by immunocytochemistry and prostaglandin production. *Histochemistry* 1991; **96**: 149–52.

59. Keirse MJNC, van Oppe M. Comparison of prostaglandins and oxytocin for inducing labour. In: Chalmers I, Enkin M, Keirse MJNC (eds), *Effective Care in Pregnancy and Childbirth*, vol 2. Oxford: Oxford University Press, 1989: 1080–11.

60. Calder AA. The unripe cervix. *57th William Blair Bell Memorial Lecture, June 1977*. London: Royal College of Obstetricians and Gynaecologists.

61. Mellows HJ, Sims C, Craft IL. Prostaglandin E_2 in tylose for induction of labour in patients with a favourable cervix. *Proc R Soc Med* 1977; **70**: 537–8.

62. Miller JF, Welply GA, Elstein M. Prostaglandin E_2 tablets compared with intravenous oxytocin in induction of labour. *BMJ* 1975; **1**: 14–16.

63. Gordon-Wright AP, Elder MG. The routine use of oral prostaglandin E_2 tablets for induction or augmentation of labour. *Acta Obstet Gynecol Scand* 1978; **58**: 23–6.

64. Gordon-Wright AP, Elder MG. Prostaglandin E_2 tablets used intravaginally for the induction of labour. *Br J Obstet Gynaecol* 1979; **86**: 32–6.

65. Gordon-Wright AP, Elder MG. Systemic absorption from the vagina of PGE_2 administered for the induction of labour. *Prostaglandins* 1979; **18**: 153–60.

66. Castle BM, Bellinger J, Brennecke S, Embrey MP, MacKenzie IZ. *In vivo* studies using the bicyclo PGE M assay to assess release of PGE$_2$ from vaginal preparations used for labour induction. *Abstracts British Congress of Obstetrics and Gynaecology, Birmingham, July 1983*.

67. Kennedy JH, Gordon-Wright AP, Stewart P, Calder AA, Elder MG. Induction of labour with a stable based prostaglandin E$_2$ vaginal tablet. *Eur J Obstet Gynaecol Reprod* 1982; **13**: 203–8.

68. Lilienthal C, Ward J. Medical induction of labour. *J Obstet Gynaecol Br Commonwlth* 1971; **78**: 317–22.

69. Frydman R, Baton C, Lelaidier C, Vial M, Bourget Ph, Fernandez H. Mifepristone for induction of labour. *Lancet* 1991; **337**: 488–9.

70. Keirse MJNC, Flint APF, Turnbull AC. F prostaglandins in amniotic fluid during pregnancy and labour. *Obstet Gynaecol Br Commonwlth* 1974; **81**: 131–5.

71. Johnston TA, Greer IA, Kelly RW, Gallacher A, Calder AA. Plasma prostaglandin metabolites in human labour. *7th International Conference on Prostaglandins and Related Molecules, Florence 1990*, p 165.

72. Greer IA, McLaren M, Calder AA. Plasma prostaglandin E$_2$ and prostaglandin F$_{2\alpha}$ metabolite levels following vaginal administration of prostaglandin E$_2$ for induction of labor. *Acta Obstet Gynecol Scand* 1990; **69**: 621–5.

73. Calder AA, Embrey MP, Tait T. Ripening of the cervix with extraamniotic prostaglandin E$_2$ in viscous gel before induction of labour. *Br J Obstet Gynaecol* 1977; **84**: 264–8.

74. MacKenzie IZ, Embrey MP. Cervical ripening with intravaginal PGE$_2$ gel. *BMJ* 1977; **2**: 1381.

75. Ulmsten U, Kirstein-Pedersen A, Stenberg P, Wingerup L. A new gel for intracervical application of PGE$_2$. *Acta Obstet Gynecol Scand* 1979; **84** (suppl): 19–21.

76. Johnston TA, Greer IA, Calder AA. Prostaglandins and the induction of labour. *Curr Obstet Gynaecol* 1991; **1**: 221–8.

77. Kennedy JH, Stewart P, Barlow DH, Hillan E, Calder AA. Induction of labour: a comparison of a single prostaglandin E$_2$ vaginal tablet with amniotomy and intravenous oxytocin. *Br J Obstet Gynaecol* 1982; **89**: 704–7.

78. Calder AA. Reasons for and methods of induction. *J Obstet Gynaecol* 1991; **11** (suppl 1): S2–S5.

79. Gordon D, Myatt L, Gordon-Wright A, Hanson J, Elder MG. Radioimmunoassay of 15-keto-prostaglandin E$_2$ in peripheral plasma after oral administration of prostaglandin E$_2$ tablets used for induction of labour. *Prostaglandins* 1977; **13**: 399–408.

80. Massil HY, Baker AC, O'Brien PMS. A comparison of oral prostaglandin E$_2$ tablets with intravenous oxytocin for stimulation of labour after premature rupture of membranes at term. *Acta Obstet Gynecol Scand* 1988; **67**: 703–9.

81. Mahmood TA. A prospective comparative study on the use of prostaglandin E$_2$ gel (2 mg) and prostaglandin E$_2$ tablet (3 mg) for the induction of labour in primigravid women with unfavourable cervices. *Eur J Obstet Gynaecol Reprod* 1989; **33**: 169–75.

82. Oosterbaan HP, Corbey RSACM, Keirse MJNC. Induction of labour and cervical priming with vaginal prostaglandin E$_2$ gel. In: Keirse MJNC, Elder MG (eds), Special issue proceedings of a satellite symposium, *2nd European Congress on Prostaglandins in Reproduction, The Hague, 1991*. Amsterdam: Excerpta Medica, 1991: 13–22.

83. MacKenzie IZ. Prostaglandin induction and the scarred uterus. In: Keirse MJNC, Elder MG (eds), Special issue of a satellite symposium, *2nd European Congress on Prostaglandins in Reproduction, The Hague, 1991*. Amsterdam: Excerpta Medica, 1991: 29–39.

84. Magos AL, Noble MB, Wong Chen Yuen A, Rodeck CH. Controlled study comparing vaginal PGE$_2$ pessaries with intravenous oxytocin for the stimulation of labour after spontaneous rupture of the membranes. *Br J Obstet Gynaecol* 1983; **90**: 726–31.

85. Lamont RF, Neave S, Baker AC, Steer PJ. Intrauterine pressures in labours induced by amniotomy and oxytocin or vaginal prostaglandin gel compared with spontaneous labour. *Br J Obstet Gynaecol* 1991; **98**: 441–7.

8 Prostaglandins in erectile dysfunction

Otto I Linet

Erectile dysfunction (male impotence) is a fairly common and complex syndrome which involves many psychological and pathophysiological factors. Among the multitude of definitions, probably the most relevant is the inability to achieve and/or maintain an erection necessary for sexual intercourse.[1] According to one estimate there are about 10–20 million American men with erectile insufficiency.[2] Another assessment, from Germany, indicates that about 10% of sexually active men suffer from chronic disturbances of erection.[3] In the past two decades the evaluation, management and treatment of patients with erectile dysfunction (ED) have evolved greatly because of increased understanding of both the physiology of erection and the pathophysiology of erectile dysfunction. For many years, psychological factors were implicated as the main cause of impotence. However, in the 1970s it was increasingly recognized that an organic cause of ED is much more common than a psychological one. Today, an organic problem is considered to be the cause of 50–70% of cases of chronic impotence rather than the 10% range as it was believed in the early 1950s.[1] As an example, in one report including 1500 men with ED, more than 70% of these patients were diagnosed as having organic impotence.[4] In a follow-up of patients impotent for longer than 1 year a contributing organic abnormality was documented in 85% of them when sophisticated diagnostic testing was used.[2] In another report, 75% of patients with ED were found to have compromised arterial capability.[5] In general,

ED is a common problem in patients with diabetes, atherosclerosis, chronic renal failure and neurological diseases. Equally important in achieving and maintaining erection is a competent venous drainage system.[6] There is also a long list of drugs that may cause sexual dysfunction;[1] medications have been estimated to be responsible for impotence in up to 25% of patients.[7]

One of the most dramatic changes in urology in the past decade has been the introduction of intracavernous injection of vasoactive agents for both the treatment and diagnosis of erectile dysfunction.[8] The first report on pharmacologically induced penile erection with intracavernous injection of papaverine came from Virag.[9] The following year Brindley[10] induced erection with phenoxybenzamine. Self-injection of a combination of papaverine and phentolamine by patients in their homes followed.[11]

The first clinical experience concerning prostaglandins (PGs) was with alprostadil (prostaglandin E_1, PGE_1), which was reported by Ishii *et al.* during the Second World Meeting on Impotence in Prague, Czechoslovakia, in 1986; the paper followed in 1987.[12] Soon after this first report, another experience with PGE_1 was reported.[13] Numerous studies related to the use of intracavernosal alprostadil have since been published world wide.

Although only the combination of papaverine and phentolamine (Androskat®) was recently approved by regulatory agencies in Austria and the Netherlands, the use of vasoactive agents including alprostadil for

ED is widespread and several reviews have already been devoted to this subject.[14-17]

PGE$_1$ is the only prostaglandin at present that enjoys wide use for ED, and a considerable amount of clinical material related to its use has been accumulated.

Mechanism of erection

Studies of animal models and human volunteers have clarified many aspects of the haemodynamics and mechanism of erection.[18-21] During the flaccid state, the smooth cavernous muscle and sinusoids are contracted and the arterioles are constricted. Only small amounts of arteriolar blood enter corpora cavernosa and the venules between the sinusoidal wall and tunica albuginea drain freely to the emissary veins. During erection the smooth cavernosal muscles of the sinusoids and arterioles relax and the peripheral resistance decreases to a minimum. This induces a large and instantaneous increase in arterial blood flow. The sinusoidal compliance increases and the blood is trapped in the sinusoids. The relaxed trabecular walls are expanded against relatively indistensible tunica albuginea which compresses the subtunical venules, reduces venous outflow, elevates sinusoidal pressure and induces rigidity. The complementary phase consists of contraction of the bulbocavernous and ischiocavernous muscles, resulting in compression of the proximal part of the distended corpora cavernosa, leading to additional rigidity and further congestion of the glans penis. Thus, three factors – increased flow in cavernous arteries, relaxation of cavernous smooth muscle and restriction of venous outflow – are crucial for attainment of erection. However, the smooth muscle in the arteriolar wall and trabeculae surrounding the sinusoids is the controlling mechanism of penile erection.[19]

Both flaccidity and erection are controlled by the release of neurotransmitters, and this is an area that is still undergoing investigation.[20-22] The state of flaccidity is primarily the result of continuous firing of adrenergic neurotransmitters which exercise their effect via the α-receptors. *In vitro* pharmacological studies have shown that agents other than sympathomimetic amines are capable of contracting the cavernosal smooth muscle. Hence, prostaglandins such as PGF$_{2\alpha}$ as well as epoprostenol (prostacyclin, PGI$_2$) and PGE$_2$ at certain concentrations have contractant effects.[23] However, their actual role in the physiological mechanisms of flaccidity is unclear.

Control of relaxation of the cavernosal smooth muscle is more complex. The principal phenomenon appears to be inhibition of α-adrenergic tone. It is exercised by cholinergic and non-adrenergic, non-cholinergic neurotransmitters.[20,22] Vasoactive intestinal polypeptide (VIP), acetylcholine and histamine (acting on H$_2$-receptors) relax the smooth muscle.[21] In addition, various substances produced by endothelium may have either contractant or relaxation effects. Among factors with the latter effect belongs endothelium-derived-relaxing factor (EDRF), identified as nitric oxide or a related molecule and possibly prostaglandins.[20,22] The physiological regulation of the release of these vasoactive factors is unknown.

Adaikan and Ratnam[20] have postulated three interactive stages in the erectile process: (1) inhibition of the α-adrenoceptor activity by release of endogenous substances (e.g. VIP) and prostaglandins; (2) activation of non-adrenergic, non-cholinergic relaxant neurotransmission (e.g. EDRF); and (3) direct relaxation of cavernosal smooth muscle by other endogenous substances.

Physiology and pharmacology of prostanoids in erectile process

The potential role of prostaglandins in the mechanism of erection has been supported by findings that penile tissue is capable of generating prostaglandins and thromboxanes. Using [^{14}C]arachidonic acid as the substrate, it was found that human corpora cavernosa muscle homogenates produced substantial amounts of PGE$_2$, PGF$_{2\alpha}$, PGD$_2$, 6-keto-PGF$_{1\alpha}$ and thromboxane B$_2$ (TXB$_2$) *in vitro*. 6-keto-PGF$_{1\alpha}$ and TXB$_2$ are stable metabolites of epoprostenol (prostacyclin, PGI$_2$) and thromboxane A$_2$ (TXA$_2$), respectively.[24] Another study[25] confirmed that human corpus cavernosum tissue releases PGI$_2$; this release occurred in response to cholinergic but not to adrenergic agonists. 6-keto-PGF$_{1\alpha}$, PGE$_2$ and PGF$_{2\alpha}$ were also produced by human corpus cavernosum endothelial cells in culture.[26] Presence of prostaglandin 15-hydroxydehydrogenase, an enzyme that catalyses the initial reaction in the metabolic degradation of prostaglandins, was documented in human corpora cavernosa homogenate.[27] Different affinities of several prostaglandins for this enzyme were observed, indicating possible role of 15-hydroxydehydrogenase in the control of prostaglandin tissue levels. So far, there appears to be a lack of evidence that human penile tissue can synthesize PGE$_1$.[28]

Physiology and pharmacology of individual prostaglandins

Thromboxane A$_2$ (TXA$_2$)

A synthetic TXA$_2$ agonist as well as PGF$_{2\alpha}$ contracted isolated preparations of human corpus cavernosum and spongiosum strips and segments of cavernous artery at resting tension *in vitro*.[23] Using the same *in vitro* model and the same TXA$_2$ agonist, it was concluded that the main contraction-mediating prostanoid in human penile erectile tissues is a TXA$_2$ sensitive receptor.[29] It is of interest that the same TXA$_2$ agonist was studied on the electrically stimulated isolated rabbit vas deferens and found to potentiate adrenergic neurotransmission.[30] The actual role of natural TXA$_2$ as well as PGF$_{2\alpha}$ in the physiology of penile tissue needs further investigation, however.

Epoprostenol (prostacyclin, prostaglandin I$_2$, PGI$_2$)

The potential role of PGI$_2$ in the pathogenesis of impotence has been recently reviewed.[31] The penis of normal and diabetic rats was studied because the fine structure of the human penis is similar to that of the rat.[32,33] Diabetes is a major risk for ED: in diabetic human patients the estimated prevalence of ED is high – from 35% to 75% (for review, see reference 34). Penile tissues from normal (control), acute ketotic and chronic diabetic (streptozocin) rats were incubated and 6-keto-PGF$_{1\alpha}$ measured. The released quantities of this PGI$_2$ metabolite were the same in the control and the acute diabetic animals, whereas penile tissue from long-term diabetic rats produced significantly less 6-keto-PGF$_{1\alpha}$. Treatment with insulin reversed this diminished release of 6-keto-PGF$_{1\alpha}$.[35] Smoking is also one of the risks for ED.[1] Incubation of penile tissue from normal or diabetic rats with smoke extract resulted in significant inhibition of methacholine-stimulated 6-keto-PGF$_{1\alpha}$ production.[36] These findings support the concept that PGI$_2$ may play a role in the pathogenesis of impotence.

Results from the following studies indicate that the physiological role of PGI$_2$ in penile tissue deserves further investigation. In the *in vitro* study discussed above,[23] PGI$_2$ contracted both human corpus cavernosum and spongiosum strips at resting tension and did not relax these tissue preparations when precontracted by noradrenaline. On the other hand,

PGI$_2$ did not contract the cavernous artery segments at resting tension and it relaxed noradrenaline-contracted artery segment preparations. In an *in vivo* study on pigtail monkeys,[37] intracavernosal injections of PGI$_2$ in doses of 100 or 200 μg did not increase the cavernous arterial blood flow and a large reduction of the cavernosal compliance due to smooth muscle contraction was recorded. The authors concluded that PGI$_2$ will most probably not be beneficial in the diagnosis and treatment of ED. PGI$_2$ has not yet been explored in patients with ED. It cannot be excluded that PGI$_2$ may serve as a vasodilator in the initial phase of penile erection.[23] Furthermore, because PGI$_2$ is a potent inhibitor of platelet aggregation, the local release of PGI$_2$ may prevent thrombosis during erection.[31]

Alprostadil (prostaglandin E$_1$, PGE$_1$)

PGE$_1$ is present in a wide range of mammalian tissues and fluids, including the semen of fertile men,[38] and possesses a wide variety of pharmacological actions. The most important pharmacological action includes vasodilatation, inhibition of platelet aggregation, inhibition of gastric secretion, and stimulation of intestinal and uterine smooth muscle. Several reviews dealing with the pharmacology of PGs including PGE$_1$ are available.[39–42]

The *in vitro* effects of a number of drugs including PGE$_1$ and PGE$_2$ on retractor penis and corpus cavernosum urethrae have been studied in 12 different species of animals.[43] In most of them, both these prostaglandins had relaxant actions. In another *in vitro* investigation,[23] PGE$_1$ and PGE$_2$ relaxed human corpus cavernosum and spongiosum contracted by noradrenaline and PGF$_{2\alpha}$. PGE$_1$ was more effective in this respect. PGE$_1$ (but not PGE$_2$) relaxed noradrenaline and PGF$_{2\alpha}$-contracted cavernous arterial segments. An interesting experimental approach was used in another *in vitro* study.[44] After addition of PGE$_1$ (and also papaverine) to the human cavernous tissue specimens, the distance between the nuclei of epithelial cells was measured and found to increase in a dose-related fashion. This was interpreted as a relaxation effect.

In vivo changes in penile haemodynamics induced by PGE$_1$ were investigated by ultrasound and pulsed Doppler technique in 11 pigtail monkeys.[37] After intracavernous injection of PGE$_1$, in doses of 5, 10 and 20 μg, the cavernous arterial blood flow increased and cavernous smooth muscle relaxed; the degree and duration of this effect were dose-dependent. Thus, both *in vitro* and *in vivo* data document the relaxant properties of PGE_1 on smooth cavernosal muscle.

Safety along with clinical efficacy of PGE_1 were addressed in animal studies. The effects of six different vasoactive agents including PGE_1 on erectile response and histological change of corpora cavernosa were investigated after five injections given over a 6- to 12-week period in five rabbits at each dose level.[45] Though PGE_1 did not induce erections, there was no inflammation in the corpus cavernosum in four animals and only moderate inflammation in one. In contrast to PGE_1, injection of phenobenzamine or papaverine induced a greater severity and frequency of inflammatory reactions. In pigtail monkeys, papaverine (10 mg) was compared to alprostadil (20 μg) in a 9-month trial using 75 intracavernosal injections.[46] Elevated liver enzymes *in vivo* and marked histological changes with loss of normal architecture (fibrosis, increased amount of collagenous tissue, oedema, degeneration and atrophy of smooth muscle) were observed in the corpora cavernosa of animals treated with papaverine. No changes in liver enzymes and no evidence of fibroses at the injection site occurred in the PGE_1 group. Slight hypertrophy of smooth muscle was revealed, but to a lesser degree than seen in the papaverine-injected cavernosal bodies. These findings were confirmed by transmission electron microscopy. Papaverine induced an initially strong erectile response, which was maintained in two out of three animals. PGE_1 induced tumescence that was maintained in all three monkeys studied. In another safety-related study,[47] motility, fructose utilization and total ATPase activity of human spermatozoa were investigated after addition of PGE_1, PGE_2, $PGF_{1\alpha}$ and $PGF_{2\alpha}$ in a 100 μg dose each *in vitro*. Only PGE_1 had no effect on any of the parameters studied.

Systemic distribution, metabolism and excretion of alprostadil have been extensively studied both in animals and in man, and several reviews are available.[48–51] The levels of PGE_1 in mammalian tissues and plasma are low and reliable quantitative measurements are difficult to obtain. When administered intravenously to man, PGE_1 is transformed rapidly to relatively inactive metabolites. In healthy men 70–90% of PGE_1 is extensively extracted and metabolized in a single pass through the lungs, resulting in a metabolic half-life of less than 1 minute.[52]

In contrast, the pharmacokinetics of PGE_1 in penile tissue has been explored in only one study[53]. Twelve patients were injected intracavernosally with 20 μg of alprostadil. PGE_1 concentrations were measured in cavernosal blood 5, 15, 30 and 60 minutes after administration. PGE_1 levels were increased up to 900 000 pg/ml but decreased rapidly. The concentration of the metabolite 15-keto-13,14-dihydro-PGE_1 increased also and declined slightly during the study. No significant increases of PGE_1 or its metabolites were detected in the systemic venous blood. This finding is consistent with local PGE_1 metabolism. Lack of increase of PGE_1 or its metabolites in the peripheral circulation correlates both with the extensive metabolization of PGE_1 in the lungs[52] and with lack of systemic side effects in the vast majority of clinical trials after intracavernosal PGE_1 (see below).

It is presumed that the pharmacological effect of PGE_1 is mediated by inhibition of α_1-adrenergic activity in penile tissue and by the relaxant effect on cavernosal smooth muscle.[23,43,44] Inhibition of noradrenaline release from adrenergic nerve endings and inhibition of effector responses which result from adrenergic nerve stimulation have also been postulated in studies exploring PGE_1 in organs and organ systems other than penile tissue (e.g. reference 54).

Prostaglandin E_2

As compared to PGE_1, PGE_2 was shown to have similar, perhaps weaker, relaxing capabilities on corpus cavernosum preparation *in vitro*.[23,43] Only one clinical study appears to be reported which indicates that transcutaneous application of PGE_2 to patients was not associated with a therapeutic benefit.[28]

Clinical use of alprostadil in patients with erectile dysfunction

As alluded to above, alprostadil (PGE_1) has not been approved by drug regulatory agencies for the ED indication anywhere as yet. The current approved indications are: palliative therapy to temporarily maintain the patency of ductus arteriosus until corrective or palliative surgery can be performed in neonates who have congenital heart defects and who depend upon patent ductus for survival; in Germany and Japan, PGE_1 has been approved for treatment of peripheral vascular disease. Based on its diverse pharmacology, PGE_1 has also been explored with a varying degree of success in other clinical situations such as coronary heart disease, adult respiratory distress syndrome, pulmonary disease, organ transplantation and hepatitis; none of these later indications is yet approved by regulatory agencies.

Several different formulations of PGE_1 have been used in the ED studies that are reviewed here. For example, when investigators used alprostadil manufactured by Sanol Schwarz GmbH in Germany, they dealt with a freeze-dried formulation of 20 μg of PGE_1 per ampoule in a complex formation with α-cyclodextrin. Another formulation, manufactured by the Upjohn Company, consists of PGE_1 sterile solution (Prostin VR© Pediatric Sterile Solution), containing 500 μg of PGE_1 in 1 ml of dehydrated alcohol. In Japan, PGE_1 is manufactured by at least four companies. In most of the clinical studies of ED, the origin of the PGE_1 formulation is not given and, consequently, all data from published studies are discussed together.

Short-term studies

Short-term studies are divided into those with PGE_1 versus placebo and those comparing PGE_1 with other intracavernosal agents. The nature of ED in these trials varied and patients with psychogenic/psychiatric, neurogenic, vasculogenic, hormonal, drug-induced, anatomical or mixed causes were included. The causes of ED were diverse: bowel tumour resection, pelvic and low back surgery, cerebral infarction, spinal cord injury, hyperlipidaemia, arteriosclerosis, hypertension, venous incompetence, diabetes, hyperthyroidism, hypogonadism, alcoholism, antihypertensive drugs, smoking, Peyronie's disease and urethral injury. Besides the published data, undocumented use of PGE_1 for ED appears to be widespread.

The causes of ED were, in some studies, identified by medical history and physical examination or by additional non-invasive or invasive laboratory testing. Among the non-invasive tests nocturnal penile tumescence, penile biothesiometry, bulbocavernous reflex, penile brachial index and duplex sonography were used. Invasive tests included the intracavernous injection of vasoactive agents; rarely, more complex procedures such as arteriography were employed. Determinations of serum testosterone, luteinizing hormone, follicle-stimulating hormone and prolactin levels were made on occasion, together with routine laboratory tests.

The age of the patients is not given in all these studies. From the available data, the mean age was calculated as 56.6 (16–83) years. The duration of ED was given in only about half of the studies and it varied between 0.3 and 7.6 years.

The results of the short-term studies presented in Tables 8.1 and 8.2 were summarized as follows: for calculation of mean dose per study for all drugs, individual doses reported for each study were added and the mean calculated. In a study where dose ranges were given, the highest dose was always taken. The response to PGE_1 was defined as the percentage of patients who developed full erection capable of penetration and consequently of intercourse. The quality of erection was usually assessed by observation and palpation: in one study, the penile length, circumference and angle were measured.[79] The highest grade of erection was described usually as 'complete erection', 'full erection', 'capable of intercourse', 'completely functional', 'good response' or a grading of 4–5 on scale from 1 to 5 (from 'none' to 'full erection'). These descriptions were all considered as 'full erection' and used for calculation of 'percentage of patients responding'. Responses such as 'partial erection' or 'incomplete tumescence' were excluded from these calculations. In terms of side effects, if they were not reported (NR) this was regarded as a missing value. However, where it was expressly stated that no side effects were observed, this was considered as 'none' and zero was included into the calculation of averages and ranges. The definition of prolonged erection/priapism by individual investigators varied widely in terms of duration (hours) – see Tables 8.1 and 8.2. However, all reported cases of prolonged erection/priapism were taken into consideration regardless of the actual duration.

Short-term studies with PGE_1 and placebo
The results are summarized in Table 8.1. With the exception of one double-blind, placebo-controlled study,[64] all the rest of the studies were open-label with PGE_1 only. The total number of patients included was 2063. However, the actual number could have been smaller, as it is not clear whether some of the authors, after publishing their first experience, added further patients to the original count in subsequent reports (e.g. references 55, 71). The doses of PGE_1 varied from 2.5 μg to 100 μg, with an average of 20 μg per injection. In terms of efficacy the percentage of patients responding to PGE_1 (regardless of the PGE_1 dose), ranged from 33% to 100%, with a mean of 70.9%. (The 3.8% response to a 40 μg dose was excluded from calculations because this very low response occurred in patients who already had not responded to 20 μg of PGE_1.[55]) On close examination, patients who responded to PGE_1 did not show any greater response to doses greater than 20 μg. It is of interest that patients who initially did

Table 8.1   Short-term studies with PGE_1

No. of patients	Drug and dose	No. of intracavernosal injections	Patients responding (%)	Side effects (% of patients)				Reference
				Pain	Haematomas, ecchymosis	Prolonged erection/ priapism	Other	
71	PGE_1 – 20 µg	1	72	None	None	None	None	12
6	PGE_1 – 2.5 µg	1	33	NR	NR	NR	NR	13
6	PGE_1 – 15 µg	1	83	NR	NR	NR	NR	
210	PGE_1 – 20 µg	1	68.1	16.7 (8.1 at injection site; 3.8 during erection; 4.8 both)	4.8	0.95 (5 h or >)	NR	55
67 (not responding to 20 µg)	PGE_1 – 40 µg	1	3.8	NR	NR	NR	NR	
12 (failed PAP)	PGE_1 – 5–10 µg	1	100	8.3	NR	None	None	56
135	PGE_1 – 20 µg	1	62	'Limited number'	None	None	None	57
8	PGE_1 – 2.5–10 µg	3	100	None	NR	NR	NR	58
15 (failures on PAP + PHE)	PGE_1 – 50–100 µg	3	33	40	NR	NR	None	
120	PGE_1 – 5–15 µg	1	NR	NR	NR	9.1 (2 h or >)	NR	59
11	PGE_1 – 5–20 µg	1	100	None	NR	None	None	60
14	PGE_1 – 20, 40 µg	1–2	92.3	50	None	None	None	61
47	PGE_1 – 10 µg	1	80:1	4.2	6.4	None	None	62
447	PGE_1 – 10 or 20 µg	1	72	9.4	None	4.9 (3–6 h)	None	63
20	Saline	1	0	5	None	None	None	64
	Preservative		0	5	None	None	None	
	PGE_1 – 5 µg		55	55	None	None	None	
	PGE_1 – 10 µg		85	70	None	None	None	
67	PGE_1 – 10–40 µg	1–2	73	5.9	None	None	Dizziness 1.5% Collapse 1.5%	65
35 (pelvic surgery)	PGE_1 – 10 µg	1	100	5.7	5.7	None	None	66
41 diabetics	PGE_1 – 20 µg	1	70.8	24.4	None	2.4 (18 h)	None	67

Table 8.1   *Contd.*

No. of patients	Drug and dose	No. of intracavernosal injections	Patients responding (%)	Side effects (% of patients)					Reference
				Pain	*Haematomas, ecchymosis*	*Prolonged erection/ priapism*	*Other*		
32	PGE$_1$ – 20 µg	1	56	NR	NR	NR	NR		68, 69
149	PGE$_1$ – 5– 40 µg	1–2	79	40 total (24 unpleasant sensation, 16 severe discomfort)	None	2.7 (7–16 h)	None		70
550	PGE$_1$ – 20 µg	1 (24 patients with psychogenic impotence, 3 injections – 5, 10 and 20 µg)	70	22 (7 from injection, 11 during erection, 4 both)	3	1.1	None		71

NR = not reported; PAP = papaverine; PHE = phentolamine.

Table 8.2   Short-term studies comparing PGE$_1$ with other intracavernosal agents

Study design	No. of patients	Drug and dose	No. of intracavernosal injections	Patients responding (%)	Side effects (% of patients)				Reference
					Pain	*Haematomas, ecchymosis*	*Priapism*	*Other*	
Crossover	6	PGE$_1$ – 20 µg PAP – 40 mg PAP 80 mg + phentramine 0.8–1.0 mg	1	33 0 0	NR NR NR	NR NR NR	NR NR NR	None None None	72
Double-blind crossover	15	PGE$_1$ – 10 µg, 20 µg PAP – 30 mg, 60 mg	1	40 40	None 40	6.6 None	None None	None None	73
Double-blind crossover	61	PGE$_1$ – 10 or 20 µg PAP – 25 or 50 mg PAP 50 mg + PHE 2 mg	1	67.2 32.8 32.8	37.7 Tension (13.1 painful) 75 'Rare'	None None 1.6	None 9.8 (6–22 h) 1.6 (6–22 h)	NR NR NR	74
Double-blind crossover	12	PGE$_1$ – 20 µg PAP – 7.5 mg + PHE – 0.25 mg	1	91.7 50	75 None	NR NR	8.3 (11 h) None	None None	75
Double-blind crossover	25	PGE$_1$ – up to 50 µg PAP – 30 mg + PHE – 1 mg	4	100 100	80 41	NR NR	NR NR	None None	58
Double-blind crossover	15	PGE$_1$ – 10 µg, 20 µg PAP 30 mg, 60 mg	1	22 25	33 None	None None	None None	None None	76

Table 8.2   *Contd.*

Study design	No. of patients	Drug and dose	No. of intracavernosal injections	Patients responding (%)	Side effects (% of patients)				Reference
					Pain	Haematomas, ecchymosis	Priapism	Other	
Open-label	80	PGE$_1$ – 20 μg	1	78.8	23.8	5.0	None	SC injection – 2.5	77
	300	PAP – 9–60 mg		NR	None	None	17.0 (1 h or >)	Dizziness – 3 Hypotension – 0.3	78
Open-label crossover	12 (incl. 5 normal volunteers)	PGE$_1$ – 10 μg	1	100	'Some, more with PAP'	16.7 Drug not given	None	None	79
		PAP – 60 mg		100			8.3 (6 h)	None	
Single-blind crossover	129	PGE$_1$ – 5 μg	1	26	NR	NR	None	NR	80
		PAP – 18 mg		13	NR	NR	None	NR	
Open-label crossover	50	PGE$_1$ – 20 μg	1	PAP = PGE$_1$ in 58; PGE$_1$ > PAP in 30; PAP > PGE$_1$ in 12	38	None	4 (> 2 h)	Late pain – 2	81
		PAP – 60 mg			54	None	8 (> 2 h)	Late pain – 2 Dysuria – 2	
Open-label	10 13 11	PGE$_1$ – 20 μg PAP – 40 mg or less PAP – 40 mg or more	5 or >	80 53.8 72.7	40* 100 100	1 patient – drug not specified	None 7.7 (h NR) None	NR NR NR	82
Crossover design	38	PGE$_1$ – 20 μg	1	52.6	NR	NR	None	NR	44
		PAP – 40 mg		28.9	NR	NR	2.6 (hNR)	NR	
Randomized double-blind	43 76	PGE$_1$ – 10, 20 μg	Several	79.1	'A few'	'Several'	None	NR	83
		PAP – 7.5–60 mg + PHE – 0.25–2 mg		67.1	None	'Several'	5.3 (4 h or >)	NR	
NR	64	PGE$_1$ – 15 μg	1	65 of patients preferred E$_1$ vs	56	NR	NR	24 ↓ BP, 14 ↑ BP	84
		PAP + PHE – dose NR		25 of patients PAP + PHE	20	NR	NR	17 ↓ BP, 9 ↑ BP, Cardiac arrhythmias, 6 PGE$_1$ and 5 PAP + PHE	
Double-blind crossover	50	PGE$_1$ – 20 μg	1	46	45 'mild'	None	None	2 dizziness & headache	85
		PAP – 60 mg		14	44 'mild'	None	None	4 dizziness & headache	
Open-label crossover	34	PGE$_1$ – 20 μg	1	52.9	Present, but not specified	'Rare' (drug not specified)	None	Dizziness – 'rare' (drug not specified)	86
		PAP – 60 mg		58.8			5.9 (hNR)		

*Moderate perineal pain.
NR, not reported; PAP, papaverine; PHE, phentolamine.

not respond to papaverine[56] or the combination of papaverine and phentolamine[58] responded to PGE$_1$. There was no response to vehicle (placebo).[64]

Penile pain was the most frequently reported side effect. It was reported in from zero to up to 70% of patients in twelve studies.[55,56,58,61–67,70,71] It was reported as absent in two[12,60] and not reported in three observations[13,59,68] each. Excluding the not reported and 'limited number'[57] of cases, pain occurred in an average of 22% of patients. Haematomas/ecchymosis were reported as absent in eight trials,[12,57,61,63–65,67,70] not reported in six[13,56,58–60,68] and reported in four.[55,62,66,71] Thus, from the available data, the average number of patients with haematomas/ecchymosis was 1.7% (0–6.4%). Prolonged erection/priapism was not observed in nine,[12,56,57,60–62,64–66] not reported in four[13,55,58,69] and reported in five studies.[55,59,63,67,70] Accordingly, the average proportion of patients with prolonged erection/priapism was 1.4% (0–4.9%). With the exception of one trial[65] in which dizziness and collapse were reported in one patient each (out of 67 patients), no other local or systemic adverse reactions were observed or they were 'not reported'.

Short-term studies comparing PGE₁ to other intracavernosal agents

These results are summarized in Table 8.2. The design for the vast majority of these trials was a crossover design, either double-blind or open-label. The number of patients exposed to PGE_1, papaverine, or papaverine and phentolamine was 639, 691 and 276, respectively; this includes 5 normal volunteers who received single injections of both PGE_1 and papaverine.[79] Six patients were injected with a combination of papaverine and phentramine [?phentolamine] mesylate.[72] With regard to dose, the averages and ranges were as follows: PGE_1 – 18.4 µg (5–50 µg); papaverine – 43.8 mg (18–60 mg); and in combination treatment, papaverine – 31 mg (7.5–60 mg) plus phentolamine – 1.1 mg (0.25–2 mg). In terms of efficacy, the averages and ranges of responses (percentages of patients) were as follows: alprostadil – 62.1% (26–100%); papaverine – 43.9% (13–100%); and combination of pa-

paverine plus phentolamine – 62.4% (32.8–100%). PGE_1 had higher efficacy rates than papaverine in seven[44,72,74,80–82,85] comparisons, equal in two[76,79] and a little bit worse in two.[76,86] PGE_1 was better than the combination of papaverine plus phentolamine in four[74,75,83,84] and equal in one comparison.[58] Thus, it appears that alprostadil is at least as effective as both papaverine and papaverine plus phentolamine.

Side effects

Pain was encountered in ten[58,73–77,81,82,84,85] out of 16 studies. The average percentage and range of patients reporting pain were as follows: PGE_1 – 42.3% (0–80%); papaverine – 45.9% (0–100%); and papaverine and phentolamine – 15.3% (0–41%). Haematomas/ecchymosis were rare, being encountered in only six studies.[73,74,76,77,81,85] None was reported in patients injected with papaverine; on average they were observed in 1.9% (0–6.6%) of patients with PGE_1 and in 1.6% of patients with papaverine plus phentolamine[74] (this is the only available value). In contrast, prolonged erection/priapism were counted in the majority of the trials.[44,73–77,79–83,85,86] The average proportions of patients with this side effect were 0.95% (0–8.3%), 4.9% (0–17%) and 1.73% (0–5.3%) for PGE_1, papaverine and papaverine plus phentolamine, respectively. Systemic adverse reactions were reported only in three studies[84–86] and their incidences were low. A brief overview summarizing the short-term studies is given in Table 8.3.

The comparisons shown in Table 8.3 are crude because, as pointed out above, in a number of instances the data were not reported or the drug was not specified. The number of patients per study varied widely and in some studies the numbers were low; thus, incidents that occurred in just a few of

Table 8.3 A summary of all the short-term studies*

Studies	No. of patients	Mean doses	Efficacy (%)	Pain (%)	Haematomas (%)	Priapism (%)
PGE₁ only	2063	20 µg	70.9	22	1.70	1.40
PGE₁	639†	18.4 µg	62.1	42.3	1.90	0.95
PAP	691†	43.8 mg	43.9	45.9	None	4.90
PAP + PHE	276	PAP: 31 mg PHE: 1.1 mg	62.4	15.3	1.60	1.73

*The mean values are expressed in percentages of patients for both efficacy and side effects.
†Includes 5 normal subjects.
PAP, papaverine; PHE, phentolamine.

them translate into a high percentage. More patients were exposed to PGE$_1$ than to papaverine or papaverine plus phentolamine and it is not certain that doses used for all these agents were equipotent. Therefore, any conclusion must be reached with caution and one can get at best only an overall impression in regard to the efficacy and safety of these vasoactive agents.

Although the most frequently used dose of PGE$_1$ was 20 µg, it is not clear whether this is an optimal one because a formal dose–response study with several fixed doses of PGE$_1$ was not done. The only dose–response study exploring placebo (vehicle), 5 µg and 10 µg of PGE$_1$ suggests that doses lower than 20 µg could be sufficient with regard to duration of erection.[64] This study also showed that the latency between injection and onset of erection, as well as duration of erection, was dose dependent. Clearly, a dose–response study with several doses of PGE$_1$ in a well-defined patient population is warranted. On the other hand, some patients required up to 40 µg to obtain an adequate response[55,61,65,70] or even higher.[58] Over all the onset to erection was about 5–10 minutes and the duration of erection varied widely (see below).

In some studies it was shown that the response to PGE$_1$ in terms of quality and length of erection was dependent on the type of ED. The best responses seemed to occur in neurogenic and psychogenic causes of ED followed by cases with a milder form of arterial dysfunction.[12,55–58,64,65,70,71,75,86] ED in diabetic patients appears to be less responsive,[57] especially in those with diabetes lasting over 10 years and with a history of ED longer than 5 years.[67] ED due to venous leakage usually has a poor response to PGE$_1$ as well as to other vasoactive agents.[63,68,79,83] Patients with neurogenic ED seem to have a higher tendency to develop prolonged erection;[55,60,70,71] therefore, lower initial doses of PGE$_1$ are warranted. Patients with a history of endocrine disorders[57] and long-term heavy smoking[77] had a poor response to PGE$_1$.

Pain following intracavernous injection of PGE$_1$ is the most frequently reported side effect; however, it occurs also after papaverine and a combination of papaverine and phentolamine (see Tables 8.1 and 8.2). Pain after PGE$_1$ was usually described as a 'burning sensation' or 'tightness' and was reported to be generally mild and transient. In some cases, however, it may be of increased severity.[70,74,81] In one study,[70] patients with arterial pathology or venous incompetence had the lowest incidence of pain; the possibly low intracavernous concentrations

of PGE$_1$ were seen as a reason for lack of pain. The cause of the penile discomfort and/or pain is unclear. It is viewed by some as dose-[58] or concentration-dependent[75] whilst one group suggests that the PGE$_1$ molecule itself is responsible.[64,70] With regard to the latter, it is of interest that PGE$_1$ was shown to cause hyperalgesia in man after subdermal infusion[87] and also in experimental animal models.[88]

The haematomas/ecchymoses generally result from faulty injection technique; digital compression to the needle puncture site for several minutes may help to reduce the incidence of this side effect.[8,67]

Priapism constitutes the most serious concern with intracavernosal injection of vasoactive substances. The true incidence of this side effect with PGE$_1$ is difficult to assess because the investigators used different criteria for what constitutes prolonged erection or priapism and what is the acceptable duration of erection. The duration that was considered as neither prolonged erection nor priapism was as follows: up to 1,[78] 2,[59,81] 3,[10,63,79] 4,[61,67,83] 5[55,62,74] and 6 hours.[58,65] For example, in one study,[78] any erection lasting 60 minutes or more was immediately treated with blood aspiration and α-adrenergic agents. The majority of cases with prolonged erection/priapism occurred at PGE$_1$ doses of 20 µg or less. Taking all the available data from Tables 8.1 and 8.2 into consideration, regardless of the duration of prolonged erection/priapism, the overall incidence of prolonged erection/priapism was lower for PGE$_1$ than for papaverine or combination of papaverine and phentolamine. This observation is supported by data from Zentgraf *et al.*,[89] who reviewed the incidence of prolonged erection after papaverine and phentolamine from studies with large numbers of patients. The frequency of prolonged erection in studies involving groups of 100 patients or more was 10.5% (9.1–12.1) for papaverine alone and 5.4% (4.5–6.4%) for the combination of papaverine plus phentolamine. A prolonged erection was defined as one lasting for 3–6 hours.

Systemic side effects were rare and of low incidence: dizziness (1.5%,[65] 2%[85] and 'rare'[86]), collapse (1.5%[65]) and headache (2%[85]). In one abstract[84] undefined cardiac arrhythmias of short duration and both increases and decreases in blood pressure (unclear whether in systolic, diastolic or mean arterial pressure) were reported after both PGE$_1$ and papaverine plus phentolamine in several patients.

Over all, the values of routine laboratory tests were not significantly altered by PGE$_1$.

Table 8.4 Self-injection treatment with alprostadil (PGE$_1$)

No. of patients	No. selecting self-injection (%)	PGE$_1$ dose (µg)	Maximum no. of injections	Duration of self-injection (months)	Pain	Haematomas	Priapism	Other	Reference
210	112 (53.3)	5–40	Up to 90	Up to 8	None	9.8	None	10.7% faulty injection	55
47	30 (63.8)	Personalized	Up to 30	Up to 6	None	10	None	None	62
—	187*	13.1 (mean)	24	Up to 6	16.6	2.7	None	Haemosiderosis: 1 Deviation: 1 Fibrosis: 1	92
35 pelvic surgery	28 (80)	10–20	Up to 100	NR	None	None	None	None	66
—	11	10–40	25–70	3–16	9.1 unpleasant sensation	None	None	None	70
41	29 (70.7)	10–40	4–50 (estimate)	1–20	21	14.6	None	None	67
52	26 (50)	2.5–25.2	NR	3.8 (mean)	40 mild/ transient	None	None	None	93
550	275 (50)	5–60	More than 400	NR	None	None	None	Faulty injection: 'some'	71
72	35† (49)	10–40	Up to 180 (estimate)	2–28	2.9	None	None	None	94

Side effects (% of patients): Pain, Haematomas, Priapism, Other

*24 patients dropped out for various reasons.
†15 patients dropped out for various reasons within 2–12 months.
NR, not reported.

Experience with self-injection of PGE$_1$

Thorough instructions for patients who decide to enter a self-injection treatment programme with vasoactive agents have been developed and described,[14,15,17,90,91] and audiovisual programmes accompanied by printed material have become available for the patient. Initially, the patient will usually learn how to self-inject at the urologist's office, and at that time the optimum dose is established. At home the usual number of injections is one or two per week. The patient returns to the physician's office at regular intervals. At that time effectiveness and side effects of the intracavernosal treatment are assessed and the dose adjusted if necessary. Most importantly, patients should be strongly advised to call their physician if an erection lasts more than 4–6 hours.[17]

The results of nine studies reporting on self-injection therapy with PGE$_1$ are summarized in Table 8.4. In the majority of these reports the patients were at first treated with short-term PGE$_1$ in their physician's office and then decided to go on to self-injection treatment. Two reports deal with the self-injection phase only.[70,92] The mean percentage of patients who went on to the self-injection programme[55,62,66,67,71,93,96,97] was 59.5, with a range of 49–80%. Similar results were reported for other intracavernosal agents.[95,97] The dropout rate was mentioned in only two studies:[92,94] in one it was

12.8%,[92] and in the second one, 42.9%.[94] With the exception of one investigation,[92] the dose of PGE$_1$ was given in ranges. This indicates that the dose was tailored to the desirable expectation and need of the patients; it ranged from 2.5 µg to 60 µg. In one study[92] the development of subjective tolerance to PGE$_1$ was explored. At the beginning of the self-injection therapy, the average dose of PGE$_1$ was 13.5 µg and at 6 months it was 12.8 µg. This difference was statistically significant. In another report,[65] only 2 out of 25 patients developed certain tolerance to PGE$_1$ and the dose had to be increased. One of these patients had to be switched to papaverine. Over all, development of tolerance to PGE$_1$ does not appear to be a problem.

The duration of erection was dose-dependent and patients adjusted it according to their sexual desire.[55,71] The actual duration of erection with self-treatment is given in only two studies – as 1.1 hours (0.5–3 hours)[67] and 0–3 hours,[66] respectively. However, some investigators did aim for a duration of erection that mimics the physiological length of erection, i.e. about 45–60 minutes (T. Lue, 1991, personal communication; and[78,93]).

Discontinuation of the self-injection programme by some patients because of the return of spontaneous erection was reported from two studies.[92,94]

The number of intracavernosal injections per patient ranged from 24[92] to more than 400,[71] with a duration of self-injection from 1[67] to 28 months.[94] The incidence of side effects was small. The mean proportion of patients reporting pain was 10% (0–40%). An incidence of severe pain leading to 17% dropout was reported in one study with 72 patients.[94] In contrast, in a follow-up of 187 patients, no dropout was related to pain.[92] The overall incidence of haematoma was 4.1% (0–14.6%). In five out of nine studies, no haematomas were reported. A relatively high incidence of haematoma (9.8%) reported in one trial was due to a faulty injection technique in 10.7% of patients.[55] Not a single case of priapism occurred; this attests to the importance of determining the optimal dose in the physician's office before commencing the self-injection programme.

Multiple intracavernosal injections of papaverine plus phentolamine lead to fibrosis, nodular thickening or hardening of tunica albuginea and penile deviation.[89,98] Fibrosis was observed in only one study with PGE$_1$ and at a low incidence of 1%.[92] Fibrotic changes after papaverine and phentolamine were reported more frequently in patients,[89] and they were also documented in primates after papaverine.[46]

Based on the data presented in Table 8.4, PGE$_1$ appears to be suited for self-injection therapy. The side effect profile seems to be acceptable, but local pain was reported frequently after intracavernosal injection and long-term safety was not investigated systematically.

Alprostadil (PGE$_1$) in the diagnosis of ED

Many laboratory approaches, both non-invasive and invasive, are used for the diagnosis of ED.[1,4,6,8] One invasive procedure is the direct injection of vasoactive agents, including PGE$_1$, into the corpora cavernosa which is considered a dynamic test for vascular integrity. The injected drug bypasses the autonomic nerve system, acts locally as a substitute for normal neurogenic stimulation and affects the cavernous smooth muscles and arterioles. An erection results if arterial inflow is sufficient and venous leakage is absent. Penile vascularity is assumed to be normal if a firm erection results within 10 minutes of injection. Partial tumescence and rigidity in response to vasoactive agents usually indicates mild to moderate arterial or venous disease, or both. Excessive venous outflow may be suspected in a case of incomplete erection with early loss of rigidity.[79] In other words, if a patient develops a sustained rigid erection after intracavernosal vasoactive drugs, significant arterial or venous problems are unlikely

and further vascular testing is not warranted. In the event of a partial response, addition of sexual stimulation may potentiate the response to intracavernosal injection.[8,99] However, false negative results were reported in both venous and arterial abnormalities.[44]

A substantial number of short-term studies summarized in Tables 8.1 and 8.2 addressed the feasibility of using PGE$_1$ for diagnosis of ED either when studied alone[55,63,65,68–71,77] or in comparison to papaverine[74,76–79,81,86] or in comparison to papaverine plus phentolamine.[74,75]

PGE$_1$ was also explored in more sophisticated tests. Intracavernous injection of 9–60 mg of papaverine (300 patients) or 20 µg of PGE$_1$ (80 patients) combined with duplex ultrasonography was employed in a study of penile blood flow.[78] Results using onset of response, increase in diameter of cavernous arteries and peak velocity favoured PGE$_1$ in the diagnosis of impotence. In another study, the effects of PGE$_1$ (20 µg) and papaverine (60 mg) on penile blood flow was studied by colour duplex sonography in 34 men with ED. The results demonstrated that PGE$_1$ was at least as effective as papaverine in inducing increase in penile blood flow. The effect of PGE$_1$ on penile blood flow was also measured in 120 patients after 5–15 µg of PGE$_1$.[59] Functional changes in the penile arteries following intracavernosal injection of PGE$_1$ permitted accurate assessment of inflow disease and indirect assessment of venous drainage. The average peak blood flow velocity for the paired cavernosal arteries ranged from 7 to 58 cm per second. An average peak velocity of 22 cm per second following PGE$_1$ was designated as severe arterial insufficiency. These patients indeed had uniformly poor erectile responses to PGE$_1$.

Two groups of investigators combined the intracavernosal injection of PGE$_1$ with a ^{133}Xe penile washout test. Hwang *et al.*[100,101] conducted skin and corporal ^{133}Xe penile washout tests before and after intracavernosal injection of 20 µg of PGE$_1$ in 2 normal subjects and 8 patients with ED. Half-time clearance and blood flow were the main endpoints. These authors concluded that this approach may help in assessing the haemodynamics of both cavernosal and dorsal arteries and in evaluating the severity of penile vascular impairment. However, penile venous competence may not be readily demonstrated. Others[68,69] employing a similar technique and the same dose of PGE$_1$ also could not distinguish venogenic cases from others using the Xe-133 washout approach. However, they showed that cavernosography after intracavernosal injection of PGE$_1$ can be used to determine venous incompetence.

In conclusion, the use of PGE_1 in the diagnosis of erectile dysfunction appears to be well established, and its scope is being broadened. PGE_1 appears to be as suitable for the diagnosis of ED as papaverine and/or phentolamine.

Conclusion

Naturally occurring prostaglandins may play a role in the physiology and mechanism of erection. Both synthetic and natural prostaglandins in pharmacological doses affect the cavernosal smooth muscle. Several prostaglandins were tested in pharmacological doses *in vitro* as smooth muscle relaxants and *in vivo* in animal experiments as inductors of erection. PGE_1 induced relaxation of cavernosal smooth muscle and cavernosal artery from human penile preparations *in vitro*. In an *in vivo* primate model, the cavernous arterial blood flow increased and cavernous smooth muscle relaxed after PGE_1. PGE_1 is also the only prostaglandin that demonstrated significant clinical efficacy in treatment and diagnosis of ED when given by intracavernosal route. It has been extensively studied in both short-term studies and in self-injection therapy for ED. In short-term studies, PGE_1 induced full erection in 60–70% of patients. The dose used most was 20 µg though the only dose–response study done so far[64] indicates that lower doses could be sufficient. In crossover trials, PGE_1 appears to be at least as effective as papaverine or combination of papaverine plus phentolamine. Two studies[56,58] showed that patients who failed on papaverine and/or phentolamine responded to PGE_1, but the converse has also been reported.[65] In terms of side effects, penile pain (usually transient and mild) occurred in 20–40% of patients; however, pain was also reported after both papaverine alone and its combination with phentolamine. Haematomas/ecchymosis were reported in less than 2% of patients after PGE_1 in short-term trials, and were apparently due to faulty injection techniques. Haematomas also occurred after papaverine plus phentolamine.

The definition of prolonged erection/priapism in terms of duration varied considerably from author to author. Regardless of the actual duration of this adverse reaction, this side effect was observed, on average, in 0.95% and 1.40% of patients exposed to PGE_1 whereas after papaverine and papaverine plus phentolamine the mean was 4.90% and 1.73%, respectively (see Table 8.3). Even higher incidences of priapism after the latter two agents were reported

in the literature.[89] The systemic side effects were rare, which supports the concept of local metabolism of PGE_1.

Nine studies report on the use of PGE_1 in self-injection. Before the start of this treatment, the optimal dose of PGE_1 was established in the physician's office and the patient was instructed in self-injection technique. The PGE_1 dose was usually tailored to the sexual desire of the patient. The length of self-injection treatment was up to 28 months,[94] number of injections reaching over 400.[71] There was no development of tolerance in one large study;[92] in another one,[65] however, in 2 out of 25 patients the dose of PGE_1 had to be increased with time. The incidence of side effects was low. There was no report of priapism and only 2 cases of penile fibrosis were reported.[92] This compares favourably to the experience with papaverine/phentolamine.[89] The proportion of patients who opted for self-injection treatment varied between 49% and 80%. The dropout rate from self-injection was not systematically studied with the exception of two reports.[92,94] In one[92] the dropout was 24 out of 187 patients (12.8%), and in the other one[94] 15 out of 35 (42.9%).

The requisites for an ideal intracavernosal drug were proposed and indeed it was concluded that PGE_1 is a potential candidate for such an ideal drug.[14] It is also of interest that a panel of 23 experts[102] concluded that PGE_1 is a useful addition to the family of vasoactive agents for ED: the efficacy of PGE_1 was considered by 52% to be established and by 39% to be promising. Safety was judged to be established by 43.5% and promising by 39%.

There is, however, a multitude of issues related to intracavernosal use of PGE_1 that must be addressed in the future, especially if one considers the wide use of this PG outside its licensed indications. Long-term safety must be established in controlled trials. Formal dose–response studies with several fixed doses of PGE_1 both in naïve patients and in patients experienced with self-injection treatment are desirable. Comparison of PGE_1 to papaverine or to papaverine plus phentolamine must be carried out at equipotent doses and in consistently defined patient populations. For future studies, it would be helpful to have a broadly accepted definition as to what constitutes 'prolonged erection' and what is priapism. Subgroups of patient populations with ED who are more or less sensitive to intracavernosal PGE_1 should be recognized and investigated so that proper dose adjustments can be made. New types of formulations applied topically on the skin of the penis could be of great advantage. A combination of vasoactive drugs including PGE_1[103,104] may offer a better side effect profile and should be explored in more detail. Combination of sex therapy and intracavernosal injection of vasoactive agents[105] may offer better therapeutic results and a more comprehensive approach to the treatment of ED. Finally, a targeted drug development programme is needed for PGE_1 to obtain necessary efficacy and safety data for regulatory approval. This should be followed by development of training and information programmes for both physicians and patients for proper use of PGE_1 to assure patients' safety. Last, but not least, clinical exploration of other prostaglandins such as stable analogues of prostacyclin (PGI_2) should be considered.

Acknowledgements

The author expresses his sincere thanks to Byron D. McLees, MD, PhD, for critical review of the manuscript and to Arlene F. Behie and Cindy L. Shattuck for skilful secretarial help.

References

1. Whitehead ED, Klyde BJ, Zussman S, Salkin P. Diagnostic evaluation of impotence. *Postgrad Med* 1990; **88:** 123–36.
2. Padma-Nathan H, Payton T, Goldstein I. *Treatment of Organic Impotence: Alternatives to the Penile Prosthesis.* American Urological Association, Inc. AUA Update Series, 1987; 2–6.
3. Porst H. Die erektile Dysfunktion. Praxis-orientierte Diagnostik der erektilen Dysfunktion (ED) und therapeutische Konsequenzen. *Z Allgemeinmed* 1988; **64:** 325–33.
4. Padma-Nathan H, Goldstein I, Krane RJ. Evaluation of the impotent patient. *Semin Urol* 1986; **4:** 225–32.
5. Lue TF. Evaluation and treatment of impotence – where are we going? *West J Med* 1985; **142:** 546.
6. Mueller SC, Lue TF. Evaluation of vasculogenic impotence. *Urol Clin North Am* 1988; **15:** 65–76.
7. Lue TF. Pharmacology of erection and impotence. In: Tanagho EA, Lue TF, McClure RD (eds), *Contemporary Management of Impotence and Infertility.* Baltimore: Williams & Wilkins, 1988: 51–4.
8. Lue TF. Intracavernous drug administration: its role in diagnosis and treatment of impotence. *Semin Urol* 1990; **8:** 100–6.
9. Virag R. Intracavernous injection of papaverine for erectile failure. *Lancet* 1982; **2:** 938.
10. Brindley GS. Cavernosal alpha-blockage: a new technique for investigating and treating erectile impotence. *Br J Psychiatry* 1983; **143:** 322–37.
11. Zorgniotti AW, Lefleur RS. Auto-injection of corpus cavernosum with a vasoactive drug combination for vasculogenic impotence. *J Urol* 1985; **133:** 39–41.
12. Ishii N, Watanabe H, Irisawa C, *et al.* Studies on male sexual impotence report 18: therapeutic trial with prostaglandin E_1 for organic impotence. *J Japanese Soc Urol* 1986; **77:** 954–62.
13. Virag R, Adaikan PG. Effects of prostaglandin E_1 on penile erection and erectile failure. *J Urol* 1987; **137:** 1010.
14. Wein AJ, Malloy TR, Hanno PM. Intracavernosal injection programs. *Probl Urol* 1987; **1:** 496–506.
15. Sidi AA. Vasoactive intracavernous pharmacotherapy. *Urol Clin North Am* 1988; **15:** 95–101.
16. Jünemann K-P, Alken P. Pharmacotherapy of erectile dysfunction: a review. *Int J Impotence Res* 1989; **1:** 71–93.
17. Bénard F, Lue TF. Self-administration in the pharmacological treatment of impotence. *Drugs* 1990; **39:** 394–8.
18. Lue TF, Tanagho EA. Physiology of erection and pharmacological management of impotence. *J Urol* 1987; **137:** 829–36.
19. Lue TF, Tanagho EA, McClure RD. Functional anatomy and mechanism of penile erection. In: Lue TF, Tanagho EA, McClure RD (eds), *Contemporary Management of Impotence and Infertility.* Baltimore: Williams & Wilkins, 1988; 39–51.
20. Adaikan PG, Ratnam SS. Pharmacology of penile erection in humans. *Cardiovasc Intervent Radiol* 1988; **11:** 191–4.
21. Buvat J. Intrapenile neurotransmission. *Ann Urol* 1989; **23:** 359–66.
22. Krane RJ, Goldstein I, Saenz de Tejada I. Impotence. *N Engl J Med* 1989; **321:** 1648–59.
23. Hedlund H, Andersson K-E. Contraction and relaxation induced by some prostanoids in isolated human penile erectile tissue and cavernous artery. *J Urol* 1985; **134:** 1245–50.
24. Roy AC, Tan SM, Kottegoda SR, Ratnam SS. Ability of human corpora cavernosa muscle to generate prostaglandins and thromboxanes *in vitro*. *IRCS J Med Sci* 1984; **12:** 608–9.
25. Jeremy JY, Morgan RJ, Mikhailidis DP, Dandona P. Prostacyclin synthesis by the corpora cavernosa of the human penis: evidence for muscarinic control and pathological implications. *Prostaglandins Leukot Med* 1986; **23:** 211–16.
26. Saenz de Tejada I, Carson MP, Taylor L, Polgar P, Goldstein I. Prostaglandin production by human corpus cavernosum endothelial cells (HCC EC) in culture. *J Urol* 1988; **139:** 252A.
27. Roy AC, Adaikan PG, Sen DK, Ratnam SS. Prostaglandin 15-hydroxy-dehydrogenase activity in human penile corpora cavernosa and its significance in

prostaglandin-mediated penile erection. *Br J Urol* 1989; **64**: 180–2.

28. Mikhailidis DP, Jeremy JY, Shoukry K, Virag R. Eicosanoids, impotence and pharmacologically induced erection. *Prostaglandins, Leukot Essent Fatty Acids* 1990; **40**: 239–42.

29. Hedlund H, Andersson K-E, Fovaeus M, Holmquist F, Uski T. Characterization of contraction-mediating prostanoid receptors in human penile erectile tissues. *J Urol* 1989; **141**: 182–6.

30. Trachte GJ. Thromboxane agonist (U46619) potentiates norepinephrine efflux from adrenergic nerves. *J Pharmacol Exp Ther* 1986; **237**: 473–7.

31. Jeremy JY, Mikhailidis DP. Prostaglandins and the penis: possible role in the pathogenesis and treatment of impotence. *Sexual Marital Ther* 1990; **5**: 155–65.

32. Crowe R, Lincoln J, Blacklay PF, *et al.* Vasoactive intestinal polypeptide-like immunoreactive nerves in diabetic penis. A comparison between streptozotocin-treated rats and man. *Diabetes* 1983; **32**: 1075–7.

33. Benson GS, McConnel J, Lipshultz LI. Neuromorphology and neuropharmacology of the human penis. *J Clin Invest* 1980; **65**: 506–13.

34. McCulloch DK, Campbell IW, Wu FC, Prescott RJ, Clarke BF. The prevalence of diabetic impotence. *Diabetologia* 1980; **18**: 279–83.

35. Jeremy JY, Thompson CS, Mikhailidis DP, Dandona P. Experimental diabetes mellitus inhibits prostacyclin synthesis by the rat penis: pathological implications. *Diabetologia* 1985; **28**: 365–8.

36. Jeremy JY, Mikhailidis DP, Thompson CS, Dandona P. The effect of cigarette smoke and diabetes mellitus on muscarinic stimulation of prostacyclin synthesis by the rat penis. *Diabetes Res* 1986; **3**: 467–9.

37. Bosch RJLH, Benard F, Aboseif SR, *et al.* Changes in penile hemodynamics after intracavernous injection of prostaglandin E_1 and prostaglandin I_2 in pigtailed monkeys. *Int J Impotence Res* 1989; **1**: 211–21.

38. Templeton AA, Cooper I, Kelly RW. Prostaglandin concentrations in the semen of fertile men. *J Reprod Fertil* 1978; **52**: 147–50.

39. Bergström S, Carlson LA, Weeks JR. The prostaglandins: a family of biologically active lipids. *Pharmacol Rev* 1968; **20**: 1–48.

40. Higgins CB, Braunwald E. The prostaglandins. Biochemical, physiologic and clinical considerations. *Am J Med* 1972; **53**: 92–112.

41. Weeks JR. Prostaglandins. *Annu Rev Pharmacol* 1972; **12**: 317–36.

42. Horton EW. Prostaglandins. In: Gilliland I, Peder M (eds), *The Scientific Basis of Medicine Annual Reviews*. London: Athlone Press, 1973: 58–79.

43. Klinge E, Sjöstrand NO. Comparative study of some isolated mammalian smooth muscle effectors of penile erection. *Acta Physiol Scand* 1977; **100**: 354–67.

44. Tamura M, Hasine K, Kimura K, Kawanishi Y, Imagawa A. Comparison of the effect of papaverine hydrochloride and prostaglandin E_1 on human corpus cavernosum. *Int J Impotence Res* 1990; **2**, suppl 1: 141–5.

45. Stackl W, Loupal G, Holzmann A. Intracavernous injection of vasoactive drugs in the rabbit. *Urol Res* 1988; **16**: 455–8.

46. Aboseif SR, Breza J, Bosch RJLH, *et al.* Local and systemic effects of chronic intracavernous injection of papaverine, prostaglandin E_1, and saline in primates. *J Urol* 1989; **142**: 403–8.

47. Didolkar AK, Roychowdhury D. Effects of prostaglandins E-1, E-2, F-1a and F-2a on human sperm motility. *Andrologia* 1980; **12**: 135–40.

48. Piper PJ. Distribution and metabolism. In: Cuthbert MF (ed), *The Prostaglandins*. London: Heinemann Medical, 1973: 125–50.

49. Granström E, Samuelsson B. Quantitative measurement of prostaglandins and thromboxanes: general considerations. In: Frölich JC (ed), *Advances in Prostaglandin and Thromboxane Research*, vol 5. New York: Raven Press, 1978: 1.

50. Green K, Hamberg M, Samuelsson B, Smigel M, Frölich JC. Measurement of prostaglandins, thromboxanes, prostacyclin and their metabolites by gas liquid chromatography–mass spectrometry. In: Frölich JC (ed), *Advances in Prostaglandin and Thromboxane Research*, vol 5. New York: Raven Press, 1978: 39–94.

51. Rosenkranz B, Fischer C, Boeynaems J-M, Frölich JC. Metabolic disposition of prostaglandin E_1 in man. *Biochim Biophys Acta* 1983; **750**: 231–6.

52. Hammon GL, Cronau LH, Whittaker D, Gillis CN. Fate of prostaglandins E_1 and A_1 in the human pulmonary circulation. *Surgery* 1977; **81**: 716–22.

53. Van Ahlen H, Peskar BA, Sticht G. Pharmakokinetik vasoaktiver Substanzen bei der Schwellkorperinjektionstherapie. *11th International Symposium.* February 22–24, 1990, Vienna, Austria, Abstracts.

54. Kadowitz PJ, Sweet CS, Brody MJ. Blockade of adrenergic vasoconstrictor responses in the dog by prostaglandins E_1 and A_1. *J Pharmacol Exp Ther* 1971; **170**: 563–72.

55. Stackl W, Hasun R, Marberger M. Intracavernous injection of prostaglandin E_1 in impotent men. *J Urol* 1988; **140**: 66–8.

56. Reiss H. Use of prostaglandin E_1 for papaverine-failed erections. *Urology* 1989; **33**: 15–16.

57. Ishii N, Watanabe H, Irisawa C, *et al.* Intracavernous injection of prostaglandin E_1 for the treatment of erectile impotence. *J Urol* 1989; **141**: 323–5.

58. Lee LM, Stevenson RWD, Szasz G. Prostaglandin E_1 versus phentolamine/papaverine for the treatment of erectile impotence: a double-blind comparison. *J Urol* 1989; **141**: 549–50.

59. Broderick GA, Lue TF. Penile blood flow study and the diagnostic use of prostaglandin E₁: a review of 120 patients. *J Urol* 1989; **141**: 288A.

60. Puppo P, DeRose AF, Pittaluga P. La farmacoerezione con PGE₁; studio preliminare. *VI Congresso Nazionale Società Italian di Andrologia*, May 13, 1989, Florence, Italy, Abstracts, 179–84.

61. Quadraccia A, Castellani R, Salvini A, Baresi A. La prostaglandina E₁ nei disturbi dell'erezione. *VI Congresso Nazionale Società Italian di Andrologia*, May 13, 1989, Florence, Italy, Abstracts, 185–91.

62. Beretta G, Zanollo A, Ascani L, Re B. Prostaglandin E₁ in the therapy of erectile deficiency. *Acta Eur Fertil* 1989; **20**: 305–8.

63. Porst H. Prostaglandin E₁ in erectile dysfunction. *Urologe [A]* 1989; **28**: 94–8.

64. Schramek P, Waldhauser M. Dose-dependent effect and side-effect of prostaglandin E₁ in erectile dysfunction. *Br J Clin Pharmacol* 1989; **28**: 567–71.

65. Rauchenwald M, Petritsch PH, Stenzl A. Unsere Erfahrungen mit dem Prostaglandin E₁-SKAT-TEST. Eine neue Form der Skat-Applikation. *11th International Symposium*, 1990, Vienna, Austria, Abstracts.

66. Stackl W, Hasum R. Impotenztherapie mit Prostaglandin E₁ nach Operationen im kleinen Becken. *11th International Symposium*, 1990, Vienna, Austria, Abstracts.

67. Ravnik-Oblak M, Oblak C, Vodušek DB, Kristl V, Ziherl S. Intracavernous injection of prostaglandin E₁ in impotent diabetic men. *Int J Impotence Res* 1990; **2**: 143–50.

68. Ishigooka M, Irisawa C, Watanabe H, Kubota Y, Ishii N. Intracavernous injection of prostaglandin E₁: the diagnosis of venogenic impotence. *Int J Impotence Res* 1990; **2**, suppl 1: 123–5.

69. Ishigooka M, Irisawa C, Watanabe H, Adachi M, Ishii N, Nakada T. Intracavernous injection of prostaglandin E₁: the application to cavernosography and penile blood flow measurement for the diagnosis of venogenic impotence. *Urologia Int* 1991; **46**: 193–6.

70. Schramek P, Dorninger R, Waldhauser M, Konecny P, Porpaczy P. Prostaglandin E₁ in erectile dysfunction. Efficiency and incidence of priapism. *Br J Urol* 1990; **65**: 68–71.

71. Stackl W, Hasun R, Marberger M. The use of prostaglandin E₁ for diagnosis and treatment of erectile dysfunction. *World J Urol* 1990; **8**: 84–6.

72. Yasumoto R, Asakawa M, Kawashima H, *et al.* Intracavernous injection of vasoactive drugs for treating erectile impotence. *Arch Urol (Japan)* 1988; **34**: 301–4.

73. Hudnall CH, Erickson DR, Sarosdy MF. Evaluation of intracorporeal prostaglandin E-1 in the treatment of impotence – a pilot study. *J Urol* 1988; **139**: 252A.

74. Porst H. Comparative usefulness of prostaglandin E₁, papaverine and papaverine/phentolamine for the diagnosis of erectile dysfunction in 61 patients. *Urologe [A]* 1988; **27**: 22–6.

75. Waldhauser M, Schramek P. Efficiency and side effects of prostaglandin E₁ in the treatment of erectile dysfunction. *J Urol* 1988; **140**: 525–7.

76. Sarosdy MF, Hudnall CH, Erickson DR, Hardin TC, Novicki DE. A prospective double-blind trial of intracorporeal papaverine versus prostaglandin E₁ in the treatment of impotence. *J Urol* 1989; **141**: 551–3.

77. Hwang TI-S, Yang C-R, Wang S-J, *et al.* Impotence evaluated by the use of prostaglandin E₁. *J Urol* 1989; **141**: 1357–9.

78. Hwang TI-S, Lue TF, Yang C-R, *et al. J Formosan Med Ass* 1989; **88**: 1038–41.

79. Siraj QH, Akhtar MA. Intracavernosal injection of pharmacological agents in the diagnosis and treatment of impotence. *J Pakistan Med Ass* 1991; **41**: 181.

80. Earle CM, Keogh EJ, Wisniewski ZS, *et al.* Prostaglandin E₁ therapy for impotence, comparison with papaverine. *J Urol* 1990; **143**: 57–9.

81. Chiang H-S, Wen T-C, Wu C-C, Chiang W-H. Prostaglandin E₁ versus papaverine for diagnosis of erectile dysfunction. *Int J Impotence Res* 1990; **2**, suppl 1: 127–30.

82. Imagawa A, Miyamoto T, Tamura M, Yuasa M. Therapeutic intracavernous injection of a vasoactive drug for mild arterial impotence. *Int J Impotence Res* 1990; **2**, suppl 1: 131–4.

83. Liu SM-C, Lin JS-N. Treatment of impotence: comparison between the efficacy and safety of intracavernous injection of papaverine plus phentolamine (regitine) and prostaglandin E₁. *Int J Impotence Res* 1990; **2**, suppl 1: 147–57.

84. Raboy A, Combs A, Godec CJ, Irwin M, Grunberger I. Comparison of papaverine and prostaglandin E₁ (PGE₁) in impotent patients. *J Urol* 1990; **143**, suppl 1: 303A.

85. Kattan S, Collins JP, Mohr D. Double-blind, cross-over study comparing prostaglandin E₁ and papaverine in patients with vasculogenic impotence. *Urology* 1991; **37**: 516–18.

86. Liu L-C, Wu C-C, Liu L-H, *et al.* Comparison of the effects of papaverine versus prostaglandin E₁ on penile blood flow by color duplex sonography. *Eur Urol* 1991; **19**: 49–53.

87. Ferreira SH. Prostaglandins, aspirin-like drugs and analgesia. *Nature New Biol* 1972; **240**: 200–3.

88. Ferreira SH. Prostaglandins: peripheral and central analgesia. In: Bonica JJ (ed), *Advances in Pain Research and Therapy*. New York: Raven Press, 1983: 627–34.

89. Zentgraf M, Ludwig G, Ziegler M. How safe is the treatment of impotence with intracavernous auto-injection? *Eur Urol* 1989; **16**: 165–71.

90. Porst H, Ebeling L. Erektile Dysfunktion. Übersicht

and aktueller Stand von Diagnostik und Therapie. *Fortschr Med* 1989; **107:** 44–53.

91. Lakin MM. Therapeutic pharmacologic erections. In: Doody DJ (ed), *Disorders of Male Sexual Function.* Chicago: Year Book Medical, 1988: 223–9.

92. Porst H, Van Ahlen H, Block T, *et al.* Intracavernous self-injection of prostaglandin E₁ in the therapy of erectile dysfunction. *VASA* 1989; suppl 28: 50–6.

93. Hirsch IH, Bagley DH, Christinzio J. Dosage considerations in the self-administration of PGE-1 for erectile dysfunction. 85th Annual Meeting of the American Urological Association, 1990, New Orleans LA, 305A.

94. Gerber GS, Levin LA. Pharmacological erection program using prostaglandin E₁. *J Urol* 1991; **146:** 786–9.

95. Zorgniotti AW, Lefleur RS. Auto-injection of the corpus cavernosum with a vasoactive drug combination for vasculogenic impotence. *J Urol* 1985; **133:** 39–41.

96. Sidi AA, Cameron JS, Duffy LM, Lange PH. Intracavernous drug-induced erections in the management of male erectile dysfunction: experience with 100 patients. *J Urol* 1986; **135:** 704–6.

97. Sidi AA, Reddy PK, Chen KK. Patient acceptance of and satisfaction with vasoactive intracavernous pharmacotherapy for impotence. *J Urol* 1988; **140:** 293–4.

98. Larsen EH, Gasser TC, Brus-Kewitz RC. Fibrosis of corpus cavernosum after intracavernous injection of phentolamine/papaverine. *J Urol* 1987; **137:** 292–3.

99. Lue TF. Recent advances in the diagnosis and treatment of erectile dysfunction. *11th International Symposium*, February 22–24, 1990, Vienna, Austria, Abstracts.

100. Hwang TI-S, Lin M-S, Yang C-R. Evaluation of vasculogenic impotence using dynamic penile washout test. *J Formosan Med Ass* 1990; **89:** 992–6.

101. Hwang TI-S, Lin M-S, Yang C-R. Dynamic penile washout test. Xe-133 washout study after prostaglandin E₁ intracavernous injection. *Int J Impotence Res* 1990; **2**, suppl 1: 111–17.

102. Diagnostic and Therapeutic Technology Assessment (DATTA). Questions and answers. Vasoactive intracavernous pharmacotherapy for impotence: intracavernous injection of prostaglandin E₁. *JAMA* 1991; **265:** 3321–3.

103. Bennett AH, Carpenter AJ. An improved vasoactive drug combination for a pharmacological erection program (PEP). *J Urol* 1990; **143**, suppl 1: 317A.

104. Floth A, Schramek P. Intracavernous injection of prostaglandin E₁ in combination with papaverine: enhanced effectiveness in comparison with papaverine plus phentolamine and prostaglandin E₁ alone. *J Urol* 1991; **145:** 56–9.

105. Kaplan HS. The combined use of sex therapy and intrapenile injections in the treatment of impotence. *J Sex Marital Ther* 1990; **16:** 195–207.

9 Prostaglandins in the management of gastroduodenal ulceration

CJ Hawkey and BJR Whittle

Epidemiology

Although the incidence of peptic ulcer is declining, it remains a significant cause of morbidity and mortality. In 1988 the Office of Population Censuses and Surveys recorded 4302 deaths as being due to peptic ulceration and its complications in the UK.[1] Of these, 4026 were in the elderly, with about half recorded as due to bleeding. More men than women get peptic ulcers, though the incidence is rising in elderly women, who are also the major recipients of non-steroidal anti-inflammatory drugs (NSAIDs), whilst falling in all other groups.[2]

The organism *Helicobacter pylori* is recognized to be a major cause of duodenal ulcer with nearly all patients infected. The prevalence of *Helicobacter* in gastric ulcer patients is raised, though to a lesser degree. Smoking is associated with a two- to three-fold enhancement of the risk of gastric and duodenal ulcer and reduction in ulcer healing rates. NSAIDs are also associated with a three- to fourfold enhancement of uncomplicated gastric (but not duodenal) ulcers,[3-7] gastric and duodenal ulcer bleeding, perforation and death, and account for 25–30% of all ulcer disease in the elderly in the UK. Whilst uncomplicated and complicated gastric ulceration are both more common with NSAID use, there appears to be an increased risk of duodenal ulcer bleeding but not of uncomplicated duodenal ulcer. This discrepancy has led to the proposal that NSAIDs may in part provoke ulcer bleeding by an antihaemostatic effect.[3,8]

The importance of NSAIDs in peptic ulcer disease has focused attention on the possibility of a more general role for prostaglandin deficiency in all types of peptic ulceration.

Prostaglandin levels in ulcer patients

Many studies have addressed the question of whether ulcer patients have reduced mucosal production of NSAID, with impairment of prostaglandin-related mucosal protection mechanisms. As seen in Tables 9.1 and 9.2, the results are widely divergent.[9-23] Although some studies have reported reduced prostanoid production, others have not. Moreover, there are a number of problems with the studies. Firstly, it is almost impossible to be certain that changes in prostaglandin formation seen are not secondary; for example, to differences in mucosal inflammation, metaplasia or pH changes associated with Helicobacter infection. Secondly, it can be difficult to be certain that these patients are not taking aspirin or even other NSAIDs. Thirdly, protocols for measuring prostaglandin production vary widely and there has been no systematic investigation of how this might affect the results. Fourthly, interpretation

Table 9.1   Mucosal PGE_2 in gastric ulcer patients

Author	Gastric mucosa		Comment
	Unbroken	Ulcer edge	
Schlegel et al., 1977[8]	↑	—	—
Wright et al., 1982[10]	↓ (B/A)	N	—
Kobayashi et al., 1982[11]	N	N	—
Konturek et al., 1984[12]	↓	—	—
Hawkey, 1986[13]	N (B/A)	N	↑ + gastritis ↓ + NSAIDs
Pugh, 1986[14]	↓ (A)	↓	—
Crampton et al., 1987[15]	↓	—	—

Results for PGE_2 shown because this is the major eicosanoid reported in gastric mucosa in humans.
A, antrum; B, body.

Table 9.2   Mucosal PGE_2 in duodenal ulcer patients

Author	Gastric mucosa	Duodenal mucosa		Comment
		Unbroken	Rim	
Cheung et al., 1975[16]	↑ *	—	—	—
Konturek et al., 1981[17]	N	N	N	—
Aly et al., 1982[18]	↑ (A)	N	—	—
Ahlquist et al., 1983[19]	—	↑	—	—
Sharon et al., 1983[20]	↓	N	—	—
Hillier et al., 1985[21]	—	N	N	Other eicosanoids ↓
Pugh, 1989[22]	N	↓	↓	—

Results with PGE_2 shown because this is the main prostaglandin identified in human duodenal mucosa.
Results with other eicosanoids have been generally, they are not precisely the same. The Ahlquist results refer to fasting levels – they report a blunted post-cibal rise (see text).
*Gastric juice measurements.

of the data may vary. Thus, one study claimed a prostaglandin deficiency in duodenal ulcer disease largely on the basis that the ratio of post-cibal to anti-cibal prostaglandins was reduced.[19] However, this was due to increased prostaglandin production in the anti-cibal (fasting) condition. Finally, the concept of local prostaglandin deficiency, a primary abnormality localized to a restricted area of the gastrointestinal tract, could be regarded as biologically implausible. The current data do not support the notion of prostaglandin deficiency in patients not taking NSAIDs, though they do not exclude the possibility.

Effect of predisposing factors on prostaglandin synthesis

Age and sex

In the above studies no sex- or age-related differences in prostaglandin synthesis have been reported. More recently, Feldman and colleagues have suggested that levels of prostaglandin synthesis seen in the elderly may be inappropriate to the increased acid output they have demonstrated in some of these patients.[24] It is difficult to be certain that this relative fall in prostaglandin levels is, as claimed by the authors, independent of mucosal atrophy.

Helicobacter pylori

Three studies have reported trends towards increased prostaglandin synthesis with *H. pylori* infection, presumably secondary to the associated gastritis,[25-27] whilst another has suggested prostaglandin synthesis is inhibited.[28]

Smoking

Three short-term studies on the effects of smoking have all suggested that synthesis of gastric mucosal prostaglandin is inhibited.[29-31] The mechanism for these interesting results is unclear. Smoking is known to enhance the activity of mixed function oxidases which can subserve thromboxane synthesis,[32] raising the possibility that reduced prostaglandin synthesis might occur by substrate diversion. However, concurrently enhanced synthesis of local thromboxane has not been demonstrated.

Aspirin and non-steroid anti-inflammatory drugs

Many studies have shown that these drugs can inhibit the synthesis of gastric mucosal prostaglandin,[33,34] synthesis in humans being inhibited by doses of aspirin as low as 75 mg.[34]

Other eicosanoids

Two studies have shown enhanced synthesis of LTC_4 (but not LTB_4) with *H. pylori* infection.[35,36] Smoking does not appear to affect LTB_4 production.[27] Long-standing NSAID therapy is associated with enhanced LTB_4 synthesis, particularly where there is type C gastritis.[36]

Experimental anti-ulcer actions

Inhibition of gastric acid secretion

It is now well established that prostaglandins, particularly of the E series, inhibit the formation of gastric erosions and ulcers induced by a wide variety of experimental techniques, including pyloric ligation, administration of steroid or non-steroid anti-inflammatory drugs, stress and treatment with reserpine, serotonin or bile salts.[23,37-42] The pioneering studies conducted by Robert in the late 1960s demonstrated the anti-ulcer activity of the naturally occurring prostanoids, particularly prostaglandins of the E series. The methylated synthetic analogues of these prostanoids were subsequently shown to have more potent anti-ulcer activity, as has also been

demonstrated with prostacyclin and its stable analogues.[40,41]

However, many of these anti-ulcer prostaglandins are potent inhibitors of gastric acid secretion. Because an acidic environment in the gastric lumen is a prerequisite in the development of many types of gastric damage, it is important to distinguish the anti-ulcer activity resulting from antisecretory properties from other potential protective mechanisms. In an early study of many synthetic and naturally occurring prostanoids, Robert demonstrated a dissociation between the doses of these compounds required for antisecretory and for the anti-ulcer activities and used the all-embracing term 'cytoprotection' to describe the additional protective properties.[37] Similarly, an early comparison of the doses of several prostaglandins and a histamine H_2-receptor antagonist required to prevent acid output and to reduce gastric erosions in rats suggested that the prostaglandins had protective properties distinct from their antisecretory actions.[38]

Cytoprotection, protection or anti-ulcer?

Additional early evidence of these protective mechanisms came from studies in which prostaglandin analogues substantially reduced the gross gastric damage induced by acidified bile salts, either alone or in combination with indomethacin.[38] Intragastric administration of exogenous acid in the gastric lumen was employed to reduce any antisecretory component in the overall protective process. A striking demonstration of the protective phenomena was the finding that the macroscopically visible gastric damage induced by topical application of strong acids, bases, hypertonic solutions or ethanol in rats could be reduced by co-administration of various prostaglandins. The methyl analogues of PGE_2 were effective in low, apparently non-antisecretory dose and within 2 minutes of oral administration.[39] Likewise, oral and intravenous administration of PGE_2 and its 16,16-dimethyl analogue inhibited mucosal injury induced by challenge with acidified ethanol (Fig. 9.1).

The description of the gastric protective properties of prostaglandins against such injurious agents has evoked much discussion, and experimental verification. Thus, a detailed histological analysis of the effects of pretreatment with the potent synthetic prostanoid 16,16-dimethyl PGE_2 on the rat gastric mucosa, 10 minutes following exposure to absolute ethanol was conducted by Lacy and Ito.[43] Extensive damage to the superficial mucosal cell layers fol-

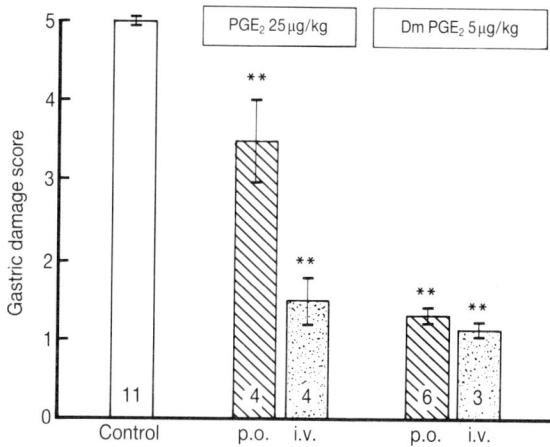

Fig. 9.1 Inhibition by oral (p.o.) or intravenous (i.v.) administration of PGE₂ or 16,16-dimethyl PGE₂ (Dm PGE₂) of macroscopically apparent rat gastric mucosal damage induced by a 10-minute intragastric challenge with acidified ethanol (40% ethanol in 100 mmol HCl). Results, shown as a score that takes into account both the incidence and severity of the haemorrhagic necrotic injury, are the mean ± SE mean of (*n*) experiments, where significant difference from the control level of damage is given as **$p<0.01$.

lowing ethanol application was observed, even in rats receiving the prostaglandin. Although prostaglandin pretreatment in these doses failed to reduce the total area of damage to the surface epithelial cell, it did cause a small reduction in the depth damage, and, interestingly, substantially reduced the severity of the deep necrotic lesions, characterized by haemorrhagic sites with focal accumulation of blood.

In a further study, local application of PGE₂ reduced the haemorrhagic lesions and vasocongestion following topical application of ethanol and acid, but likewise failed to prevent damage to the surface cells.[44] These histological findings have been confirmed by other groups.[45] The deep haemorrhagic lesions are clearly observed on macroscopic observation as red and black streaks, and therefore a reduction in such damage gives the mucosa the appearance of being grossly normal, accounting for the early definition of cytoprotection. From the histological studies, although inhibition of the macroscopic necrotic damage by these prostanoids was clearly confirmed, protection of all gastric cells and hence general cytological protection (cytoprotection) was not observed.

Other studies demonstrated that some protection was afforded with higher doses of the dimethyl prostaglandin analogue, against the surface cell

damage as well as the deeper haemorrhagic necrosis induced by a 10-minute exposure to ethanol (Fig. 9.2), as estimated by both histological and enzyme-marker techniques.[46] In further studies, significant protection of gastric epithelial cells by this prostanoid against aspirin- or indomethacin-induced damage was observed using scanning electron microscopy.[47] It is likely that the nature and extent of the mucosal cellular protection may well depend on the severity and character of the challenging agent. However, prostanoid-induced protection of the cells lying deep in the glandular mucosa from necrotic damage is a consistent finding from all the histological studies and thus the term 'cytoprotection', if used at all, may more correctly be applied to the preservation of these subepithelial mucosal cells.

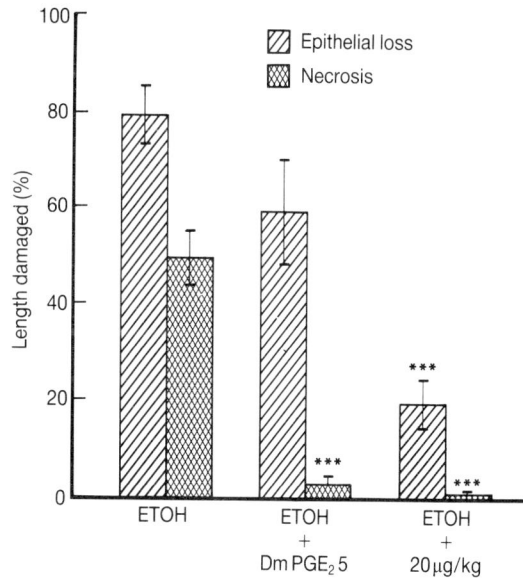

Fig. 9.2 Protection of the rat gastric mucosa by oral pretreatment with 16,16-dimethyl PGE₂ (Dm PGE₂) against damage induced by a 10-minute challenge with ethanol (1 ml, by oral route). Results are from histological evaluation and show the epithelial cell loss and disruption and the deep necrosis, expressed as percentage of length of tissue section exhibiting such damage. The data are the mean ± SE mean of 7–10 experiments per group, where the level of statistical significance from control is shown by ***$p<0.001$. Data adapted from Whittle and Steel (1985).[46]

Mechanisms of mucosal protection

The mechanisms underlying the gastric anti-ulcer and protective actions of prostaglandins are not yet clearly defined, apart from their ability to inhibit acid secretion. However, actions on several gastric processes have been proposed to be involved.

Luminal factors

Much attention has been directed to the actions of prostanoids in promoting luminal protective factors. One such factor is gastric mucus, which is a viscoelastic polymeric gel secreted from surface epithelial cells. The major components of mucus consist of large molecular weight glycoproteins. These so-called mucins exist in polymeric form of a number (usually four) of glycoprotein subunits joined by disulphide bonds. The central protein backbone is surrounded by a large number of branched carbohydrate chains, each composed of 12–19 sugar residues. This surface gel layer is continuously formed and degraded, the biosynthesis and release of glycoproteins from the surface mucous cells being balanced by enzymic proteolysis and disruptive shear forces in the gastric lumen.[48,49]

The mucus layer itself offers little buffering capacity and appears to be readily permeable to acid. However, mucus can act as a lubricant, and forms a barrier to physical damage such as that induced by contact of local tissue with fragments of food or tablets. Other than acting simply as a barrier, mucus could act to trap an unstirred layer of alkali secreted by gastroduodenal surface epithelial cells and hence help to neutralize hydrogen ions diffusing back from the lumen. The active secretion of bicarbonate by both gastric and duodenal mucosae and its stimulation by prostanoids have been characterized in a number of models.[50–52] Evidence for a pH gradient from the gastric lumen to the surface epithelial cells, in support of this mucus–bicarbonate layer, has also been reported.[53,54]

The unstirred-layer effect for surface neutralization is only likely to offer a protective action to the gastric mucosa with luminal acidity of pH 2 or above.[52] Such effects may have physiological relevance but cannot explain protection by prostanoids under conditions of high acidity in the gastric lumen. Furthermore, it is doubtful whether the mucus–bicarbonate complex could protect against injury induced by such topical gastric irritants as ethanol which would disrupt such layers. The net secretion of fluid into the lumen may, in addition, contribute to protection by diluting any topical irritant to non-damaging concentrations in the micro-milieu of the mucosal cells.[46]

The stimulation of mucus, bicarbonate and fluid secretion by prostanoids could also be important in epithelial restitution, the process which rapidly follows mucosal damage that allows recovery of epithelial continuity within 20–30 minutes. Thus, the formation of a mucus cap, rich in bicarbonate and plasma exudate, over areas of mucosal damage would create a local environment suitable for cellular migration and subsequent re-epithelialization of the damaged mucosa.[54–56] Such encouragement of the rapid repair process by prostanoids could thus contribute to their overall mucosal protective processes.[57] The rapid epithelial repair may also account for the apparently intact mucosa when determined by histological techniques in gastric tissue taken at least 30 minutes after ethanol challenge.[45]

An increased diffusion of luminal hydrogen ions back into the mucosal tissue, which is accompanied by a fall in transmucosal potential difference (PD), has been implicated in the gastric damage induced by topical irritants such as bile salts, salicylates and ethanol, the so-called 'barrier breakers'. Thus, another mechanism by which prostaglandins could protect the gastric mucosa could be by reducing acid back-diffusion in damaged mucosa, and such an action has indeed been found both in experimental models and in humans.[42] In addition to changes in hydrogen ion back-diffusion, studies *in vitro* have suggested that prostaglandin analogues can directly alter the transmucosal flux of sodium and chloride ions, but as yet the contribution and importance of these latter ionic flux changes to the protective mechanisms of these prostaglandins *in vivo* are not known.[42]

Changes in surface-active phospholipids at the surface apical membranes have also been suggested to be involved in altered gastric 'barrier' function and in the protective processes of prostaglandins.[58] In studies in the dog isolated mucosa, the local application of aspirin reduced surface hydrophobicity and therefore could allow more readily the passage of hydrogen ions back into the tissue. The dimethyl prostaglandin analogues inhibited this change in hydrophobicity induced by aspirin, and, under non-challenged conditions, actually enhanced this hydrophobicity.[58] More recently, the hydrophobic nature of the gastric mucosa has been shown to be largely dependent on surface mucus gel.[59] Although surface-active properties of the luminal layer may have a physiological role in preventing back-diffusion of acid, it is not clear how such effects could account for the protective actions of various prostanoids against other topical irritants such as bile salts or ethanol, which would disrupt directly this luminal layer, or against systemically acting ulcerogenic agents.

Microvascular actions

Prostaglandins of the E series, prostacyclin and their analogues are generally potent vasodilators in the gastric mucosal circulation.[60,61] Increases in gastric mucosal blood flow would be beneficial in maintaining the functional integrity of the gastric tissue by supplying essential nutrients and by preventing the intramucosal accumulation of hydrogen ions and other potentially damaging products.[60]

Although net mucosal vasodilatation could be an important component of the protective actions of many of the prostanoids, more local changes in the gastric microcirculation may also be of major significance. Thus, prevention of ethanol-induced vascular damage and vasocongestion by these prostanoids has been observed in histological studies.[43,44] Furthermore, the deep necrotic damage and vascular engorgement were correlated with stasis of flow in the damaged area, observed by *in vivo* fluorescent microscopy of the mucosa. Pretreatment with the dimethyl PGE_2 analogue prevented these microcirculatory changes, which may be an underlying mechanism of the protection against the deep necrotic lesions.[62–64] By preventing stasis, the prostanoids would allow intramucosal dilution and washout of the damaging agent in the microcirculation and help preserve the integrity of the deeper mucosal tissue. Such vascular actions of prostaglandins may be especially important under conditions where relative ischaemia or a primary injury to the microvasculature initiates or contributes to gastric damage. Thus protection of the gastric microvasculature, either by direct actions on endothelial cell integrity or by the prevention of the release of vasoconstrictor or cytotoxic mediators,[65] may therefore be an important mechanism that underlies the protective actions of the prostanoids. The anti-ulcer drugs that are thought to act through the stimulation of endogenous prostaglandin biosynthesis may likewise operate through actions on the microcirculation.

Interactions between prostanoids and other protective mediators

Local neuronal mechanisms are also thought to be involved in the local modulation of mucosal integrity and function. Of particular importance is the involvement of primary afferent neurons that can release sensory neuropeotides such as calcitonin gene-related peptide. Evidence for such a role comes from the findings that chronic pretreatment with capsaicin, an extract of red peppers that brings about

function ablation of primary sensory neurons, augments the gastric damage induced by a number of pro-ulcerogenic agents, including indomethacin.[66,67] In addition, acute mucosal application of capsaicin, which releases sensory neuropeptides, can protect against gastric damage.[68]

Apart from the vasodilator prostanoid, prostacyclin, endothelial cells also form and release the labile vasodilator substance, nitric oxide.[69] Using the selective inhibitor of nitric oxide synthesis, N^G-monomethyl-L-arginine (L-NMMA), a role has been established for endogenous nitric oxide in the local modulation of gastric mucosal blood flow.[70] Although short-term administration of L-NMMA alone did not lead to any detectable gastric damage, concurrent administration of indomethacin to inhibit cyclo-oxygenase led to the rapid appearance of mucosal lesions.[67] Administration of L-NMMA to rats pretreated with capsaicin to deplete their neuropeptide content led to extensive mucosal haemorrhage; this was exacerbated by indomethacin, such that it involved virtually all of the mucosal surface, including the antral region.[67] These findings indicate a close interaction between the protective mediators prostaglandins, sensory neuropeptides and nitric oxide in the regulation of tissue integrity.[67]

As can be seen, many divergent mechanisms evoking changes in a wide range of gastric parameters have been proposed to explain the potent protective properties of the prostaglandins. It is likely that no single action can account for 'cytoprotective' process, and it is possible that many of the properties act in concert or synergistically to produce the overall phenomenon. Indeed, the contribution of each may well depend on the type of gastric damage under investigation and the nature of the prostaglandin being investigated. As protection of the cells lying deep in the mucosa against damage is a consistent histological observation following prostanoid administration, and preservation of such cells allows the physiological process of a mucosal repair, future studies at the cellular level will be of importance. The observations that aspirin-induced disruption of rat gastric epithelial cells in culture can be attenuated by prostanoids suggest that direct cellular protection can occur under certain conditions.[71] Whether prostanoids can induce fundamental alterations in the biochemical make-up of the cell membrane is an intriguing but unanswered question. Furthermore, not only do endogenous prostanoids interact with endogenous nitric oxide and sensory neuropeptides in the regulation of mucosal integrity, but recent studies have also demonstrated that the full protective actions of exogenous prostanoids are dependent on intact sensory neuronal processes.[72,73]

Clinical studies

Available prostaglandin analogues

The demonstration of the potent protective properties of a number of prostaglandins on the gastric mucosa against experimental challenge pointed to a potential therapeutic use in the treatment of ulcer disease. Indeed, it was anticipated that such protective properties in addition to their antisecretory action would provide a significant advantage over agents acting solely by inhibiting acid secretion for healing and prevention of ulcer relapse. However, results have been disappointing and, moreover, compromised by a high level of adverse drug reactions.

Natural prostaglandins which are available for obstetric use were evaluated in ulcer disease,[23,42] but abandoned because they were rapidly metabolized *in vivo*, and because of a high incidence of side effects, principally diarrhoea. A number of more stable ana-

Table 9.3   Prostaglandin analogues assessed in ulcer disease

PGE$_2$ derivatives	*PGE$_1$ derivatives*
Arbaprostil	Misoprostol
Enprostil	Rioprostil

logues were developed, usually by substitution at the 15 or 16 position to prevent metabolism, some of which are shown in Table 9.3. Of these, only misoprostol is currently widely available for the treatment of peptic ulceration.

Ulcer healing with prostaglandin analogues

A curious oversight of clinical trial evaluation has had a significant effect on drug development in this area. Traditionally, patients taking NSAIDs are excluded from ulcer healing trials, and the early evaluations of prostaglandin analogues in the 1980s were no exception despite the fact that such patients represent the logical target for prostaglandin treatment. Ulcer

Table 9.4   Four-week ulcer healing with arbaprostil

Author	*Placebo*		*Arbaprostil 100 μg or less*					*Arbaprostil 600 μg*			
	n	*Healing*	*Dose*	n	*Healing*	*Therapeutic gain**	*Healing index†*	n	*Healing*	*Therapeutic gain**	*Healing index†*
Duodenal ulcer											
A. VanTrappen *et al.*, 1982[74]		39%	—	—	—	—	—	—	67%	28%	1.79
B. Euler *et al.*, 1987[76]	40	45%	40 μg	38	50%	—	—	—	—	—	—
C. Wengrower *et al.*, 1989[75]	53	40%	100 μg	52	31%	−9%	0.78	—	—	—	—
NSAIDs – gastric ulcer											
C. Euler *et al.*, 1990[107]	24	8%	10 μg	8	75%	67%	9.0	—	—	—	—
	30	3%	25 μg	31	45%	42%	13.5	—	—	—	—
	34	15%	10 μg	32	38%	23%	2.55	—	—	—	—
	—	—	25 μg	28	43%	28%	2.92	—	—	—	—
	—	—	50 μg	23	52%	37%	3.55	—	—	—	—
Average values‡											
Duodenal ulcer – cytoprotective doses (B + C)	**93**	**42%** (32–52%)		**90**	**39%** (29–49%)	**−3%**	**0.93** (0.65–1.32)				
NSAID associated gastric ulcer – cytoprotective doses (C)	**88**	**9%** (3–15%)		**122**	**46%** (37–58%)	**36.81**	**4.80** (2.77–8.31) ($p < 0.00001$)				

*Healing on prostaglandin minus healing on placebo.
†Odds ratio for healing compared to placebo.
‡Mantel Haenzel technique for cohorts. Mean (95% confidence limits) are shown. Healing index is the adjusted odds ratio.

Table 9.5   Four-week ulcer healing with misoprostol

Author	Placebo		Misoprostol 400 µg				Misoprostol 800 µg			
	n	Healing	n	Healing	Therapeutic gain*	Healing index†	n	Healing	Therapeutic gain*	Healing index†
Duodenal ulcer										
A. Sontag et al., 1985[78]	116	47%	111	65%	18%	1.38	—	—	—	—
	144	38%	142	51%						
B. Bright-Asare et al., 1986[79]	90§	42%	104§	53%	11%	1.26	81§	65%	23%	1.55
	111	34%	118	47%	13%	1.38	101	52%	18%	1.53
C. Brand et al., 1985[77]	100	51%	—	—	—	—	107	77%	26%	1.51
D. Lam et al., 1986[80]	76§	36%	—	—	—	—	77§	61%	25%	1.69
Gastric ulcer										
E. Agrawal et al., 1985[97]	103	36%	104	36%	0	1	—	—	—	—
Aspirin – duodenal ulcer										
G. Roth et al., 1989[108]	8	38%	—	—	—	—	10	50%	12%	1.32
Aspirin – gastric ulcer										
Roth et al., 1989[108]	28	29%	—	—	—	—	29	62%	33%	2.13
Average values, duodenal ulcer										
Misoprostol 800 µg (B–D)	**287**	**40%**	—	—	—	—	**285**	**64% (58–69)%**	**24%**	**1.58 (1.33–1.83)**
Misoprostol 400 µg (A–B)	**255**	**36% (33–39%)**	**260**	**49% (46–52%)**	**13%**	**1.34 (1.10–1.64)**	—	—	—	—

*Healing on prostaglandin minus healing on placebo.
†Odds ratio for healing compared to placebo.
§Calculated values.
‡Mantel Haenzel technique for cohorts. Mean (95% confidence limits) are shown. Healing index is the adjusted odds ratio.
Where papers report results for evaluable patients, these are shown first, with subsequent results calculated on an intention to treat basis, and used for meta analysis.

Table 9.6   Four-week ulcer healing with misoprostol – comparisons with H_2-antagonists

Author	Comparator			Misoprostol 400 µg				Misoprostol 800 µg			
	Identity/dose	n	Healing	n	Healing	Therapeutic gain*	Healing index†	n	Healing	Therapeutic gain*	Healing index†
Duodenal ulcer											
Nicholson et al., 1985[81]	Cimetidine 1200 mg	236	67%	226	41%	−26%	0.61	231	60%	−7%	0.90
Gastric ulcer											
Rachmilewitz et al., 1986[98]	Cimetidine 1200 mg	218	58%	178	39%	−19%	0.76	218	51%	−7%	0.88

*Healing on prostaglandin minus healing on comparator.
†Odds ratio for healing compared to comparator.

healing by prostaglandins in patients continuing to take NSAIDs has subsequently been the subject of a surprisingly small number of further trials. This is because these studies were carried out at a time when therapeutic emphasis was switching to prophylaxis of ulceration.

Duodenal ulcer healing

Arbaprostil
Arbaprostil (150 μg q.i.d.) in an antisecretory dose healed 67% of ulcers at 4 weeks compared to 39% with placebo[74] (Table 9.4). However, 39% of patients developed diarrhoea. Lower doses of arbaprostil were not effective.[75,76]

Misoprostol
Several large studies have shown misoprostol (800 μg daily) to enhance duodenal ulcer healing, on average by 1.58 times (95% confidence limits 1.33–1.83) compared to placebo[77–80] (Table 9.5). Comparison with the histamine H_2-receptor antagonist cimetidine has shown no significant difference; there was certainly no evidence for superiority over cimetidine[81] (Table 9.6). Indeed, in most of these studies the therapeutic gain and healing index favoured cimetidine. There are, as yet, no comparisons with the H_2-receptor antagonist ranitidine or the proton pump inhibitor omeprazole. An early meta-analysis of trials showed that only antisecretory doses of misoprostol enhanced ulcer healing.[82]

Enprostil
In clinical trials enprostil (70 μg daily) caused an enhancement of about 2.20 (1.56–3.11) times ulcer healing compared to placebo[83,84] (Table 9.7). Comparisons with H_2-receptor antagonists show that enprostil is of similar potency[85,87] to cimetidine but less effective than ranitidine (Table 9.8). Lower, non-antisecretory, doses of enprostil have not been evaluated.

Rioprostil
One study achieved 57% healing of duodenal ulcers with rioprostil (600 μg daily) at 4 weeks compared to 33% with placebo.[88] Most studies have involved comparisons with H_2-antagonists (Table 9.9). Rioprostil (in the dose range 400–600 μg daily) has generally achieved healing rates comparable to cimetidine (800 mg) or ranitidine (300 mg) daily, but without evidence of any specific advantage.[89–95] Indeed, all studies showed a slight advantage for H_2-antagonists compared to rioprostil although this did not reach significance in individual studies. Meta-analysis suggests 89% (83–95%) of the effectiveness of ranitidine 300 mg daily at 4 weeks (Table 9.9).

Duodenal ulcer maintenance

There have been no comparisons of arbaprostil, misoprostol and trimoprostil with H_2-antagonists as maintenance treatment for healed duodenal ulcers. Enprostil (35 μg nocte) has been shown to be significantly less effective than ranitidine (150 mg nocte).[86]

Table 9.7   Four-week ulcer healing with enprostil – comparison with placebo

Author	Placebo		Enprostil 70 μg				Enprostil 140 μg			
	n	Healing	n	Healing	Therapeutic gain*	Healing index†	n	Healing	Therapeutic gain*	Healing index†
Duodenal ulcer										
A. Thomson *et al.*, 1986[83]	36	14%	40	65%	51%	4.68	36	78%	64%	5.60
B. Tesler *et al.*, 1986[84]	37	49%	33	70%	21%	1.43	—	—	—	—
Gastric ulcer										
C. Navert, 1986[99]	34	35%	41	54%	19%	1.52	40	53%	18%	1.49
NSAIDs – gastric ulcer (6 weeks)										
D. Sontag *et al.*, 1900[109]	24	21%	31	61%	40%	2.45	31	65%	44%	2.58
Average values‡										
Duodenal ulcer (A & B)	**73**	**32%** (**21–42%**)	**73**	**67%** (**56–78%**)	**36%**	**2.20** (**1.56–3.11**)	—	—	—	—

*Healing on prostaglandin minus healing on placebo.
†Odds ratio for healing compared to placebo.
‡Mantel Haenzel technique for cohorts. Mean (95% confidence limits) are shown. Healing index is the adjusted odds ratio.

Table 9.8 Four-week ulcer healing with enprostil – comparison with H_2-antagonists

Author	Comparator			Enprostil 800 µg			
	Identity/dose	n	Healing	n	Healing	Therapeutic gain*	Healing index†
Duodenal ulcer							
A. Winters et al., 1986[85]	Cimetidine 800 mg	161	77%	166	75%	−2%	0.97
B. Lauritsen et al., 1986[86]	Ranitidine 300 mg	87	89%	82	74%*	−15%	0.84
		90	86%	90	71%	−15%	0.79
C. Walt et al., 1987[87]	Ranitidine 300 mg	51	76%	51	51%	−24%	0.66
Gastric ulcer							
Dammann et al., 1986[100]	Ranitidine 300 mg	46	66%	43	58%	−8%	0.89
Average values‡ – duodenal ulcer							
Ranitidine vs enprostil (B + C)			**84%** (78.0–90.2)		**65.4%** (57.3–73.5%)	**−18.6%**	**0.78** (0.68–0.90)

*Healing on prostaglandin minus healing on comparator.
†Odds ratio for healing compared to comparator.
‡Mantel Haenzel technique for cohorts. Mean (95% confidence limits) are shown. Healing index is the adjusted odds ratio.
Where papers report results for evaluatable patients, these are shown first, with subsequent results calculated on an intention to treat basis, used in the meta analysis.

Table 9.9 Four-week ulcer healing with rioprostil

Author	Comparator			Rioprostil (600 µg)			
	Identity/dose	n	Healing	n	Healing	Therapeutic gain*	Healing index†
Duodenal ulcer							
A. Bianchi Porro et al., 1989[89]	Cimetidine 800 mg	121	60%	123	55%	−5%	0.90
B. Lavignolle et al., 1989[90]	Ranitidine 300 mg	87	79%	80	73%	−6%	0.92
C. Coremans et al., 1989[91]	Ranitidine 300 mg	177	72%	178	62%	−9%	0.88
D. Dammann et al., 1989[92]	Ranitidine 300 mg	104	90%	104	84%	−6%	0.93
E. Miglio et al, 1989[93]	Ranitidine 300 mg	130	69%	125	63%	−6%	0.91
F. Whorwell, 1989[94]	Ranitidine 300 mg	105	77%	101	61%	−16%	0.79
Gastric ulcer							
G. Quinton et al, 1989[101]	Ranitidine 300 mg	47	50%	41	44%	−6%	0.88
H. Rutgeerts et al., 1989[102]	Ranitidine 300 mg	95	54%	87	47%	−7%	0.87
Average values‡							
Duodenal ulcer							
Rioprostil vs ranitidine (B–F)		603	76.3 (72.7–80.0)	588	67.7 (63.9–71.5)	−8.4%	0.89 (0.83–0.95)
Gastric ulcer							
Rioprostil vs ranitidine (G, H)		142	52.5 (44.3–60.7)	128	46.1 (37.0–55.2)	−6.4%	0.86 (0.69–1.12)

*Healing on prostaglandin minus healing on comparator.
†Odds ratio for healing compared to comparator.
‡Mantel Haenzel technique for cohorts. Mean (95% confidence limits) are shown. Healing index is the adjusted odds ratio.

In three studies, relapse rates with rioprostil (300 µg or 600 µg daily) have tended to be higher than with ranitidine (150 mg nocte) although differences did not achieve significance in individual trials.[95,96]

Gastric ulcer healing

Misoprostol
Four-week healing rates with misoprostol (100 or 400 µg daily) were not significantly different from placebo (see Table 9.5) but the higher dose increased

healing from 44.7% to 62.0% at 8 weeks.[97] In another study, a 4-week healing rate of 51% with misoprostol (800 µg daily) was not significantly different from 58% seen with cimetidine (1200 mg daily).[98] The healing rate of 39% with misoprostol (400 µg daily) was significantly lower (see Table 9.6).

Enprostil
Enprostil (70 µg daily) healed 54% of ulcers compared to 35% with placebo at 4 weeks (not significant), and 82% compared to 52% ($p<0.05$) at 6 weeks[99] (see Table 9.7). A higher dose of enprostil (140 µg daily) showed no advantage. In another study, 58% of ulcers healed at 4 weeks with enprostil (70 µg daily) compared to 66% with ranitidine, with no significant difference between the treatments[100] (see Table 9.8).

Rioprostil
In the studies with the prostanoids, there are no reported comparisons with placebo. Table 9.9 depicts results of studies with rioprostil that show no significant difference from ranitidine for the healing of gastric ulcer.[101,102]

Special groups

Smokers
It is well recognized that smoking impairs ulcer healing by placebo and H_2-antagonists. One study showed that differences between smokers and non-smokers seen under placebo conditions were partially overcome during misoprostol treatment. It was suggested that prostaglandin analogues might have a specific role in patients who continue to smoke,[80] a proposition that was biologically plausible granted the reductions in prostaglandin synthesis seen with smoking[29–31], but which has not in fact been borne out by published results (Tables 9.10 and 9.11). As Table 9.11 shows, the therapeutic gain (loss) and healing index for prostaglandins in smokers compared to non-smokers are indistinguishable from those for both placebo and H_2-antagonists.

Non-steroidal anti-inflammatory drugs
Prostaglandins represent logical treatment for patients who develop or are prone to ulceration while taking NSAIDs.[103] However, a number of considerations make evaluation very difficult in this group. Virtually all patients who take aspirin or NSAIDs develop mucosal lesions, ranging from superficial erosions to deep chronic ulcers. The frequency and

range of their impact on the gastric mucosa are encompassed in the term 'NSAID gastropathy', which acknowledges a pathogenesis different from that of classic peptic ulceration.[104] This difference is reflected in differences in the prevalence of smoking, *H. pylori* and symptoms, and a higher level of injury in the stomach than duodenum (a reversal of the pattern seen in patients not taking NSAIDs), compared to classic peptic ulcers.

Although the majority of patients given NSAIDs develop NSAID gastropathy, epidemiological studies suggest that the risk of ulcer complications is much lower, with only a three- to fourfold enhancement.[3] It is not known which endoscopic features of NSAID gastropathy are predictive of complications, or which are intrinsically harmless. Moreover, endoscopists find it difficult to distinguish superficial erosions from NSAID-associated ulcers.[105] There is good evidence that NSAIDs may reactivate *H. pylori*-associated ulcers in both stomach and duodenum by mechanisms that may be different to those causing *de novo* ulceration,[106] and it is also possible that they may provoke bleeding in pre-existing ulcers, perhaps by interfering with platelet function.[8]

Healing of NSAID-associated ulcers and gastropathy

Arbaprostil
Daily doses of arbaprostil (in the range 10–50 µg), which have no or limited effects on acid secretion have been shown to accelerate resolution of NSAID-associated gastropathy and to increase the rate of healing of gastric ulcer[107] (see Table 9.4). This effectiveness of supposedly cytoprotective doses of arbaprostil in healing NSAID-associated gastric ulcers is in interesting contrast to the lack of efficacy of such doses in non-NSAID-associated duodenal ulcers.[75]

Misoprostol
One study has shown that misoprostol (800 µg daily) reduces the level of gastric mucosal injury compared to placebo in patients with pre-existing aspirin-induced damage, with 62% compared with 29% healing of gastric ulcers[108] (see Table 9.5).

Enprostil
One abstract reports 61% and 80% healing of NSAID-associated gastric ulcers at 6 and 9 weeks with enprostil treatment (70 µg daily), compared to

Table 9.10 Effect of smoking on duodenal ulcer healing rates with placebo and prostaglandins

| | Placebo | | | | | | Misoprostol 800 µg | | | | |
| | Non-smoker | | Smoker | | | | Non-smoker | | Smoker | | | |
	n	Heal	n	Heal	Therapeutic gain*	Healing index†	n	Heal	n	Heal	Therapeutic gain*	Healing index†
Misoprostol												
A. Brand et al., 1985[77]	47	65%	60	43%	−22%	0.66	37	79%	63	73%	−6%	0.92
B. Sontag et al., 1985[78]	37	51%	79	46%	−5%	0.88	36	81%	75	51%	−30%	0.71
C. Bright-Asare et al., 1986[79]	39	44%	51	41%	−2%	0.94	41	73%	44	59%	−24%	0.81
D. Lam et al., 1986[80]	51	51%	25	12%	−39%	0.26	42	69%	35	54%	−15%	0.79
Enprostil												
E. Bright-Asare et al., 1986[79]	16	50%	21	48%	−2%	0.96	14	86%	19	58%	−28%	0.67
Average values‡												
Misoprostol studies (A–D)	123	54% (46–63%)	190	44% (37–51%)	−11%	0.80 (0.63–1.01)	117	75% (8–82%)	134	62% (55–68%)	−13%	0.82 (0.71–0.95)
All studies (A–E)	190	53% (49–57%)	236	41% (34–47%)	−12%	0.72 (0.58–0.90)	170	76% (69–82%)	236	61% (55–68%)	−14%	0.80 (0.69–0.91)

*Healing in smokers minus healing in non-smokers.
†Odds ratio for healing in smokers compared to non-smokers.
‡Mantel Haenzel technique for cohorts. Means (95% confidence limits) are shown. Healing index is adjusted odds ratio.

Table 9.11 Effect of smoking on duodenal ulcer healing rates with prostaglandins and H_2-receptor antagonists

| | Comparator | | | | | | | | | | | | |
| | | Non-smoker | | Smoker | | | | | Non-smoker | | Smoker | | | |
	Identity	n	Heal	n	Heal	Therapeutic gain*	Healing index†	Prostaglandin	n	Heal	n	Heal	Therapeutic gain*	Healing index†
A. Nicholson et al., 1985[81]	Cimetidine 1200 mg	82	74%	154	63%	−11%	0.85	Misoprostol 800 µg	93	71%	138	53%	−18%	0.75
B. Lauritsen et al., 1986[86] (2 weeks)	Ranitidine 300 mg	22	82%	67	60%	−22%	0.73	Enprostil 70 µg	21	67%	62	45%	−22%	0.68
C. Walt et al., 1987[87]	Ranitidine 300 mg	27	81%	24	71%	−10%	0.87	Enprostil 70 µg	23	56%	28	46%	−10%	0.82
D. Businger et al., 1989[96]	Ranitidine 300 mg	49	90%	70	90%	0	1.00	Rioprostil 600 µg	54	93%	64	83%	−10%	0.91
Average values‡													
Enprostil vs ranitidine (B + C)		49	82% (66–97%)	91	63% (52.3–72.6%)	−19%	0.79 (0.63–0.99)		44	61% (47–76%)	90	46% (35–56%)	−16%	0.74 (0.52–1.04)
All (A–D)		184	79% (73–85%)	315	69% (64–74%)	−10%	0.90 (0.81–1.00)		192	74% (68–81%)	292	57% (52–63%)	−17%	0.80 (0.70–0.91)

*Healing in smokers minus healing in non-smokers.
†Odds ratio for healing in smokers compared to non-smokers.
‡Mantel Haenzel technique for cohorts. Means (95% confidence limits) are shown. Healing index is adjusted odds ratio.

21% and 23% with placebo.[109] Comparative figures for enprostil (140 µg daily) are 65% and 72%[108] (see Table 9.7). These data, therefore, do not support dose-dependent actions of this prostanoid. The effects of non-antisecretory doses of enprostil have not been reported.

Rioprostil

One small study reports 10 out of 12 NSAID-associated gastric ulcers healing with 12 weeks of rioprostil (400 µg or 450 µg daily) compared to 1 out of 5 with placebo.[110]

Table 9.12   Incidence of diarrhoea with misoprostol

Author	Placebo	Misoprostol				
		100 μg	*200* μg	*400* μg	*800* μg	*1200* μg
Brand *et al.*, 1985[77]	5.0%	—	4.0%	—	13.1%	—
Sontag *et al.*, 1986[78]	3.5%	—	—	—	8.5%	—
Bright-Asare *et al.*, 1986[79]	1.8%	—	—	5.9%	8.9%	—
Lam *et al.*, 1986[80]	2.0%	—	—	—	24.7%	34.2%
Agrawal *et al.*, 1985[97]	1.9%	9.8%	—	7.7%	—	—
Graham *et al.*, 1988[112]	13.1%	—	—	26.1%	39.0%	—

Adverse drug reactions

Prostaglandins have a higher level of adverse drug reactions than other anti-ulcer agents, diarrhoea being particularly prominent. Misoprostol (800 μg per day) causes an approximate threefold increase in diarrhoea (Table 9.12). With rioprostil, four times as many patients complained of diarrhoea as those treated by ranitidine.[95,111] Similar increases in the incidence of diarrhoea are seen with other prostaglandins.[83–87]

Both misoprostol and enprostil have been shown to induce second trimester abortion in a substantial number of women who receive the drug.[82] Some studies have shown a somewhat lower incidence of central nervous system side effects such as headache for prostaglandins compared to H_2-antagonists.

Conclusion

It is extremely difficult to identify an advantage for prostaglandins over other agents in the treatment of established peptic ulcers whether associated with NSAID usage or not. Constipated patients who develop headaches on H_2-antagonists might prefer prostaglandin treatment but it is doubtful that others generally would. Although prostaglandin analogues should be logical treatment for NSAID-associated ulcers, where NSAIDs continue to be taken, there is a surprising dearth of studies, and particularly of studies investigating ulcers rather than more minor mucosal damage and/or involving comparisons with other agents. It is well recognized that other ulcer healing agents can heal NSAID-associated ulcers while these drugs are continued, and informal comparisons between different trials suggest no special benefit for prostaglandins.[111] In particular, high doses of omeprazole have been reported to heal NSAID-associated gastric ulcers at a rate that prostaglandin analogues are unlikely to better.

Prophylaxis against NSAID associated ulcers

The situation, however, is different for prophylaxis. There are abundant data about the prophylactic effects of misoprostol in preventing gastric and duodenal ulcers in patients who take NSAIDs.[111–118] Most of these have involved comparisons with placebo. The main studies are shown in Tables 9.13 and 9.14. These data can be summarized as follows. All studies have shown that misoprostol can retard the development of acute gastric ulcers on average by 74% (50–87%) compared to placebo (tablets). Whether the same was true for duodenal ulcers was less clear from early studies but subsequent studies have shown a therapeutic effect here, too, with an average 82% (64–91%) reduction compared to placebo (Table 9.14). However, despite the large size of these studies, no data have yet emerged on the critical question of whether ulcer complications are prevented. This is important for two reasons. Firstly, NSAID-associated ulcers can be difficult to distinguish from erosions and may thus encompass a number of relatively benign lesions.[105] Secondly, NSAID ulcers are often silent and, where this is so, the only purpose of preventing them is to reduce the morbidity and mortality associated with ulcer complications.[3]

Informal comparisons with other trials involving H_2-antagonists also suggest that there may be a difference in the pattern of protection for prostaglandins and H_2-antagonists. Ranitidine has consistently been shown to be effective in the prevention of duodenal ulcer development in patients taking NSAIDs, but its potency against gastric ulcer appears to be less. Recently, one study reported in abstract form comparing misoprostol and ranitidine directly showed that misoprostol was more effective in the prevention of gastric ulcers over 12 weeks.[117] As yet, the only other published comparative study was

Table 9.13   Gastric ulcer prophylaxis with misoprostol

	Placebo				Misoprostol											
					400 mg/day				400–600 mg/day				800 mg/day			
	n	3 m	6 m	12 m	n	3 m	6 m	12 m	n	3 m	6 m	12 m	n	3 m	6 m	12 m
A. Graham *et al.*, 1988[112]	138	21.7	—	—	143	5.6%	—	—	—	—	—	—	139	1.4%	—	—
B. Agrawal *et al.*, 1990[113]	131	16.0	—	—	—	—	—	—	—	—	—	—	122	1.6%	—	—
C. Elliott *et al.*, 1990[115]	38	18.4	26.3%	34.2%	—	—	—	—	32	3.1%	12.5%	12.5%	—	—	—	—
D. Geiss *et al.*, 1991[114]	99	8.3	11.1%	—	—	—	—	—	96	4.7%	9.2%	—	—	—	—	—
E. Graham *et al.*, 1991[116]	311	7.7%	—	—	—	—	—	—	308	1.9%	—	—	—	—	—	—
F. Vendikt *et al.*, 1991[118]	153	3.9%	—	—	—	—	—	—	137	2.9%	—	—	—	—	—	—

Average values over 3 months (A, C–F)	Placebo (n = 763) **9.9%** (7.8–12.0%)	Misoprostol (n = 716)	Therapeutic gain **6.6%** **3.3%** (2.0–4.6%)	Effectiveness **73%** (50–87%)

Cumulative percentage of patients developing gastric ulcers is shown.   m = month.
Calculated by Mantel Haenzel technique for cohorts. Mean (95% confidence limits) are shown.
Placebo ulcer rate minus misoprostol ulcer rate.
(1 − adjusted odds ratio for misoprostol compared to placebo) × 100.

Table 9.14   Duodenal ulcer prophylaxis with misoprostol

	Placebo				Misoprostol											
					400 mg/day				400–600 mg/day				800 mg/day			
	n	3 m	6 m	12 m	n	3 m	6 m	12 m	n	3 m	6 m	12 m	n	3 m	6 m	12 m
A. Graham *et al.*, 1988[112]	138	3.6%	—	—	143	2.1%	—	—	—	—	—	—	139	2.9%	—	—
B. Agrawal *et al.*, 1990[113]	131	0.8%	—	—	—	—	—	—	—	—	—	—	122	1.6%	—	—
C. Geiss *et al.*, 1991[114]	99	8.1%	9.7%	—	—	—	—	—	96	0%	1.4%	—	—	—	—	—
D. Graham *et al.*, 1991[116]	311	4.8%	—	—	—	—	—	—	308	0.6%	—	—	—	—	—	—
E. Vendikt *et al.*, 1991[118]	153	7.8%	—	—	—	—	—	—	137	1.5%	—	—	—	—	—	—

Average values over 3 months (A, C–E)	Placebo (n = 701) **5.7%** (4.0–7.4%)	Misoprostol (n = 684)	Therapeutic gain **4.7%** **1.0%** (0.3–1.8%)	Effectiveness **82%** (64–91%)

Cumulative percentage of patients developing duodenal ulcers is shown.   m = month.
Calculated by Mantel Haenzel technique for cohorts. Mean (95% confidence limits) are shown.
Placebo ulcer rate minus misoprostol ulcer rate.
(1 − adjusted odds ratio for misoprostol compared to placebo) × 100.

between misoprostol and sucralfate, and this also showed misoprostol to be better (than sucralfate) in preventing gastric ulcers.[113]

Concluding comment

There is no doubt about the efficacy of prostaglandin analogues, particularly misoprostol, in NSAID-associated gastric and duodenal ulcer prophylaxis,[119–122] but prescribers have been reluctant to use these drugs widely. There would appear to be several reasons for this. Efficacy against ulcer complications has not yet been established. Universal prophylaxis would be very expensive although it has been argued that this would be balanced by savings in hospital costs. The available prostanoids cannot be considered ideal prophylactic drugs for wide-spread use because of the high incidence of complications, principally diarrhoea and, in women of child-bearing age, their ability readily to cause uterine contraction and abortion. It is not clear whether the clinical experience with other anti-ulcer agents compared with existing prostaglandins will encourage the development of a second generation of synthetic prostanoids devoid of such side effects, even if potent antisecretory actions and potentially beneficial protective properties could be demonstrated.

References

1. Office of Population Censuses and Surveys. *Mortality Statistics for the United Kingdom 1988.* London: HMSO, 1991.

2. Walt R, Katschinski B, Logan R, Ashley J, Langman M. Rising frequency of ulcer perforation in elderly people in the United Kingdom. *Lancet* 1986; **2:** 489–92.

3. Hawkey CJ. Non-steroidal anti-inflammatory drugs and peptic ulcers. Facts and figures multiply, but do they add up? *BMJ* 1990; **300:** 278–84.

4. Somerville K, Faulkner G, Langman MJS. Non-steroidal anti-inflammatory drugs and bleeding peptic ulcer. *Lancet* 1986; **1:** 462–4.

5. Carson JL, Strom BL, Soper KA, West SL, Morse ML. The association of non-steroidal anti-inflammatory drugs with upper gastrointestinal tract bleeding. *Arch Intern Med* 1987; **147:** 85–8.

6. Griffin MR, Ray WA, Schaffner W. Non-steroidal anti-inflammatory drug use and death from peptic ulcer in elderly persons. *Ann Intern Med* 1988; **109:** 359–63.

7. Griffin MR, Piper JM, Daugherty JR, Snowden M, Ray WA. Non-steroidal anti-inflammatory drug use and increased risk for peptic ulcer disease in elderly persons. *Ann Intern Med* 1991; **114:** 257–63.

8. Hawkey CJ, Hawthorne AB, Hudson N, Cole AT, Mahida YR, Daneshmend TK. Separation of aspirin's impairment of haemostasis from mucosal injury in the human stomach. *Clin Sci* 1991; **81:** 565–73.

9. Schlegel W, Wenk W, Dollinger HC, Raptis S. Concentrations of prostaglandin A, E and F like substances in gastric mucosa of normal subjects and patients with various gastric diseases. *Clin Sci Mol Med* 1977; **52:** 255–8.

10. Wright JP, Young GO, Klaff LJ, Weers LA, Price SK, Marks IN. Gastric mucosal prostaglandin E levels in patients with gastric ulcer disease and carcinoma. *Gastroenterology* 1982; **82:** 263–7.

11. Kobayashi K, Arakawa T, Nakamura H, *et al.* Role of prostaglandin E_2 on human gastric ulcers. *Gastroenterol Jpn* 1982; **17:** 21–4.

12. Konturek SJ. Actions of non-steroidal anti-inflammatory compounds on gastric mucosal integrity and prostaglandin formation in healthy subjects and peptic ulcer patients. *Adv Inflam Res* 1984; **6:** 29–37.

13. Hawkey CJ. Influence of gastritis on gastric mucosal prostaglandin synthesis. *Gastroenterology* 1984; **86:** 1108.

14. Pugh S. Prostaglandins: is deficiency a pathophysiological influence in peptic ulcer disease? *GI Futures* 1986; **1** (3): 11–14.

15. Crampton JR, Gibbons LC, Rees WDW. Simultaneous measurement of *in vitro* gastroduodenal prostaglandin E_2 synthesis and degradation in peptic ulcer disease. *Scand J Gastroenterol* 1987; **22:** 425–30.

16. Cheung LY, Jubiz W, Moore JG, Frailey J. Gastric prostaglandin E output during basal and stimulated acid secretion in normal subjects with peptic ulcer. *Gastroenterology* 1975; **16:** 873.

17. Konturek SJ, Ostulowicz W, Sito E, Olesky J, Wilkon S, Kiec-Dembinska A. Distribution of prostaglandin in gastric and duodenal mucosa of healthy subjects and duodenal ulcer patients: effects of aspirin and paracetamol. *Gut* 1981; **22:** 283–9.

18. Aly A, Green K, Johansson C, Slezak P. Prostaglandin synthesis in gastroinestinal mucosa in man. *Scand J Gastroenterol Suppl* 1982; **78:** A179.

19. Ahlquist DAS, Dozois RR, Zinsmeister AR, Malagelad JR. Duodenal prostaglandin synthesis and acid load in health and in duodenal ulcer disease. *Gastroenterology* 1983; **85:** 522–8.

20. Sharon P, Cohen F, Ziffroni A, Karmeli F, Ligumsky M, Rachmilewitz D. Prostanoid synthesis by cultured gastric and duodenal mucosa. Possible role in the pathogenesis of duodenal ulcer. *Scand J Gastroenterol* 1983; **18:** 1045–9.

21. Hillier K, Smith CL, Jewell R, Arthur MJP, Ross G. Duodenal mucosa synthesis of prostaglandins in duodenal ulcer disease. *Gut* 1985; **26:** 237–40.

22. Pugh S, Williams SE, Lewin MR, *et al.* Duodenal and antral mucosal prostaglandin E_2 synthesis in a study of normal subjects and all stages of duodenal ulcer disease treated by H_2 receptor antagonists. *Gut* 1989; **30** (2): 161–5.

23. Hawkey CJ, Rampton DS. Prostaglandins and the gastrointestinal mucosa: are they important in its function, disease and treatment. *Gastroenterology* 1985; **89:** 1162–88.

24. Cryer B, Redfern JS, Lee E, Feldman M. Decline in gastroduodenal mucosal prostaglandins (PGs) with aging in humans: relationship with gastric acid secretion. *Gastroenterology* 1991; **100:** A518.

25. Taha AS, Boothman P, Holland P, *et al.* Gastric mucosal prostaglandin synthesis in the presence of *Campylobacter pylori* in patients with gastric ulcers and non-ulcer dyspepsia. *Am J Gastroenterol* 1990; **85:** 47–50.

26. Avunduk C, Suliman M, Gang G, Polakowski N, Eastwood GL. Gastroduodenal mucosal prostaglandin generation in patients with *Helicobacter pylori* before and after treatment with bismuth subsalicylate. *Dig Dis Sci* 1991; **36:** 431–4.

27. Hudson N, Everitt SJ, Filipowicz B, Hawkey CJ. Effect of *Helicobacter pylori* colonisation on gastric mucosal eicosanoid synthesis in patients using non-steroidal anti-inflammatory drugs. *Gut* 1991; **32:** A1257.

28. Goren A, Fotherby KJ, Shorthouse M, Wright DGD, Hunter JO. *Campylobacter pylori* and acid secretion. [letter] *Lancet* 1989; **2:** 212.

29. McCready DR, Clark L, Cohen MM. Cigarette smoking reduces human gastric luminal prostaglandin E_2. *Gut* 1985; **26:** 1192–6.

30. Quimby GF, Bonnice CA, Burstein SH, Eastwood GL. Active smoking depresses prostaglandin synthesis in human gastro-duodenal mucosa. *Gastroenterology* 1985; **88:** A1548.

31. Hudson N, Daneshmend TK, Hurst S, Bhaskar NK, Brown NS, Hawkey CJ. Effect of smoking on prostaglandin, thromboxane and leukotriene synthesis by human gastric mucosa. In: Samuelsson B, Paoletti R, Ramwell P (eds), *Advances in Prostaglandin, Thromboxane and Leukotriene Research*. New York: Raven Press, 1991.

32. Haurand M, Ullrich V. Isolation and characterisation of thromboxane synthase from human platelets as a cytochrome P-450 enzyme. *J Biol Chem* 1985; **260**: 15059–67.

33. Whittle BJR. The mechanisms of gastric damage by non-steroid anti-inflammatory drugs. In: Cohen M (ed), *Biological Protection with Prostaglandins*. Boca Raton FL: CRC Press, 1986: 1–27.

34. Hudson N, Cole AT, Murray FE, *et al.* Low dose aspirin: an unrecognised cause of gastric mucosal damage. *Gut* 1991; **32**: A1245.

35. Ahmed A, Vaira D, Cairns SR, *et al.* Increased formation of leukotriene C₄ in *Campylobacter pyloridis*. *Gut* 1987; **28**: A1405.

36. Hudson N, Balsitis M, Everitt S, Hawkey CJ. Enhanced gastric mucosal leukotriene B₄ synthesis in patients taking non-steroidal anti-inflammatory drugs. *Gut* 1993 (in press).

37. Robert A. Antisecretory, anti-ulcer, cytoprotective and diarrhoegenic properties of prostaglandins. In: Samuelson B, Vane JR (eds), *Advances in Prostaglandin and Thromboxane Research*, vol 2. New York: Raven Press, 1976: 507–20.

38. Whittle BJR. Relationship between the prevention of rat gastric erosions and the inhibition of acid secretion by prostaglandins. *Eur J Pharmacol* 1976; **40**: 233–9.

39. Robert A, Nezamis JE, Lancaster C, Hanchar AJ. Cytoprotection by prostaglandins in rats – prevention of gastric necrosis produced by alcohol, HCl, NaOH, hypertonic NaCl and thermal injury. *Gastroenterology* 1979; **77**: 433–43.

40. Miller TA. Protective effects of prostaglandins against gastric mucosal damage: current knowledge and proposed mechanisms. *Am J Physiol* 1983; **245**: G601–G623.

41. Robert A. Prostaglandins and the gastrointestinal tract. In: Johnson LR (ed), *Physiology of the Gastrointestinal Tract*. New York: Raven Press, 1981: 1407–34.

42. Whittle BJR, Vane JR. Prostanoids as regulators of gastrointestinal function. In: Johnson LR (ed), *Physiology of the Gastrointestinal Tract*, 2nd ed. New York: Raven Press, 1987: 601–38.

43. Lacy ER, Ito S. Microscopic analysis of ethanol damage to rat gastric mucosa after treatment with a prostaglandin. *Gastroenterology* 1982; **83**: 619–25.

44. Wallace JL, Morris GP, Krausse EJ, Greaves SE. Reduction by cytoprotective agents of ethanol-induced damage to the rat gastric mucosa: a correlated morphological and physiological study. *Can J Physiol Pharmacol* 1982; **60**: 1686–99.

45. Tarnawski A, Hollander D, Stachura J, Krause WL, Gergely H. Prostaglandin protection of the gastric mucosa against alcohol injury – a dynamic time-related process. Role of the mucosal proliferative zone. *Gastroenterology* 1985; **88**: 334–52.

46. Whittle BJR, Steel G. Evaluation of the protection of rat gastric mucosa by a prostaglandin analogue using cellular enzyme marker and histological techniques. *Gastroenterology* 1985; **88**: 315–27.

47. Ohno T, Ohtuski H, Okabe S. Effects of 16,16-dimethyl prostaglandin E₂ on ethanol-induced and aspirin-induced gastric damage in rat. Scanning electron microscopic study. *Gastroenterology* 1985; **88**: 353–61.

48. Allen A, Hunter AC, Leonard AJ, Pearson JP, Sellers LA. Peptic activity and the mucus-bicarbonate barrier. In: Garner A, Whittle BJR (eds), *Advances in Drug Therapy of Gastrointestinal Ulceration*. Chichester: John Wiley, 1989: 139–55.

49. Allen A, Garner A. Mucus and bicarbonate secretion in the stomach and their possible role in mucosal protection. *Gut* 1980; **21**: 249–62.

50. Flemstrom G, Garner A. Gastroduodenal HCO₃ transport: characteristics and proposed role in acidity regulation and mucosal protection. *Am J Physiol* 1982; **242**: G183–G193.

51. Kauffman GL, Reeve JJ, Grossman MI. Gastric bicarbonate secretion, effect of topical and intravenous 16,16-dimethyl prostaglandin E₂. *Am J Physiol* 1980; **239**: G44–G48.

52. Flemstrom G. Gastroduodenal mucosal secretion of bicarbonate and mucus: physiological control and stimulation by prostaglandins. *Am J Med* 1986; **81**: 18–22.

53. Turberg LA, Ross IN, Bahari HMM. pH gradient across gastric mucus. In: Allen A, Flemstrom G, Garner A, Silen W, Turnberg LA (eds), *Mechanisms of Mucosal Protection in the Upper Gastrointestinal Tract*. New York: Raven Press, 1984: 223–6.

54. Wallace JL, McKnight GW. The mucoid cap over superficial gastric damage in the rat. A high-pH microenvironment dissipated by non-steroidal anti-inflammatory drugs and endothelin. *Gastroenterology* 1990; **99**: 295–304.

55. Morris GP, Harding PL. Mechanisms of mucosal recovery from acute gastric damage: roles of extracellular mucus and cell migration. In: Allen A, Flemstrom G, Garner A, Silen A, Turnberg LA (eds), *Mechanisms of Musocal Protection in the Upper Gastrointestinal Tract*. New York: Raven Press, 1984: 209–13.

56. Wallace JL, Whittle BJR. Role of mucus in the repair of gastric epithelial damage in the rat. *Gastroenterology* 1986; **91**: 603–11.

57. Wallace JL, Whittle BJR. Acceleration of recovery of gastric epithelial integrity by 16,16-dimethyl

prostaglandin E$_2$. *Br J Pharmacol* 1985; **86**: 837–42.

58. Lichtenberger LM, Richards JE, Hills BA. Effect of 16,16-dimethyl prostaglandin E$_2$ on the surface hydrophobicity of aspirin-treated canine gastric mucosa. *Gastroenterology* 1985; **88**: 308–14.

59. Goddard PJ, Kao YJ, Lichtenberger LM. Luminal surface hydrophobicity of canine gastric mucosa is dependent on a surface mucous gel. *Gastroenterology* 1990; **98**: 361–70.

60. Whittle BJR. Action of prostaglandins on gastric mucosal blood flow. In: Fielding LP (ed), *Gastrointestinal Mucosal Blood Flow*. Edinburgh, New York: Churchill Livingstone, 1980: 180–91.

61. Konturek SJ, Robert A, Hancher AJ, Nezamis JE. Comparison of prostacyclin and prostaglandin E$_2$ on gastric acid secretion, gastrin release and mucosal blood flow in dogs. *Dig Dis Sci* 1980; **25**: 673–9.

62. Guth PH, Paulsen G, Nagata H. Histologic and microcirculatory changes in alcohol-induced gastric lesions in the rat. Effect of prostaglandin cytoprotection. *Gastroenterology* 1984; **87**: 1083–90.

63. Pihan G, Majzoubi D, Haudenschild C, Trier JS, Szabo S. Early microcirculatory stasis in acute gastric mucosal injury in the rat and prevention by 16,16-dimethyl prostaglandin E$_2$ or sodium thiosulfate. *Gastroenterology* 1986; **91**: 1415–26.

64. Oates PJ, Hakkinen JP. Studies on the mechanism of ethanol-induced gastric damage in rats. *Gastroenterology* 1988; **94**: 10–21.

65. Boughton-Smith NK, Whittle BJR. Inhibition by 16,16-dimethyl PGE$_2$, of ethanol-induced gastric mucosal damage and leukotriene B$_4$ and C$_4$ formation. *Prostaglandins* 1988; **35**: 945–7.

66. Holzer P, Sametz W. Gastric mucosal protection against ulcerogenic factors in the rat mediated by capsaicin-sensitive afferent neurones. *Gastroenterology* 1986; **91**: 975–81.

67. Whittle BJR, Lopez-Belmonte J, Moncada S. Regulation of gastric mucosal integrity by endogenous nitric oxide: interactions with prostanoids and sensory neuropeptides in the rat. *Br J Pharmacol* 1990; **99**: 607–11.

68. Holzer P, Pabst MA, Lippe ITh, *et al.* Afferent nerve-mediated protection against deep mucosal damage in the rat stomach. *Gastroenterology* 1990; **99**: 838–48.

69. Moncada S, Palmer RMJ, Higgs EA. Nitric oxide: physiology, pathophysiology and pharmacology. *Pharmacol Rev* 1991; **43**: 109–42.

70. Pique JM, Whittle BJR, Esplugues JV. The vasodilator role of endogenous nitric oxide in the rat gastric microcirculation. *Eur J Pharmacol* 1989; **174**: 293–6.

71. Terano A, Mach T, Stachura A, Tarnawski A, Ivey KJ. Effect of 16,16-dimethyl prostaglandin E$_2$ on aspirin induced damage to rat gastric epithelial cells in tissue culture. *Gut* 1984; **25**: 19–25.

72. Esplugues JV, Whittle BJR. Peripheral opioid-sensitive mechanisms of mucosal injury and protection. In: Garner A, O'Brien PE (eds), *Mechanisms of Injury, Protection and Repair of the Upper Gastrointestinal Tract*. Chichester: John Wiley, 1991: 115–25.

73. Esplugues JV, Whittle BJR, Moncada S. Modulation by opioids and by afferent sensory neurones of prostanoid protection of the rat gastric mucosa. *Br J Pharmacol* 1992; **106**: 846–52.

74. Van Trappen G, Janssens J, Popiela T, *et al.* Effect of 15(R)-15-methyl prostaglandin E$_2$ (arbaprostil) on the healing of duodenal ulcer. A double-blind multicentre study. *Gastroenterology* 1982; **83**: 357–63.

75. Wengrower D, Fich A, Goldin E, Eliakim R, Ligumsky M, Rachmilewitz D. Cytoprotective doses of arbacet with minimal antisecretory properties are not effective in duodenal ulcer healing. *Dig Dis Sci* 1987; **32**: 857–60.

76. Euler AR, Tytgat G, Berenguer J, *et al.* Failure of a cytoprotective dose of arbaprostil to heal acute duodenal ulcers. Results of a multi clinic trial. *Gastroenterology* 1987; **92**: 604–7.

77. Brand DL, Roufail WM, Thomson AB, Tasser EJ. Misoprostol, a synthetic PGE$_1$ analog, in the treatment of duodenal ulcers. A multicentre double blind study. *Dig Dis Sci* 1985; **30** (suppl 11): 147S–158S.

78. Sontag SJ, Mazure PA, Pontes JF, Beker SG, Dajani EZ. Misoprostol in the treatment of duodenal ulcer: a multicentre double-blind, placebo controlled study. *Dig Dis Sci* 1985; **30** (suppl): 159–63.

79. Bright-Asare P, Sontag SJ, Gould RJ, Brand DL, Roufail WM. Efficacy of misoprostol (twice daily dosage) in acute healing of duodenal ulcer: a multicentre double-blind controlled trial. *Dig Dis Sci* 1986; **31** (suppl): 63–7.

80. Lam SK, Lau WY, Choi EK, *et al.* Prostaglandin E$_1$ (misoprostol) overcomes the adverse effect of chronic cigarette smoking on duodenal ulcer healing. *Dig Dis Sci* 1986; **31** (suppl): 68–74.

81. Nicholson PA. A multicentre international controlled comparison of two dosage regimens of misoprostol and cimetidine in the treatment of duodenal ulcer in outpatients. *Dig Dis Sci* 1985; **30** (suppl): 171–7.

82. Herting RL, Nissen CH. Overview of misoprostol clinical experience. *Dig Dis Sci* 1986; **31** (2): 47S–54S.

83. Thomson ABR, Archambault AP, Halvorsen L, *et al.* Comparison of enprostil and placebo in active duodenal ulcer. *Am J Med* 1986; **81** (suppl 2A): 59–63.

84. Bright-Asare P, Krejs CJ, Sannangelo WC, *et al.* Treatment of duodenal ulcer with enprostil, a prostaglandin E$_2$ analogue. *Am J Med* 1986; **81** (suppl 2A): 64–8.

85. Winters L, Willcox R, Ligny G, *et al.* Comparison of enprostil and cimetidine in active duodenal ulcer: summary of pooled European studies. Protective and therapeutic effects of gastrointestinal prostaglandins. *Am J Med* 1986; **81** (suppl 2A): 69–74.

86. Lauritsen K, Laursen LS, Havelund T, Bytzer P, Svendsen LB, Rask-Masden J. Enprostil and ranitidine in duodenal ulcer healing: double blind comparative trial. *BMJ* 1986; **292**: 864–6.

87. Walt RP, Pounder RE, Hawkey CJ, *et al.* Twenty-four hour intragastric acidity and clinical trial of bedtime enprostil 70 μg compared with ranitidine 300 mg in duodenal ulcer. *Aliment Pharmacol Therap* 1987; **1**: 161–6.

88. Boucekkine T, Meknini B, Bitoun A, *et al.* Treatment of duodenal ulcer with rioprostil: a randomised multicentre double-blind study. *Scand J Gastroenterol* 1989; **24** (suppl 164): 191–5.

89. Bianchi Porro G, Parente F, Hentschel E, *et al.* Rioprostil in the short-term treatment of duodenal ulcer: a multicentre double-blind trial vs cimetidine. *Scand J Gastroenterol* 1989; **24** (suppl 164): 219–23.

90. Lavignolle A, Raillat A, Slama JL, *et al.* Rioprostil vs ranitidine in duodenal ulcer healing: a double-blind multicentre trial. *Scand J Gastroenterol* 1989; **24** (suppl): 194–7.

91. Coremans G, Vantrappen G, Businger JA, *et al.* Efficacy and safety of rioprostil, 300 μg bd in the treatment of duodenal ulcer: a double blind, controlled multicentre clinical study vs ranitidine. *Scand J Gastroenterol* 1989; **24** (suppl 164): 198–206.

92. Dammann HG, Dreyere M, Muller P, Simon P, Demol P. A single evening dose of rioprostil 600 μg in the treatment of acute duodenal ulcers. *Scand J Gastroenterol* 1989; **24** (suppl 164): 215–18.

93. Businger A, Miglio F, Gasbarrini T, Vismans FJ, Geraedts AAM, Stocker H. Rioprostil, a new prostaglandin E₁ analogue, in the once daily treatment of acute duodenal ulcer: a comparison with ranitidine. *Scand J Gastroenterol* 1989; **24** (suppl 164): 161–8.

94. Whorwell PJ. Rioprostil in the healing of duodenal ulceration: a short report. *Scand J Gastroenterol* 1989; **24** (suppl 164): 214.

95. Dammann HG, Dreyer M, Muller P, Simon B. Rioprostil in the acute and long-term treatment of peptic ulcers: a review. *Scand J Gastroenterol* 1989; **24** (suppl 164): 207–13.

96. Businger JA, Fumagalli I, Michel H, Delas N, Stocker H. Rioprostil, a new prostaglandin E₁ analogue in the once daily treatment for the prevention of duodenal ulcer recurrence: a comparison with ranitidine. *Scand J Gastroenterol* 1989; **24** (suppl 164): 152–60.

97. Agrawal NM, Saffouri B, Kruss DM, Callison DA, Dajani EZ. Healing of benign gastric ulcer: a placebo controlled comparison of two dosage regimens of misoprostol, a synthetic analog of prostaglandin E₁. *Dig Dis Sci* 1985; **30** (suppl): 164–70.

98. Rachmilewitz D, Chapman JW, Nicholson PA. A multicenter international controlled comparison of two dosage regimens of misoprostol with cimetidine in treatment of gastric ulcer in outpatients. *Dig Dis Sci* 1986; **31**: 75S–80S.

99. Navert H. Treatment of gastric ulcer with enprostil. *Am J Med* 1986; **81**: 75–9.

100. Dammann HG, Hutteman W, Kalek HD, Rohner HG, Simon B. A comparative clinical trial of enprostil and ranitidine in the treatment of gastric ulcer. *Am J Med* 1986; **81** (suppl): 80–4.

101. Quinton A, Goldfain D, Weber F, *et al.* Treatment of benign gastric ulcer: a comparative clinical trial of rioprostil and ranitidine. *Scand J Gastroenterol* 1989; **24** (suppl 164): 178–83.

102. Rutgeerts P, Vantrappen G, Businger JA, Demol P, Simon B, Barbier P. Efficacy and safety of rioprostil, 300 μg bd in the treatment of gastric ulcer: a comparison vs ranitidine, 150 mg bd in a randomised multicentre study. *Scand J Gastroenterol* 1989; **24** (suppl 164): 184–90.

103. Hawkey CJ, Walt RP. Prostaglandins in peptic ulceration – a promise unfulfilled. *Lancet* 1986; **2**: 1084–7.

104. Roth SH, Bennett RE. Nonsteroidal anti-inflammatory drug gastropathy. Recognition and response. *Arch Intern Med* 1987; **147**: 2093–100.

105. Hudson N, Everitt SJ, Hawkey CJ. Inter-observer variability in assessment of gastric lesions by video endoscopy. *Gut* 1991; **32**: A1256.

106. Graham DY, Lidsky MD, Cox AM, *et al.* Long term non steroidal anti-inflammatory drug use and *Helicobacter pylori* infection. *Gastroenterology* 1991; **100**: 1653–7.

107. Euler AR, Safdi M, Rao J, *et al.* A report of three multiclinic trials evaluating arbaprostil in arthritic patients with ASA/NSAID gastric mucosal damage. *Gastroenterology* 1990; **98**: 1549–57.

108. Roth S, Agrawal N, Mahowald M, *et al.* Misoprostol heals gastroduodenal injury in patients with rheumatoid arthritis receiving aspirin. *Arch Intern Med* 1989; **149**: 755–9.

109. Sontag SJ, Schnell TG, Mak K, *et al.* Enprostil heals NSAID induced gastric ulcers. *Gastroenterology* 1990; **98**: A129.

110. Paladini G, Fabiani MG, Tosato F, Maggiozo F. Prophylactic and therapeutic role of misoprostol in NSAID induced gastroduodenal lesions. *Scand J Gastroenterol* 1989; **24** (suppl 164): 242–6.

111. Mahida YR, Perkins AC, Frier M, Wastie ML, Hawkey CJ. Monoclonal antigranulocyte antibody imaging in inflammatory bowel disease: a preliminary report. *Nucl Med Commun* (in press).

112. Graham DY, Agrawal N, Roth SH. Prevention of NSAID-induced gastric ulcer with misoprostol: multicentre, double-blind, placebo-controlled trial. *Lancet* 1988; **2**: 1277–80.

113. Agrawal N, Stromatt S, Brown J. Comparative study of misoprostol and sucralfate in the prevention of NSAID-induced gastric ulcers. *Gastroenterology* 1990; **98**: A14.

114. Geiss S, Stead H, Wallemark C-B, Nicholson PA. Prevalence of mucosal lesions in the stomach and

duodenum due to chronic use of NSAID in patients with rheumatoid arthritis or osteoarthritis, an interim report on prevention by misoprostol of diclofenac associated lesions. *J Rheumatol* 1991; **18** (suppl 28): 11–14.

115. Elliott SL, Yeomans ND, Buchanan RRC, *et al.* Long term effects of misoprostol on gastropathy induced by nonsteroidal anti-inflammatory drugs (NSAID). *Gastroenterology* 1990; **98:** A40.

116. Graham DY, Stromatt SC, Jaszewski R, White RH, Triadafilopoulos G. Prevention of duodenal ulcer in arthritics who are chronic NSAID users: a multicentre trial of the role of misoprostol. *Gastroenterology* 1991; **100:** A75.

117. Raskin J, White R, Jaszewski R. Double-blind comparative study of the efficacy and safety of misoprostol and ranitidine in the prevention of NSAID-induced gastric ulcers and upper GI symptoms: preliminary findings. *Digestion* 1991; **49** (suppl 1): 50–1.

118. Verdickt W, Moran C, Hantzschel H, Fraga AM, Stead H, Geiss GS. A double-blind comparison of the gastroduodenal safety and efficacy of diclofenac and a fixed dose combination of diclofenac and misoprostol in the treatment of rheumatoid arthritis. *Scand J of Rheumatology* 1992; **21** (2): 85–9.

119. Hillman AL, Bloom BS. Economic effects of prophylactic use of misoprostol to prevent gastric ulcer in patients taking nonsteroidal anti-inflammatory drugs. *Arch Intern Med* 1989; **149:** 2061–55.

120. Knill-Jones R, Drummond M, Kohli H, Davies L. Economic evaluation of gastric ulcer prophylaxis in patients with arthritis receiving non-steroidal anti-inflammatory drugs. *Postgrad Med J* 1990; **66:** 639–46.

121. Edelson JT, Tosteson ANA, Sax ScD. Cost-effectiveness of misoprostol for prophylaxis against nonsteroidal anti-inflammatory drug-induced gastrointestinal tract bleeding. *JAMA* 1990; **264:** 41–7.

122. Carrin GJ, Torfs KE. Economic evaluation of prophylactic treatment with misoprostol in osteoarthritis patients treated with NSAIDs. The case of Belgium. *Rev Epidemiol Sante Publique* 1990; **38:** 187–99.

10 Prostaglandins in the treatment of heart and lung disease in infants

Elliot A Shinebourne and Andrew Bush

Therapeutic uses of prostaglandins E$_1$ and E$_2$, D$_2$ and prostacyclin (PGI$_2$) have been explored in a large number of heart and lung diseases of babies and small infants. Their impact in clinical practice has been variable. The use of the E series prostaglandins to reopen or prevent closure of the arterial duct ranks with cross-sectional echocardiography as one of the two innovations most radically to have changed the practice of paediatric cardiology in the last 20 years. It is difficult to think of another compound that has had such a major impact on any specialty. The word 'breakthrough' is freely bandied about, usually in a context of triviality; in the case of the E series prostaglandins and the ductus, this hackneyed description is fully justified. The use of prostaglandins in lung disease is less securely based. PGI$_2$ has been widely prescribed as a pulmonary vasodilator, and its short half-life and safety make it an ideal agent for this purpose; however, comparative studies with other agents are scarce and it is not selective, causing systemic as well as pulmonary vasodilatation. PGD$_2$, on theoretical grounds an even better pulmonary vasodilator, has not been found useful. The E series prostaglandins have also been used as pulmonary vasodilators, although less widely than PGI$_2$. The ideal pulmonary vasodilator has yet to be dis-covered, and prostaglandins are one of several agents available for use in the intensive care unit.

The newborn child/infant exhibits unique cardio-pulmonary physiology. Any therapeutic intervention in this group must be interpreted in the light of the profound physiological changes in the cardiopulmonary unit at birth. The lungs switch from being of trivial importance, receiving only 10% or less of the right ventricular output, to being the only organ of gas exchange; the switchover must be swift if extrauterine life is to be sustained. The immediate functional changes are followed in the ensuing weeks by corresponding, equally essential, structural alterations. Disease processes can interfere with either function or structure, and this affects responses to therapy. Different insults must not be assumed to have identical effects on the maturing lung. This makes it unwise to extrapolate uncritically from adulthood to infancy, and from one disease to another. This chapter therefore begins with a brief review of the maturation of the cardiopulmonary unit in the early weeks of life with particular relevance to the role of prostaglandins, before a more detailed consideration of the therapeutic roles of the individual prostaglandins.

Development of the cardiopulmonary unit

Development of the pulmonary circulation

In week 4 of gestation, the lung bud develops at the distal end of the laryngotracheal sulcus, and then divides into two sacs, eventually to form the right and left lungs. By 6 weeks' gestation the lobar pattern is formed and the subsegmental bronchi are recognizable.[1] The intrapulmonary blood vessels develop from the splanchnic mesoderm of the ventral surface of the foregut which envelopes the lung buds. The central pulmonary arteries are derived from the sixth branchial arches.[2] The proximal pulmonary veins form as an outgrowth of the left atrium.[3]

Lung development follows three simple precepts.[4,5] The bronchial tree is developed by week 16 of intrauterine life. By contrast, mature alveoli develop after birth; they increase rapidly in number thereafter, but alveolar multiplication is probably largely complete by 2 years, rather earlier than previously thought.[6,7] Alveoli continue to increase in size until chest wall growth finishes in adulthood. The proximal vessels follow the development of airways, the intra-acinar that of the alveoli.

Along the arterial path, proximally the muscular coat is complete, more distally giving way to a spiral of muscle (partially muscular artery) and eventually a non-muscular artery, which is larger than the capillaries. In the adult and the fetus, the larger partially muscular artery is 150 μm whereas in the child, because muscularization lags behind elongation, the largest partially muscular artery is 450 μm.[8] In the fetus, the muscular arteries have thicker walls than those of the same size in the adult.[8]

The physiology of the prenatal circulation

The right ventricle ejects two-thirds of the combined ventricular output into the main pulmonary artery.[9] However, only 4–10% of the combined output goes through the lungs because of the high pulmonary vascular resistance (PVR), the rest passing through the arterial duct to the descending aorta.[10] Thus the two major areas of physiological control are the maintenance of a patent arterial duct and the sustained elevation of PVR.

In the fetus, PGE_2 (and, to a lesser extent, PGI_2)

are produced in the placenta and vascular endothelium. It is clear that patency of the arterial duct *in utero* is maintained by PGE_2 and to a lesser extent by PGI_2.[11] The immature duct is particularly sensitive to these prostaglandins.[12] Circulating levels of PGE_2 are markedly elevated, both because of high placental production and because of low lung blood flow and hence reduced opportunity for catabolism by the pulmonary vascular endothelial tree.[11] However, despite the high concentrations of vasodilator prostaglandins, PVR remains high until birth. There is some evidence that vasoconstrictor leukotrienes are responsible for overriding the effects of prostaglandins within the pulmonary vascular bed.[13]

Recent evidence suggests that the minimal intrauterine pulmonary blood flow is not uniform through the lungs with time but that there are zonal cyclical changes in flow.[14] The control of these changes, and their physiological significance, is not clear.

Changes in the cardiopulmonary unit at birth

The rapid adaptation of the pulmonary circulation, its control mechanisms and heightened sensitivity to different stimuli in the perinatal period are wholly dissimilar to anything pertaining in later life. On cessation of flow in the umbilical vessels, usually due to clamping of the umbilical cord, the lungs switch from being an almost vestigial organ to the sole means of ventilatory support. PVR drops, pulmonary blood flow rises, there is a functional cessation of flow in the intrauterine shunts (arterial duct, oval foramen) and gas exchange in the lungs commences. The pulmonary artery pressure falls from a mean of 60 mmHg to 30 mmHg within the first 10 hours of life.[15]

The mechanisms controlling this profound fall in resistance are uncertain. Mechanical traction on the vessels transmitted from the expanding chest wall, increasing diameter and reducing wall thickness are undoubtedly important; even ventilation with pure nitrogen lowers PVR.[16,17] The vasodilator effects of oxygen in the first breath are important,[18] but whether by a direct action on the smooth muscle cells or by the release of mediators is controversial. The release of chemical mediators such as bradykinin[19] or PGD_2[20–22] from perivascular mast cells may have a role, but the definitive mechanisms remain undiscovered. Animal experiments suggest that PGD_2, released from perivascular mast cells, is a mediator of central importance in this process.[20–22]

Whatever the fundamental mechanisms may be,

it is clear that there is much greater reactivity of the newborn compared with the adult pulmonary circulation to mediators such as bradykinin and acetylcholine.[23,24] Animal experiments also suggest that autonomic control may be much more important than in adults.[25,26]

Subsequently, the pulmonary circulation undergoes a phase of structural stabilization with deposition of connective tissue and maturation of smooth muscle cells. Finally, progressive growth and remodelling of the circulation takes place.[27] There are other major circulatory changes, in addition to the fall in PVR at birth. The duct constricts, partly in response to a rise in blood oxygen tension[28] and partly due to the fall in endogenous PGE_2 levels.[29] There is a twofold mechanism of fall in PGE_2: exclusion of the placenta reduces synthesis; and increased exposure to the pulmonary endothelium increases catabolism.[29] Furthermore, the duct itself becomes progressively less sensitive to the effects of PGE_2.[30,31] In the early days of life, the duct is merely constricted and can reopen if hypoxaemia or acidaemia develops. Subsequently, anatomical closure precludes reopening of this shunt. The oval foramen, the other main shunt bypassing the fetal lungs, closes first functionally due to passive pressure effects (left atrial rising above right atrial pressure) and then (in most normal people) structurally. In 30% of normal people, probe patency of the oval foramen persists throughout life.

Effects of abnormal perinatal progress on the pulmonary circulation

Cardiac diseases can increase or decrease pulmonary vascular smooth muscle and vessel number, depending on the haemodynamic effects of the lesion. Postnatal reduction in pulmonary blood flow will lead to hypoplasia of the lung and its circulation.[32,33] High pressures and high flow lead to progressive wall thickening and vascular obstruction (see later). The combined effects of lung immaturity (hyaline membrane disease) and its treatment (positive pressure ventilation, oxygen) increase muscularization of arteries and arterioles, but also causes profound hypoplasia of the pulmonary circulation.[34] Congenital diaphragmatic hernia causes ipsilateral and contralateral vascular hypoplasia, and the circulation may react briskly to many stimuli.[35] Prolonged hypoxia leads to development of muscle in pre-

capillary vessels which would normally be non-muscular.[24] The crude anatomical changes associated with different diseases are relatively well studied. Little is known about the functional correlates of the structural changes. The baseline tone and reactivity of the pulmonary vasculature is undoubtedly the result of complex interactions between circulating platelets and white cells, endothelial cells, smooth muscle cells and fibroblasts with each other and local neurohormonal control mechanisms. There is the potential for different disease patterns to affect different components in separate ways, and so it should never be assumed that, because (say) a compound is a good vasodilator in congenital heart disease, it is equally good in bronchopulmonary dysplasia.

Prostaglandins and the ductus arteriosus: fetus, neonate and infant with congenital heart disease

That the ductus arteriosus remains open after birth is essential for survival in a number of different congenital cardiac anomalies. Conversely, its patency in premature infants or persistence in babies born at term may cause breathlessness, heart failure and ventilator dependence. In the first weeks of life the ability to manipulate the ductus arteriosus pharmacologically has transformed the practice of paediatric cardiology and has led directly to a reduction in infant mortality.

Ductus arteriosus in the fetus

Ductal patency in the fetus was for a long time considered to be a passive process. In 1973, however, Coceani and Olley[36] proposed that patency was maintained by active relaxation induced by a prostaglandin, most probably PGE_2. PGE_2 is produced locally within the wall of the ductus although circulating PGE_2 or PGI_2 may also play a part in maintaining patency.[37] PGE_2 synthetic activity develops early in the developing ductus and is greater in immature than mature tissues. Low oxygen tensions cause the ductus arteriosus to constrict, mature ducts responding more vigorously to lesser falls in oxygen tension than immature ducts.[38] Ductus sensitivity to PGE_2 is greatly diminished by exposure to oxygen.

Glucocorticoids inhibit the release of arachidonic acid (the precursor for PGE_1 or PGE_2) from cell membranes. Experimentally, fetal ductal constriction can be produced by injecting steroids into pregnant rats.[39] Clyman *et al.*[40] studied women treated with betamethasone prior to premature labour to prevent respiratory distress syndrome in their babies. They found that, among infants delivered more than 24 hours after treatment, the overall frequency of ductal patency was lower than in controls. This suggests that endogenous steroids, plasma levels of which increase towards term, may prime the ductus for closure.[41]

Blockade of prostaglandin synthesis by cyclooxygenase inhibitors such as indomethacin or ibuprofen cause constriction of the ductus both *in vitro*[42] and *in vivo*[43] in animals, whilst aspirin and indomethacin are used therapeutically to close the ductus in preterm infants.[44] The ability of the ductus arteriosus to constrict appears also to be dependent on cytochrome P450, inactivation of which inhibits ductal constriction even in the presence of indomethacin.[45] Likewise in lambs, reactive oxygen metabolites generated by the combination of hypoxanthine and xanthine oxidase relax the ductus arteriosus, although the vasoactive effects appear to be mediated entirely through increased generation of PGE_2.[46]

The ductus arteriosus frequently remains patent in preterm infants, resulting in a large left-to-right shunt of blood from aorta to pulmonary artery. More commonly than in term infants, this results in heart failure for two main reasons. The first is that the myocardium of premature infants has fewer contractile elements and a higher water content than more mature myocardium, so the cardiac reserve or ability of the left ventricle to increase its output in response to increased preload is less well developed, and left ventricular end-diastolic pressure rises with heart failure and pulmonary oedema. Secondly there is less muscle in the smaller pulmonary arteries, so the magnitude of the left-to-right shunt cannot be as well limited by pulmonary vasoconstriction as in term infants. Fluid restriction and diuretics are first line treatment but when heart failure cannot be controlled, indomethacin, a prostaglandin synthetase inhibitor, is used. It is given orally or by retention enema in a dose of 0.1–0.2 mg/kg 6-hourly for up to three doses. Toxic effects include oliguria or anuria with nitrogen retention, a bleeding tendency, and gastrointestinal effects such as diarrhoea and vomiting. Pre-existent clotting abnormalities, necrotizing enterocolitis (a not uncommon complication of a large ductus in a premature baby) and jaundice are contraindications to the use of indomethacin. As with many new forms of therapy, initial reports of treatment were enthusiastic but it soon became apparent that the drug was frequently ineffective or that initial ductal constriction was insufficient or not sustained.[47–49]

In some very small-for-dates infants insufficient smooth muscle in the wall of the ductus was the underlying cause of an inadequate response.[50] There is some evidence that elevated circulating levels of prostaglandins distinguish those premature infants with ductal patency in which indomethacin will be effective in inducing ductal closure. Hammerman *et al.*[51] showed that responsiveness was higher in these preterm infants in whom the circulating levels of 6-keto-$PGF_2\alpha$, a stable metabolite of PGE_2, were greater than 500 pg/ml (the upper limit of the normal range) whereas those with normal levels tended not to respond. Finally, white male infants seem to be more prone to persistence of a symptomatic ductus arteriosus after indomethacin administration than females or black infants.[52]

Other circumstances in which an increase in the frequency of ductal patency may be found include the use of the diuretic frusemide in infants with respiratory distress syndrome.[53] Frusemide is known to stimulate renal synthesis of PGE_2. Of 33 infants with respiratory distress syndrome treated with frusemide, 18 had a persistent ductus arteriosus, 11 requiring surgical ligation. This contrasted with persistent ductus in only 8 of 33 treated with chlorothiazide, of which 7 required ligation.[53]

The use of topical PGE_2 gel to induce labour has also been associated with a significantly prolonged ductal closure time in full-term babies, compared with a control group.[54]

Use of prostaglandins to maintain patency of the ductus arteriosus

In contrast to infants with otherwise structurally normal hearts, those with certain congenital cardiac anomalies are dependent on ductal patency for survival. It is here, as much if not more than in any other branch of medicine, that the therapeutic use of prostaglandins has proved of inestimable value. We shall first consider the conditions in question.

Ductus-dependent pulmonary circulation

The causes of ductus-dependent pulmonary circulation are:

- Pulmonary atresia with intact ventricular septum
- Severe (critical) pulmonary stenosis with intact ventricular septum (neonate)
- Pulmonary atresia with ventricular septal defect
- Severe tetralogy of Fallot
- Any other complex congenital heart disease with pulmonary atresia or critical pulmonary stenosis; e.g.
  Double inlet right ventricle
  Double inlet left ventricle
  Double inlet indeterminate ventricle
  Complete transposition with ventricular septal defect
  Corrected transposition with ventricular septal defect
  Absent right atrioventricular connection (tricuspid atresia)
  Absent left atrioventricular connection (mitral atresia)
  Double outlet right ventricle
  Double outlet left ventricle

During intrauterine development, gas exchange takes place at the placenta and the lungs have no role in maintaining adequate oxygenation of the fetus.

In the mature fetus, antegrade flow of blood from right ventricle to pulmonary artery largely passes via the ductus arteriosus to descending aorta, flow to the lungs themselves being only about 8% of the combined fetal cardiac output. Organ flow in the fetus is dependent on local vascular resistance and, as already discussed, this is high in the fetal pulmonary circulation. When there is pulmonary atresia or critical pulmonary stenosis in the fetus, what flow the lungs do receive is via the ductus arteriosus although the direction is the reverse of normal, from aorta to pulmonary artery. At birth the systemic venous return passes across a foramen ovale or ventricular septal defect to the left sides of the heart and then to the aorta.

In double inlet or double outlet ventricles, the systemic venous return may pass directly from ventricle to aorta but, in all these congenital cardiac anomalies, pulmonary blood flow is dependent on blood passing from aorta via the ductus arteriosus to the lungs. If or as the duct closes, pulmonary blood becomes inadequate, with increasing arterial desaturation, cyanosis, metabolic acidosis and death.

Left-sided obstructive lesions

The causes of ductus-dependent systemic circulation are:

- Hypoplastic left heart syndrome (aortic atresia)
- Critical aortic stenosis
- Interrupted aortic arch
- Severe coarctation of the aorta

When there is aortic atresia or critical aortic stenosis in the fetus, placental blood flow and hence metabolic gas exchange in the fetus are maintained by blood passing from the pulmonary artery through the ductus arteriosus to descending aorta. Less of the inferior vena caval venous return to the heart crosses the foramen ovale, and in the extreme case all the fetal cardiac output passes from right ventricle to pulmonary artery, none leaving the heart antegradely from aorta. At birth, systemic blood flow is dependent on a right-to-left shunt across the ductus arteriosus whilst coronary perfusion is dependent on blood passing retrogradely from ductus back through the aortic arch and ascending aorta. When the ductus closes, the systemic cardiac output falls, renal, coronary and cerebral perfusion become inadequate and the patient succumbs with progressive acidosis. When there is interruption of the aortic arch, lower body and particularly renal perfusion are dependent on ductal patency. Coarctation of the aorta becomes manifest when the ductus closes. As long as it remains patent, no significant obstruction develops but in the neonate when the ductus closes rapid deterioration with heart failure results.

Transposition of the great arteries

Complete transposition of the great arteries (atrioventricular concordance, ventriculoarterial discordance) consists of an abnormal ventriculoarterial connection in which the aorta is connected to the morphologically right ventricle and the pulmonary artery to the morphologically left ventricle. Consequently there are two circuits running in parallel, not in series as in the normal, with desaturated blood passing from right atrium to right ventricle, aorta and then back to the right atrium, while fully oxygenated blood passes from left atrium, to left ventricle and pulmonary artery, returning from the lungs via pulmonary veins to left atrium. For survival there has to be mixing of the two circulations, usually through a foramen ovale or atrial septal defect, through a ventricular septal defect if present, or through the ductus arteriosus. In the absence of a ventricular septal defect and with little or no mixing at atrial level (the situation before a balloon septostomy or Rashkind procedure), mixing may be principally dependent on the ductus arteriosus.

Treatment protocols

PGE$_1$ was first used in the mid-1970s, given by continuous intravenous infusion in a dose of 0.05–0.10 μg/kg per minute.[55–57] The most dramatic results were in infants with cyanotic heart disease, such as pulmonary atresia or severe tetralogy, where within 5–10 minutes there could be a dramatic increase in arterial Po$_2$. Efficacy in treating left-sided obstructive lesions was soon demonstrated with a similar dosage regimen.[58] The major side effect was apnoea, so facilities for intubation and ventilation need also to be available. Whilst the initial work was carried out with PGE$_1$, PGE$_2$ seems equally effective, is more widely available because of its use in obstetric practice, cheaper and can also be given orally.[59,60] In the USA collaborative study[61] doses of 0.05–1.0 μg/kg per minute PGE$_1$ intravenously were given but a comparative study by Silove *et al.*[62] established the equal efficacy of PGE$_2$ in a dose of 0.003–0.005 μg/kg per minute. Occasionally this infusion rate was increased to 0.01–0.02 μg/kg per minute but higher doses were found to be no more effective and to be more likely to cause side effects, particularly apnoea. These workers also persisted with the use of oral PGE$_2$ in which a dosage regimen of 20–25 μg/kg hourly was used. If the initial response was poor, this dose could be doubled. Having said this, the majority of units would still use intravenous administration as front line treatment. Indeed, lack of response to oral therapy as well as diarrhoea or circumstances in which absorption from the gastrointestinal tract would be expected to be poor are all indications for intravenous therapy. If long-term therapy with oral PGE$_2$ is used, the frequency of dosage may be reduced in time, but even so an hourly dosage regimen amounts to a considerable burden on the carers if home usage is contemplated.

A recent report describes the use of a new oral PGE$_1$ derivative given in a dose of 1.5–2.0 μg/kg per day but on a 6-hourly basis. The authors[63] suggest that this agent may be as effective as intravenous PGE$_1$, and the need for less frequent dosage is clearly advantageous in a clinical context. More reports are needed.

Complications of PGE therapy

As already discussed, apnoea requiring ventilation is the most important acute effect of PGE therapy. The response is to some extent dose-dependent, and hence the lowest dose that is effective should be used. Jitteriness, pyrexia, diarrhoea and vomiting are not uncommon, reversible cortical hyperostosis of long bones,[64] soft-tissue swelling[65] and pseudo-widening of cranial suture[66] are also found. Perhaps the most interesting and clinically important longer term complication in neonatal heart disease is failure of the ductus arteriosus to close after PGE$_1$ or PGE$_2$ administration even after relatively short periods of time.

Of the first 50 neonates with pulmonary atresia we treated with intravenous PGE$_2$ for falling arterial Po$_2$ secondary to ductal constriction, 3 stayed in congestive heart failure from excessive pulmonary blood flow following a modified Blalock–Taussig shunt between subclavian and pulmonary artery. They all required surgical ductal closure, clearly indicating that a ductus, previously closing spontaneously, following PGE$_1$ therapy then showed impaired ability to constrict. Whilst this is a disadvantage in patients with a ductus-dependent pulmonary circulation,[67] it may be an advantage in patients with coarctation of the aorta where persistent ductal patency may obviate the need for emergency surgery in the neonate.[68]

Impaired ability of the ductus arteriosus to constrict following PGE infusion is reflected in histological changes. Most workers agree that there is an increase in histopathological features after the drug, namely medial oedema, mural thrombosis and interruption of the internal elastic lamina at sites not beneath intimal cushion.[69,70] The effects are dose-dependent, those receiving more than 0.05 μg/kg per minute showing more severe effects.[71] There appeared to be no relationship to duration of treatment, age of onset of treatment or total dose of prostaglandin, although histological changes were more marked in infants with a gestational age greater than 40 weeks. Calder *et al.*[69] found intimal tears and haemorrhage into the media in some of the treated patients, but not in controls. These workers thought such lesions to be specific for a prostaglandin effect. Gittenberger-de Groot *et al.*,[70] however, suggested that the differences in histopathology between controls and prostaglandin treated were only of degree. An additional consequence of prostaglandin therapy may be increased friability of the ductus such that if surgical closure is required, risk of haemorrhage may be greater. Aneurysm formation in the ductus has also been found at operation, but to our knowledge spontaneous rupture has not been reported.

Clinical consequences of prostaglandin therapy to maintain patency of the ductus arteriosus

A consequence of long-term PGE therapy in pulmonary atresia whether given intravenously[67] or orally[59] is that, if the ductus remains widely open because of increased pulmonary blood flow, the pulmonary arteries may grow over a period of weeks, thus facilitating subsequent surgery.

Some authors believe that the increased growth of pulmonary arteries facilitates performing a modified Blalock–Taussig shunt, i.e. insertion of a graft between subclavian and pulmonary arteries. We are not completely convinced of this, as the apparent increase in size with increased flow may simply reflect distension rather than growth. Furthermore, many surgeons would not consider the small size of central pulmonary arteries as a major contraindication for shunt surgery at any age.

Infants with pulmonary atresia and intact ventricular septum pose a difficult clinical problem, and there is no real consensus on management approach. Conventionally, balloon atrial septostomy (to facilitate right-to-left shunting at atrial level) is performed at cardiac catheterization and a surgical systemic pulmonary artery anastomosis carried out to increase pulmonary blood flow. This is because small size, lack of contractility and morphology of the right ventricle frequently preclude direct relief of obstruction as sole therapy. Nowadays, in virtually all paediatric cardiology units prostaglandin E_1 or E_2 is commenced on diagnosis – or even on suspected diagnosis, confirmation of which is by cross-sectional echocardiography. Several groups[72,73] have elected to undertake direct relief of right ventricular outflow tract obstruction in all or the majority of patients while maintaining them on prostaglandin postoperatively. This allows the right ventricle to recover from open heart surgery and many days or weeks later PGE is discontinued. Definitive repair can usually be carried out successfully if certain criteria are met: the right ventricle is tripartite, i.e. has an inflow portion, a trabecular portion and an outflow tract; the tricuspid valve annulus is more than 70% of mitral valve size and severe tricuspid regurgitation is not present; the right ventricle exhibits some systolic contraction; and the coronary arteries are not filled primarily from the right ventricular cavity via coronary venous sinusoids. When the right ventricle is thought to be contracting adequately, prostaglandin is discontinued. Should arterial saturation fall precipitously, the drug can be restarted to reopen

the duct if necessary, allowing a surgical shunt to be carried out electively.

Another circumstance in which long-term PGE may be used is hypoplastic left heart syndrome. In this condition, characterized by a grossly hypoplastic left ventricle and aortic atresia, systemic blood flow has to be sustained via the ductus arteriosus. The treatment options are a first-stage Norwood procedure (anastomosis of main pulmonary artery to aorta, right modified Blalock–Taussig anastomosis and atrial septectomy), infant heart transplantation or provision of support to the family while the baby dies. Prostaglandin administration may buy time while a donor is found – if one believes or the family agree that transplantation is a worthwhile option.

In transposition of the great arteries, by keeping the ductus arteriosus open, prostaglandin infusion facilitates shunting of desaturated blood from aorta to pulmonary artery. The increase in effective pulmonary blood flow then results in an increase in systemic arterial saturation.[74] Whilst this is clinically beneficial, the concomitant increase in pulmonary venous return causes a rise in left atrial pressure which may lead to closure of the flap valve of the foramen ovale, further elevating left atrial pressure. The respiratory rate may then rise alarmingly, necessitating an urgent balloon septostomy.

Ductus venosus

In the fetus the ductus venosus connects the portal vein to inferior vena cava, thus allowing highly oxygenated blood returning from the placenta via umbilical veins to bypass the liver. It has usually been assumed that patency of the ductus venosus is dependent on passive distension but Coceani and Olley[75] have presented evidence that, as with the arterial duct, prostaglandins E_2 and I_2 cause active dilatation, contraction being dependent on an endogenous cytochrome P450 mechanism. So far there has been no important clinical implication for this finding although one condition in which management could conceivably be affected is infradiaphragmatic total anomalous pulmonary venous connection to portal vein. In this condition, when the ductus venosus closes, acute pulmonary venous obstruction causes pulmonary oedema. Theoretically, dilator prostaglandins should open the ductus venosus, alleviating pulmonary oedema. To our knowledge, however, this has not as yet been demonstrated in clinical practice.

Prostaglandin inhibitors and pregnancy

Administration of prostaglandin inhibitors such as indomethacin to the mother of a fetus with a potentially ductus-dependent neonatal circulation might be expected to precipitate symptoms postnatally. Menaham[76] reported two patients delivered by emergency caesarean section at 34 weeks for fetal distress, who also had a ductus-dependent pulmonary or systemic circulation. He suggested that, although such instances are rare, fetal cross-sectional echocardiography should be carried out before prostaglandin inhibitors are prescribed during pregnancy.

The role of prostaglandins in the treatment of lung disease

The therapy of pulmonary hypertension in infants has been dominated by the search for a selective agent – i.e. a drug that will dilate the pulmonary vascular bed while having no effect, or even constricting, the systemic circulation. To date, 100% oxygen[77] and inhaled nitric oxide[78] are the only agents that have been found to be selective. Non-selective agents can cause dangerous hypotension, reduced myocardial perfusion and a fall in cardiac output which may even be fatal.[79] Fig. 10.1 shows the effects of giving PGI_2 to an infant after cardiac surgery, who was already receiving intravenous dopamine and isoprenaline (Bush *et al.*, 1984, unpublished observations). There is a profound fall in cardiac output, on the face of it the opposite effect to that which would be expected. Presumably, systemic venodilatation and a fall in myocardial perfusion were responsible. Data such as these underscore the need for careful monitoring when potent cardiovascular drugs are given to sick infants. Approaches to the search for other selective agents include giving compounds that are completely cleared in one pass by the pulmonary capillary bed, in the hope that they would dilate the pulmonary arteriolar bed but not spill into the systemic circulation; and combining a mixed systemic/pulmonary vasodilator with a systemic vasoconstrictor such as noradrenaline or oxygen.

A further general problem with pulmonary vasodilators relates to the physiological purpose of pulmonary vasoconstriction. In normal circumstances, pulmonary gas exchange is optimized by matching ventilation to perfusion. The most powerful local control mechanism is vasoconstriction of arterioles supplying unperfused alveoli.[80] It is only when generalized hypoxia results in global elevation in PVR that the reflex ceases to be beneficial. When a pulmonary vasodilator is given, 'beneficial' hypoxic vasoconstriction is reversed,[81] resulting in a fall in

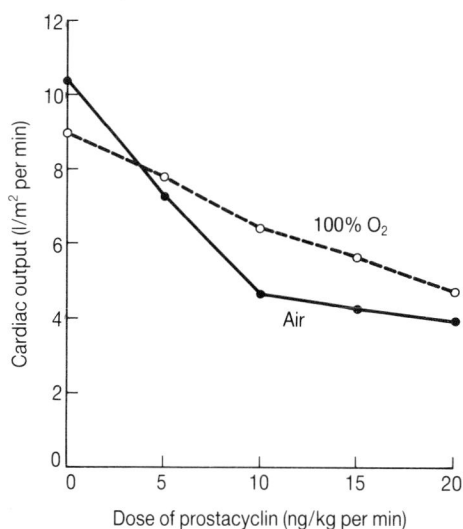

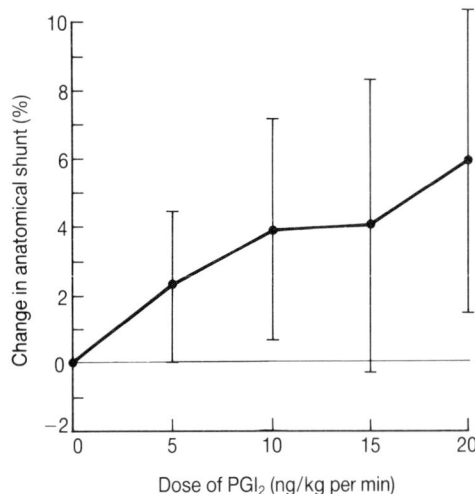

Fig. 10.1 Effect of increasing doses of prostacyclin (PGI_2) on cardiac output in an infant after cardiac surgery. There is a marked fall in cardiac output both on air and on 100% oxygen.

Fig. 10.2 Change in percentage anatomical shunt with prostacyclin (PGI_2). The mean and 95% confidence intervals are plotted. (Reproduced, with permission, from *Clin Sci*[81])

pulmonary venous P_{O_2} from increased intrapulmonary right-to-left shunting. This is not clinically significant if the P_{O_2} is high[34] (flat part of oxygen dissociation curve) but may be of major importance if oxygenation is precarious. The effects of PGI_2 on anatomical shunt are shown in Fig. 10.2.

This section details attempts to use prostaglandins as pulmonary vasodilators, with particular regard for specificity for the pulmonary circulation, and effects on gas exchange.

Therapeutic use of PGD$_2$

Speculation that the pulmonary vasodilatation seen at birth may be due in part to a release of PGD_2 from perivascular mast cells has led to its evaluation as a pulmonary vasodilator, initially in animals and then in infants with persistent fetal circulation (PFC). Studies in fetal and newborn lambs showed that PGD_2 in a dose of 5 ng/kg per minute reduced mean pulmonary artery pressure by one-third, with an increase in systemic vascular resistance (SVR), in the first 3 days of life.[20, 21] This combination of physiological properties would make PGD_2 a very attractive therapeutic agent. However, beyond 3 days of age the effects of PGD_2 become progressively less selective for the pulmonary circulation. The net circulatory effects of PGD_2 in animals depend on age, dose and presence or absence of hypoxaemia.[20-22] Clinical observations in six newborn infants with PFC were disapointing.[82] PGD_2 did not alter pulmonary artery pressure nor improve oxygenation. The authors speculate that this may be due to the underlying pathophysiology, namely insensitivity to naturally occurring vasodilators. This may be so, but the narrow therapeutic window in animals and the disappointing results in infants do not encourage further trials. Indeed, the evidence that PGD_2 may be of physiological importance in humans is tenuous.

Therapeutic use of PGI$_2$

PGI_2 is the prostaglandin most widely used in recent years as a pulmonary vasodilator. It appears to be relatively free of side effects, but is very expensive.

Pharmacokinetics of PGI$_2$

Initial studies relied on changes in heart rate to assess the cardiovascular effects of PGI_2.[83] We used an inert gas method (argon and freon-22) to determine effective pulmonary blood flow[84] which is virtually identical to cardiac output.[85] Preliminary experiments showed that there was a lower coefficient of

variation using rebreathing as opposed to single breath methods.[84, 86] Ideally we would have studied infants, but it was considered unethical to give PGI_2 to normal children. We therefore studied six normal adults, administering doses of 5 and 10 ng/kg per minute and studying the effects of increasing and decreasing the dose. The results are shown in Figs. 10.3 and 10.4, from which it can be seen that each

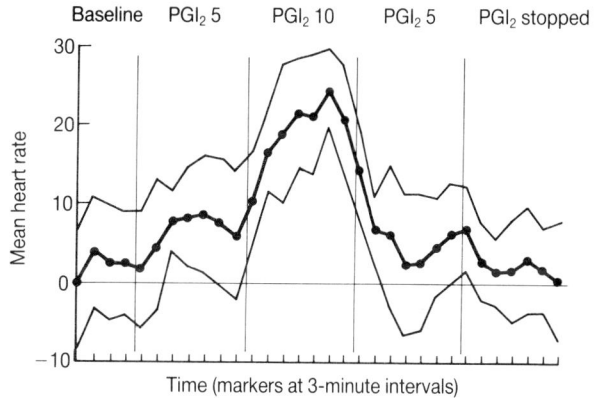

Fig. 10.3 The difference between the drug and placebo study days for heart rate is plotted against time, as prostacyclin (PGI_2) is infused in increasing and then decreasing doses (ng/kg per minute). The mean and 95% confidence intervals for this difference are shown. (Reproduced, with permission, from *Br J Clin Pharmacol*[84])

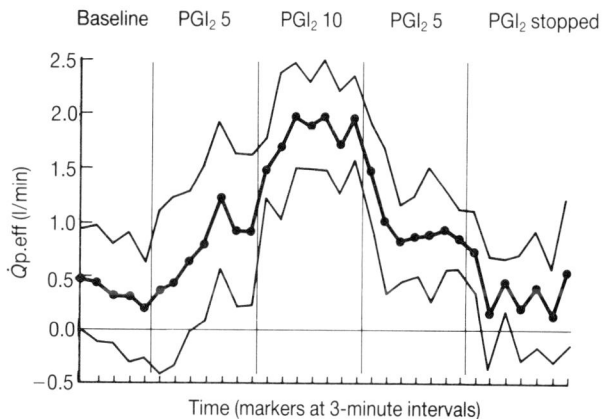

Fig. 10.4 The difference between the drug and placebo study days for effective pulmonary blood flow ($\dot{Q}$p.eff) is plotted against time, as prostacyclin (PGI_2) is infused in increasing and then decreasing doses (ng/kg per minute). The mean and 95% confidence intervals for this difference are shown. (Reproduced, with permission, from *Br J Clin Pharmacol*[84])

dose caused a mean 20% rise in effective pulmonary blood flow and a 15% rise in heart rate. The effects appeared to reach a plateau within 10 minutes of starting or increasing the rate of infusion, and to reach a new steady state within 5 minutes of reducing or stopping the infusion. At these doses there was no significant effect on systolic or diastolic blood pressure. In another study, we were able to make measurements suggesting that, in infants and children with cardiac disease, the pharmacokinetics of PGI_2 were similar.[87] The rapidity of onset and short duration of action are potential advantages of PGI_2 therapy in fragile infants. There is some evidence that sick babies may metabolize prostaglandins faster than normal, underscoring the importance of not extrapolating from normal health to disease states. Rapid metabolism would be a further advantage, but the possible need for adjustment in dosage should be remembered.

Therapeutic use in children with pulmonary vascular disease secondary to congenital heart disease

Initial experience of PGI_2 in children with pulmonary circulatory disease was largely on anecdotal reports.[88–90] We attempted to systematize knowledge of its properties by constructing dose–response curves in 20 infants and children with pulmonary vascular disease secondary to congenital heart disease. We studied the effects of PGI_2 in doses of 5–20 ng/kg per minute on the pulmonary and systemic circulations while the children were intubated and ventilated on air and then on 100% oxygen.[87] The physiological methods in this and other studies summarized here[34,81,87,91–96] are similar. In all cases, cardiac output was measured using the direct Fick principle (cardiac output = oxygen consumption/arteriovenous oxygen content difference). Oxygen consumption was measured by the argon dilution method.[77,97,98] It is important not to assume oxygen consumption, which is abnormal in children with cardiac disease[99] and chronic lung disease.[100] Blood oxygen content was measured using Kelman's subroutine with allowance for dissolved oxygen.[101] PVR was calculated as (pressure drop across the pulmonary circulation [mmHg])/(cardiac index). The normal range for our laboratory is less than 3 Wood units (mmHg·l^{-1}·min·m^2). The results are summarized in Figs. 10.5 and 10.6. When the subjects breathed air, PGI_2 caused a dose-dependent fall in PVR (11.1 to 8.1, standard error of difference (SED)=0.5, $p<0.01$). At the highest levels infused (20 ng/kg per minute), PGI_2 produced the same

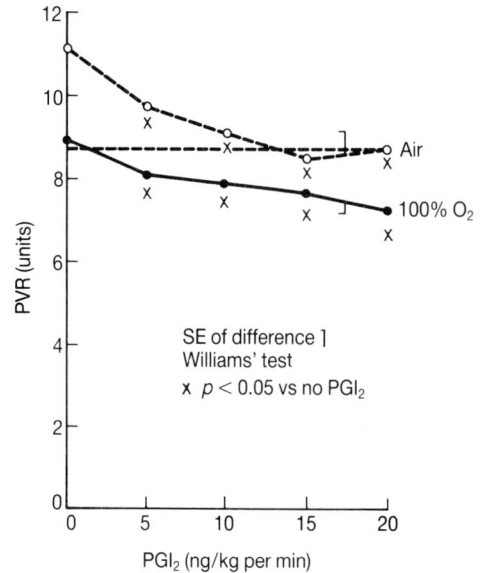

Fig. 10.5 Effects of increasing doses of prostacyclin (PGI_2) on pulmonary vascular resistance (PVR), the children breathing both air and 100% oxygen (O_2). The units of PVR are mmHg·min·l^{-1}·m^2. (Reproduced, with permission, from *Am Rev Respir Dis*[95])

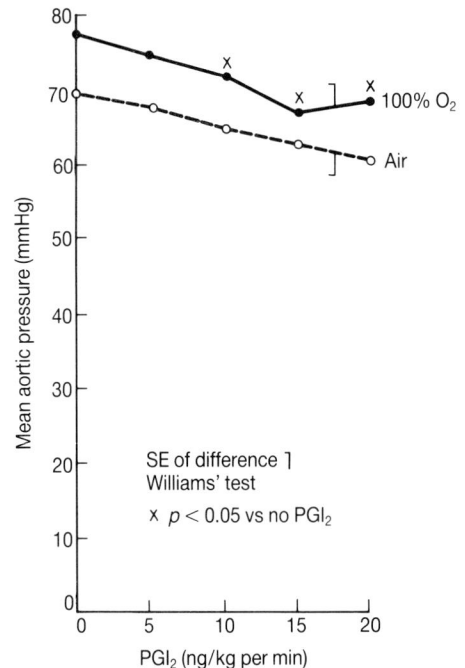

Fig. 10.6 Effects of increasing doses of prostacyclin (PGI_2) on mean aortic pressure, the children breathing both air and 100% oxygen (O_2). (Reproduced, with permission, from *Am Rev Respir Dis*[95])

levels of PVR that were reached by breathing 100% oxygen (8.7 to 8.9, SED=0.6, p=NS). PGI_2, however, caused additional dose-dependent pulmonary vasodilatation when infused while the subjects breathed oxygen (PVR 8.9 to 7.2, SED=0.3, $p<0.01$). PGI_2 was not selective for the pulmonary circulation, but caused a dose-dependent fall in aortic pressure (Fig. 10.6). Systemic vascular resistance (SVR) could not be calculated on most of the subjects because intracardiac shunting rendered impossible the obtaining of a true mixed systemic venous sample. Note that aortic pressure was higher when 100% oxygen was breathed than for the corresponding dose of PGI_2 on air, for all levels of PGI_2. Oxygen, unlike PGI_2, causes systemic vasoconstriction and pulmonary vasodilatation.[87] In children with congenital heart disease, 100% oxygen does not maximally vasodilate the pulmonary circulation; further vasodilatation can be obtained with a blood-borne agent.

Therapy of chronic lung disease

The aggressive intensive care of very premature babies has salvaged many who would otherwise have died, but some survivors are left chronically oxygen-dependent, with pulmonary hypertension and cor pulmonale. The structural features of their chronic lung disease (bronchopulmonary dysplasia) (BPD) include increased bronchial smooth muscle, reduced number of alveoli, pulmonary vascular hypoplasia and increased muscularization of the pulmonary arterial tree. The functional correlates include bronchial hyperreactivity, hyperinflation, an elevation in PVR and a reactive pulmonary circulation.[102] We compared oxygen and PGI_2 in five children with severe BPD.[34] Oxygen caused no change in PVR (cf. congenital heart disease[72] and other studies in less severe BPD[103,104]) but PGI_2 caused a mean 23% fall in PVR (Fig. 10.7). These individual differences, presumably reflecting different diseases and different stages of the same disease, underscore the importance of not extrapolating uncritically between infants. Hypotension (Fig. 10.8) and a fall in arterial Po_2 (Fig. 10.9) were noted. The infants studied were all very ill, and only one eventually survived. Earlier use of PGI_2 in hyaline membrane disease (the acute lung injury that is the common antecedent of BPD) could reduce ventilatory requirements and hence barotrauma by reducing lung stiffness secondary to pulmonary hypertension,[105] as well as improving oxygen dispatch[102] from the lung (pulmonary blood flow × blood oxygen content). Conversely, the fall in arterial Po_2 could adversely affect peripheral tissue

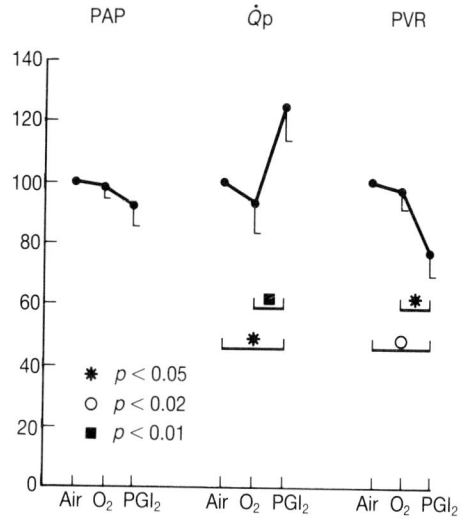

Fig. 10.7 Percentage changes over baseline (vertical axis) in pulmonary haemodynamics with 100% oxygen (O_2) and the dose of prostacyclin (PGI_2) resulting in the lowest pulmonary vascular resistance. There was no significant change in pulmonary artery pressure; cardiac output rose, and pulmonary vascular resistance fell, when prostacyclin was given. (Reproduced, with permission, from *Arch Dis Child*[34])

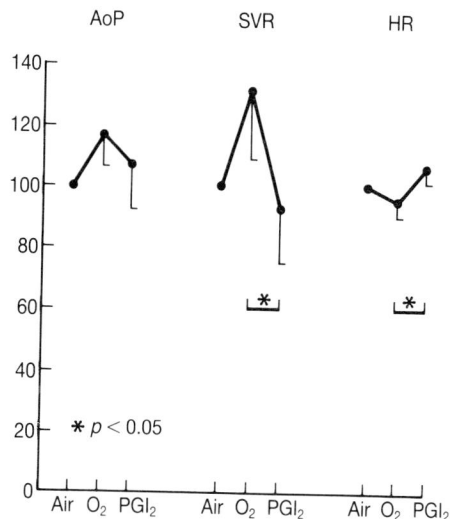

Fig. 10.8 Percentage change over baseline (vertical axis) in systemic haemodynamics with 100% oxygen (O_2) and the dose of prostacyclin (PGI_2) resulting in the lowest pulmonary vascular resistance. There was no significant change in aortic pressure; systemic vascular resistance fell, and heart rate rose, when prostacyclin was given. (Reproduced, with permission, from *Arch Dis Child*[34])

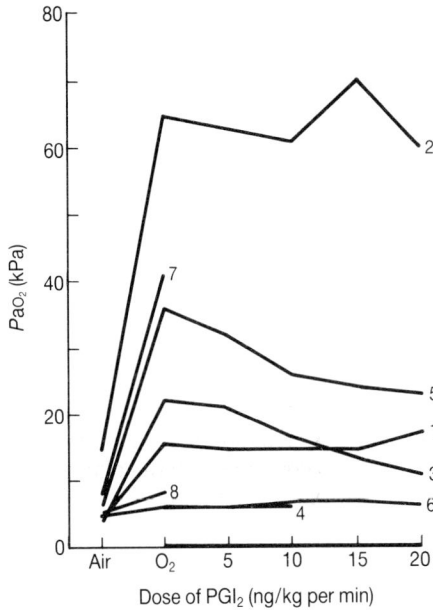

Fig. 10.9 Changes in systemic arterial oxygen tension (Pa_{O_2}) with 100% oxygen (O_2) and prostacyclin (PGI_2). The baseline for cases 6 and 7 was not air but fractional inspiratory oxygen of 0.6 and 0.3 respectively. (Reproduced, with permission, from *Arch Dis Child*[34])

metabolism to perfusion matching. However, the role of PGI_2 other than in acute pulmonary hypertension in BPD remains controversial.

Therapy of other lung diseases

Persistent fetal circulation (PFC) has numerous septic, developmental and other causes.[106] Different causes have different pathogenetic mechanisms. For example, there are high levels of thromboxane A_2 in septic PFC, but not in that due to meconium aspiration,[107] confirming animal work.[108] In one series, two of five infants with PFC benefited from intravenous PGI_2.[109] A further variable in determining the response is the possibility of the abnormal metabolism of prostanoids in sick, septic infants,[110] underscoring the need to titrate doses to the individual baby. It cannot be assumed to be useful in all cases, and its use should be assessed on an individual basis.

Congenital diaphragmatic hernia is associated with pulmonary hypoplasia and PFC,[106] which are major factors in determining management. Surgery is associated with a rise in thromboxane B_2 levels.[111] There are anecdotes of good responses to PGI_2, but no systematic trial; possibly extracorporeal mem-

brane oxygenation, although much more invasive, will be the treatment of choice for both PFC and congenital diaphragmatic hernia, whilst inhalation of nitric oxide, now identified as endothelium-derived relaxing factor, remains a further possibility.

Comparisons with other vasodilators

Tolazoline is an α-adrenergic antagonist, H_2-agonist agent that has been widely used in the treatment of pulmonary hypotension in children. It is cheap but serious side effects are common.[112–114] These include hypotension, thrombocytopenia, pulmonary and gastrointestinal bleeding, fits, oliguria and renal failure, and hyponatraemia. The half-life of tolazoline has been measured as 90 minutes to more than 40 hours, being prolonged by oliguria and renal failure.[115] We compared its effects with those of PGI_2 in 11 children with pulmonary vascular disease.[92] PGI_2 was always given first, because of the differences in half-life. For the group as a whole, both drugs caused systemic (Fig. 10.10) and pulmonary (Fig. 10.11) vasodilatation, and there were no significant differences between the two. Some individuals appeared to respond more favourably to one drug or the other. Side effects are unlikely with single doses of tolazoline, but, if multiple doses of a vasodilator are required, PGI_2 is likely to be safer than tolazoline.

PGI_2 and PGE_2 have been compared in children after cardiac surgery (see below); otherwise, detailed comparisons between vasodilators have not been made. In general, there is no reason to believe that any blood-borne agent is ideal.

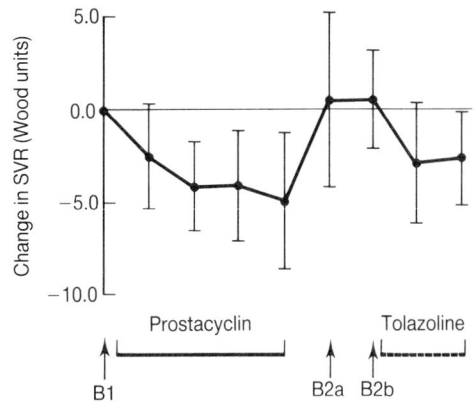

Fig. 10.10 Change (mean, 95% confidence limits) in systemic vascular resistance (SVR) with prostacyclin and tolazoline infusions; 6 patients studied. B1, B2a, B2b are baseline measurements. (Reproduced, with permission, from *Br Heart J*[92])

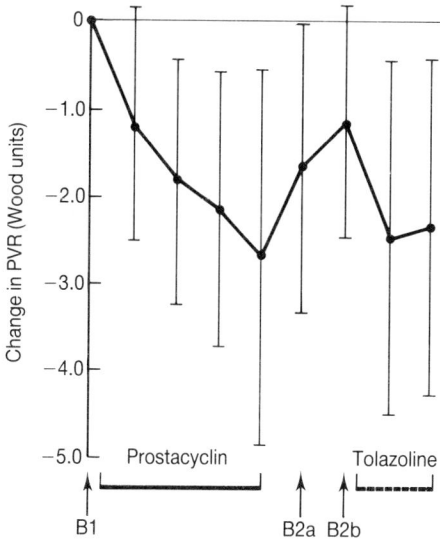

Fig. 10.11 Change (mean, 95% confidence limits) in pulmonary vascular resistance (PVR) with prostacyclin and tolazoline; 11 patients studied. (Reproduced, with permission, from *Br Heart J*[92])

Diagnostic use of PGI_2

Abnormally high pressure and flow within the pulmonary circulation produces structural damage which eventually becomes irreversible even if the underlying cause can be corrected. This damage can be assessed invasively using open lung biopsy, the sample being examined qualitatively[116–118] or quantitatively.[119,120] Physiologically, the damage is characterized by an elevation in PVR. This comprises two elements – a fixed irreversible component due to structural damage and vasoconstriction, which might be expected to reverse after a corrective operation. If the reversible component is not identified by using appropriate vasodilators, the extent of damage may be overestimated, and the child denied appropriate treatment.[87] Prompted by our observation that 100% oxygen and PGI_2 are additive,[87,92] we now give both agents in order to assess reversibility.[95] We have reviewed our experience[93] and shown that a lowest PVR (on PGI_2 and oxygen) of 6.0 Wood units or greater, predicts a bad prognosis. In some patients this is due to late stage pulmonary vascular disease (Heath Edwards late grade III or worse); in others there are no 'irreversible' changes (Heath Edwards grade I or II) but very marked medial muscle hypertrophy; many of the latter group die after a stormy postoperative course. The haemodynamic profile of PGI_2 makes it an ideal agent for this kind of diagnostic evaluation.

Therapeutic use of PGE₁ and PGE₂

The major use of PGE₁ and PGE₂ has been the maintenance of ductal patency in duct-dependent systemic or pulmonary circulation (see previous sections). An early report described the use of PGE₁ in an 11-year-old with an acute pulmonary hypertensive crisis superimposed on primary pulmonary hypertension.[121] Nitroglycerin failed to reduce the suprasystemic pulmonary artery pressures, and PGE₁, in a dose of 30 ng/kg per minute reduced pulmonary artery pressure from 85 to 56 mmHg, wedge pressure from 18 to 4 mmHg, and increased arterial Po_2 (on 100% O_2) from 193 to 216 mmHg. The effect on oxygenation may seem paradoxical in view of previous comments on the effect of vasodilatation on hypoxic vasoconstriction. However, in primary pulmonary hypertension there is minimal ventilatory disturbance, so local hypoxic vasoconstriction is unlikely to be important, and the increase in oxygenation can be explained by an increase in pulmonary blood flow disproportionate to peripheral oxygen consumption, thus elevating mixed venous saturation and improving pulmonary gas exchange in alveolar compartments with gas exchange limited by transit time. There has been some more recent interest in the role of the E series prostaglandins as pulmonary vasodilators; as the authors of the original case report noted, they are rapidly metabolized by the pulmonary circulation. A recent paper[122] compared the effects of PGE₁ (up to 100 ng/kg per minute) with PGI_2 (up to 25 ng/kg per minute) in 20 infants who had undergone corrective cardiac surgery. Both agents were effective pulmonary vasodilators, and neither was selective for the pulmonary circulation. Cost was the only thing to choose between them, PGE₁ being much cheaper. All the patients had been given phenoxybenzamine, an α-adrenergic blocking agent, and so possibly the results should not be generalized to all patients. In a further study, Rubin et al.[123] administered PGE₁ to 26 children in doses of 0.1–1.0 µg/kg per minute and compared it with sodium nitroprusside (0.59–8.7 µg/kg per minute). The vasodilator effects with PGE₁ were less predictable, and in 5 children it had to be discontinued. When this was done, the adverse effects (tachycardia, $n=2$; reduced cardiac index, headache and agitation, abdominal pain and agitation, $n=1$ each) subsided within 15 minutes.

Side effects of prostaglandins

Immediate side effects

The largest series studied to ascertain side effects of PGE_1 was 492 infants from 56 centres.[124] The overall incidence of PGE_1-related side effects was about 20%; cardiovascular problems included cutaneous vasodilatation, oedema, hypotension and arrhythmia; next commonest was seizure-like activity. Respiratory depression was seen in 12% over all, rising to 42% in babies whose birth weight was less than 2 kg. There was no convincing increase in the incidence of sepsis. There is no doubt that repiratory depression immediately after commencing PGE_1 is common, especially in small babies, and facilities to begin assisted ventilation should be to hand. It is wise to allow a period of stabilization after starting PGE_1 rather than immediately transferring the baby to the cardiac surgical centre for further management.

The general problems of vasodilator agents have been addressed in previous sections, namely worsening of ventilation to perfusion matching in the lungs causing hypoxaemia,[81] and hypotension and a fall in cardiac output due to effects on the systemic circulation.[87,92] Problems specific to PGI_2 in infants are flushing and erythema along the course of the vein into which the drug is being infused. Anecdotally, their effects appear to be antagonized by hypercapnia;[125] it is thus important to optimize ventilation before using these agents, and probably the same is true for other blood-borne vasodilators also. The theoretical risk of bleeding due to effects on platelets has not been encountered in our practice. PGI_2 appears to be remarkably free from other acute side effects, which constitutes a major advantage.

Long-term side effects

PGI_2 has not been used other than for relatively short periods (days) in intensive care units in infants. PGE_1 and PGE_2 and oral derivatives have been used long term, and concerns have arisen, chiefly over effects on the pulmonary circulation and the bones.

Effects of E prostaglandins on the pulmonary circulation

There is controversy in the literature as to the effects of E prostaglandins on the pulmonary circulation, and these probably vary depending on the underlying cardiac lesion. Haworth, studying infants with pulmonary atresia after up to 12 days' treat-ment, found reduction in arterial medial thickness, failure of muscle to extend distally and localized aneurysmal dilatations of pre-acinar vessels.[126] The intra-acinar arteries were abnormally small, but more numerous than in untreated controls. There was widespread lymphatic distension. By contrast, three infants with hypoplastic left heart syndrome had more peripheral extension of smooth muscle than normal, and alveolar wall thickening, inter-lobular septal oedema and fibrosis with chronic passive congestion, presumably reflecting chronic increases in pulmonary blood flow. One child had a necrotizing pulmonary vasculitis;[127] in an animal model, vasculitis was not confined to the lungs.[128,129] Suggestions that this may be related to an effect on neutrophils[128] remain speculative, and vasculitis is not a problem in clinical practice.

Effects of E prostaglandins on the bones

Bony changes have been described after prolonged treatment. They may appear as early as 9 days, but usually take more than 30 days to appear. The lesions may be painful, and radiologically consist of layered periosteal new bone formation, which is symmetrical (a helpful point in differentiating them from osteomyelitis), and particularly affect the lower limbs, with sparing of the mandible. There is no specific feature distinguishing the lesions from other infectious, inflammatory or neoplastic causes of periosteal new bone formation. There may also be pseudo-widening of the cranial sutures. The appearances are reversible, and progress can be followed by repeated measurements of serum alkaline phosphatase.[129–134]

Miscellaneous effects of E prostaglandins

Hypokalaemic alkalosis (pseudo-Bartter's syndrome) has been described after prolonged treatment with E prostaglandins.[135] The mechanism is presumably due to glomerular sodium loss and secondary increased reabsorption with increased exchange for potassium in the distal tubules, due to renal prostaglandin effects. The electrolyte derangement is worsened by concomitant diuretic therapy, but is reversible on stopping therapy with prostaglandin.

Conclusions

Without question, PGE_1 and PGE_2 will continue to be used in an attempt to buy time to stabilize the child with duct-dependent pulmonary or systemic circulation. Their use enables the child with complex abnormalities to be assessed and sent for operation in good condition instead of deeply cyanosed, cold or peripherally shut down. They will continue for the foreseeable future to have a major role in paediatric cardiology.

The future therapeutic role of prostaglandins in the pulmonary circulation is more debatable. There seems to be little to choose between PGI_2 and the E series prostaglandins. There is more experience with the former, but the financial cost is higher. One could speculate that the antiplatelet effects of PGI_2, and its possible actions on endothelial/smooth muscle interactions, may offer benefit over and above its vasodilator actions in preventing worsening of established pulmonary vascular disease. In this context, the orally active analogue of PGI_2, iloprost, might be worth trying as a long-term oral treatment in children with inoperable pulmonary vascular disease complicating congenital heart lesions. The whole field of therapeutic manipulation of microvascular interactions is very much in its infancy, and at the moment one can only speculate.

The advantages of prostaglandins as pulmonary vasodilators are relative safety and short half-life, but these must be set against cost (particularly for PGI_2) and the likelihood of hypotension and of deterioration in gas exchange. They are not ideal, and, unlike the E series prostaglandins for the arterial duct, are likely to be superseded by newer, more selective agents. While they continue in clinical use, it is essential to optimize ventilation, monitor arterial blood pressure and arterial oxygenation during infusion, and preferably measure cardiac output as well.

References

1. Wells LJ, Boyden EA. The development of the bronchopulmonary segments in human embryos of horizons XVII to XIX. *Am J Anat* 1954; **95:** 163–201.
2. Congdon ED. Transformation of the aortic-arch system during the development of the human embryo. *Contrib Embryol* 1922; **14:** 47–110.
3. Butler H. Some derivatives of the foregut venous plexus of the albino rat, with reference to man. *J Anat* 1952; **86:** 95–109.
4. Hislop A, Reid L. Growth and development of the respiratory system: anatomical development. In: Davis JA, Dobbin J (eds), *Scientific Foundations of Paediatrics*, 2nd edn. London: Heinemann Medical, 1981: 390–431.
5. Reid LM. Lung growth in health and disease. *Br J Dis Chest* 1984; **78:** 113–34.
6. Dunnill MS. The problem of lung growth. *Thorax* 1982; **37:** 561–3.
7. Thurlbeck WM. Postnatal human lung growth. *Thorax* 1982; **37:** 564–71.
8. Hislop A, Reid L. Intrapulmonary arterial development during fetal life-branching pattern and structure. *J Anat* 1972; **113:** 35–48.
9. Rudolph AM, Heymann MA. The circulation of the fetus in utero. Methods for studying distribution of blood flow, cardiac output and organ blood flow. *Circ Res* 1967; **21:** 163–84.
10. Rudolph AM, Heymann MA. Circulatory changes during growth in the fetal lamb. *Circ Res* 1970; **26:** 289–99.
11. Heymann MA. Arachidonic acid derivatives in the perinatal period. *Adv Pediatr* 1989; **36:** 151–76.
12. Clyman RI, Mauray F, Rudolph AM, *et al.* Age-dependent sensitivity of the lamb ductus arteriosus to indomethacin and prostaglandins. *J Pediatr* 1980; **96:** 94–8.
13. Schreiber MD, Heymann MA, Soifer SJ. Leukotriene inhibition prevents and reverses hypoxic pulmonary vasoconstriction in newborn lambs. *Pediatr Res* 1985; **19:** 437–41.
14. Lipsett J, Gannon B. Regional cycles of perfusion and non-perfusion in the lung of the term fetal rabbit. *Pediatr Pulmonol* 1991; **11:** 153–60.
15. Yao AC. Cardiovascular changes during the transition from fetal to neonatal life. In: Gootman N, Gootman PM (eds), *Perinatal Cardiovascular Function*. New York: Marcel Dekker, 1983.
16. Cassin S, Dawes GS, Mott JC, Ross BB, Strang LB. The vascular resistance of the foetal and newly ventilated lung of the lamb. *J Physiol* 1964; **171:** 61–79.
17. Lauer RM, Evans JA, Aoki M, Kittle CF. Factors controlling pulmonary vascular resistance in fetal lambs. *J Pediatr* 1965; **67:** 568–77.
18. Dawes GS, Mott JC, Widdicombe JG, Wyatt DG. Changes in the lungs of the newborn lamb. *J Physiol* 1953; **121:** 141–62.
19. Heymann M, Rudolph A, Nies A, *et al.* Bradykinin production associated with oxygenation of the fetal lamb. *Circ Res* 1969; **25:** 521–34.
20. Soifer SJ, Morin FC, Heymann MA. Prostaglandin D_2 reverses induced pulmonary hypertension in the newborn lamb. *J Pediatr* 1982; **100:** 458–63.
21. Soifer SJ, Morin FC, Kaslow DC, Heymann MA. The developmental effects of prostaglandin D_2 on the pulmonary and systemic circulations in the newborn lamb. *J Dev Physiol* 1983; **5:** 237–50.
22. Drummond WH, Carter RL. Cardiac depressant and circulatory effects of prostaglandin D_2 in developing lambs. *Am J Physiol* 1987; **252:** H374–83.
23. Campbell AGM, Dawes GS, Fishman AP, Hyman AI, Perks AM. The release of a bradykinin-like pulmonary vasodilator substance in foetal and new-born lambs. *J Physiol* 1968; **195:** 83–96.

24. Hislop A, Reid L. New findings in pulmonary arteries of rats with hypoxia-induced pulmonary hypertension. *Br J Exp Pathol* 1976; **57:** 542–54.

25. Campbell AGM, Cockburn F, Dawes GS, Milligan JE. Pulmonary vasoconstriction in asphyxia during cross-circulation between twin foetal lambs. *J Physiol* 1967; **192:** 111–21.

26. Campbell AGM, Dawes GS, Fishman AP, Hyman AI. Pulmonary vasoconstriction and changes in heart rate during asphyxia in immature foetal lambs. *J Physiol* 1967; **192:** 93–110.

27. Haworth SG. Pulmonary vascular development. In: Long WA (ed), *Fetal and Neonatal Cardiology*. Philadelphia: WB Saunders, 1990.

28. McMurphy DM, Heymann MA, Rudolph AM, Melmon KL. Developmental change in the constriction of the ductus arteriosus: response to oxygen and vasoactive substances in the isolated ductus arteriosus of the fetal lamb. *Pediatr Res* 1972; **6:** 231–8.

29. Clyman RI, Mauray F, Roman C, et al. Circulating prostaglandin E_2 concentrations and patent ductus arteriosus in fetal and neonatal lambs. *J Pediatr* 1980; **97:** 455–61.

30. Clyman RI. Developmental responses to oxygen, arachidonic acid and indomethacin in the fetal lamb ductus arteriosus *in vitro*. *Prostaglandins Med* 1978; **1:** 167–74.

31. Clyman RI, Mauray F, Rudolph AM, et al. Age-dependent sensitivity of the lamb ductus arteriosus to indomethacin and prostaglandins. *J Pediatr* 1980; **96:** 94–8.

32. De Troyer A, Yernault J-C, Englert M. Lung hypoplasia in congenital pulmonary valve stenosis. *Circulation* 1977; **56:** 647–51.

33. Fletcher BD, Garcia EJ, Colenda C, Borkat G. Reduced lung volume associated with acquired pulmonary artery obstruction in children. *Am J Roentgenol* 1979; **133:** 47–52.

34. Bush A, Busst CM, Knight WB, et al. Changes in pulmonary circulation in severe bronchopulmonary dysplasia. *Arch Dis Child* 1990; **65:** 739–45.

35. Geggel RL, Murphy JD, Langleben D, Crone RK, Vacanti SP, Reid LM. Congenital diaphragmatic hernia: arterial structural changes and persistent pulmonary hypertension after surgical repair. *J Pediatr* 1985; **107:** 457–64.

36. Coceani F, Olley PM. The response of the ductus arteriosus to prostaglandins. *Can J Physiol Pharmacol* 1973; **51:** 220–5.

37. Olley PM, Coceani F. Prostaglandins and the ductus arteriosus. *Annu Rev Med* 1981; **32:** 375–85.

38. McMurphy DM, Heymann MA, Rudolph AM, Melmon KL. Developmental changes in constriction of the ductus arteriosus: responses to oxygen and vasoactive agents in the isolated ductus arteriosus of the fetal lamb. *Pediatr Res* 1972; **6:** 231–8.

39. Momma K, Nishihara S, Ota Y. Constriction of the fetal ductus arteriosus by glucocorticoid hormones. *Pediatr Res* 1981; **15:** 19–21.

40. Clyman RL, Ballard PL, Sniderman S, et al. Prenatal administration of betamethasone for prevention of patent ductus arteriosus. *J Pediatr* 1981; **98:** 123–6.

41. Clyman RL, Mauray F, Roman C, Rudolph AM, Heymann MA. Glucocorticoids alter the sensitivity of the lamb ductus arteriosus to prostaglandin E_2. *J Pediatr* 1981; **98:** 126–8.

42. Sharpe GL, Thalme B, Larsson KS. Studies on closure of the ductus arteriosus. Ductal closure in utero by a prostaglandin synthesis inhibitor. *Prostaglandins* 1974; **8:** 363–8.

43. Olley PM, Bodach E, Heaton J, Coceani F. Further evidence implicating E-type prostaglandins in the patency of the lamb ductus arteriosus. *Eur J Pharmacol* 1975; **34:** 247–50.

44. Friedman WF, Hirschklan MJ, Printz MP, Pitlick PT, Kirkpatric SE. Pharmacologic closure of patent ductus arteriosus in premature infant. *N Engl J Med* 1992; **295:** 526–9.

45. Olley PM, Coceani F. Lipid mediators in the control of the ductus arteriosus. *Am Rev Respir Dis* 1987; **136:** 218–19.

46. Clyman RI, Saugstad OD, Mauray F. Reactive oxygen metabolites relax the lamb ductus arteriosus by stimulating prostaglandin production. *Circ Res* 1989; **64:** 1–8.

47. Neal WA, Kyle JM, Mullet MD. Failure of indomethacin therapy to induce closure of patent ductus arteriosus in premature infants with respiratory distress syndrome. *J Pediatr* 1977; **91:** 621–3.

48. Cooke RWI, Pickesing D. Poor response to oral indomethacin therapy for persistent ductus arteriosus in very low birthweight infants. *Br Heart J* 1978; **41:** 301–3.

49. Ivey HH, Kattwinkel J, Park TS, Krovetz LH. Failure of indomethacin to close persistent ductus arteriosus in infants weighing less than 1000 grams. *Br Heart J* 1978; **41:** 304–7.

50. Danilowicz D, Rudolph AM, Hoffman JIE. Delayed closure of the ductus arteriosus in premature infants. *Pediatrics* 1966; **37:** 74–8.

51. Hammerman C, Aramburo MJ, Bui KC. Endogenous dilator prostaglandins in congenital heart disease. *Pediatr Cardiol* 1987; **8:** 155–9.

52. Cotton RB, Haywood JL, FitzGerald GA. Symptomatic patent ductus arteriosus following prophylactic indomethacin. A clinical and biochemical appraisal. *Biol Neonate* 1991; **60:** 273–82.

53. Green TP, Thompson TR, Johnson DE, Lock JE. Furosemide promotes patent ductus arteriosus in premature infants with the respiratory-distress syndrome. *N Engl J Med* 1983; **308:** 743–8.

54. Sung RY, Yin JA, Loong EP, Fok TF, Lau J. Topical prostaglandin E_2 gel for cervical ripening and closure of the ductus arteriosus in the newborn. *Arch Dis Child* 1990; **65:** 703–4.

55. Olley PM, Coceani F, Bodach E. A new emergency therapy for certain cyanotic congenital heart malformations. *Circulation* 1976; **53**: 728–31.

56. Heymann MA, Rudolph AM. Ductus arteriosus dilatation by prostaglandin E₁ in infants with pulmonary atresia. *Pediatrics* 1977; **59**: 325–9.

57. Neutze JM, Starling MB, Elliott RB, Barratt-Boyes BG. Palliation of cyanotic congenital heart disease in infancy with E-type prostaglandins. *Circulation* 1977; **55**: 238–41.

58. Heymann MA, Berman W Jr, Rudolph AM, Whitman V. Dilatation of the ductus arteriosus by prostaglandin E₁ in aortic arch abnormalities. *Circulation* 1979; **59**: 169–73.

59. MacMahon P, Gorham PF, Arnold R, Wilkinson JL, Hamilton DI. Pulmonary artery growth during treatment with oral prostaglandin E₂ in ductus dependent cyanotic congenital heart disease. *Arch Dis Child* 1983; **58**: 187–9.

60. Fujiseki Y, Yamamoto H, Hattori M, Yamawaki Y, Goto M, Shimada M. Oral administration of prostaglandin E₂ in the hypoplastic left heart syndrome. *Jpn Heart J* 1983; **24**: 481–7.

61. Lewis AB, Freed MD, Heymann MA, Roehl SL, Keusey RC. Side effects of therapy with prostaglandin E₁ in infants with critical congenital heart disease. *Circulation* 1981; **64**: 893–8.

62. Silove ED, Roberts DGV, de Giovanni JV. Evaluation of oral and low dose intravenous prostaglandin E₂ in management of ductus dependent congenital heart disease. *Arch Dis Child* 1985; **60**: 1025–30.

63. Saji T, Matsuura H, Hoshino K, Yamamoto S, Ishikita T, Matsuo N. Oral prostaglandin E₁ derivative (OP-1206) in an infant with double outlet ventricle and pulmonary stenosis. Effect on ductus-dependent pulmonary circulation. *Jpn Heart J* 1991; **32**: 735–40.

64. Hist A, Halken S, Andersen PE Jr. Reversibility of cortical hyperostosis following long-term prostaglandin E₁ therapy in infants with ductus-dependent congenital heart disease. *Pediatr Radiol* 1988; **18**: 149–53.

65. Jureidini S, Chase NA, Alpert BS, Vanderzalm T, Sheneflet RE. Soft-tissue swelling in two neonates during prostaglandin E₁ therapy. *Pediatr Cardiol* 1986; **7**: 157–60.

66. Beitzke A, Stein J. Pseudo-widening of cranial sutures as a feature of long-term prostaglandin E₁ therapy. *Pediatr Radiol* 1986; **16**: 57–8.

67. Yokota M, Muraoka R, Aoshima M, *et al.* Modified Blalock–Taussig shunt following long-term administration of prostaglandin E₁ for ductus-dependent neonates with cyanotic congenital heart disease. *J Thorac Cardiovasc Surg* 1985; **90**: 399–403.

68. Sidi D, Duval-Arnould M, Kachaner J, Villain E, Pedroni E, Piechaud JF. Treatment by prostaglandin E₁ of isolated coarctations in newborn infants with acute cardiac failure. *Arch Fr Pediatr* 1987; **44**: 21–5. [in French]

69. Calder AL, Kirker JA, Neutze JM, Starling MB. Pathology of the ductus arteriosus treated with prostaglandins: comparisons with untreated cases. *Pediatr Cardiol* 1984; **5**: 85–92.

70. Gittenberger-de Groot AC, Strengers JL. Histopathology of the arterial duct (ductus arteriosus) with and without treatment with prostaglandin E₁. *Int J Cardiol* 1988; **19**: 153–66.

71. Silove ED, Roberts DG, de Giovanni JV. Evaluation of oral and low dose intravenous prostaglandin E₂ in management of ductus dependent congenital heart disease. *Arch Dis Child* 1985; **60**: 1025–30.

72. Foker JE, Braunlin EA, St Cyr JA, *et al.* Management of pulmonary atresia with intact ventricular septum. *J Thorac Cardiovasc Surg* 1986; **92**: 706–15.

73. McCaffrey FM, Leatherbury L, Moore HV. Pulmonary atresia and intact ventricular septum. Definitive repair in the neonatal period. *J Thorac Cardiovasc Surg* 1991; **102**: 617–23.

74. Beitzke A, Suppan CH. Use of prostaglandin E₂ in management of transposition of great arteries before balloon atrial septostomy. *Br Heart J* 1983; **49**: 341–4.

75. Coceani F, Olley PM. The control of cardiovascular shunts in the fetal and perinatal period. *Can J Physiol Pharmacol* 1988; **66**: 1129–34.

76. Menahem S. Administration of prostaglandin inhibitors to the mother; the potential risk to the fetus and neonate with duct-dependent circulation. *Reprod Fertil Dev* 1991; **3**: 489–94.

77. Davies NJH, Shinebourne EA, Scallan MJ, Sopwith TA, Denison DM. Pulmonary vascular resistance in children with congenital heart disease. *Thorax* 1984; **39**: 895–900.

78. Pepke-Zaba J, Higenbottam TW, Dinh-Xuan AT, Stone D, Wallwork J. Inhaled nitric oxide as a cause of selective pulmonary vasodilatation in pulmonary hypertension. *Lancet* 1991; **338**: 1173–4.

79. Packer M, Greenburg B, Massie B, Dash H. Deleterious effects of hydralazine in patients with pulmonary hypertension. *N Engl J Med* 1982; **306**: 1326–31.

80. von Euler US, Liliestrand G. Observations on the pulmonary arterial blood pressure in the cat. *Acta Physiol Scand* 1946; **12**: 301–20.

81. Bush A, Busst CM, Knight WB, Shinebourne EA. Effects of infusion of prostacyclin on anatomical intrapulmonary right to left shunt: a useful model of human hypoxic vasoconstriction? *Clin Sci* 1989; **76**: 143–9.

82. Soifer SJ, Clyman RI, Heymann MA. Effects of prostaglandin D₂ on pulmonary arterial pressure and oxygenation in newborn infants with persistent pulmonary hypertension. *J Pediatr* 1988; **112**: 774–7.

83. O'Grady J, Warrington S, Moh MJ, *et al.* Effects of

intravenous infusions of prostacyclin (PGI₂) in man. *Prostaglandins* 1980; **19**: 319–32.

84. Bush A, Busst CM, Millar A, Syrett N. Time course of the effects of epoprostenol on effective pulmonary blood flow in normal volunteers. *Br J Clin Pharmacol* 1988; **25**: 341–8.

85. Davidson FF, Glazier JB, Murray JF. The components of the alveolar–arterial oxygen tension difference in normal subjects and in patients with pneumonia and obstructive lung disease. *Am J Med* 1972; **52**: 754–62.

86. Bush A. Functional Assessment of Pulmonary Circulation in Man. MD Thesis, University of Cambridge, 1987.

87. Bush A, Busst CM, Booth K, Knight WB, Shinebourne EA. Does prostacyclin enhance the selective pulmonary vasodilator effect of oxygen in children with congenital heart disease? *Circulation* 1986; **74**: 135–44.

88. Lock SE, Olley PM, Coceani F, Swyer PR, Rowe RD. Use of prostacyclin in persistent fetal circulation. *Lancet* 1979; **1**: 1343.

89. Watkins WD, Peterson MB, Crone RK, Shannon DC, Levine L. Prostacyclin and prostaglandin E₁ for severe idiopathic pulmonary artery hypertension. *Lancet* 1980; **1**: 1083.

90. Barst RJ, Stalcup SA, Steeg CN, *et al.* Relation of arachidonate metabolites to abnormal control of the pulmonary circulation in a child. *Am Rev Respir Dis* 1985; **131**: 171–7.

91. Bush A, Busst CM, Shinebourne EA. The use of oxygen and prostacyclin as pulmonary vasodilators in congenital heart disease. *Int J Cardiol* 1985; **9**: 267–74.

92. Bush A, Busst CM, Knight WB, Shinebourne EA. Comparison of the haemodynamic effects of epoprostenol (prostacyclin) and tolazoline. *Br Heart J* 1988; **60**: 141–8.

93. Bush A, Busst CM, Haworth SG, *et al.* Correlations of lung morphology, pulmonary vascular resistance, and outcome in children with congenital heart disease. *Br Heart J* 1988; **59**: 480–5.

94. Bush A, Busst CM, Knight WB, Shinebourne EA. Cardiopulmonary interactions in bronchopulmonary dysplasia (BPD). In: Daum S (ed), *Interaction between Heart and Lung*. Stuttgart: Thieme Medical, 1989.

95. Bush A, Busst CM, Knight WB, Shinebourne EA. Modification of pulmonary hypertension secondary to congenital heart disease by prostacyclin therapy. *Am Rev Respir Dis* 1987; **136**: 767–9.

96. Shinebourne EA, Bush A, Busst CM, *et al.* Oxygène et prostacycline dans l'appréciation et le traitement de la maladie vasculaire pulmonaire. *Coeur* 1988; **19**: 297–301.

97. Davies NJH, Denison DM. The measurement of metabolic gas exchange and minute volume by mass spectrometry alone. *Respir Physiol* 1979; **36**: 261–7.

98. Davies NJH, Denison DM. The uses of long sampling probes in respiratory mass spectrometry. *Respir Physiol* 1979; **36**: 335–46.

99. Abdul-Rasool IH, Chamberlain JH. Respiratory gas exchange before and after cardiac operations. *J Thorac Cardiovasc Surg* 1985; **85**: 856–63.

100. Weinstein MR, Oh W. Oxygen consumption in infants with bronchopulmonary dysplasia. *J Pediatr* 1981; **99**: 958–61.

101. Kelman GR. Digital computer subroutine for the conversion of oxygen tension into oxygen saturation. *J Appl Physiol* 1966; **21**: 1375–6.

102. Bush A, Shinebourne EA. Cardiac implications of bronchopulmonary dysplasia. In: Long WA (ed), *Fetal and Neonatal Cardiology*. Philadelphia: WB Saunders, 1989: 401–18.

103. Berman W, Yabek SM, Dillon T, Burstein R, Corlew S. Evaluation of infants with bronchopulmonary dysplasia using cardiac catheterization. *Pediatrics* 1982; **70**: 708–12.

104. Abman SH, Wolfe RR, Accurso FJ, Koops BL, Bowman CM, Wiggins JW. Pulmonary vascular response to oxygen in infants with severe bronchopulmonary dysplasia. *Pediatrics* 1985; **75**: 80–4.

105. Bancalari E, Jesse MJ, Gelband H, Garcia O. Lung mechanics in congenital heart disease with increased and decreased pulmonary blood flow. *J Pediatr* 1977; **90**: 192–5.

106. Long WA. Persistent pulmonary hypertension of the newborn (PPHNS). In: Long WA (ed), *Fetal and Neonatal Cardiology*. Philadelphia: WB Saunders, 1989: 627–55.

107. Kuhl PG, Cotton RB, Schweer H, Seybirth HW. Endogenous formation of prostanoids in neonates with persistent pulmonary hypertension. *Arch Dis Child* 1989; **64**: 949–52.

108. Hammerman C, Komar K, Abu-Khudair H. Hypoxic vs septic pulmonary hypertension. Selective role of thromboxane mediation. *Am J Dis Child* 1988; **142**: 319–25.

109. Kaapa P, Koivisto M, Ylikorkala O, Kouvalainen K. Prostacyclin in the treatment of neonatal pulmonary hypertension. *J Pediatr* 1985; **107**: 951–3.

110. Schweer H, Seyberth HW, Kuhl PG, Meese CO. Unusual metabolism of prostacyclin in infants with persistent septic pulmonary hypertension. *Eicosanoids* 1990; **3**: 237–42.

111. Bos AP, Tibboel D, Hazebroek FW, Stijnen T, Molenaar JC. Congenital diaphragmatic hernia: impact of prostanoids in the perioperative period. *Arch Dis Child* 1990; **65**: 994–5.

112. McIntosh N, Walters RO. Effects of tolazoline in severe hyaline membrane disease. *Arch Dis Child* 1979; **54**: 105–10.

113. Stevens DC, Schreiner RL, Bull MJ, *et al.* An analysis of tolazoline therapy in the critically ill neonate. *J Pediatr Surg* 1980; **15**: 964–70.

114. Trompeter RS, Chantler C, Haycock GB. Tolazoline

and acute renal failure in the newborn. [letter] *Lancet* 1981; **1:** 1219.

115. Ward RM, Daniel CH, Kendig JW, Wood MA. Oliguria and tolazoline pharmacokinetics in the newborn. *Pediatrics* 1986; **77:** 307–15.

116. Heath D, Edwards JE. The pathology of hypertensive pulmonary vascular disease. *Circulation* 1958; **18:** 533–47.

117. Heath D, Helmholz HF, Burchell HB, Du Shane JW, Edwards JE. Graded pulmonary vascular changes and hemodynamic findings in cases of atrial and ventricular septal defect and patent ductus arteriosus. *Circulation* 1958; **18:** 1155–66.

118. Heath D, Helmholz HF, Burchell HB, Du Shane JW, Kirklin JW, Edwards JE. Relation between structural changes in the small pulmonary arteries and the immediate reversibility of pulmonary hypertension following closure of ventricular and atrial septal defects. *Circulation* 1958; **18:** 1167–74.

119. Rabinovitch M, Haworth SG, Castaneda AR, Nadas AS, Reid LM. Lung biopsy in congenital heart disease: a morphometric approach to pulmonary vascular disease. *Circulation* 1978; **58:** 1107–22.

120. Haworth SG, Hislop AA. Pulmonary vascular development: normal values of peripheral vascular structure. *Am J Cardiol* 1983; **52:** 578–83.

121. Kermode J, Butt W, Shann F. Comparison between prostaglandin E_1 and epoprostenol (prostacyclin) in infants after heart surgery. *Br Heart J* 1991; **66:** 175–8.

122. Swan PK, Tibballs J, Duncan AW. Prostaglandin E_1 in primary pulmonary hypertension. *Crit Care Med* 1986; **14:** 72–3.

123. Rubin LJ, Stephenson LW, Johnston MR, Nagaraj S, Edmunds LH. Comparison of effects of prostaglandin and nitroprusside on pulmonary vascular resistance in children after open heart surgery. *Ann Thorac Surg* 1981; **32:** 563–70.

124. Lewis AB, Freed MD, Heymann MA, Roehl SL, Kensey RC. Side-effects of therapy with prostaglandin E_1 in infants with critical congenital heart disease. *Circulation* 1981; **64:** 893–8.

125. Bush A, Busst CM, Knight WB, Shinebourne EA. Interactions between alveolar hypercapnia and epoprostenol on the pulmonary circulation: clinical and pharmacological implications. *Pulm Pharmacol* 1990; **3:** 167–70.

126. Haworth SG, Sauer U, Buhlmeyer K. Effect of prostaglandin E_1 on pulmonary circulation in pulmonary atresia: a quantitative morphometric study. *Br Heart J* 1980; **43:** 306–14.

127. Heffelfinger S, Hawkins EP, Nihill M, Langston C. Pulmonary vascular changes associated with prolonged prostaglandin E_1 treatment. *Pediatr Pathol* 1987; **7:** 165–73.

128. Goddard-Feingold J, Langston C, Hawkins EP, Michael LH, Ou CN. Prostaglandin E_1-associated pathology of pulmonary microvasculature in newborn pups: similarity to findings in prostaglandin E_1-treated human newborns. *Pediatr Pathol* 1989; **9:** 251–60.

129. Issekutz AC, Movat HZ. The effect of vasodilator prostaglandins on polymorphonuclear leukocyte infiltration and vascular injury. *Am J Pathol* 1982; **107:** 300–9.

130. Ueda K, Saito A, Nakano H, *et al.* Cortical hyperostosis following long-term administration of prostaglandin E_1 in infants with cyanotic congenital heart disease. *J Pediatr* 1980; **97:** 834–6.

131. Sone K, Tashiro M, Fujinaga T, Tomoasat T, Tokuyama K, Kuroume T. Long term low-dose prostaglandin E_1 administration. [letter] *J Pediatr* 1980; **97:** 866–7.

132. Ringel RE, Brenner JI, Haney PJ, Burns JE, Moulton AI, Berman MA. Prostaglandin-induced periostitis: a complication of long-term PGE_1 infusion in an infant with congenital heart disease. *Radiology* 1982; **142:** 657–8.

133. Abe K, Shimada Y, Takezawa J, Oka N, Yoshiga I. Longterm administration of prostaglandin E_1. *Crit Care Med* 1982; **10:** 155–8.

134. Hoevels-Guerich H, Haferkorn L, Persigehl M, Hofstetter R, von Bernuth G. Widening of cranial sutures after longterm prostaglandin E_2 therapy in two newborn infants. *J Pediatr* 1984; **105:** 72–4.

135. Langhendries JP, Thiry V, Bodart E, *et al.* Exogenous prostaglandin administration and pseudo-Bartter syndrome. *Eur J Pediatr* 1989; **149:** 208–9.

11 Prostaglandins in myocardial infarction and angina

Åke Wennmalm

Current concepts in the aetiology of angina and acute myocardial infarction

Cardiovascular disease (CVD) is the major cause of death in developed countries. Ischaemic heart disease is its most common manifestation, with its clinical presentations of angina pectoris (AP) and acute myocardial infarction (AMI). In round numbers every second adult person in a developed country will eventually die from CVD, and among these victims at least every third will do so due to a myocardial infarction. Beside its fatal outcome in a substantial proportion of cases, ischaemic heart disease also causes considerable human suffering and high costs for society's health care systems.

The pathophysiological basis of ischaemic heart disease is usually defined in terms of an imbalance between myocardial oxygen supply and demand. It was previously assumed that an increase in demand under conditions of a restricted supply would be sufficient to elicit not only angina pectoris but also an AMI. This view has changed and most investigators now favour the idea that an increase in cardiac work (e.g. in response to physical effort) is not alone capable of eliciting an infarction. Mechanisms restricting myocardial supply are therefore the subject of increasing interest.

Atherosclerosis of the coronary vessels is the usual morphological cause for an inadequate myocardial oxygen supply. Because atherosclerosis is usually not restricted to the coronary vessels, ischaemic heart disease is in most cases a manifestation of a generalized involvement of the vascular system. This is an important aspect, in that some of the manifestations of coronary disease may thereby influence other organs. For instance, left ventricular incompetence based on coronary insufficiency may lower cardiac output such that perfusion of other organs with atherosclerotic vessels (kidneys, legs, brain) is further impaired. In addition, systemic vascular disease may have a negative impact on the coronary circulation; for example, hypertension which increases left ventricular afterload and thereby promotes the development of left ventricular hypertrophy. Similarly, with respect to the activity of the platelets, which play a key role in acute coronary occlusion with subsequent AMI, the systemic aspect of atherosclerosis should be kept in mind. Platelets are activated by irregular vessel walls, and it is well known that there is a correlation between the severity of the atherosclerotic disease and the activity of the platelets.

The development of atherosclerosis has been established from basic, clinical, epidemiological and pathological studies. With onset well before adolescence there is a gradual incorporation of fatty acids in the vessel walls, constituting the so-called fatty streaks. This is an early sign, harmless from a mechanical point of view. Fatty streaks have been demonstrated at an early age, even in apparently healthy teenagers. The further development of atherosclerosis comprises smooth muscle hypertrophy and formation of plaque, the latter materializing as irregular protuberances of the vessel wall into the lumen. Promoting or risk factors in this atherosclerotic process are high plasma lipids (particularly low density lipoprotein (LDL) cholesterol), hypertension and cigarette smoking. Each of the risk factors may alone more than double the risk for AMI, and in conjunction with each other the accumulated increase in risk may be considerable.

The limitation of the luminal area in the atherosclerotic coronary vessel is certainly unfavourable from a haemodynamic point of view, since it will be paralleled by an impairment of flow at a fixed pressure gradient. However, the morphological obstruction has wider implications, since its appearance is accompanied by several unfavourable phenomena, related or unrelated to the atherosclerotic process as such. Among these, the impaired flow-dependent vasodilation in hypercholesterolaemic, irregular or stenotic vessels is the most recently recognized phenomenon, usually explained in terms of an attenuation of endothelium-derived vascular relaxation.

The other factors aggravating the functional significance of the atherosclerotic plaque are the steal phenomenon and the risk of acute occlusion of the stenotic coronary vessel. 'Coronary steal' is the term used to indicate that a poststenotic coronary vessel, maximally dilated by metabolic factors to maintain sufficient perfusion in the basal state, may actually be less perfused when the myocardial demand is increased. The haemodynamic prerequisite for this is that an adjacent branch of the same poststenotic vessel, not maximally dilated by metabolic factors in the basal state, will be so dilated when the myocardial demand is increased and thereby take an increased fraction of the blood passing the stenosis.

The risk for an acute occlusion, finally, is intimately related to the degree of platelet–vessel wall interaction at the stenotic site. It is well known from experimental studies that a fixed coronary occlusion, even in an otherwise normal vessel, will be a preferred site for platelet thrombus formation provided that the degree of obstruction is sufficiently large. It is hardly surprising that this phenomenon is even more pronounced when the endothelium is injured. The endothelial cells play a key role in the defence against platelet adhesion and aggregation in healthy vessels, via their continuous formation of the antiplatelet mediators nitric oxide and prostacyclin. Impaired or abolished formation of these mediators has been recognized as an important aggravating factor in ischaemic heart disease.

Angina pectoris and AMI are occasionally regarded as quantitatively but not qualitatively different manifestations of the same primary pathological process. This is correct only to some extent. No more than a fraction of patients with stable angina pectoris develop an AMI. Furthermore, most patients appearing in the emergency department with their first AMI have no previous history of angina. The current view to explain this is that coronary atherosclerosis, not necessarily pronounced enough to manifest itself as effort-induced angina, is a prerequisite for coronary thrombosis and AMI. However, the atherosclerotic lesion obstructing part of the vessel lumen must be completed to a full occlusion to result in an AMI, whether by thrombus formation at the site of the plaque, by a rupture of the plaque or by a bleeding in the vessel wall underlying the plaque. More than 70% of patients with a fatal AMI display signs of coronary occlusion upon autopsy.[1] However, patients with stable coronary disease and angina based on a limitation of coronary perfusion that restricts their capacity to increased cardiac work, may never get an AMI because an occlusion never develops. On the other hand, patients with a subclinical coronary occlusion, for example with a plaque giving no significant limitation of myocardial supply during increased work, may well develop AMI due to a sudden occlusion at the site of the plaque, thrombus formation, rupture or bleeding into the plaque.

Possible mechanisms of action of prostacyclin in angina and acute myocardial infarction

Vasodilation

The basic physiological actions of prostacyclin in the cardiovascular system are based on its ability to activate adenylyl cyclase and thereby to increase cyclic AMP.[2] In the coronary vessels such activity leads to relaxation of smooth muscle. A dilator influence in the coronary vessels might, at first glance, seem ideal therapy for a disease characterized by restriction of coronary flow. This is, however, true only if there is insufficient endogenous dilator influence on the vessel wall in a section of the coronary tree. There is little reason to assume that the metabolic dilator tone in the coronary resistance vessels would be lowered in patients with ischaemic heart disease; the contrary is more likely the case. Hence, addition of an exogenous vasodilator should be of little or no help in cases of myocardial hypoperfusion without spasm, because the endogenous vasodilator system can be assumed to be operating fully. In fact, addition of a vasodilator might even worsen regional myocardial perfusion, due to induction of coronary steal.

Recent data concerning the impact of the vascular endothelium on coronary tone *in vivo* have, however, changed this view somewhat. It is well known that, under healthy conditions, an increase in coronary flow rate leads to coronary dilation. Such dilation is impaired in irregular or stenotic sections of the coronary vessels, when flow is increased by increased physical activity,[3] cold stress,[4] drugs[5,6] or mental stress.[7] The common denominator to the vascular dysfunction in these cases is probably an impaired endothelium-dependent dilation, because the response to local infusion of acetylcholine is attenuated.[8] The relative importance of such endothelium-dependent vasodilation to the total and regional myocardial blood flow cannot be fully appreciated at present. However, if endothelium-dependent vasodilation turns out to be a major factor in determining coronary perfusion, the need for direct-acting vasodilator drugs might need to be reconsidered.

Antiplatelet activity

Prostacyclin is a powerful antiplatelet agent, limiting platelet aggregation and even reversing existing aggregation by activation of adenylyl cyclase. Prostacyclin should consequently be potentially efficient in the treatment of clinical states characterized by increased platelet activity and aggregation.

In stable angina there is no evidence of increased platelet activity. In a recent study in our laboratory, patients with stable coronary disease did not excrete more thromboxane metabolite in the urine following leg exercise to a level at which ECG signs of myocardial ischaemia materialized, in comparison to the basal state.[9] Furthermore, there was no difference in thromboxane metabolite excretion following leg exercise in patients with and without ECG signs of myocardial ischaemia.[9] Hence, stable coronary disease with effort-induced angina pectoris is hardly a good target for an antiplatelet drug such as prostacyclin.

In patients with unstable coronary disease there is both direct and indirect evidence of platelet activation. Lewis *et al.*[10] demonstrated that aspirin, the antiplatelet drug most commonly used currently, reduced AMI in patients with unstable angina by more than 50%. The observation indicates that increased platelet activity with facilitation of thromboxane formation plays an important role in the development of AMI in unstable angina, and, hence, that antiplatelet drugs should be active in this setting. More direct evidence for the involvement of platelets in unstable angina was obtained in a study on excretion of thromboxane metabolite in such patients. There was a marked increase in metabolite excretion, and, furthermore, the increased excretion occurred during the periods of ischaemic pain.

AMI is characterized by augmented excretion of both thromboxane and prostacyclin metabolite.[11,12] This evidence has been taken to indicate that patients with AMI have a coronary occlusion[1] that, to a large extent, is of platelet origin. As such, this type of occlusion should also be a suitable target for antiplatelet therapy, provided that the drug administered can penetrate the site of the occlusion. Regrettably, this is not easily achieved because the occlusion by definition halts perfusion not only in the tissue distal to the thrombus but presumably also in a direction proximal to the level of the nearest previous branching. Hence, the possibility that any antiplatelet drug administered systematically is efficient in AMI is critically dependent on its ability to penetrate into the platelet thrombus at the site of the occlusion. Furthermore, the drug must do so before the platelet thrombus has begun to be organized by incorporation of fibrin.

Other possible mechanisms (cytoprotection, effects on neutrophils)

If the coronary occlusion is maintained for more than a certain critical time – which varies with respect to a number of factors such as collateral supply, metabolic state, and myocardial oxygen demand – there is a gradual development of irreversible tissue injury in the unperfused area.

Prostacyclin has been claimed to have a role in conditions in which its vasodilator or antiplatelet actions are no longer relevant. In principle, two different mechanisms may be of interest here. Firstly, interference with the inflammatory and tissue repair processes in the damaged myocardium might limit the size of the area eventually becoming fibrotic, thereby favourably moving the border between the infarct mass and the area at risk. There is some evidence that such an effect, usually referred to as cytoprotection, can be achieved via impairment of the migration of inflammatory cells into the jeopardized myocardium.

Secondly, if reperfusion of the ischaemic area is obtained – spontaneously or as a result of pharmacological or surgical intervention – any drug that limits the so-called reperfusion injury may be beneficial. Reperfusion injury is a complex phenomenon involving disturbance of mitochondrial function and distribution of ionic calcium, rapid formation of free radicals, and possibly also other factors. Any intervention that can limit the consequences of these harmful functional derangements can be assumed to have a beneficial effect on the size of the final myocardial infarction.

Evidence from animal experiments

Studies in isolated hearts

The effect of prostacyclin and its analogues has been studied in isolated hearts from a number of species. Several aspects of cardiac function have been evaluated in these studies, including coronary patency, arrhythmias, atrioventricular conduction, myocardial performance, nucleotide preservation, general metabolic status and membrane stability.

In isolated mongrel dog hearts, maintained *in situ* and subjected to cardioplegic arrest under moderate hypothermia, prostacyclin given immediately prior to induction of ischaemia counteracted the substantial platelet deposition found upon reperfusion.[13] The authors concluded that prostacyclin is capable of preventing and disaggregating ischaemia-induced intracoronary platelet deposition during and after cardioplegic arrest. Although this observation is primarily of interest to cardiac surgeons and anaesthesiologists, it may bear some significance also for other events in the coronary vessels such as unstable angina, as discussed later.

Several studies have dealt with the effect of prostacyclin and its analogues on ischaemia-induced arrhythmias. In isolated perfused hearts from rats pretreated *in vivo* with the prostacyclin analogue iloprost and with vehicle control ventricular arrhythmias developing during reperfusion following 30 minutes of global ischaemia were significantly in-

hibited by pretreatment with the active drug.[14] In another study of isolated rat hearts the prostacyclin analogue CG-4203, added in nanomole concentrations to the perfusing medium prior to induction of hypoxia, attenuated the occurrence of ventricular arrhythmias to less than 50% of that observed in control.[15] However, PGI_2 was found to prolong atrioventricular conduction when given to isolated guinea-pig hearts prior to induction of ischaemia.[16]

Ventricular performance and nucleotide levels in ventricular myocytes following ischaemia or hypoxia have been studied. In isolated rat hearts low flow perfusion for 30 minutes reduced tension development and lowered the myocyte content of energy-rich phosphates; these effects were reversed upon reperfusion.[17] Prostacyclin given from the onset of low flow counteracted the decline in tension development and hastened the recovery of contractions upon reperfusion. The effects were, however, not due to improved supply of ATP since the nucleotide levels were not affected by PGI_2.[17]

Pissarek and co-workers[18–20] studied the prostacyclin analogue iloprost, alone or in combination with PGE_1, on nucleotide levels in isolated rat hearts subjected to 20 minutes of ischaemia followed by reperfusion. Eicosanoids were given prior to the ischaemia. The creatine phosphate to inorganic phosphate ratio in the myocardial cells was improved by iloprost, but only during the early phase of the reperfusion.[18] In a later study using the same model, the combination of iloprost and PGE_1 was more efficient in preserving inorganic phosphate levels during reperfusion than either of these eicosanoids alone,[19,20] but again the beneficial effect was seen only during the early phase of the reperfusion.

The effect of prostacyclin, given prior to or shortly after the ligation of a coronary artery in rabbit Langendorff hearts, was studied in our laboratory.[21] Reperfusion was not induced in this study. Although coronary flow and oxygen uptake were elevated by prostacyclin, no change in lactate or purine turnover was observed following ligation. Furthermore, the weight of the non-perfused myocardium was not affected by prostacyclin, and there was no improvement in adenine nucleotide, creatine phosphate or lactate levels in the ischaemic zone of the myocardium.

Mechanical recovery during reperfusion following ischaemia has also been investigated in several studies. Iloprost given prior to 60 minutes of ischaemia followed by reperfusion improved the functional recovery of the myocardium and improved the metabolic state in rabbit isolated hearts.[22] In contrast, prostacyclin given before and during low flow ischaemia in isolated guinea-pig hearts caused a decline in recovery upon reperfusion.[16] The deleterious effect of prostacyclin was counteracted by verapamil and by lowering the level of external calcium, suggesting that prostacyclin exerted a negative effect in this preparation through a mechanism involving slow calcium channels.[16] Similar data were reported by Karmazyn and Neely.[23] They found that prostacyclin given to isolated rat hearts at low concentrations might depress left ventricular recovery during reperfusion following total ischaemia. The effect was more pronounced as the ischaemia duration was prolonged. Also in this study there was some indication that the effect was associated with the function of the slow calcium channels.[23]

Some data on the beneficial effects of prostacyclin or its analogues have also been reported. Iloprost improved the recovery of myocardial function, limited the extent of myocardial damage and counteracted arrhythmias in isolated rat hearts subjected to 24 hours of hypothermic cardiac arrest.[24] In another study the same analogue was reported to improve membrane integrity in isolated rabbit hearts subjected to low flow ischaemia.[25]

Taken together, these observations do not provide any simple, homogenous view on the action of prostacyclin in isolated heart models of ischaemia. In most studies prostacyclin or its analogue was given prior to induction of ischaemia or hypoxia. This is certainly a factor to consider when evaluating the significance of the reports in a clinical perspective. There are no data to indicate that prostacyclin given before or during ischaemia would be beneficial if reperfusion were not induced. Some, but not all, studies indicate that prostacyclin might elicit a moderate beneficial effect on myocardial functional recovery during reperfusion. There are, however, no biochemical data to support such an effect, as analyses of nucleotide levels have not provided any functional basis for an improved mechanical performance following administration of prostacyclin. Hence, available information provides a mixed view, suggesting that the overall actions of prostacyclin in isolated hearts are of no more than minor relevance.

In vivo infarction models

Prostacyclin and its analogues have also been studied in several *in vivo* models of acute myocardial infarction, and in different species. A major difference between these models is whether drug was administered prior to or after occlusion. Administration of

prostacyclin prior to occlusion may yield important information about mechanisms involved in the development of AMI; from a clinical and therapeutic point of view, infusion of prostacyclin after coronary occlusion must, however, be more relevant. Another important difference relates to whether reperfusion has been induced; the effect of prostacyclin and its analogues has been investigated in both of these states.

Studies in which prostacyclin or an analogue was given prior to coronary occlusion will be discussed first. In an open-chest pig model the time required to elicit an electrically induced coronary thrombosis was prolonged by iloprost,[26] obviously as a result of the antiaggregatory effect of the analogue. In mongrel dogs subjected to 2 hours of coronary occlusion mitochondrial dysfunction and leakage of lysosomal enzymes from the ischaemic area were counteracted by infusion of prostacyclin maintained from 25 minutes before and to the end of the occlusion.[27] In another study, infusion of iloprost starting 30 minutes before a 20-minute ligation of a coronary artery in open-chest dogs did not improve collateral blood flow to the ischaemic region or myocardial high energy phosphate content during reperfusion, but improved functional recovery during reperfusion.[28] A similar beneficial effect was obtained in open-chest pigs in which iloprost, given before coronary occlusion, improved recovery of regional myocardial function during reperfusion.[29] Iloprost given 30 minutes before coronary occlusion and maintained during a 30-minute occlusion followed by 2 hours of reperfusion also diminished infarct size, from 29.5% to 5.5% of area at risk, in open-chest pigs.[30]

Studies on the effect of prostacyclin or analogues given prior to coronary occlusion have also been performed in closed-chest animals. In resting conscious dogs prostacyclin, given during and following electrical induction of a coronary thrombosis, reduced thrombus weight and myocardial ischaemia but had no consistent effect on left ventricular performance.[31] Infarct size was not reported. In another study in conscious dogs, balloon occlusion of a coronary artery induced 30 minutes after onset of prostacyclin infusion, was found to reduce infarct size from 18% to 10% of the left ventricular mass.[32] Border zone myocardial function and blood flow were also improved in prostacyclin-treated animals. In pigs, iloprost, given from 30 minutes before to 30 minutes after coronary microembolization, counteracted early ventricular fibrillation and development of myocardial infarction.[33] An antiarrhythmogenic action of prostacyclin was also obtained in conscious rats subjected to coronary occlusion.[34] Infarct size was, however, not affected by the drug.

Some analogues differ considerably in activity from prostacyclin. Thus, in open-chest dogs subjected to 90 minutes of coronary ligation followed by reperfusion for 6 hours, prostacyclin given for 4 hours starting 30 minutes before occlusion reduced infarct mass by 59%, whilst the PGI_2 analogue SC-39902 was no better than vehicle in this respect.[35] In the same study prostacyclin, but not SC-39902, was found to inhibit neutrophil migration and production of free radicals, suggesting that the cytoprotective action of prostacyclin is related to inhibition of the local inflammatory response in the injured myocardium.[35]

Turning to the effect of prostacyclin or analogues given after coronary ligation, a number of studies have been reported. In experiments with permanent coronary occlusion (i.e. without reperfusion), the effect of prostacyclin or analogues given from 10 minutes to 4 hours after occlusion has been studied. Intravenous infusion of prostacyclin (20–40 ng/kg per minute) given 10 minutes after coronary occlusion in open-chest dogs did not affect regional myocardial blood flow but reduced infarct size by about 50%.[36] A favourable effect of iloprost on infarct size with a reduction in necrotic zone by about 50% was also found in rats subjected to coronary ligation with onset of drug infusion 3–4 hours after the occlusion.[37] However, in dogs given a clinically relevant dose of prostacyclin for 72 hours starting 35–60 minutes after coronary ligation, no improvement of regional myocardial blood flow or infarct size was obtained.[38]

Several studies have estimated more indirect indices of myocardial injury and claimed beneficial effects of prostacyclin and analogues. Nileprost, a mixed PGI_2/PGE_2 agonist, protected against myocardial injury (as shown by reduction in ECG changes and myocardial enzyme leakage) in open-chest cats subjected to 5 hours of coronary occlusion when given from 30 minutes after ligation of the coronary vessel.[39] In the same preparation, similar effects were obtained with iloprost given 30 minutes after ligation; prolongation of the interval between ligation and onset of infusion to 4 hours resulted in a progressive loss of beneficial effect of iloprost.[40,41] In another series, prostacyclin and vehicle, infused from 1 hour after coronary ligation, was studied in an open-chest dog model in which the occlusion was maintained for 3 hours. Prostacyclin was found to elevate creatine phosphate in ischaemic as well as non-ischaemic areas of the myocardium,[42] and a

similar effect was obtained with iloprost.[43] Iloprost was also claimed to have favourable effects on the plasma lipoprotein pattern in this model.[44] Prostacyclin did not affect occlusion-induced swelling of the mitochondria or dilation of the sarcoplasmic reticulum.[45] A favourable metabolic effect of iloprost was also seen in rats subjected to coronary ligation for 6 hours, iloprost being infused from 30 minutes after the occlusion.[46] Coronary ligation was associated with loss of phospholipids in the ischaemic myocardium, and this was partly counteracted by the drug. The authors concluded that the observed effects might be an important component of the cytoprotective action of iloprost.[46]

The experiments on prostacyclin and its analogues in infarct models with permanent coronary occlusion referred to above provide heterogeneous results, as did the studies in isolated perfused hearts. Some claim an effect on infarct size, while others do not. The discrepancies cannot fully be explained in terms of differences in species and technique. There is some evidence that prostacyclin or its analogues may preserve mitochondrial function and nucleotide levels in the ischaemic area, but there are also results contradicting such an action of the drug. There is no information that myocardial function, in terms of left ventricular performance, would be better maintained by administration of prostacyclin or analogues. Hence, available data do not fully support the idea that prostacyclin or its analogues would be beneficial in preserving myocardial integrity or function following permanent coronary occlusion.

Data from reperfusion models of AMI provide a somewhat different view. In open-chest dogs iloprost, given from 5–10 minutes after ligation and continued during the occlusion and the initial part of the reperfusion periods, reduced infarct area by almost 50% and reduced the accumulation of neutrophils in the ischaemic myocardium.[47] The authors suggested that the ability of iloprost to reduce infarct size was related both to a reduction in blood pressure and to a modulation of neutrophil infiltration and activation at the site of injury. A similar effect on infarct size was obtained in a reperfusion model of AMI in open-chest rabbits. Iloprost, given from 15 minutes after a coronary ligation that was maintained for 1 hour and followed by reperfusion for 5 hours, reduced infarct size from 89% to 54% of the area at risk without causing any major haemodynamic effects.[48] Another PGI_2 analogue, taprostene, given from 30 minutes after coronary ligation that was maintained for 1.5 hours and followed by reperfusion for 4.5 hours, decreased infarct size, diminished neutrophil invasion and counteracted coronary endothelial damage in open-chest cats.[49] Hence, prostacyclin and analogues do seem to counteract the development of ischaemic injury if given after coronary occlusion but well before onset of reperfusion in various open-chest animal models of AMI.

A different reperfusion model of AMI was reported by Nicolini *et al.*[50] They infused tissue-type plasminogen activator (t-PA) with or without iloprost in open-chest dogs with an electrically induced coronary arterial thrombus. The time to thrombolysis was almost doubled by iloprost, duration of reperfusion was shorter and reocclusion occurred in all iloprost-treated animals. The authors assumed that iloprost was detrimental because it enhanced plasma degradation of t-PA.[50] The possible clinical impact of this observation is discussed later in this chapter.

Clinical experience with prostacyclin and its analogues

Prostacyclin in angina

Angina pectoris (i.e. chest pain or discomfort caused by myocardial ischaemia) may be based on a number of factors that induce a transient imbalance between myocardial oxygen supply and demand. A fixed stenosis, usually of atherosclerotic origin, is probably the most common cause of angina. Such occlusion does, in uncomplicated cases, elicit myocardial ischaemia when demand is increased by, for example, an increase in physical activity. When the demand is lowered the angina disappears, to materialize again when new increases in myocardial work appear. Hence, in the most typical cases, the disease pattern in reproducible and therefore characterized as stable angina or effort-induced angina.

Unstable angina is defined as transient, repeated periods of chest pain appearing in the absence of an increase in demand. Unstable angina may appear to be very similar to an AMI but lacks the objective laboratory findings typical of the injured myocardium (Q wave in the ECG, plasma enzyme pattern, etc.). However, a period of unstable angina, often with increasing severity of symptoms (crescendo angina), may eventually end with the development of a true AMI. Unstable angina is thought to be based on accumulation of adhering and aggregating platelets forming a transient thrombus at the site of an atherosclerotic coronary occlusion. Unstable angina consequently elicits repeated periods of increasing

coronary occlusion and myocardial ischaemia, which are followed by periods of normalized flow and myocardial energy supply. With such an aetiological basis for unstable angina it is hardly surprising that the setting eventually may proceed to a fully developed AMI.

Variant angina, initially described by Prinzmetal in 1959, is caused by coronary spasm in a segment of an epicardial artery. Prinzmetal's angina occurs almost exclusively at rest, and it cannot be precipitated by exercise. Its most prominent clinical feature is the ST elevation appearing in the ECG during an angina attack. Variant angina occurs in patients with angiographically normal arteries, which at the time of an attack display a typical segmental spasm. The endogenous factor responsible for the spasm has not been characterized.

Stable coronary disease (effort angina)
Prostacyclin and iloprost have been studied in patients with stable coronary disease at rest, during cold pressor testing and during physical exercise. The variables studied include platelet aggregability, haemodynamics, physical capacity and appearance of angina.

In patients with angiographically confirmed stable coronary disease, iloprost (1–6 ng/kg per minute) given during leg exercise displayed potent antiaggregatory activity in platelet-rich plasma and also reversed platelet hyperaggregation occurring in whole blood after exercise.[51]

The effect of prostacyclin or iloprost on the appearance of angina at rest in patients with stable coronary disease has been studied by two groups. Bugiardini *et al.*[52,53] gave prostacyclin (2–10 ng/kg per minute) and iloprost (1–6 ng/kg per minute) to patients with severe coronary obstruction. Prostacyclin lowered systemic blood pressure and induced flushing in all patients, and in addition elicited chest pain and ECG changes typical of myocardial ischaemia in six of them. Iloprost also lowered the systemic pressure, and provoked chest pain and ECG changes in three patients. Myocardial blood flow was augmented both by prostacyclin and by iloprost. It was concluded that the mechanism of myocardial ischaemia developing during drug infusion was coronary steal. Similar findings were reported by the same group in a separate study in 33 patients.[54] In another study, 17 patients with stable angina and coronary artery disease given prostacyclin (2.5–10 ng/kg per minute) displayed flushing, increased heart rate and cardiac index, and a lowering of systemic blood pressure.[55] There was no change in pulmonary arterial pressure or capillary wedge pressure, and no change in coronary sinus blood flow. None of the patients experienced any chest pain. The apparent discrepancy between these studies[52,55] in the appearance of chest pain may be explained by the difference between them in the effect of the infused prostacyclin on myocardial blood flow. It is hardly surprising that a dose of a vasodilator that elicits a significant increase in myocardial blood flow[52] also may induce a steal phenomenon if coronary artery disease is present, whilst no such effect is obtained if myocardial blood flow is unobstructed.[55]

Prostacyclin and iloprost have also been studied with respect to their effect during physical exercise in patients with stable coronary disease. In 28 patients with effort angina and proven coronary artery narrowing, iloprost (6 ng/kg per minute) was given prior to and during leg exercise.[56] Four patients were excluded because of chest pain and ST segment depression during iloprost infusion. In the others, iloprost prolonged exercise duration and time to onset of ST depression. Both angina and ST depression occurred at a greater heart rate and rate–pressure product with iloprost compared to placebo. It was concluded that iloprost may improve exercise capacity in patients with stable angina and that the improvment is independent of changes in the major determinants of myocardial oxygen demand.[56] Ganz et al.[57] studied whether prostacyclin (4–10 ng/kg per minute) influenced the coronary vasomotor response to a cold pressor test in 11 patients with stable angina pectoris. Prostacyclin lowered systemic and coronary vascular resistances and increased heart rate, as expected. Of the 11 patients, 7 displayed a coronary vasoconstrictor response to cold exposure in the basal state; this response was not affected by prostacyclin. They concluded that, although prostacyclin caused marked coronary and systemic vasodilation, there was no evidence of a selective effect in the coronary vessels.

Hence, in patients with stable coronary disease, prostacyclin and iloprost, when infused in doses sufficient to lower coronary vascular resistance, may elicit chest pain and myocardial ischaemia, probably as a consequence of coronary steal elicited by their vasodilator activity.

Unstable angina (crescendo angina)
Prostacyclin has been given to patients with unstable angina in both open and double-blind placebo-controlled studies. Szczeklik et al.[58] infused prostacyclin (4 ng/kg per minute) for 48 hours in 18 patients

with coronary atherosclerosis and spontaneous ischaemic attacks. It may be questioned whether these patients really were representative of unstable angina, and the authors did not claim this. Nevertheless, in these patients prostacyclin consistently diminished both frequency of anginal attacks and nitroglycerin consumption. The authors suggested that healing of endothelial damage by prostacyclin could explain the favourable therapeutic response.

In a randomized double-blind study in 27 patients with unstable angina given a 72-hour infusion of prostacyclin at a dose of 5 ng/kg per minute active drug was not superior to placebo in preventing recurrence of angina during infusion or protecting against development of AMI. It was concluded that prostacyclin, despite favourable effects upon platelet aggregation and systemic haemodynamics, failed to improve the clinical evolution of unstable angina.[59] Similar data were reported by Lichstein et al.[60] who studied 63 patients with unstable angina, each given prostacyclin or placebo in a double-blind design. They found no significant differences between the placebo and prostacyclin groups for levels of cardiac enzymes throughout the hospitalization period, severity of angina, number of patients with congestive heart failure, new myocardial infarction, balloon pump insertion, coronary artery bypass grafting or percutaneous coronary angioplasty. They assumed that the lack of clinical benefit of prostacyclin might be explained by the heterogeneous mechanisms behind the disease, by the multiple standard medications their patients were exposed to by the inability of prostacyclin to prevent or lyse coronary thrombus in an advanced stage of unstable angina, or simply by its pharmacological ineffectiveness in the disease.[60]

From these data it may be concluded that prostacyclin is not effective in the treatment of unstable angina (crescendo angina).

Variant angina (Prinzmetal's angina)
Only a few studies have been reported on the effects of prostacyclin or analogues in patients with variant angina. Szczeklik observed that prostacyclin given for 48 hours at an average dose of 4 ng/kg per minute decreased the number of ischaemic attacks in only one of four patients with Prinzmetal's angina.[58] Chierchia et al.[61] infused prostacyclin (8–20 ng/kg per minute) in five patients with spontaneous ischaemic episodes due to coronary vasospasm and in three with ergonovine-induced spasm. Although one patient consistently appeared to respond to the infusion of prostacyclin, the drug did not affect the

number, severity and duration of the episodes in the entire group of patients with spontaneous attacks. In addition, prostacyclin caused no apparent differences in severity and duration of ECG changes in two patients with ergonovine-induced spasm. Another study involved five men who had more than five episodes daily of transient ischaemia with ST segment elevation at rest with or without symptoms. Iloprost was administered in single-blind fashion for four periods of 6 hours each, alternated with placebo.[62] Iloprost had no effect on the total number of episodes of ST segment elevation, but did in fact increase the number of symptomatic episodes and the consumption of nitroglycerin in these subjects. This unfavourable result was suggested to be based on induction of coronary steal, similar to that described with dipyridamole and prostacyclin.[62]

On the basis of these results, it may be concluded that prostacyclin and iloprost are not effective in the treatment of variant angina.

Prostacyclin in acute myocardial infarction

The possible effects of prostacyclin and its analogues in AMI have been investigated both in small open studies and in more comprehensive randomized double-blind investigations. In general, it may be concluded that prostacyclin[63-65] and iloprost[66] can be given safely to patients with AMI, provided that the dose during prolonged infusion is kept below 5 ng/kg per minute. This dose has been claimed sufficient to elicit profound inhibition of ADP-induced *ex vivo* platelet aggregation.[66]

In preliminary reports Uchida *et al.*[67,68] infused prostacyclin at a dose of 8 ng/kg per minute in six patients with AMI who experienced reocclusion following successful thrombolysis with urokinase. Recanalization was obtained in all six patients and, in addition, in three patients who did not receive urokinase. It was suggested that prostacyclin is effective in recanalization of the obstructed coronary artery in patients with AMI.[67] These promising results could not, however, be confirmed by others. Thus, in five patients with AMI and given prostacyclin at a dose of 8–20 ng/kg per minute for 90 minutes, starting on average 3 hours after onset of chest pain, total occlusion of the infarct-related artery persisted in four of the patients at the end of the infusion; in only one subject was partial recanalization achieved at 90 minutes of infusion.[69] Similar results were reported recently by Hackett *et al.*[70] They infused prostacyclin at a dose of up to 10 ng/kg per minute in

17 patients within 5 hours of the onset of continuous ischaemic chest pain, and were unable to demonstrate any general dilation of the infarct-related stenosis or coronary recanalization in response to the infusion of drug.

Studies aimed to reveal an effect of prostacyclin on the evolution of the infarct process, that is on the size of the infarct, on possible extension of the necrotic zone and on the occurrence of reinfarction, have also been performed. The experience from our own laboratory may serve as an example. In an initial pilot study we administered prostacyclin at a dose of 2–5 ng/kg per minute over 72 hours to five patients, within 16 hours after onset of symptoms of AMI. We were surprised to find that all five patients returned to our coronary care unit with status anginosus within 8–25 days after the first admission.[71] These preliminary findings seemed to indicate that prostacyclin might have limited the size of the infarct, thereby leaving more myocardium at risk after the end of the infusion. However, in a controlled double-blind placebo study in 30 patients we were unable to confirm the preliminary observations that patients receiving prostacyclin would be more prone to develop reinfarction.[65] On the other hand, there was a strong tendency that patients receiving active drug would benefit more from the treatment the earlier after onset of symptoms of AMI it was initiated.[72] In fact, patients receiving prostacyclin within 6 hours after onset of chest pain developed significantly lower plasma levels of myocardial-specific creatine kinase (CK-MB) and lactate dehydrogenase (LD) than those receiving placebo, indicating that their infarctions were smaller.[65] Furthermore, none of the patients given prostacyclin displayed infarct extension during the course of the infusion, compared with four patients given placebo. Based on this positive evidence, the study was extended. The study was closed when a total of 76 AMI patients had been included. The results of the final study confirmed the previously observed difference in infarct extension during the course of infusion, in that none of the patients given prostacyclin developed extension during the infusion whilst six patients given placebo did.[73] However, in contrast to the previous study, there was no difference in plasma enzymes indicating myocardial injury or ECG score indicating infarct size between the prostacyclin and placebo groups, irrespective of the duration of symptoms at the time of onset of infusion. Plasma levels of enzymes in the prostacyclin and placebo groups are shown in Fig. 11.1. Hence, it appeared that prostacyclin was unable to limit the size of the

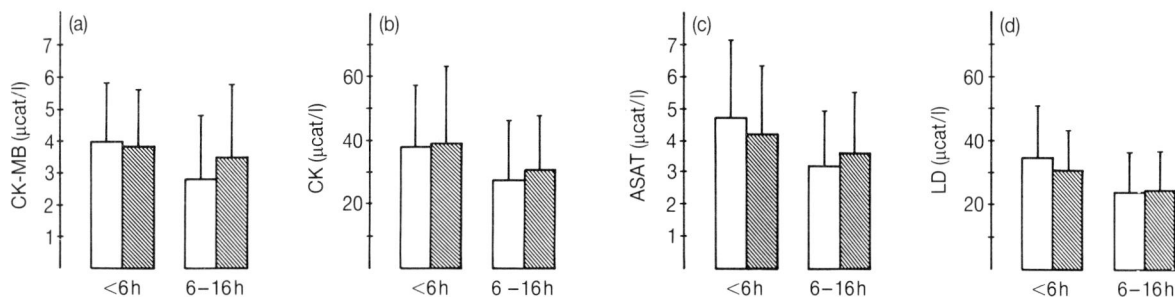

Fig. 11.1 Peak activities of (*a*) myocardial-specific creatine kinase (CK-MB), (*b*) total creatine kinase (CK), (*c*) aspartate aminotransferase (ASAT), and (*d*) lactate dehydrogenase (LD) in patients with acute myocardial infarction treated with placebo (open columns) or prostacyclin 6 ng/kg per minute for 72 hours (shaded columns) within 6 hours (<6 h) and between 6 and 16 hours (6–16 h) after onset of pain.

infarct, although offering protection against infarct extension during the course of the infusion.

In a study with similar design, Kiernan *et al.*[63] infused prostacyclin in 23 and placebo in 22 patients with AMI. Infusion was given at 5 ng/kg per minute for 72 hours. Although prostacyclin was well tolerated in all patients, there was no benefit from active drug treatment compared to placebo, whether in terms of infarct size, left ventricular function or complications during the hospital period. Hence, two studies with identical protocol[63,73] gave the same results with respect to infarct size but divergent results with respect to infarct extension in the group of patients given active drug. At present there is no obvious explanation for this discrepancy.

One other study deserves to be mentioned in this context. Armstrong *et al.*[64] gave prostacyclin and placebo at a rate of ≤ 5 ng/kg per minute for 24 hours in a random study of 54 patients with AMI. They were also unable to demonstrate any beneficial effect of prostacyclin, as evidenced by measurements of infarct size, time to peak plasma creatine kinase, wall motion abnormality and ejection fraction. Infarct extension during the hospital stay, postinfarction angina and fatal outcome during the first 6 months following the AMI did not display any difference between the groups, either.

Hence, three different randomized studies[63,64,73] yielded similar results, demonstrating that prostacyclin at a dose of ≤5 ng/kg per minute does not limit infarct size in patients with AMI. A meta-analysis of these three studies is hardly indicated, since none of them displayed data of borderline significance that could be assumed to change with a larger number of study subjects. The positive finding concerning protection against infarct extension during the course of the infusion observed by us[73] was not con-

firmed in the other studies,[63,64] and should probably be regarded as accidental.

Effect of prostacyclin in conjunction with other therapies

Prostacyclin and/or analogues have been evaluated as complementary therapies in both angina and AMI. Firstly, prostacyclin has been given to patients undergoing percutaneous transluminal coronary angioplasty, in an attempt to counteract subsequent restenosis of the dilated coronary vessel; such restenosis is the major drawback related to this type of therapy. Secondly, prostacyclin and analogues have been administered in parallel with different types of thrombolytic therapies. The findings in these studies are preliminary, and provide no concluside evidence. Nevertheless, a brief review of these studies is indicated.

A prospective single-blind randomized trial was recently presented on the short-term effect of prostacyclin on the incidence of restenosis after coronary angioplasty.[74] The trial comprised 134 patients given prostacyclin and 136 given placebo prior to and for 48 hours following successful coronary dilatation. At follow-up after 6 months, restenosis was present in 27% in the prostacyclin group compared with 32% in the control group (not significant). It was concluded that short-term administration of prostacyclin did not significantly lower the risk of restenosis after coronary angioplasty.

In 1983 a report was presented on simultaneous administration of streptokinase and prostacyclin in two patients with AMI.[75] No controls were presented to these cases, but thrombolysis was successful in both cases without any complications. This preliminary study has been followed by both animal experiments and clinical studies. The ability of heparin and prostacyclin to improve streptokinase-induced recanalization of a coronary artery in open-chest dogs subjected to thrombotic occlusion was studied by Schumacher *et al.*[76] They gave streptokinase alone, with heparin, or with heparin and prostacyclin (intermittently during reperfusion). The percentage of animals recanalized and the time to successful recanalization did not differ between the groups, but reflow volume was lower in animals given streptokinase only than in the other groups. Furthermore, the intermittent reocclusions that persisted during reperfusion were diminished during the infusion of prostacyclin. Infarct size was not reported. It was proposed that heparin and prostacyclin were effective in increasing coronary flow during recanalization achieved with thrombolytic therapy.[76]

In a similar open-chest model, thrombolytic therapy with fibrin-specific recombinant single-chain urokinase-type plasminogen activator (r-scu-PA) was given following induction of an occlusive thrombus in the left anterior circumflex artery.[77] In conjunction with the thrombolytic therapy, two different doses of the prostacyclin analogue taprostene were tested. Infarct size was not diminished by taprostene, but the plasma levels of creatine kinase following recanalization were lower in animals given the higher dose of taprostene. The authors concluded, somewhat surprisingly, that treatment with taprostene as an adjunct to r-scu-PA yielded significantly enhanced myocardial salvage compared with thrombolytic treatment alone.

Kerins *et al.*[78] were less enthusiastic in a paper reporting on the effect of iloprost combined with tissue plasminogen activator (t-PA) in a closed chest canine model of coronary thrombosis. Iloprost was found to increase the time to reperfusion by 50%, in comparison with control, whilst a thromboxane receptor antagonist reduced it by 47%. This somewhat unexpected result was explained by an increased plasma clearance of t-PA in the presence of iloprost. Unfavourable results were also reported in a study of patients with AMI given t-PA alone or in combination with iloprost.[79] Infarct-related vessel patency at 90 minutes after drug administration was not improved by iloprost, and reocclusion at 1 week was not lowered. Ejection fraction increased significantly from baseline to 1 week in patients given t-PA alone, but decreased in patients given t-PA plus iloprost. It was concluded that the combination of t-PA plus iloprost did not improve immediate or follow-up coronary artery patency or left ventricular functional recovery compared with that achieved with t-PA alone.

The above studies provide a heterogeneous view, as do a number of reports in this field. Initial experiments in animals or small open uncontrolled clinical trials tended to present positive findings, which could not be confirmed in larger blind randomized and properly controlled studies in patients. With the currently available information, there is little reason to expect any dramatic effect with prostacyclin or its analogues in conjunction with thrombolytic therapy in patients with AMI.

Concluding remarks

Prostacyclin is an endogenous mediator with enormous clinical potential. It has been pointed out repeatedly that its biological properties might make it an ideal agent in the treatment of ischaemic heart disease. Yet, after 10 years of laboratory studies and repeated clinical trials, prostacyclin has no established position in the treatment of such disease. This may seem paradoxical, and the basis for it is complex and multifactorial.

For reasons discussed in the first section of this chapter, stable coronary disease is hardly a suitable setting for treatment with an antiplatelet vasodilator such as prostacyclin. On the other hand, unstable angina, presumed to be related to intermittent occlusions and reperfusions of a semioccluded vessel, could be expected to be successfully counteracted by the antiplatelet and vasodilator actions of prostacyclin. Yet, carefully conducted controlled trials have failed to document such an action of prostacyclin. We have to accept the results obtained in these trials, although we do not understand the basis for their negative outcome. Perhaps less surprising is the lack of effect of prostacyclin or analogues in variant angina; because this state is characterized by coronary vasospasm, only a selective receptor antagonist may be effective. The data available indicate that prostacyclin is not such a compound.

Turning to the studies of prostacyclin and analogues in AMI, the lack of favourable effects may seem more surprising. This assumption is not primarily based on the positive results obtained in preliminary animal studies, but rather on the pharmacological profile of prostacyclin. A condition characterized by thrombus formation might seem ideal for an antiplatelet drug. That this is not the case is apparent from the clinical studies available. Hence what factors may have contributed to prevent the antiplatelet effect of prostacyclin from providing positive benefit in these studies? Several possible factors need to be considered:

1. Prostacyclin cannot be given in adequate amounts to patients with AMI. In the bedside situation the vasodilator action of the drug must always be taken into account, and any tendency to lowering of the patient's systemic blood pressure by more than 10–15 mmHg must be countered by lowering of the infusion rate. If prostacyclin is given intravenously, the antiplatelet action might then be too limited to be efficient. Unlike thrombolytic drugs such as streptokinase and t-PA, prostacyclin affects not just one target, the coronary thrombus, but the entire cardiovascular system. This is a disadvantage that is hard to overcome.

2. Prostacyclin does not reach the target. Although this is an obvious possibility, it must be considered in the light of the fact that other thrombolytic agents, such as streptokinase and t-PA, efficiently penetrate the thrombus. Another alternative must therefore be considered; namely that

3. Prostacyclin has no pharmacological effect in AMI. This may be true if the drug is given when the coronary thrombus is no longer of platelet origin only. The more fibrinogen that is incorporated into the platelet thrombus, the less thrombolytic effect can be expected from prostacyclin. Considering this, it is not surprising that drugs primarily affecting the fibrin network in the thrombus, such as streptokinase and t-PA, are more effective.

4. Prostacyclin interacts with other drugs, thereby disguising an intrinsic positive effect. The data demonstrating an increased clearance of t-PA by iloprost in dogs[78] give a hint that such an action of prostacyclin is not entirely unlikely. In this connection it may be of interest to note that the half-life of prostacyclin is lowered in patients with unstable angina and AMI.[80,81]

However, it cannot be excluded that future prostacyclin analogues with selective antiplatelet activity may prove efficient in the treatment of unstable coronary disease, either alone or in conjunction with other therapies. The prerequiste for this is probably that a functionally significant difference in vascular and platelet prostacyclin receptor structure can be demonstrated and utilized pharmacologically. But even in the absence of success in this respect, prostacyclin will always be one of the important physiological and pathophysiological cardiovascular mediators – and for one particular reason: its discovery was the first step in the field of endothelial

research, an area that may turn out to be one of the major contributors in our understanding of cardiovascular disease.

References

1. Davies MJ, Thomas A. Thrombosis and acute coronary-artery lesions in sudden cardiac ischemic death. *N Engl J Med* 1984; **310:** 1137–40.
2. Tateson JE, Moncada S, Vane JR. Effects of prostacyclin (PGX) on cyclic AMP concentrations in human platelets. *Prostaglandins* 1977; **13:** 389–98.
3. Gordon JB, Ganz P, Nabel EG, *et al.* Atherosclerosis influences the vasomotor response of epicardial coronary arteries to exercise. *J Clin Invest* 1989; **83:** 1946–52.
4. Nabel EG, Ganz P, Gordon JB, Alexander RW, Selwyn AP. Dilation of normal and constriction of atherosclerotic coronary arteries caused by the cold pressor test. *Circulation* 1988; **77:** 43–52.
5. McFadden EP, Clarke JG, Davies GJ, Kaski JC, Haider AW, Maseri A. Effect of intracoronary serotonin on coronary vessels in patients with stable angina and patients with variant angina. *N Engl J Med* 1991; **324:** 648–54.
6. Golino P, Piscione F, Willerson JT, *et al.* Divergent effects of serotonin on coronary-artery dimensions and blood flow in patients with coronary atherosclerosis and control patients. *N Engl J Med* 1991; **324:** 641–8.
7. Yeung AC, Vekshtein VI, Krantz DS, *et al.* The effect of atherosclerosis on the vasomotor response of coronary arteries to mental stress. *N Engl J Med* 1991; **325:** 1551–6.
8. Ludmer PL, Selwyn AP, Shook TL, *et al.* Paradoxical vasoconstriction induced by acetylcholine in atherosclerotic coronary arteries. *N Engl J Med* 1986; **315:** 1046–51.
9. Wennmalm Å, Nowak J, Bjurö T. Excretion of thromboxane A_2 and prostacyclin metabolites before and after exercise testing in patients with and without signs of ischemic heart disease. *Circulation* 1990; **82:** 1737–43.
10. Lewis HD Jr, Davis JW, Archibald DG, *et al.* Protective effects of aspirin against acute myocardial infarction and death in men with unstable angina. *N Engl J Med* 1983; **309:** 396–403.
11. Henriksson P, Wennmalm Å, Edhag O, Vesterqvist O, Green K. *In vivo* production of prostacyclin and thromboxane in patients with acute myocardial infarction. *Br Heart J* 1986; **55:** 543–8.
12. Fitzgerald DJ, Roy L, Catella F, FitzGerald GA. Platelet activation in unstable coronary disease. *N Engl J Med* 1986; **315:** 983–9.
13. Aherne T, Price DC, Yee ES, Hsieh WR, Ebert PA. Prevention of ischemia-induced myocardial platelet

deposition by exogenous prostacyclin. *J Thorac Cardiovasc Surg* 1986; **92**: 99–104.

14. Tosaki A, Koltai M, Paubert-Braquet M. Effect of iloprost on reperfusion-induced arrhythmias and myocardial ion shifts in isolated rat hearts. *Eur J Pharmacol* 1990; **191**: 69–81.

15. Müller B, Schneider J, Hennies HH, Flohé L. Cardioprotective action of the new stable epoprostenol analogue CG 4203 in rat models of cardiac hypoxia and ischemia. *Arzneimittelforschung [Drug Research]* 1984; **34** (II): 1506–9.

16. Moffat MP. Concentration-dependent effects of prostacyclin on the response of the isolated guinea pig heart to ischemia and reperfusion: possible involvement of the slow inward current. *J Pharmacol Exp Ther* 1987; **242**: 292–9.

17. Nayler WG, Purchase M, Dusting GJ. Effect of prostacyclin infusion during low-flow ischaemia in the isolated perfused rat heart. *Basic Res Cardiol* 1984; **79**: 125–34.

18. Pissarek M, Gründer W, Keller T. ^{31}P-NMR-spectroscopy on ischemic and reperfused rat hearts: effects of iloprost. *Biomed Biochim Acta* 1987; **46** (8/9): S564–7.

19. Pissarek M, Gründer W, Keller T, Goos H, Mest HJ, Krause EG. Action of iloprost and PGE$_1$ on global ischemic and reperfused myocardium: a ^{31}P-NMR-study. *Biomed Biochim Acta* 1988; **47** (10/11): S121–4.

20. Pissarek M, Gründer W, Keller T, Lindenau KF, Krause EG. PGE$_1$ and iloprost affect the high energy phosphates in the global ischemic and reperfused rat heart: a ^{31}P-NMR study. *Biomed Biochim Acta* 1989; **48**: 43–50.

21. Edlund A, Sahlin K, Wennmalm Å. Effect of prostacyclin on the severity of ischaemic injury in rabbit hearts subjected to coronary ligation. *Mol Cell Cardiol* 1986; **18**: 1067–76.

22. Ferrari R, Cargnoni A, Curello S, Boffa GM, Ceconi C. Effects of iloprost (ZK 36374) on glutathione status during ischaemia and reperfusion of rabbit isolated hearts. *Br J Pharmacol* 1989; **98**: 678–84.

23. Karmazyn M, Neely JR. Inhibition of post-ischemic ventricular recovery by low concentrations of prostacyclin in isolated working rat hearts: dependency on concentration, ischemic duration, calcium and relationship to myocardial energy metabolism. *Mol Cell Cardiol* 1989; **21**: 335–46.

24. Van Gilst WH, Boonstra PW, Terpstra JA, Wildevuur ChRM, de Langen CDJ. Rapid communication: improved functional recovery of the isolated rat heart after 24 hours of hypothermic arrest with a stable prostacyclin analogue (ZK 36374). *Mol Cell Cardiol* 1983; **15**: 789–92.

25. Smith EF III, Kloster G, Stöcklin G, Schrör K. Effect of iloprost (ZK 36374) on membrane integrity in ischemic rabbit hearts. *Biomed Biochim Acta* 1984; **43** (8/9): S155–8.

26. van der Giessen WJ, Mooi WJ, Rutteman AM, Berk L, Verdouw PD. The effect of the stable prostacyclin analogue ZK 36374 on experimental coronary thrombosis in the pig. *Thromb Res* 1984; **36**: 46–51.

27. Hieda N, Toki Y, Sugiyama S, Ito T, Satake T, Ozawa T. Prostaglandin I$_2$ analogue and propranolol prevent ischaemia induced mitochondrial dysfunction through the stabilisation of lysosomal membranes. *Cardiovasc Res* 1988; **22**: 219–25.

28. Farber NE, Pieper GM, Thomas JP, Gross GJ. Beneficial effects of iloprost in the stunned canine myocardium. *Circ Res* 1988; **62**: 204–15.

29. van der Giessen WJ, Schoutsen B, Tijssen JGP, Verdouw PD. Iloprost (ZK 36374) enhances recovery of regional myocardial function during reperfusion after coronary artery occlusion in the pig. *Br J Pharmacol* 1986; **87**: 23–7.

30. Stürzebecker S, McDonald FM, Grundmann G, Hartmann S, Lammert C. Myocardial ischaemia and reperfusion in the anaesthetised pig: reduction of infarct size and myocardial enzyme release by the stable prostacyclin analogue iloprost. In: *Prostaglandins in Clinical Research: Cardiovascular System.* New York: AR Liss, 1989: 155–9.

31. Fiedler VB, Mardin M. Influence of prostacyclin on coronary thrombosis and myocardial ischemia in conscious canine experiments. *Arch Int Pharmacodyn Ther* 1985; **278**: 114–27.

32. Lupinetti FM, Starnes VA, Laws KA, Collins JC, Hammon JW Jr. Prostacyclin reduction of regional ischemic injury in the canine myocardium. *J Surg Res* 1986; **41**: 146–57.

33. de Langen CDJ, van Gilst WH, Wesseling H. Sustained protection by iloprost of the porcine heart in the acute and chronic phases of myocardial infarction. *J Cardiovasc Pharmacol* 1985; **7**: 924–8.

34. Johnston KM, MacLeod BA, Walker MJA. Effects of aspirin and prostacyclin on arrhythmias resulting from coronary artery ligation and on infarct size. *Br J Pharmacol* 1983; **78**: 029–37.

35. Simpson PJ, Mitsos SE, Ventura A, et al. Prostacyclin protects ischemic reperfused myocardium in the dog by inhibition of neutrophil activation. *Am Heart J* 1987; **113**: 129–37.

36. Melin JA, Becker LC. Salvage of ischemic myocardium by prostacyclin during experimental myocardial infarction. *J Am Coll Cardiol* 1983; **2**: 279–86.

37. Mueller B, Maass B, Krause W, Witt W. Limitation of myocardial unperfused area and necrotic zone 24 hours and eight days after coronary artery ligation in rats by the stable prostacyclin analogue iloprost. *Prostaglandins Leukot Med* 1986; **21**: 331–40.

38. Herbaczynska-Cedro K, Karwatowska-Prokopczuk E, Michalowski J, Wennmalm Å. Prostacyclin and regional coronary blood flow in experimental myocardial infarction. *Clin Physiol* 1988; **8**: 255–66.

39. Darius H, Thomsen T, Schrör K. Cardiovascular actions *in vitro* and cardioprotective effects *in vivo*

of nileprost, a mixed type PGI$_2$/PGE$_2$ agonist. *J Cardiovasc Pharmacol* 1987; **10**: 144–52.

40. Thiemermann C, Schrör K. Comparison of the thromboxane synthetase inhibitor dazoxiben and the prostacyclin mimetic iloprost in an animal model of acute ischaemia and reperfusion. *Biomed Biochim Acta* 1984; **43** (8/9): S151–4.

41. Smith EF III, Gallenkämper W, Beckmann R, Thomsen T, Mannesmann G, Schrör K. Early and late administration of a PGI$_2$-analogue, ZK 36374 (iloprost): effects of myocardial preservation, collateral blood flow and infarct size. *Cardiovasc Res* 1984; **18**: 163–73.

42. Goos H, Krause EG, Beyerdörfer I, *et al.* Improved protection in myocardial ischemia by combined prostacyclin administration and intraaortic balloon pumping. *Biomed Biochim Acta* 1984; **43** (8/9): S159–62.

43. Pissarek M, Goos H, Nöhring J, *et al.* Prostacyclin and iloprost: equal efficiency in preserving high energy phosphate in the dog heart following coronary artery ligation. *Basic Res Cardiol* 1987; **82**: 566–75.

44. Beitz A, Taube Ch, Beitz J, *et al.* Influence of iloprost on eicosanoid generation and lipid levels in experimental myocardial ischemia in dogs. *Prostaglandins Leukot Essent Fatty Acids* 1989; **35**: 141–5.

45. David H, Goos H, Nöhring J, Lindenau KF, Behrisch D. Ultrastructural morphometric examinations on the protection provided by prostacyclin against myocardial ischaemia. *Exp Pathol* 1985; **27**: 163–9.

46. Darius H, Osborne JA, Reibel DK, Lefer AM. Protective actions of a stable prostacyclin analog in ischemia induced membrane damage in rat myocardium. *Mol Cell Cardiol* 1987; **19**: 243–50.

47. Simpson PJ, Mickelson J, Fantone JC, Gallagher KP, Lucchesi BR. Iloprost inhibits neutrophil function *in vitro* and *in vivo* and limits experimental infarct size in canine heart. *Circ Res* 1987; **60**: 666–73.

48. Chiariello M, Golino P, Cappelli-Bigazzi M, Ambrosio G, Tritto I, Salvatore M. Reduction in infarct size by the prostacyclin analogue iloprost (ZK 36374) after experimental coronary artery occlusion–reperfusion. *Am Heart J* 1988; **115**: 499–504.

49. Johnson G III, Furlan LE, Aoki N, Lefer AM. Endothelium and myocardial protecting actions of taprostene, a stable prostacyclin analogue, after acute myocardial ischaemia and reperfusion in cats. *Circ Res* 1990; **66**: 1362–70.

50. Nicolini FA, Mehta JL, Nichols WW, Saldeen TGP, Grant M. Prostacyclin analogue iloprost decreases thrombolytic potential of tissue-type plasminogen activator in canine coronary thrombosis. *Circulation* 1990; **81**: 1115–22.

51. Grauso F, Biagi G, Puddu P, Bugiardini R, Capelli M, Coccheri S. Effects of iloprost (ZK 36374), a prostacyclin derivative, on platelet function after ischaemic exercise in patients with stable angina pectoris. *Thromb Res* 1987; **48**: 131–43.

52. Bugiardini R, Galvani M, Ferrini D, *et al.* Myocardial

ischemia during intravenous prostacyclin administration: hemodynamic findings and precautionary measures. *Am Heart J* 1987; **113**: 234–40.

53. Galvani M, Bugiardini R, Ferrini D, *et al.* Side effects of prostacyclin in patients with angina pectoris and coronary artery disease. *Ric Clin Lab* 1985; **15**: 145–9.

54. Bugiardini R, Galvani M, Ferrini D, *et al.* Myocardial ischemia induced by prostacyclin and iloprost. *Clin Pharmacol Ther* 1985; **38**: 101–8.

55. Firth BG, Winniford MD, Campbell WB, Hillis LD. Hemodynamic effects of intravenous prostacyclin in stable angina pectoris. *Am J Cardiol* 1983; **52**: 439–43.

56. Bugiardini R, Galvani M, Ferrini D, *et al.* Effects of iloprost, a stable prostacyclin analog, on exercise capacity and platelet aggregation in stable angina pectoris. *Am J Cardiol* 1986; **58**: 453–9.

57. Ganz P, Gaspar J, Colucci WS, Barry WH, Mudge GH, Alexander RW. Effects of prostacyclin on coronary hemodynamics at rest and in response to cold pressor testing in patients with angina pectoris. *Am J Cardiol* 1984; **53**: 1500–4.

58. Szczeklik A, Nizankowski R, Szczeklik J, Tabeau J, Krolikowski W. Treatment with prostacyclin of various forms of spontaneous angina pectoris not responding to placebo. *Pharmacol Res Commun* 1984; **16**: 1117–30.

59. Théroux P, Latour JG, Diodati J, *et al.* Hemodynamic, platelet and clinical responses to prostacyclin in unstable angina pectoris. *Am J Cardiol* 1990; **65**: 1084–9.

60. Lichstein E, Mendizabal R, Théroux P, *et al.* Epoprostenol (prostacyclin) in unstable angina. *J Clin Pharmacol* 1988; **28**: 300–5.

61. Chierchia S, Patrono C, Crea F, *et al.* Effects of intravenous prostacyclin in variant angina. *Circulation* 1982; **65** (3): 470–7.

62. De Caterina R, Pelosi G, Carpeggiani C, *et al.* Iloprost in Prinzmetal's angina. *Am J Cardiol* 1986; **58**: 553–4.

63. Kiernan FJ, Kluger J, Regnier JC, Rutkowski M, Fieldman A. Epoprostenol sodium (prostacyclin) infusion in acute myocardial infarction. *Br Heart J* 1986; **56**: 428–32.

64. Armstrong PW, Langevin LM, Watts DG. Randomized trial of prostacyclin infusion in acute myocardial infarction. *Am J Cardiol* 1988; **61** (1): 455–7.

65. Henriksson P, Edhag O, Wennmalm Å. Prostacyclin infusion in patients with acute myocardial infarction. *Br Heart J* 1985; **53**: 173–9.

66. Swedberg K, Held P, Wadenvik H, Kutti J. Central haemodynamic and antiplatelet effects of iloprost – a new prostacyclin analogue – in acute myocardial infarction in man. *Eur Heart J* 1987; **8**: 362–8.

67. Uchida Y, Hanai T, Hasegawa K, Kawamura K, Oshima T. Coronary recanalization induced by intracoronary administration of prostacyclin in patients

with acute myocardial infarction. *Circulation* 1982; **66**: II-261.

68. Uchida Y, Hanai T, Hasegawa K, Kawamura K, Oshima T. Recanalization of obstructed coronary artery by intracoronary administration of prostacyclin in patients with acute myocardial infarction. *Adv Prostaglandin Thromboxane Leukotriene Res* 1983; **11**: 377–83.

69. Grose R, Greenberg M, Strain J, Mueller H, Dyer A. Intracoronary prostacyclin in evolving acute myocardial infarction. *Am J Cardiol* 1985; **55**: 1625–6.

70. Hackett D, Davies G, Maseri A. Effects of prostacyclin on coronary occlusion in acute myocardial infarction. *Int J Cardiol* 1990; **26**: 53–8.

71. Edhag O, Henriksson P, Wennmalm Å. Prostacyclin infusion in patients with acute myocardial infarction (preliminary report). *N Engl J Med* 1983; **308**: 1032–3.

72. Henriksson P, Edhag O. Wennmalm Å. Limitation of myocardial infarction with prostacyclin: a double-blind study. In: Gryglewski RJ, Szczeklik A, McGiff J, *et al. Prostacyclin – Clinical Trials.* New York: Raven Press, 1985: 31–41.

73. Henriksson P, Edhag O, Wennmalm Å. Prostacyclin offers protection against early extension of acute myocardial infarction. *Adv Prostaglandin Thromboxane Leukotriene Res* 1987; **17**: 435–6.

74. Knudtson ML, Flintoft VF, Roth DL, Hansen JL, Duff HJ. Effect of short-term prostacyclin administration on restenosis after percutaneous transluminal coronary angioplasty. *J Am Coll Cardiol* 1990; **15**: 691–7.

75. Blasko G, Berentey E, Harsanyi A, Sas G. Intracoronarily administered prostacyclin and streptokinase for treatment of myocardial infarction. *Adv Prostaglandin Thromboxane Leukotriene Res* 1983; **11**: 385–90.

76. Schumacher WA, Lee EC, Lucchesi BR. Augmentation of streptokinase-induced thrombolysis by heparin and prostacyclin. *J Cardiovasc Pharmacol* 1985; **7**: 739–46.

77. Groves R, Schneider J, Friderichs E, Giertz H, Flohé L. Additional myocardial salvage by coadministration of the epoprostenol analog taprostene to recombinant single-chain urokinase-type plasminogen activator in a canine coronary thrombosis model. *Arzneimittelforschung [Drug Research]* 1989; **39** (I): 534–8.

78. Kerins DM, Shuh M, Kunitada S, FitzGerald DJ. A prostacyclin analog impairs the response to tissue-type plasminogen activator during coronary thrombolysis: evidence for a pharmacokinetic interaction. *J Pharmacol Exp Ther* 1991; **257**: 487–92.

79. Topol EJ, Ellis SG, Califf RM, *et al.* Combined tissue-type plasminogen activator and prostacyclin therapy for acute myocardial infarction. *J Am Coll Cardiol* 1989; **14**: 877–84.

80. Sinzinger H, Fitscha P, Tiso B. Decreased prostaglandin-I_2 stability in acute myocardial infarction. *Thromb Res* 1990; **57**: 677–84.

81. Aoyama T, Yui Y, Morishita H, Kawai C. Prostaglandin I_2 half-life regulated by high density lipoprotein is decreased in acute myocardial infarction and unstable angina pectoris. *Circulation* 1990; **81**: 1784–91.

12 Prostaglandins in percutaneous transluminal coronary angioplasty

Donald M Demke

The use of prostaglandins in patients undergoing percutaneous transluminal coronary angioplasty (PTCA) is reviewed in this chapter. Following an overview of the percutaneous transluminal coronary angioplasty procedure, the complications associated with it and the pathophysiological mechanisms involved, the rationale for the use of prostaglandins in PTCA patients and the results of clinical studies will be summarized.

PTCA is a therapeutic cardiac catheterization procedure in which focal atherosclerotic stenoses in coronary arteries are dilated in order to improve myocardial blood flow.[1] PTCA involves the passage and inflation *in situ* of a balloon-tipped flexible catheter at a site of arterial narrowing to dilate and recanalize the obstructed vessel (Fig. 12.1).[2] Therefore, the procedure consists of mechanically induced coronary vasodilatation and recanalization with restoration of blood flow through segmentally stenosed coronary arteries.[3] PTCA is now a well-accepted non-surgical treatment for atherosclerotic coronary artery disease. In 1990, approximately 200 000 PTCA procedures were performed in the USA and an additional 100 000 in Europe.[4]

A successful PTCA procedure can reduce the extent of coronary artery stenosis and can relieve angina pectoris and improve objective signs of myocardial ischaemia.[5] Parisi *et al.* demonstrated that PTCA results in earlier and more complete relief of angina than medical therapy in patients with single vessel coronary artery disease.[6] In addition, the patients undergoing PTCA achieved better performance on treadmill exercise testing than those receiving medical therapy.

Dotter and Judkins described the first clinical mechanical dilatation of blood vessels.[7] Initially, short stenoses of the femoropopliteal artery, and later the iliac artery,[8] were dilated using a system of serial catheters of increasing external diameter telescopically inserted through the atherosclerotic lesion to mechanically expand the obstructed area. In the early 1970s, Gruentzig developed a modified catheter system for the dilatation of atherosclerotic stenoses in blood vessels. His system utilized a double-lumen, balloon-tipped catheter. Inflation of the balloon provided the dilatation effect. Coronary angioplasty was first introduced by Gruentzig in 1977, using a miniaturized version of the balloon catheter to dilate segmentally stenosed coronary arteries in patients suffering from ischaemic heart disease.[8,9]

Originally, the clinical and angiographic selection criteria for patients undergoing PTCA were quite restrictive.[10–12] Patients were required to have angina pectoris and confirmed myocardial ischaemia. Patients were also required to have single vessel

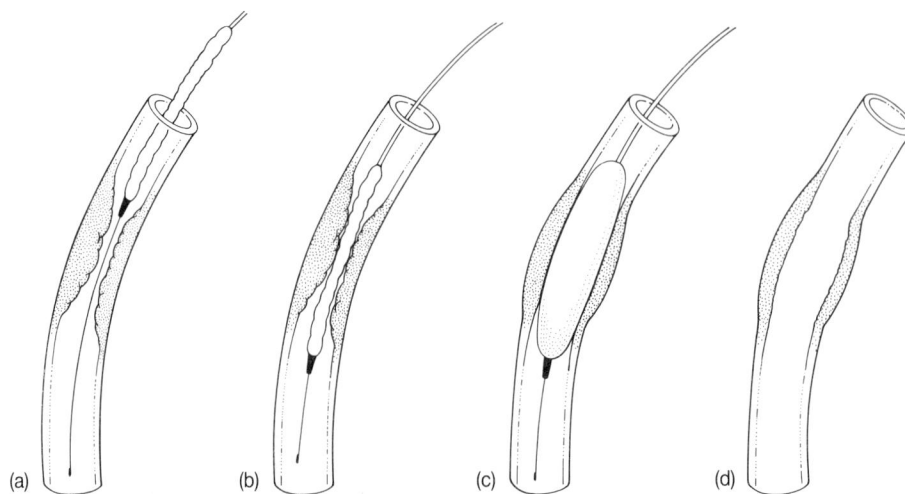

Fig. 12.1 Diagram of a PTCA procedure. (*a*) A coronary artery stenosis is represented. A guidewire has been advanced across the stenosis. (*b*) The balloon catheter (with balloon deflated) is advanced into position, across the stenoses. The balloon is inflated, one or more times, to dilate the stenosis. This results in (*c*) splitting and compression of the atherosclerotic plaque, and stretching of the vessel wall. (*d*) The balloon catheter and guidewire have been removed, and a successful dilatation is illustrated.

coronary artery disease and well-preserved left ventricular function, demonstrated angiographically. Subtotal, discrete, non-calcified, proximal coronary artery stenoses met the original angiographic selection criteria. Since the original selection criteria were so restrictive, a relatively small percentage of patients were eligible for the PTCA procedure. Gruentzig estimated in 1979/1980 that approximately 10–15% of patients having coronary artery bypass-graft surgery would be suitable candidates for PTCA.[10] In 1979, the results of PTCA in the first reported series of 50 patients was published by Gruentzig *et al.*[10] In this series, the primary success rate of the PTCA procedure was 66%; 6% of the patients had a documented myocardial infarction and 14% required emergency coronary artery bypass graft surgery following PTCA.

Since then, the primary success rate for PTCA has increased, due to improved operator experience and patient selection. In addition, many technical advances have taken place, including improvements in radiographic systems, guide catheters, balloon catheters and guidewires.[4] Some of the more important advances include the development of a large range of guiding catheters, including manoeuvrable catheters,[13] and the development of balloon catheters with a reduction in the external diameter of the catheter tip (low profile catheters).[13–15] Improved materials and coatings have resulted in stronger catheters and balloons that tolerate greater inflation

pressures.[16] These advances have allowed for the application of PTCA to a wider variety of lesions, including the accurate placement of the balloon catheter across more difficult and distal lesions, and have also resulted in a higher rate of success.[4,13] PTCA is now performed not only in single vessel coronary artery disease but also in multilesion and multivessel coronary artery disease,[1,13,17–20] stenosis of the left main coronary artery,[1] stenoses of coronary artery bypass grafts,[21–23] stenoses at bifurcations of coronary arteries,[24,25] complex lesions and total occlusions of coronary arteries.[1,26–28] Also, PTCA is now being used in 'high risk' patients, including patients with unstable angina[1] and acute myocardial infarction,[1,29–32] and in patients with poor left ventricular function.[1,26] Results from the National Heart, Lung, and Blood Institute PTCA Registry revealed a primary angiographic success rate for elective PTCA of 61% in 1977–1981 and 88% in 1985–1986.[33] In experienced centres, the primary success rate has currently improved to 90% or greater in selected subsets of patients (those with single, proximal, discrete, subtotal lesions).[4,26] In patients with multivessel disease, the primary success rate is approximately 80%.[26] In patients with chronic total vessel occlusions, the primary success rate is approximately 65–70%.[26] It is now estimated that 50% or more of patients who are candidates for coronary artery bypass graft surgery are also acceptable candidates to be treated with PTCA, instead.[13]

Complications and restenosis following PTCA

Despite the improvements in the primary success rate, major acute complications can occur as a result of PTCA. Coronary artery dissection, acute coronary artery occlusion and angioplasty-induced vasospasm are potential serious complications.[26] In patients who have undergone elective PTCA, the incidence of non-fatal myocardial infarction is approximately 4%, the need for emergency coronary artery bypass graft surgery is approximately 3% and the mortality rate is approximately 1–1.5%.[26] In addition, restenosis of the coronary artery after successful dilatation remains a persistent problem that reduces the long-term efficacy of the procedure.[26]

Restenosis is the process of renarrowing of the vessel early after PTCA. Restenosis has been reported to occur in 25–50% of patients, with an average range of 30–35% for many published series.[34–39] Restenosis is a phenomenon that usually occurs within 6 months in the majority of patients, necessitating repeat procedures.[35,37,39–41] Studies have shown that patients with the recent onset of angina prior to PTCA,[35,37,42] unstable angina,[35,37,43–45] vasospastic angina,[39,46] diabetes,[35,45,47] hypercholesterolaemia,[48,49] or smokers[48,50] may have an increased incidence of restenosis following successful PTCA. In addition, restenosis is more likely to occur when PTCA is performed on the following types of coronary lesions: totally occluded[51–53] or severely stenotic (pre-PTCA) coronary arteries,[35,42,54–56] proximal coronary artery stenoses,[47,57] stenoses of the left anterior descending coronary artery,[37,47,54,56] lesions involving vessel bifurcations,[24,25] lesions greater than 10–15 mm long,[58,59] calcified lesions,[39,54] eccentric lesions,[54] diffusely diseased vessels[54] and saphenous vein bypass grafts.[21–23] Several factors related to the result following the PTCA procedure may be associated with an increased risk of restenosis, including the presence of a severe residual stenosis[35–37,39,54] or a high pressure gradient (>20 mmHg) across the stenosis following PTCA,[35,37,60] the presence of a large dissection of the vessel wall[39] and the absence of a small intimal tear post-PTCA.[39,56,61] Also, the use of an undersized angioplasty balloon[39,62] and the need for a larger number of balloon inflations or higher balloon inflation pressures to dilate lesions may be associated with an increased incidence of restenosis.[35,37]

A variety of pharmacological and technical approaches have been studied in an attempt to reduce the restenosis rate after PTCA. Although aspirin appears to reduce the incidence of acute thrombosis, it does not appear to reduce the restenosis rate.[63–65] Most centres routinely heparinize patients during the PTCA procedure to reduce the formation of thrombi, but heparin has not been shown to reduce the restenosis rate.[66] Other pharmacological interventions, such as other antiplatelet agents (dipyridamole, sulphinpyrazone, ticlopidine),[65,67] low molecular weight dextran,[68] calcium antagonists (nifedipine, diltiazem),[69–71] oral anticoagulants (warfarin),[72] glucocorticosteroids (methylprednisolone),[73,74] omega-3 fatty acids (fish oils),[75,76] and serotonin antagonists (ketanserin)[77] have not been proven to significantly reduce the restenosis rate after PTCA. Technical procedural changes, such as changes in the duration or pressure of the balloon inflation, have not resulted in a reduction of the restenosis rate. Newer angioplasty procedures under study include the use of intravascular stents, laser-assisted angioplasty and mechanical devices such as atherectomy catheters. To date, none of these newer procedures has been shown to reduce the restenosis rate.[78]

Pathophysiological mechanisms

An understanding of the pathophysiological mechanisms involved is important in understanding why therapy with prostaglandins may prove beneficial in reducing complications and restenosis following PTCA. Several reviews of normal arterial wall and endothelial function have been published.[66,79–81] The inner surface of the arterial wall consists of a single layer of endothelial cells which has several important functions. The vascular endothelium is a selective, semipermeable membrane that separates circulating blood elements from underlying vascular structures. It forms a barrier to blood macromolecules and cells and is involved in the active transfer of metabolic substances between the blood and the tissues. The endothelium is important in the maintenance of vascular thromboresistance and in important functions related to haemostasis, thrombolysis and the vascular repair processes of cell migration and proliferation. It is also involved in the process of lipid transport from the blood into the vascular wall. In addition, the endothelium interacts with plasma proteins and formed elements in the blood, including the processing of antigens which is important for cellular immunity.[82]

The endothelium is active in the synthesis and/or metabolism of a variety of compounds involved in the interactions between blood components and the vascular wall. For instance, endothelial cells produce the prostaglandin prostacyclin (epoprostenol, PGI_2), which inhibits platelet adhesion and aggregation and also is a potent vasodilator.[79] Injury or damage to endothelial cells may result in a decrease in prostacyclin production, possibly leading to platelet aggregation, thrombosis and vasoconstriction. Endothelial cells also secrete a heparin-like compound (heparan sulphate) which is thought to be important in the coagulation system, and may also inhibit the proliferation of smooth muscle cells.[79,83] Endothelial cells synthesize a variety of factors important for blood coagulation, including factor V, factor VIII antigen (von Willebrand's factor), thrombomodulin and tissue factor.[66] Endothelial cells also possess binding sites for several coagulation factors.[66] Therefore, the endothelium plays an important role in the process of haemostasis. The endothelium also produces another compound, known as endothelium-dependent relaxing factor, that may be important for vasodilatation.[66] Since endothelial cells produce tissue-type (t-PA) and urokinase-type (u-PA) plasminogen activators, as well as an inhibitor of these plasminogen activators, the endothelium is important for the process of fibrinolysis.[84,85] Endothelial cells are also active in the synthesis of connective tissue components, such as collagen.[66] In summary, the normal endothelium prevents local platelet activation, inhibits smooth muscle cell proliferation and maintains normal vascular tone.[66]

Balloon angioplasty results in localized injury to the arterial wall.[86,87] The effects of angioplasty on the arterial wall are complex and involve a combination of several morphological alterations (Table 12.1), which have been studied in animal models as well as in man. Almost all studies reveal that balloon angioplasty results in denudation of endothelial cells from portions of the vessel wall.[85,88,89] In addition,

Table 12.1 Morphological alterations of the arterial wall following balloon angioplasty

---

Denudation of endothelial cells
Deposition of platelets and fibrin
Thrombus formation
Neointimal proliferation of smooth muscle cells
Cracking or splitting of atherosclerotic plaque
Compression of atherosclerotic plaque
Dehiscence of intima and plaque from underlying media
Intimal flap or dissection
Stretching of arterial media and adventitia with localized aneurysmal dilatation

---

cracking or splitting of the atherosclerotic plaque occurs.[85,90-96] Studies have shown that eccentric plaques tend to produce longitudinal tearing at the junction of the plaque and the arterial wall.[94,96-100] Concentric plaques are usually split at their thinnest or weakest point.[94,96-100] Dehiscence of the intima and the plaque from underlying media[90-93] often occurs and may lead to the presence of an intimal flap or dissection.[90,93,101] The split may extend down to the intimal–media border and occasionally into the media.[96,97,102] With continued inflation of the dilating balloon, the split in the atherosclerotic plaque widens, leading to circumferential stretching or tearing of the arterial media and adventitia.[89-93,103] Prolonged inflation at high pressure may produce damage or necrosis of medial muscle cells.[90] This disruption of the intima and plaque as well as the stretching of the arterial media and adventitia may result in localized aneurysmal dilatation of the vessel wall.[90,92,104] The primary mechanisms responsible for successful angioplasty appear to be splitting of the atherosclerotic plaque and stretching of the vessel wall.[90,92,97,98,104] Compression and remodelling of the atherosclerotic plaque may occur to a small degree, but these mechanisms are not of primary importance.[90] A successful balloon angioplasty results in a reduction of the arterial stenosis and a decrease in the pressure gradient across the stenosis.[1]

Responses to the arterial wall injury associated with balloon angioplasty may lead to complications, such as acute occlusion and vasospasm, and restenosis. Complex interactions involving platelet adhesion and aggregation, the coagulation system, the fibrinolytic system, vasospasm and proliferation of vascular elements may all be partly responsible for producing these complications and restenosis. With the removal or damage of endothelial cells, the vessel wall has an increased thrombotic potential due to the loss of the physical separation of the flowing blood from the deeper thrombogenic structures, exposure of the underlying connective tissue, and also the reduction in the endogenous production of antithrombotic substances such as prostacyclin.[102] This results in a rapid deposition of platelets and fibrin.[85,88,89,105,106] Several studies have demonstrated that rapid platelet deposition is one of the earliest responses following balloon angioplasty and may be an important mechanism initiating the complications of acute thrombosis and restenosis.[40,81] The amount of platelet accumulation appears to be directly related to the degree of endothelial denudation and arterial injury.[105,106] In addition to platelet aggregation, endothelial injury may also result in the activation of other cellular elements such as macrophages and smooth muscle cells.[107–109] This process results in the production of growth factors, such as platelet-derived growth factor and chemotaxins, which stimulate the proliferation of smooth muscle cells[107–109] Numerous studies have documented neointimal proliferation of smooth muscle cells following angioplasty.[89,105] In a study of restenosis in pigs, progressive intimal proliferation of smooth muscle cells was demonstrated within 14 days after angioplasty.[105] Smooth muscle cells produce connective tissue matrix[110] and also accumulate lipid, since they contain low density lipoprotein receptors.[111,112] Injury to the arterial wall and platelet accumulation also results in activation of the coagulation system, which may lead to obstructive or nonobstructive thrombus formation.[105,113–115] The presence of fibrocellular organization of previously formed thrombus has been documented in experimental studies.[116]

With denudation of the endothelium and vessel wall injury, the production of vasodilator substances, such as the prostaglandins prostacyclin and PGE_2, may be reduced.[102,117] In addition, platelet activation may result in the release of potent vasoconstrictors, such as thromboxane A_2 and serotonin.[118,119] As a result, vasoconstriction is often associated with balloon angioplasty. Vasoconstriction usually occurs proximal or distal to the angioplasty site.[105,120] It may contribute to acute occlusion or restenosis by altering blood flow and therefore contributing to thrombus formation.[121] In clinical studies, coronary artery vasospasm at the site of angioplasty has been documented and has been shown to correlate with a high incidence of restenosis.[122]

In summary, the vessel wall injury associated with balloon angioplasty results in a series of complex interactions that can lead to acute thrombosis, vasospasm and restenosis. Restenosis is a complicated process that involves platelet adhesion and aggregation, thrombosis, intimal proliferation and atherosclerosis.[123,124] Therefore, the lesion associated with restenosis is composed of fractured atheromatous plaque with superimposed smooth muscle proliferation and intimal hyperplasia of sufficient magnitude to compromise the arterial lumen.[125]

Rationale for prostaglandin use in PTCA

Prostacyclin and PGE_1 are potent inhibitors of platelet aggregation and vasodilators.[66] As discussed earlier in this chapter, platelet deposition and activation play an important role in the processes of thrombosis, vasospasm and restenosis following PTCA. Steele *et al.*[126] demonstrated that prostacyclin and PGE_1 reduced the platelet deposition and microthrombosis that occurred following angioplasty of the carotid arteries in the pig. Cragg *et al.*[117] studied the effects of angioplasty of the carotid artery in the dog. In this model, angioplasty caused significant reductions in vessel wall prostacyclin and PGE_2 production. Angioplasty also caused a significant increase in vessel wall HETE, a vasoconstrictor lipoxygenase product. Peterson *et al.*[127] described marked increases in plasma thromboxane levels in patients whose PTCA procedure was complicated by occlusion. In these patients, the increased thromboxane was not accompanied by an increase in the production of prostacyclin, the physiological antagonist of thromboxane. Therefore, angioplasty may result in the reduction of vascular vasodilator prostaglandin synthesis, while at the same time increasing the synthesis of vasoconstrictor prostaglandins and lipoxygenase products. These changes may result in vasospasm.

Following balloon angioplasty, rapid deposition of platelets on the injured surface of the vessel wall is seen. However, a process of adaptation appears to occur within a matter of hours, resulting in a less thrombogenic vessel wall.[128] This process was demonstrated in a rabbit model of balloon injury. Following arterial balloon injury in this model, immediate platelet deposition occurred in animals receiving no antiplatelet treatment. Treatment with prostacyclin prevented the rapid deposition of platelets. If the prostacyclin infusion was discontinued less than 8 hours following the angioplasty, the deposition of platelets occurred as in the control animals. However, if the prostacyclin infusion was continued for 8 hours and then discontinued, platelet deposition did not occur. Therefore, in this rabbit model of angioplasty, there appeared to be adaptation of the vessel wall resulting in reduction of platelet deposition and reduced thrombogenic potential.

The use of prostacyclin or PGE_1 in patients undergoing PTCA is logical, because the potent antiplatelet effect of these agents may reduce the processes occurring after angioplasty that may lead to acute thrombosis, vasospasm and restenosis. Preclinical studies indicate that a short duration of treatment with prostacyclin or PGE_1 (perhaps as short as 8 hours) may result in clinical benefit.[128]

At the present time, treatment with prostacyclin or PGE_1 requires intravascular administration (intra-arterial or intravenous infusion). Side effects such as nausea, vomiting, flushing and, occasionally, hypotension may occur at relatively low doses and may prevent the administration of a sufficient, potent, antiplatelet dose in many patients. Also, tachyphylaxis may occur in patients receiving continuous infusions of these drugs for more than 24–48 hours.[129]

Results of clinical studies

Few clinical studies evaluating the effects of prostaglandin administration in PTCA patients have been completed. See *et al.*[130] evaluated the effects of PGE_1 in a randomized, double-blind study of 80 patients. All patients received a standard regimen, which included aspirin, dipyridamole, heparin, nitrates and slow-channel blockers. In addition, all patients were given a bolus of PGE_1 (65 ng) into the coronary artery immediately before and after the PTCA procedure. Following PTCA, half of the patients were treated with a 12-hour intravenous (i.v.) infusion of PGE_1 (20 or 40 ng/kg per minute) while the other half received intravenous normal (physiological) saline. Patients were followed clinically for up to 6 months, although routine follow-up angiography was not performed in this study. A review of the study results indicated that the angioplasty was initially successful in 79 of 80 patients. Post-PTCA abrupt occlusion (occlusion at 24 hours or less) occurred in 3 patients in the placebo group (patients who received the intravenous normal saline infusion) and in no patients in the PGE_1 group. Restenosis occurred in 4 patients in the placebo group and in no patients in the PGE_1 group. All 4 cases of restenosis were seen at 5 months or less. The rate of symptomatic restenosis in the placebo group was statistically significantly greater than that in the PGE_1 group ($p < 0.05$). Because follow-up angiography was not completed routinely, asymptomatic restenosis was not assessed. One patient in the PGE_1 group developed hypotension which was promptly relieved with volume replacement and a second patient had peripheral venous inflammation. Nausea occurred in the placebo and PGE_1 group with equal frequency. See *et al.* concluded that the use of PGE_1 in physiological doses post-PTCA was safe and had the beneficial effects of inhibiting coronary spasm and reducing abrupt occlusions and early restenosis following PTCA.

Knudtson *et al.*[131] evaluated the effects of prostacyclin (PGI_2) administration in a single-blind, randomized study of 286 patients undergoing PTCA. Immediately before angioplasty, all patients received a standard regimen of sublingual nifedepine and nitroglycerin, intravenous heparin and intracoronary nitroglycerin. In addition, all patients received nifedipine and isosorbide dinitrate orally for 48 hours after the PTCA. Patients in the prostacyclin group received a 15-minute intracoronary infusion (0.05–7.0 ng/kg per minute) immediately before and after the PTCA procedure. Then, these patients received an intravenous prostacyclin infusion (5.0–8.0 ng/kg per minute) for 48 hours. Patients in the placebo group received an intracoronary infusion of placebo but not an intravenous infusion. Patients received repeat angiography at 6 months post-PTCA, or earlier if dictated by symptoms. The PTCA procedure was initially successful in 270 (134 of 139 prostacyclin and 136 of 147 placebo patients) of the 286 patients. Follow-up angiograms were obtained in 93% of patients in whom angioplasty was successful. Restenosis of one or more lesions was present in 27% and 32% of prostacyclin and placebo patients, respectively. Restenosis was present in 35 of 159 (22%) arteries in the prostacyclin patients and in 45 of 156 (29%) arteries in placebo patients. Neither of these differences was statistically significant. Acute vessel closure was seen in 4 of 134 (3%) patients who received prostacyclin versus 14 of 136 (10%) patients who received placebo ($p < 0.01$). The main cause of acute vessel closure in the majority of patients appeared to be vessel dissection. Ventricular tachycardia or fibrillation was seen in none of 139 (0%) patients who received prostacyclin versus 5 of 147 (3%) patients who received placebo ($p < 0.05$). Myocardial infarction occurred in 1 of 139 (1%) patients who received prostacyclin versus 3 of 147 (2%) patients who received placebo ($p = $ NS). Emergency coronary artery bypass graft surgery was performed in 2 of 139 (1%) patients who received prostacyclin versus 1 of 147 (1%) patients who received placebo. One procedure-related death occurred in a placebo patient. Adverse events of facial flushing, nausea and vomiting were frequently seen in patients receiving prostacyclin. Hypotension occurred in 5% of prostacyclin patients versus 0% of placebo patients; the hypotension always quickly responded to fluid replacement. No significant bleeding complications were noted during the course of the study. Therefore, although the incidence of restenosis was lower in prostacyclin-treated patients than in placebo-treated patients, the difference was not statistically significant. Statistically significant reductions in two clinical endpoints, acute vessel closure and ventricular arrhythmias, were seen in the prostacyclin-treated group.

Gershlick *et al.*[132] evaluated the effects of prosta-cyclin administration in 132 patients undergoing PTCA. Patients received either a 36-hour intra-venous infusion of prostacyclin (4 ng/kg per minute) or placebo following PTCA; 96% of the patients re-ceived post-PTCA angiography at 6 months, or sooner if needed. The overall incidence of restenosis was 31% in the prostacyclin group and 34% in the placebo group. Gershlick *et al.* concluded that pro-stacyclin, given in this dose and regimen, did not beneficially influence the restenosis rate following PTCA.

Demke *et al.*[133] reported the results of a study evaluating the effects of ciprostene (a stable pros-tacyclin analogue) in a multicentre, double-blind, placebo-controlled, randomized study of 659 patients undergoing PTCA. All patients received a standard heparin bolus prior to PTCA. Patients in the ciprostene group received a 15-minute intra-coronary infusion (40 ng/kg per minute) immediately prior to PTCA, followed by a 48-hour intravenous infusion (40–120 ng/kg per minute). Patients in the placebo group received similar infusions of placebo. PTCA was initially successful in 608 of 659 (92%) patients (310 of 333 ciprostene; 298 of 326 placebo). Of 608 patients, 516 (85%) had post-PTCA angio-graphy at 6 months, or sooner if needed. Angio-graphic restenosis was seen in 90 of 266 (34%) ciprostene-treated patients and 111 of 250 (44%) placebo-treated patients. This difference was stat-istically significant ($p=0.01$). In addition, one or more major clinical events (myocardial infarction, death, repeat PTCA to the study vessel, or coronary artery bypass graft surgery to the study vessel) occurred in 75 of 314 (24%) ciprostene-treated patients compared to 115 of 316 (36%) placebo-treated patients ($p=0.001$) during the 6-month study follow-up. A review of each major clinical event re-vealed that myocardial infarction occurred in 7 cipro-stene and 15 placebo patients ($p=0.085$); death occurred in no ciprostene and 5 placebo patients ($p=0.025$); repeat PTCA to the study vessel was performed in 58 ciprostene and 80 placebo patients ($p=0.038$); and coronary artery bypass graft surgery to the study vessel was performed in 17 ciprostene and 34 placebo patients ($p=0.014$). Also, an im-provement in the New York Heart Association Angina classification from class III or IV before PTCA to class I or II 6 months after PTCA was noted in 114 of 297 (38%) ciprostene-treated patients and 82 of 288 (28%) placebo-treated patients ($p=0.011$). In this study, ciprostene-treated patients had a higher incidence of nausea, vomiting and headache than did placebo-treated patients; however, the ciprostene and placebo groups were comparable with respect to all other adverse events, including hypotension and bleeding complications. The conclusion of this study was that angiographic restenosis was significantly less frequent in cipro-stene-treated patients. In addition, ciprostene-treated patients had significantly fewer major clinical events (myocardial infarctions, death, repeat PTCA or coronary artery bypass graft surgery to the study vessel) than did placebo-treated patients. Cipro-stene-treated patients also had a significantly greater improvement in the New York Heart Association Angina classification than did placebo-treated patients.

Discussion of clinical studies

A review of the clinical studies in which prostaglan-dins were evaluated in patients undergoing PTCA leads to the following conclusions. In all studies re-viewed, the restenosis rate was lower in patients receiving the prostaglandin than it was in patients receiving placebo. The difference was sometimes small and not statistically significant, but it was always present. The difference among the studies in how effectively the prostaglandin reduced the rate of restenosis may be due to the fact that different prostaglandins and different dose and regimens were used. Although treatment with prostaglandins may prove beneficial in reducing angiographic restenosis, the effect appears to be relatively small. Clearly, prostaglandin treatment alone does not eliminate the problem of restenosis following PTCA. The maximum dose of prostaglandin that could be admin-istered was limited due to the increased incidence of adverse events at higher doses. Therefore, since platelet activation and aggregation were only par-tially inhibited, this may explain the limited success in reducing restenosis.

The conclusion that prostaglandin treatment may be beneficial in patients undergoing PTCA is sup-ported by the clinical results in these studies. In one or more studies, prostaglandin-treated patients had a lower incidence of acute vessel closure, ventricular tachyarrhythmias, acute myocardial infarction and death. Prostaglandin-treated patients also had a better outcome regarding their clinical angina classi-fication in one study. In addition, prostaglandin-treated patients were less likely to require a repeat procedure (repeat PTCA or coronary artery bypass graft surgery to the study vessel) following PTCA. Therefore, although treatment with prostaglandins is clearly not the total answer to the problem of restenosis following PTCA, there does appear to be clinical benefit from the use of prostaglandins in PTCA patients.

In these four clinical studies, the intracoronary and intravenous infusion of prostaglandins appeared to be safe and well tolerated. The main adverse events to be expected with the use of prostaglandins in this clinical setting appear to be facial flushing, headache, nausea and vomiting. Hypotension may occur infrequently. In these studies, hypotension was not significantly more frequent in prostaglandin-treated patients. When hypotension occurred, it responded quickly to fluid administration. Prostaglandin-treated patients did not have an increased incidence of bleeding complications in these studies.

More clinical studies are needed to answer several questions regarding the use of prostaglandins in patients undergoing PTCA. At present, it is not possible to determine if one prostaglandin is superior to the others for the treatment of PTCA patients. Also, the dose and regimen of prostaglandins that will result in the greatest clinical benefit have yet to be determined. However, based on preclinical information, as well as the results from these clinical studies, it would appear that prostaglandin treatment should be started prior to PTCA.[121] The treatment regimen may employ an intracoronary bolus or a short intracoronary infusion of the prostaglandin, or possibly an intravenous infusion prior to the PTCA. Following this, a treatment regimen that continues prostaglandin therapy following PTCA for a minimum of 24 hours seems reasonable. It has not yet been determined if the intracoronary administration of the prostaglandin before or after the PTCA is necessary to achieve the maximum clinical benefit. It is possible that prostaglandin administration for a shorter period of time (perhaps 8–12 hours) and at a dose equal to or greater than that used in these clinical studies may result in improved clinical results or a better adverse event profile. In addition, studies combining the use of prostaglandins with other types of medications would prove useful to determine if the treatment of PTCA patients with combination drug regimens will result in enhanced reduction of the restenosis rate and an improved clinical outcome. In the future, orally active prostaglandins may become available and result in new therapeutic options such as longer term administration to reduce the rate of restenosis.

Acknowledgement

The author wishes to note the contribution of Cindy L. Shattuck for her secretarial assistance.

References

1. Erlichman M. *Patient selection criteria for percutaneous transluminal coronary angioplasty.* Health Technology Assessment Report, No 11. Rockville MD: US Dept of Health and Human Services, 1985.
2. American College of Physicians: Health and Public Policy Committee. Percutaneous transluminal angioplasty. *Ann Intern Med* 1983; **99** (6): 864–9.
3. Moore TS, Russell WF, Parent AD, *et al.* Percutaneous transluminal angioplasty in subclavian steal syndrome: recurrent stenosis and retreatment in two patients. *Neurosurgery* 1982; **11** (4): 512–17.
4. Pepine CJ, Hill JA, Lambert CR. Therapeutic cardiac catheterization. Part 1. *Modern Concepts Cardiovasc Dis* 1990; **59**: 55–60.
5. Williams DO, Gruentzig A, Kent KM, *et al.* Guidelines for the performance of percutaneous transluminal coronary angioplasty. *Circulation* 1982; **66** (4): 693–4.
6. Parisi AF, Folland ED, Hartigan P. A comparison of angioplasty with medical therapy in the treatment of single-vessel coronary artery disease. *N Engl J Med* 1992; **326** (1): 10–16.
7. Gruentzig A. Recanalization of arterial stenoses with a dilatation catheter. In: Dobbelstein D (ed), *CEPID.* Munich.
8. National Center for Health Care Technology. *Percutaneous transluminal angioplasty for treatment of stenotic lesions of a single coronary artery.* Assessment Report Series, 16. Rockville MD: US Dept of Health and Human Services, 1982: 1–23.
9. Mullin SM, Passamani ER, Mock MB. Historical background of the National Heart, Lung and Blood Institute Registry for Percutaneous Transluminal Coronary Angioplasty. *Am J Cardiol* 1984; **53**: 3c–6c.
10. Gruentzig AR, Senning A, Siegenthaler WE. Nonoperative dilatation of coronary-artery stenosis: percutaneous transluminal coronary angioplasty. *N Engl J Med* 1979; **301**: 61–8.
11. Kent KM, Bentivoglio LG, Block PC, *et al.* Percutaneous transluminal coronary angioplasty: report from the registry of the National Heart, Lung, and Blood Institute. *Am J Cardiol* 1982; **49**: 2011–20.
12. Vlietstra RE, Holmes DR Jr, Smith HC, *et al.* Percutaneous transluminal coronary angioplasty: initial Mayo Clinic experience. *Mayo Clin Proc* 1981; **56**: 287–93.
13. Roubin GS, Gruentzig AR. Coronary angioplasty: changing indications. *Prim Cardiol* 1985; **11**: 59–69.

14. Gruentzig AR, Meier B. Current status of dilatation catheters and guiding systems. *Am J Cardiol* 1984; **53**: 92C–93C.

15. Anderson HV, Roubin GS, Leimgruber PP, *et al.* Primary angiographic success rates of percutaneous transluminal coronary angioplasty. *Am J Cardiol* 1985; **56** (12): 712–17.

16. Meier B, Gruentzig A, King SB, *et al.* Higher balloon dilatation pressure in coronary angioplasty. *Am Heart J* 1984; **4**: 619–22.

17. Vlietstra RE, Holmes DR Jr, Reeder GS, *et al.* Balloon angioplasty in multivessel coronary artery disease. *Mayo Clin Proc* 1983; **58**: 563–7.

18. Vandormael MG, Chaitman BR, Ischinger T, *et al.* Immediate and short-term benefit of multilesion coronary angioplasty: influence of degree of revascularization. *J Am Coll Cardiol* 1985; **6**: 983–91.

19. Cowley MJ, Vetrovec GW, DiSciascio G, *et al.* Coronary angioplasty of multiple vessels: short-term outcome and long-term results. *Circulation* 1985; **72**: 1314–20.

20. Hartzler GO. Complex coronary angioplasty: an alternative therapy. *Int J Cardiol* 1985; **9**: 133–7.

21. Jones EL, Douglas JS, Gruentzig AR, *et al.* Percutaneous saphenous vein angioplasty to avoid reoperative bypass surgery. *Ann Thorac Surg* 1983; **36**: 389–95.

22. Dorros G, Johnson WD, Tector AJ, *et al.* Percutaneous transluminal coronary angioplasty in patients with prior coronary artery bypass grafting. *J Thorac Cardiovasc Surg* 1984; **87**: 17–26.

23. Kussmaul WG III. Percutaneous angioplasty of coronary bypass grafts: an emerging consensus. *Cathet Cardiovasc Diagn* 1988; **15**: 1–4.

24. Dangoisse V, Vap PG, David PR, *et al.* Recurrence of stenosis after successful percutaneous transluminal coronary angioplasty (PTCA). *Circulation* 1982; **68**: II-331.

25. Whitworth HB, Pilcher GS, Roubin GS, *et al.* Do proximal lesions involving the origin of the left anterior descending artery (LAD) have a higher restenosis rate after coronary angioplasty (PTCA)? *Circulation* 1985; **72**: III-398.

26. Holmes DR Jr, Vlietstra RE. Percutaneous transluminal coronary angioplasty: current status and future trends. *Mayo Clin Proc* 1986; **61**: 865–76.

27. Holmes DR Jr, Vlietstra RE, Reeder GS, *et al.* Angioplasty in total coronary artery occlusion. *J Am Coll Cardiol* 1984; **3**: 845–9.

28. Holmes DR Jr, Vlietstra RE. Angioplasty in total coronary arterial occlusion. *Herz* 1985; **10**: 292–7.

29. Holmes DR Jr, Smith HC, Vlietstra RE, *et al.* Percutaneous transluminal coronary angioplasty, alone or in combination with streptokinase therapy, during acute myocardial infarction. *Mayo Clin Proc* 1985; **60**: 449–56.

30. Papapietro SE, MacLean WAH, Stanley AWH Jr, *et al.* Percutaneous transluminal coronary angioplasty after intracoronary streptokinase in evolving acute myocardial infarction. *Am J Cardiol* 1985; **55**: 48–53.

31. O'Neill W, Timmis GC, Bourdillon PD, *et al.* A prospective randomized clinical trial of intracoronary streptokinase versus coronary angioplasty for acute myocardial infarction. *N Engl J Med* 1986; **314**: 812–18.

32. Hartzler GO, Rutherford BD, McConahay DR, *et al.* Percutaneous transluminal coronary angioplasty with and without thrombolytic therapy for treatment of acute myocardial infarction. *Am Heart J* 1983; **106**: 965–73.

33. Detre K, Holubkov R, Kelsey S, *et al.* Percutaneous transluminal coronary angioplasty in 1985–1986 and 1977–1981. The National Heart, Lung, and Blood Institute Registry. *N Engl J Med* 1988; **318**: 265–70.

34. Baim DS, Faxon DP. Coronary angioplasty. In: Grossman W (ed), *Cardiac Catheterization and Angiography*. Philadelphia: Lea & Febiger, 1986: 473–92.

35. Holmes DR Jr, Vlietstra RE, Smith HC, *et al.* Restenosis after percutaneous transluminal coronary angioplasty (PTCA): a report from the PTCA Registry of the National Heart, Lung, and Blood Institute. *Am J Cardiol* 1984; **53**: 77C–81C.

36. Levine S, Ewels CJ, Rosing DR, *et al.* Coronary angioplasty: clinical and angiographic follow-up. *Am J Cardiol* 1985; **55**: 673–6.

37. Leimgruber PP, Roubin GS, Hollman J, *et al.* Restenosis after successful coronary angioplasty in patients with single-vessel disease. *Circulation* 1986; **73**: 710–17.

38. Ernst SMPG, van der Feltz TA, Bal ET, *et al.* Long term angiographic follow up, cardiac events, and survival in patients undergoing percutaneous transluminal coronary angioplasty. *Br Heart J* 1987; **57**: 220–5.

39. Guiteras Val P, Bourassa MG, David PR, *et al.* Restenosis after successful percutaneous transluminal coronary angioplasty: the Montreal Heart Institute experience. *Am J Cardiol* 1987; **60**: 50B–55B.

40. Faxon DP, Sanborn TA, Haudenschild CC. Mechanism of angioplasty and its relation to restenosis. *Am J Cardiol* 1987; **60**: 5B–9B.

41. Joelson JM, Most AS, William DO. Angiographic findings when chest pain recurs after successful percutaneous transluminal coronary angioplasty. *Am J Cardiol* 1987; **60**: 792–5.

42. Myler RK, Topol EJ, Shaw RE, *et al.* Multiple vessel coronary angioplasty: classification, results, and patterns of restenosis in 494 consecutive patients. *Cathet Cardiovasc Diagn* 1987; **13**: 1–15.

43. Hirshfeld JW Jr, MacDonald R, Goldberg S, *et al.* Patient-related variables predictive of restenosis after PTCA – a report from the M-HEART Study. *Circulation* 1987; **76**: IV-214.

44. Meyer J, Schmitz HJ, Kiesslich T, *et al*. Percutaneous transluminal coronary angioplasty in patients with stable and unstable angina pectoris; analysis of early and late results. *Am Heart J* 1983; **106**: 973–80.

45. Rupprecht HJ, Brennecke R, Erbel R, *et al*. Early and long-term outcome after PTCA in stable versus unstable angina. *J Am Coll Cardiol* 1987; **9**: 150A.

46. Leisch F, Schutzenberger W, Kerschner K, *et al*. Influence of a variant angina on the results of percutaneous transluminal coronary angioplasty. *Br Heart J* 1986; **56**: 341–5.

47. Vandormael MG, Deligonul U, Kern MJ, *et al*. Multilesion coronary angioplasty: clinical and angiographic follow-up. *J Am Coll Cardiol* 1987; **10**: 246–52.

48. Shaw RE, Myler RK, Fishman-Rosen J, *et al*. Clinical and morphologic factors in prediction of restenosis after multiple vessel angioplasty. *J Am Coll Cardiol* 1986; **7**: 63A.

49. Hamm C, Kupper W, Thier W, *et al*. Factors predicting recurrent stenosis in patients with successful coronary angioplasty. *J Am Coll Cardiol* 1985; **5**: 518.

50. Galan KM, Deligonul U, Kern MJ, *et al*. Increased frequency of restenosis in patients continuing to smoke cigarettes after percutaneous transluminal coronary angioplasty. *Am J Cardiol* 1988; **61**: 260–3.

51. Libow MA, Leimgruber PP, Roubin GS, *et al*. Restenosis after angioplasty (PTCA) in chronic total coronary artery occlusion. *J Am Coll Cardiol* 1985; **5**: 445.

52. Holmes DR Jr, Vlietstra RE, Reeder GS, *et al*. Balloon angioplasty for total coronary occlusion not associated with evolving myocardial infarction. *J Am Coll Cardiol* 1986; **7**: 211A.

53. Wexman MP, Murphy MC, Fishman-Rosen J, *et al*. Factors predicting recurrence in patients who have had angioplasty (PTCA) of totally occluded vessels. *J Am Coll Cardiol* 1986; **7**: 20A.

54. Mata LA, Bosch X, David PR, *et al*. Clinical and angiographic assessment 6 months after double vessel percutaneous coronary angioplasty. *J Am Coll Cardiol* 1985; **6**: 1239–44.

55. DiSciascio G, Cowley MJ, Vetrovec GW. Angiographic patterns of restenosis after angioplasty to multiple coronary arteries. *Am J Cardiol* 1986; **58**: 922–5.

56. Hollman J, Galan K, Franci I, *et al*. Recurrent stenosis after coronary angioplasty. *J Am Coll Cardiol* 1986; **7**: 20A.

57. Roubin GS, King SB III, Douglas JS Jr. Restenosis after percutaneous transluminal coronary angioplasty: the Emory University Hospital experience. *Am J Cardiol* 1987; **60(B)**: 39–43.

58. Uebis R, von Essen R, vom Dahl J, *et al*. Recurrence rate after PTCA in relationship to the initial length

of coronary artery narrowing. *J Am Coll Cardiol* 1986; **7**: 62A.

59. Hall DP, Gruentzig AR. Influence of lesion length on initial success and recurrence rates in coronary angioplasty. *Circulation* 1984; **70**: II-176.

60. Hodgson JM, Reinert S, Most AS, *et al*. Prediction of long-term clinical outcome with final translesional pressure gradient during coronary angioplasty. *Circulation* 1986; **74**: 563–6.

61. Leimgruber PP, Roubin GS, Anderson V, *et al*. Influence of intimal dissection on restenosis after successful coronary angioplasty. *Circulation* 1985; **72**: 530–5.

62. Hirshfeld JW Jr, Goldberg S, MacDonald R, *et al*. Lesion and procedure-related variables predictive of restenosis after PTCA – a report from the M-HEART study. *Circulation* 1987; **76**: IV-215.

63. White CW, Chaitman B, Lasar TA, *et al*. Antiplatelet agents are effective in reducing the immediate complications of PTCA: results from the Ticlopidine Multicenter Trial. *Circulation* 1987; **76**: IV-400.

64. Barnathan ES, Schwartz JS, Taylor L, *et al*. Aspirin and dipyridamole in the prevention of acute coronary thrombosis complicating coronary angioplasty. *Circulation* 1987; **76**: 125–34.

65. Schwartz L, Bourassa MG, Lesperance J, *et al*. Aspirin and dipyridamole in the prevention of restenosis after percutaneous transluminal coronary angioplasty. *N Engl J Med* 1988; **318**: 1714–19.

66. Barnathan ES, Hirshfeld JW Jr. Adjunctive pharmacologic treatment. In: Goldberg S (ed), *Coronary Angioplasty*. Philadelphia: FA Davis, 1988: 41–78.

67. White CW, Knudtson M, Schmidt D, *et al*. Neither ticlopidine nor aspirin-dipyridamole prevents restenosis post PTCA: results from a randomized placebo-controlled multicenter trial. *Circulation* 1987; **76**: IV-213.

68. Swanson KT, Vlietstra RE, Holmes DR Jr, *et al*. Efficacy of adjunctive dextran during percutaneous transluminal coronary angioplasty. *Am J Cardiol* 1984; **54**: 447–8.

69. Faxon DP, Sandborn TA, Haudenschild CC, *et al*. The effect of nifedipine on restenosis following experimental angioplasty. *Circulation* 1984; **70**: II-175.

70. Whitworth HB, Roubin GS, Hollman J, *et al*. Effect of nifedipine on recurrent stenosis after percutaneous transluminal coronary angioplasty. *J Am Coll Cardiol* 1986; **8**: 1271–6.

71. Corcos T, David PR, Guiteras Val P, *et al*. Failure of diltiazem to prevent restenosis after percutaneous transluminal coronary angioplasty. *Am Heart J* 1985; **109**: 926–31.

72. Thornton MA, Gruentzig AR, Hollman J, *et al*. Coumadin and aspirin in prevention of recurrence after transluminal coronary angioplasty: a randomized study. *Circulation* 1984; **69**: 721–7.

73. Hartzler GO, Rutherford BD, McConahay DR, *et al*.

High-dose steroids for prevention of recurrent restenosis post-PTCA: a randomized trial. *J Am Coll Cardiol* 1987; **9:** 185A.

74. Pepine CJ, Hirshfeld JW, Macdonald RG, *et al.* A controlled trial of corticosteroids to prevent restenosis following coronary angioplasty. *Circulation* 1988; **78:** II-291.

75. Grigg LE, Kay TWH, Valentine PA, *et al.* Determinants of restenosis and lack of effect of dietary supplementation with eicosapentaenoic acid on the incidence of coronary artery restenosis after angioplasty. *J Am Coll Cardiol* 1989; **13:** 665–72.

76. Reis GJ, Sipperly ME, Boucher TM, *et al.* Results of a randomized, double-blind placebo-controlled trial of fish oil for prevention of restenosis after PTCA. *Circulation* 1988; **78:** II-291.

77. Klein W, Eber B, Fluch N, *et al.* Ketanserin prevents acute occlusion but not restenosis after PTCA. *J Am Coll Cardiol* 1989; **13** (2): 44A.

78. Pepine CJ, Hill JA, Lambert CR. Therapeutic cardiac catheterization. Part 2. *Mod Concepts Cardiovasc Dis* 1990; **59** (11): 61–6.

79. Jaffe E. Physiologic functions of normal endothelial cells. *Ann NY Acad Sci* 1985; **454:** 279.

80. Simionescu M, Simionescu N. Functions of the endothelial cell surface. *Annu Rev Physiol* 1986; **48:** 279.

81. Harker LA. Role of platelets and thrombosis in mechanisms of acute occlusion and restenosis after angioplasty. *Am J Cardiol* 1987; **60:** 20B–28B.

82. Harker LA, Schwartz SM, Ross R. Endothelium and arteriosclerosis. *Clin Haematol* 1981; **10:** 283–96.

83. Castellot JJ, Addonizio ML, Rosenbery R, *et al.* Cultured endothelial cells produce a heparin-like inhibitor of smooth muscle cell growth. *J Cell Biol* 1981; **90:** 372.

84. Levin EG, Loskutoff DJ. Cultured bovine endothelial cells produce both urokinase and tissue-type plasminogen activators. *J Cell Biol* 1982; **94:** 631.

85. Erikson LA, Ginsbergy MH, Loskutoff DJ. Detection and partial characterization of an inhibitor of plasminogen activator in human platelets. *J Clin Invest* 1984; **74:** 1465.

86. McBride W, Lange RA, Hillis LD. Restenosis after successful coronary angioplasty. *N Engl J Med* 1988; **318** (26): 1734–7.

87. Block PC, Baughman KL, Pasternak RC, *et al.* Transluminal angioplasty: correlation of morphologic and angiographic findings in an experimental model. *Circulation* 1980; **61:** 778–85.

88. Pasternak RC, Baughman KL, Fallon JT, *et al.* Scanning electron microscopy after coronary transluminal angioplasty of normal canine coronary arteries. *Am J Cardiol* 1980; **45:** 591–8.

89. Zollikofer CL, Salomonowitz E, Sibley R, *et al.* Transluminal angioplasty evaluated by electron microscopy. *Radiology* 1984; **153:** 369–74.

90. Castaneda-Zuniga WR, Formanek A, Tadavarthy M,

91. Faxon DP, Weber VJ, Haudenschild C, *et al.* Acute effects of transluminal angioplasty in three experimental models of atherosclerosis. *Arteriosclerosis* 1982; **2:** 125–33.

92. Sanborn TA, Faxon DP, Haudenschild C, *et al.* The mechanism of transluminal angioplasty: evidence for formation of aneurysms in experimental atherosclerosis. *Circulation* 1983; **68:** 1136–40.

93. Lyon RT, Zarins CK, Lu C-T, *et al.* Vessel plaque, and lumen morphology after transluminal balloon angioplasty; quantitative study in distended human arteries. *Arteriosclerosis* 1987; **7:** 306–14.

94. Kohchi K, Takebayashi S, Block PC, *et al.* Arterial changes after percutaneous transluminal coronary angioplasty: results at autopsy. *J Am Coll Cardiol* 1987; **10:** 592–9.

95. Soward AL, Essed CE, Serruys PW. Coronary artery findings after accidental death immediately after successful percutaneous transluminal coronary angioplasty. *Am J Cardiol* 1985; **56:** 794–5.

96. Sanborn TA, Faxon DP, Waugh D, *et al.* Transluminal angioplasty in experimental atherosclerosis. Analysis for embolization using an *in vivo* perfusion system. *Circulation* 1982; **66:** 917–22.

97. Block PC, Myler RK, Stertzer S, *et al.* Morphology after transluminal angioplasty in human beings. *N Engl J Med* 1981; **305:** 382–5.

98. Block PC. Mechanism of transluminal angioplasty. *Am J Cardiol* 1984; **53:** 69C–71C.

99. Laerum F, Castaneda-Zuniga WR, Rysavy J, *et al.* The site of arterial wall rupture in transluminal angioplasty: an experimental study. *Radiology* 1982; **144:** 769–70.

100. Zarins CK, Lu CT, Gewertz BL, *et al.* Arterial disruption and remodeling following balloon dilatation. *Surgery* 1982; **92:** 1086–95.

101. Holmes DR Jr, Vlietstra RE, Mock MB, *et al.* Angiographic changes produced by percutaneous transluminal coronary angioplasty. *Am J Cardiol* 1983; **51:** 676–83.

102. Chesebro JH, Lam JYT, Badimon L, *et al.* Restenosis after arterial angioplasty: a hemorrheologic response to injury. *Am J Cardiol* 1987; **60:** 10B–16B.

103. Baughman KL, Pasternak RC, Fallon JT, *et al.* Transluminal coronary angioplasty of postmortem human hearts. *Am J Cardiol* 1981; **48:** 1044–7.

104. Sanborn TA, Faxon DP, Haudenschild CC, *et al.* The mechanism of transluminal angioplasty: evidence for aneurysm formation in experimental atherosclerosis. *Circulation* 1983; **68:** 1136–40.

105. Steele PM, Chesebro JH, Stanson AW, *et al.* Balloon angioplasty; natural history of the pathophysiological response to injury in a pig model. *Circ Res* 1985; **57:** 105–12.

106. Wilentz JR, Sanborn TA, Haudenschild CC, *et al.* Platelet accumulation in experimental angioplasty:

time course and relation to vascular injury. *Circulation* 1987; **75**: 636–42.

107. Ross R, Glomset JA. The pathogenesis of atherosclerosis. *N Engl J Med* 1976; **295**: 369–77.

108. Ross R, Glomset JA. The pathogenesis of atherosclerosis. *N Engl J Med* 1976; **295**: 420–5.

109. Ross R. The pathogenesis of atherosclerosis – an update. *N Engl J Med* 1986; **314**: 488–500.

110. Burke JM, Ross R. Synthesis of connective tissue macromolecules by smooth muscle. In: Hall DA (ed), *International Review of Connective Tissue Research*, vol 8. New York: Academic Press, 1979: 119–57.

111. Chait A, Ross R, Alberg J, *et al.* Platelet-derived growth factor stimulates activity of low density lipoprotein receptors. *Proc Natl Acad Sci USA* 1980; **77**: 4084–8.

112. Witte LD, Cornicelli JA. Platelet-derived growth factor stimulates low density lipoprotein receptor activity in cultured human fibroblasts. *Proc Natl Acad Sci USA* 1980; **77**: 5962–6.

113. Mustard JF. The role of platelets and thrombosis in the development of atherosclerosis and its complications. *Ann R Coll Surg Can* 1981; **14**: 22–8.

114. Ischinger T, Zack P, Aker U. Acute coronary occlusion during balloon angioplasty due to intracoronary thrombus and coronary spasm: a reversible complication. *Am Heart J* 1984; **107**: 1271.

115. MacDonald RG, Feldman RL, Conti CR, *et al.* Thromboembolic complications of coronary angioplasty. *Am J Cardiol* 1984; **54**: 916.

116. Faxon DP, Sanborn TA, Weber VJ, *et al.* Restenosis following transluminal angioplasty in experimental atherosclerosis. *Arteriosclerosis* 1984; **4**: 189–95.

117. Cragg A, Einzig S, Castaneda-Zuniga W, *et al.* Vessel wall arachidonate metabolism after angioplasty: possible mediators of postangioplasty vasospasm. *Am J Cardiol* 1983; **51**: 1441–5.

118. Lam JYT, Chesebro JH, Badimon L, *et al.* The vasoconstrictive response following arterial angioplasty in pigs: evidence for vasoconstriction resulting from rather than causing platelet-deposition. *J Am Coll Cardiol* 1986; **7**: 12A.

119. Berk BC, Alexander RW, Brock TA, *et al.* Vasoconstriction: a new activity for platelet-derived growth factor. *Science* 1986; **232**: 87–90.

120. Lam JYT, Chesebro JH, Steele PM, *et al.* Is vasospasm related to platelet deposition? *In vivo* relationship in a pig model of arterial injury. *Circulation* 1987; **75**: 243–8.

121. Cox JL, Gotlieb AI. Restenosis following percutaneous transluminal angioplasty: clinical, physiologic and pathological features. *Can Med Ass J* 1986; **134**: 1129–32.

122. Bertrand ME, Lablanche JM, Fourrier JL, *et al.* Relation to restenosis after percutaneous transluminal coronary angioplasty to vasomotion of the dilated coronary arterial segment. *Am J Cardiol* 1989; **63**: 277–81.

123. Chesebro JH, Lam JYT, Fuster V. The pathogenesis and prevention of aortocoronary vein bypass graft occlusion and restenosis after arterial angioplasty: role of vascular injury and platelet thrombus deposition. *J Am Coll Cardiol* 1986; **8**: 57B–66B.

124. Weintraub WS. Design considerations in the study of restenosis after percutaneous transluminal coronary angioplasty. *Am J Cardiol* 1987; **60**: 3B–4B.

125. Fanelli C, Aronoff R. Restenosis following coronary angioplasty. *Am Heart J* 1990; **119** (2): 357–68.

126. Steele PM, Chesebro JH, Lamb HB, *et al.* Balloon angioplasty in pigs: effect of platelet-inhibitor drugs. *Circulation* 1983; **68**: III-264.

127. Peterson MB, Machaj V, Block PC, *et al.* Thromboxane release during percutaneous transluminal coronary angioplasty. *Am Heart J* 1986; **111** (1): 1–6.

128. Groves HM, Kinlough-Rothbone RL, Mustard JF. Development of nonthrombogenicity of injured rabbit artery despite inhibition of platelet adherence. *Arteriosclerosis* 1986; **6**: 189.

129. Sinzinger H, Silberbauer K, Horsch AK, *et al.* Decreased sensitivity of human platelets to PGI_2 during long-term intraarterial prostacyclin infusion in patients with peripheral vascular disease: a rebound phenomenon? *Prostaglandins* 1981; **21**: 49.

130. See J, Shell W, Matthews O, *et al.* Prostaglandin E_1 infusion after angioplasty in human inhibits abrupt occlusion and early restenosis. In: Samuelson B, Paoletti R, Ramwell PW (eds), *Advances in Prostaglandin, Thromboxane, and Leukotriene Research*. New York: Raven Press, 1987: 266–70.

131. Knudtson ML, Flintoft VF, Roth DL, *et al.* Effect of short-term prostacyclin administration on restenosis after percutaneous transluminal coronary angioplasty. *J Am Coll Cardiol* 1990; **15** (3): 691–7.

132. Gershlick AH, Timmis AD, Rothman MT, *et al.* Post angioplasty prostacyclin infusion does not reduce the incidence of restenosis. *Circulation* 1990; **82** (4): III-497.

133. Demke DM, for the Ciprostene Study Group. Double-blind, placebo-controlled efficacy study of ciprostene (U-61,431F) in percutaneous transluminal coronary angioplasty (PTCA). *Br J Haematol* 1990; **76** (1): 20.

13 Prostaglandins in congestive heart failure

Christy L Cooper, James W Crow, William S Wheeler and Walker A Long

Congestive heart failure

Congestive heart failure (CHF) is a clinical syndrome characterized by dyspnoea, fatigue, oedema and reduced survival. The prognosis for patients diagnosed with CHF is grave, with fewer than half of the patients surviving 5 years after diagnosis.[1] The survival of patients symptomatic at rest (New York Heart Association (NYHA) class IV) is extremely poor; mortality is at least 40% at 1 year.[2,3]

This clinical syndrome currently affects an estimated 3.5–4 million people in the USA, an estimated 2 million patients in Japan and 3.8 million in the four major Western European countries.[4] CHF is currently the most common 'hospital discharge diagnosis' (the eventual diagnosis when patient is discharged from hospital) in the USA and Europe in patients over 65 years of age. Approximately 400 000 new cases and 900 000 hospitalizations are reported each year in the USA alone.[5] Results from the Framingham Study, an epidemiological study with an average of 34 years of patient follow-up, indicate that the incidence of CHF increases with age: 0.2% of the population aged 45–54 years and

4.0% in people aged 85–94 years have been diagnosed each year with CHF.[6] The ageing of society in most developed countries in the world will probably result in larger numbers of patients diagnosed with CHF in the future.

Pathophysiology of CHF

The primary event in the development of CHF is myocardial dysfunction leading to inadequate cardiac output to meet the metabolic demands of the body. Reductions in cardiac output result in activation of compensatory mechanisms that attempt to maintain adequate tissue perfusion. Compensatory mechanisms activated in CHF include: the autonomic nervous system, renin–angiotensin system, arginine vasopressin system, atrial natriuretic factor system and the arachidonic acid metabolism pathway.[7,8] In mild CHF, these compensatory mechanisms are often able to maintain adequate tissue perfusion. However, as myocardial function deteriorates, these mechanisms can become counterproductive and can compromise myocardial function further by (1) increasing the workload of the heart and (2) directly affecting the myocardium. Many of the signs and symptoms associated with CHF are a result of both reduced cardiac output and activation of these compensatory mechanisms.[9,10]

Cardiac function is determined by contractility, preload and afterload. CHF is a syndrome characterized by reduced contractility of cardiac muscle as well as increased preload and afterload, as discussed below.

Contractility is the intrinsic ability of the myocardium to contract and is independent of both preload and afterload. *Preload* is the stretch to which the myofibrils are subjected prior to contraction, and is related to end-diastolic volume/pressure. When preload is low, myofibrils are not optimally stretched, and, as a result, strength of contraction is reduced. As preload increases, myofibril stretch is optimized and contractile strength and cardiac output are increased (Frank–Starling relationship). As the myocardium fails, peripheral compensatory mechanisms increase preload by retaining sodium and increasing intravascular volume.

Cardiac function is also determined by *afterload*, which is the resistance that the myocardium must overcome in order to contract. Systemic vascular resistance and wall stress contribute to afterload. Wall stress, expressed as stress per unit volume of myocardial wall, is increased as the ventricle dilates and can be decreased to some extent by ventricular wall thickening (ventricular hypertrophy). The normal ventricle is relatively resistant to changes in afterload. However, in patients with CHF, ventricular function becomes increasingly sensitive to small changes in afterload, further decreasing cardiac output.

In addition to the compensatory mechanisms described above, ventricular remodelling occurs in patients with severe long-standing CHF, and results in regional and global changes in the left ventricle. In addition to cardiac muscle hypertrophy, diseased ventricles dilate, due in part to changes in both the myocytes and connective tissue. Dilatation and fibrosis result in impairment of ventricular function. Although various cellular mechanisms have been proposed (myocyte necrosis, myocyte stretch and rearrangement, hypertrophy or atrophy of muscle fibres), the precise mechanisms involved in ventricular remodelling are unclear.

Classically, CHF was considered to result from systolic (contractile) dysfunction alone. However, increasing evidence reveals that ventricular dysfunction is usually related to both systolic and diastolic dysfunction. Approximately one-third of elderly patients with CHF have predominantly diastolic dysfunction that is characterized by reduced ventricular distensibility. Hypertension is the most common cause of predominantly diastolic dysfunction.[11] Coronary artery disease and idiopathic dilated cardiomyopathy are the most common causes of predominantly systolic dysfunction. Although the clinical symptoms of CHF (dyspnoea, fatigue and oedema) are similar in patients with systolic or diastolic dysfunction, the treatment varies according to the type of dysfunction that predominates.

Management of CHF

The therapeutic goals for the treatment of CHF are to improve symptoms, quality of life, exercise capacity and survival. Several different pharmacological approaches are used in the management of patients with CHF, as described below.

Positive inotropic agents

Positive inotropic agents are logical choices when CHF is characterized by systolic dysfunction and reduced contractility. Digitalis glycosides have been used for well over 200 years for the treatment and management of CHF. These agents clearly improve ventricular function by increasing cardiac contractility. In addition, digitalis glycosides have been shown to partially restore the blunted arterial baroreceptor sensitivity that is common in CHF. Improved sensitivity of the baroreceptors results in tonic inhibition of the excess sympathetic stimulation that occurs in CHF.[12]

Despite the widespread use of the digitalis glycosides in the treatment of CHF, the efficacy of these agents in patients without atrial fibrillation has been a source of major controversy for decades.[13] However, recent data obtained from large placebo-controlled trials have demonstrated that digoxin, when compared to placebo, is well tolerated and significantly improves the signs and symptoms of CHF, enhances exercise capacity, reduces the frequency of hospitalization and reduces the need for co-intervention in patients with sinus rhythm who were not receiving angiotensin-converting enzyme (ACE) inhibitors.[14–18] In another recently reported trial, these beneficial effects of digoxin were also demonstrated in patients who were receiving ACE inhibitors.[17] The effects of digoxin on survival are unknown but are currently being investigated in a large multicentre study sponsored by the National Heart, Lung, and Blood Institute (Bethesda, Maryland, USA).[19]

Non-glycoside-positive inotropic agents such as the phosphodiesterase (PDE) inhibitors have also been evaluated in patients with CHF. These agents increase intracellular cyclic AMP, and have been associated with increased cardiac output and improved exercise capacity in patients with CHF. Unfortunately, the use of these agents has been associated with an increased frequency of arrhythmias and sudden death when given to patients with severe CHF.[19,20] In a single large multicentre trial (PROMISE), the incidence of sudden death appeared to increase by approximately twofold in NYHA (New York Heart Association) class III/IV patients treated with the PDE inhibitor, milrinone.[21]

β-Adrenergic receptor agonists (e.g. dobutamine) have also been used as inotropic support in the treatment of patients with CHF. Though available only as an intravenous agent, dobutamine is frequently used and has been associated with improvements in symptoms and exercise capacity when administered intermittently or continuously to patients with severe CHF.[22] However, the use of intermittent outpatient dobutamine has been associated with an increase in the frequency of sudden death in patients with CHF. As a result, dobutamine is usually reserved for the treatment of patients with end-stage disease.[23]

Vasodilators

In general, vasodilators decrease the workload of the heart by reducing preload and/or afterload. Vasodilators used in the treatment of patients with CHF are either (1) direct-acting or (2) indirect-acting. Direct-acting vasodilators reduce preload by dilating venous capacitance vessels (e.g. isosorbide dinitrate), afterload by dilating arterioles (e.g. hydralazine) or both (sodium nitroprusside, prazosin).

V-HeFT I, a multicentre Veterans Administration Cooperative Study conducted in the USA, evaluated the effects of direct-acting vasodilators (prazosin and the combination of isosorbide dinitrate plus hydralazine) on exercise capacity and survival in 642 men with NYHA class II/III CHF. Patients who received a combination regimen (isosorbide dinitrate plus hydralazine) for 2 years demonstrated improved symptoms of CHF compared to patients who received placebo. Survival over 2 years appeared to be improved in patients who received the combination regimen compared to patients who received only placebo ($p<0.028$).[24] However, the mortality difference

over the entire follow-up period (range of 6 months to 5.7 years) was not statistically significant ($p=0.093$). In contrast, prazosin failed to improve survival when compared to placebo at any time point.

Indirect-acting vasodilators act by inhibiting vasoconstrictor systems activated in patients with CHF. The most widely used indirect-acting vasodilators are the angiotensin-converting enzyme (ACE) inhibitors that inhibit the formation of angiotensin II, a very potent vasoconstrictor. Captopril and enalapril are the most commonly used ACE inhibitors in the treatment of CHF.

Several small clinical trials have demonstrated improved haemodynamics in patients who received chronic treatment with ACE inhibitor therapy for several months to 1 year. Three large clinical trials have evaluated the effects of enalapril on survival, exercise capacity and/or symptoms of CHF. One of these large, multicentre trials, CONSENSUS, was conducted in Scandinavia, and involved 253 patients with NYHA class IV CHF. Patients entered the trial sequentially and received either enalapril or placebo for up to 1 year.[25] All patients received conventional therapy composed of diuretics, digitalis glycosides and/or direct-acting vasodilators. Survival over the 1-year observation period was significantly improved ($p=0.001$) in patients treated with enalapril compared to patients treated with placebo.

A second Veterans Administration trial (V-HeFT II) was conducted in the USA in 804 patients with predominantly NYHA class II/III CHF. Patients received diuretics, digitalis glycosides, and either enalapril or the combination of isosorbide dinitrate plus hydralazine for up to 2 years.[26] Survival over 2 years was significantly improved ($p=0.016$) in patients who received enalapril compared to those who received the combination of hydralazine plus isosorbide dinitrate.

Enalapril has also been shown to improve survival in a third large multicentre trial – Studies of Left Ventricular Dysfunction (SOLVD). In this multinational study, 2569 predominantly NYHA class II/III patients were randomized to receive either enalapril or placebo for an average follow-up time of 41 months. Background therapy consisted of digitalis glycosides, diuretics, and other vasodilators as needed. Survival was significantly improved ($p=0.0036$) in these patients with class II/III CHF who received enalapril compared to those who received placebo. The effects of enalapril on the combined endpoint of death and/or hospitalization was also evaluated. Over all, significantly more patients who received placebo died or were hospitalized than

Table 13.1   Summary of survival trials in CHF

| Study name | Treatment | Patients | | Mortality | | | |
		Number	NYHA class (predominant)	Over	Control	Active Tx	p-*value*
V-HeFT I	Iso + Hyd versus Prz versus placebo	642	II/III	2 years	34.3% (placebo or Prz)	25.6%	0.028
CONSENSUS	Enl versus placebo	253	IV	1 year	52% (placebo)	36% (Enl)	0.001
V-HeFT II	Iso + Hyd versus Enl	804	II/III	2 years	25% (Iso + Hyd)	18% (Enl)	0.016
SOLVD	Enl versus placebo	2569	II/III	3 years	41% (placebo)	35% (Enl)	0.0036

Enl, enalapril; Hyd, hydralazine; Iso, isosorbide dinitrate; Prz, prazosin.

patients who received enalapril (p=0.001).[27] Results from these three large multicentre trials are summarized in Table 13.1.

In addition to the high mortality associated with CHF, quality of life is severely restricted, especially in patients with advanced disease. In numerous small clinical trials conducted in the USA and Europe, exercise capacity and signs and symptoms associated with CHF were improved in patients who received direct- and/or indirect-acting vasodilators.[28] In CONSENSUS, symptoms of CHF were improved more frequently, as reflected in improved NYHA classification, in patients who received enalapril than in those who received placebo (p=0.001). In V-HeFT II, exercise capacity was improved in patients who received enalapril and in patients who received the combination of isosorbide dinitrate plus hydralazine.[26]

Enalapril has also been shown to reduce heart size in patients with class IV CHF[25] and to inhibit ventricular remodelling (as measured by left ventricular dilatation) that occurs after anterior myocardial infarction.[29] This latter effect of enalapril involved not only limiting expansion at the site of infarction but also dilatation in the normal area of the ventricle.[29]

Diuretics

Diuretics are commonly used in the management of patients with CHF. These agents successfully control renal salt and water retention. Because certain diuretics deplete potassium and magnesium, they may aggravate arrhythmias that commonly occur in patients with CHF.

Cardiac transplantation: the final option

Cardiac transplantation is often the final option for patients with severe CHF who are failing to respond adequately to current drug therapies. The number of transplants that can be performed is severely limited because of the complexity of the procedure, intensive follow-up and donor availability. In addition, many patients are unacceptable transplant candidates because of advanced age or co-morbid diseases such as diabetes or secondary pulmonary hypertension which is unresponsive to vasodilator therapy.

Summary

Routine medical treatment of patients with CHF includes the use of (1) a positive inotropic agent to increase cardiac contractility, (2) a diuretic to control sodium and water retention and (3) both direct- and indirect-acting vasodilators to reduce preload and afterload. Beneficial effects produced by these three classes of agents are generally additive, and they are often employed in combination in the treatment of patients with all stages of CHF. Although these agents successfully treat most patients with moderate CHF, some patients will remain symptomatic despite these therapies. In severely symptomatic patients, intravenous inotropic and vasodilator agents (e.g. dobutamine, amrinone, enoximone, dopamine, sodium nitroprusside) are used intermittently or continuously to improve symptoms. These intravenous agents are often effective short term but appear to have limited usefulness on a long-term basis because of difficulties of administration, toxicity or increased mortality.

Despite the best available therapy, approximately

40% of class IV patients die within 1 year of diagnosis. Efforts to discover and develop new therapies that effectively treat this syndrome continue. The potent vasodilatory properties of prostaglandins may offer a promising new approach to the management of CHF.

Role of endogenous prostaglandins in CHF

Plasma concentrations of several endogenous prostaglandins are elevated in patients with long-standing CHF. These higher-than-normal levels may be beneficial in CHF. Vasodilatory prostaglandins may counterbalance the effects of neurohormonal systems activated in CHF. In addition, the ability of prostaglandins to improve renal blood flow may reduce salt and water retention that occurs in CHF. Although limited data are available, prostaglandins may potentially play a role in reducing and/or preventing ventricular remodelling due to their potent antiproliferative actions.

The potent direct-acting vasodilatory actions of PGE_1 and PGI_2 counteract the potent vasoconstriction that occurs in CHF due to the activation of the autonomic nervous system and the renin–angiotensin system.[30] In addition, these agents have been shown to decrease peripheral vasoconstriction indirectly by inhibiting the release of noradrenaline from presynaptic sympathetic nerve terminals.[31,32]

Renal prostaglandins appear to play an important role in the regulation of renal blood flow and thus modulate salt and water excretion, which is reduced in CHF.[33,34] PGE_2 and $PGF_{2\alpha}$ are synthesized in the interstitial and collecting duct cells of the renal medulla. These prostaglandins are released into the interstitial fluid and renal venous blood. PGI_2 is synthesized in renal vascular smooth muscle and may counteract the renal vasoconstriction produced by noradrenaline and angiotensin II. Thus, renal prostaglandins may play a beneficial role in CHF by maintaining glomerular filtration in the presence of marked renal efferent arteriolar vasoconstriction.

Synthesis of prostaglandins is stimulated by the release of vasoconstrictor substances such as noradrenaline and angiotensin II, which are elevated in CHF.[30] Several studies have shown that metabolites of arachidonic acid, including bicyclo-PGE_2 and 6-oxo-$PGF_{1\alpha}$, are elevated in animal models of CHF as well as in patients with CHF.[30,35–37]

Not only do metabolites of arachidonic acid appear to play an important role in ventricular remodelling and in modulating the vasoconstrictor and antidiuretic effects observed in CHF; recent results also suggest that prostaglandins are involved in the mechanism of action of certain vasodilators used in the long-term treatment of CHF.[38,39] Nitrates such as nitroglycerin have been shown to increase PGI_2 synthesis in cultured human endothelial cells.[40] In addition, one study has demonstrated that plasma concentrations of bicyclo-PGE_2 and 6-oxo-$PGF_{1\alpha}$ were increased in class III/IV patients treated with the ACE inhibitor captopril.[35] It has been demonstrated that administration of cyclo-oxygenase inhibitors to patients with CHF results in worsening of symptoms. Further, the symptomatic benefit produced by administration of ACE inhibitors appears to be reduced when patients with severe CHF are also receiving cyclo-oxygenase inhibitors such as indomethacin or aspirin.[34]

Rationale for the use of exogenously administered prostaglandins in the treatment of CHF

As described above, endogenous prostaglandins may counteract the detrimental physiological events, including ventricular remodelling and vasoconstriction, that occur in patients with long-standing CHF. Further rationale for using selected prostaglandins in the treatment of patients with CHF is based primarily on their potent direct vasodilatory actions, resulting in reductions in preload as well as left and right ventricular afterload.

Left ventricular dysfunction has traditionally been viewed as a major pathophysiological determinant of exercise capacity in patients with CHF. Therefore, a major therapeutic goal in the treatment of CHF has been to improve left ventricular function. Recent evidence suggests, however, that left ventricular ejection fraction (LVEF) is not well correlated with maximal oxygen consumption measured during exercise in patients with CHF (Fig. 13.1).[41] In contrast, better correlations exist between right ventricular ejection fraction (RVEF) at rest and maximal oxygen consumption (Fig. 13.2).[42] Therapies that reduce afterload of both left and right ventricles may be useful in improving exercise capacity in patients with severe CHF.

Improvement in clinical symptoms in patients with severe CHF was shown to be greatest in patients who experienced larger relative reductions in pulmonary vascular resistance (PVR) than systemic

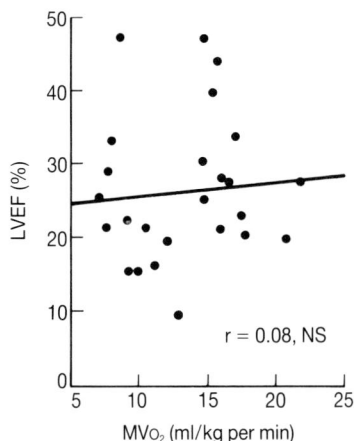

Fig. 13.1 Lack of relation between left ventricular ejection fraction (LVEF) at rest and maximal oxygen consumption (MVo$_2$) during exercise in patients with chronic left ventricular failure. NS = not significant.

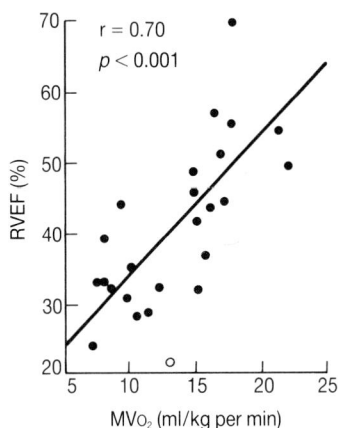

Fig. 13.2 Relation between right ventricular ejection fraction (RVEF) at rest and maximal oxygen consumption (MVo$_2$) during exercise in patients with chronic left ventricular failure.

vascular resistance (SVR) in response to the ACE inhibitor captopril.[43] Selected prostaglandins (e.g. PGI$_2$) are both very potent pulmonary vasodilators and balanced systemic venous and arterial vasodilators; these agents may prove to be particularly beneficial in treating patients with severe CHF.

As discussed previously, the antiproliferative and antiplatelet actions of prostaglandins may also prove beneficial in the treatment of CHF. Antiproliferative and antiplatelet properties may be useful in the prevention or reduction of the ventricular remodelling that occurs in CHF. The antiplatelet actions of prostaglandins may be useful in treating CHF patients with underlying coronary artery disease; however, the importance of platelet function in the aetiology and progression of CHF is unclear.

Prostaglandins that may be useful in the treatment of CHF

Of the endogenous prostaglandins, PGI$_2$ (prostacyclin), PGE$_2$ and PGE$_1$ are major prostaglandins whose pharmacological profile suggests that they may have potential beneficial effects in the treatment of patients with CHF. Only limited data are available on the usefulness of PGE$_2$ in patients with CHF. Therefore, this review focuses on the potential use of PGE$_1$ and PGI$_2$ in the treatment of CHF. PGI$_2$ is a metabolite of arachidonic acid and PGE$_1$ is a metabolic product of dihomo-γ-linolenic acid. Both prostaglandins inhibit platelet function and exhibit vasodilatory properties.[44]

It is generally accepted that both PGE$_1$ and PGI$_2$ activate the same or similar receptors on platelets.[45] Activation of platelet receptors by either PGI$_2$ or PGE$_1$ results in the stimulation of adenylate cyclase and a consequent increase in intracellular levels of cAMP.[46] Evidence suggests that there may be distinct receptors for PGE$_1$ and PGI$_2$ in other cell types (i.e. hepatocytes, polymorphonuclear leucocytes, vascular smooth muscle cells).[44]

The precise mechanism(s) responsible for the antiplatelet and vasodilatory effects of these agents is unknown; however, it has been proposed that some of the actions produced by prostaglandins may be mediated through rises in cAMP and activation of cAMP-dependent protein kinase. Other results suggest that the biological effects may be independent of increases in cAMP levels. Although the biological actions produced by PGE$_1$ and PGI$_2$ are very similar, these compounds are metabolized differently. PGE$_1$ is extensively metabolized by the lungs. PGI$_2$ is spontaneously hydrolysed at neutral pH, undergoes extensive hepatic metabolism and is not degraded by lung tissue. This difference in metabolic fate of PGI$_2$ versus PGE$_1$ leads to differences in distribution and sites of action of these agents. High concentrations of PGE$_1$ are present in the venous side of the systemic circulation, whereas concentrations of PGI$_2$ are similar in both the arterial and the venous sides of the systemic circulation.[44]

The clinical responses to infusions of PGI$_2$ and PGE$_1$ in patients with CHF have been examined in several small studies. In most cases the prostaglandin was administered only for a short period of time. The clinical trials evaluating the usefulness of selected prostaglandins in patients with CHF are described below.

Clinical studies with prostaglandins in CHF

Clinical trials with PGE₁

Several studies have examined the effects of short-term infusions of PGE$_1$ in patients with CHF. In one study, PGE$_1$ was infused at a rate of 40 ng/kg per minute for 30 minutes in five patients with class III/IV CHF with secondary pulmonary hypertension.[47] Cardiac index was increased by 20% and heart rate was slightly increased (5%). However, neither pulmonary capillary wedge pressure (PCWP) nor pulmonary artery pressure (PAP) was reduced by infusions of PGE$_1$. No side effects were reported in this study. In another study, nine patients with class III/IV CHF secondary to chronic coronary artery disease received PGE$_1$ infusions at varying doses (10–60 ng/kg per minute) for up to 1 hour.[48] Heart rate was unchanged and only a modest change in mean arterial blood pressure was noted (85 ± 6 to 76 ± 5 mmHg, $p<0.025$). PCWP fell from 19 ± 3 to 15 ± 2 mmHg ($p<0.01$). Infusions of PGE$_1$ improved the cardiac index from 1.9 ± 0.2 to 2.5 ± 0.2 l/m^2 per minute ($p<0.005$). Stroke index was also increased from 28 ± 4.4 to 35 ± 2.9 ml/m^2 per beat ($p<0.01$). No data on pulmonary artery pressure were reported in this study.

Several studies have shown that short- and long-term infusions of PGE$_1$ improve LVEF in patients with severe CHF. In one study, five of twelve patients responded to infusions of PGE$_1$ and exhibited significant improvements in LVEF (115–173% of baseline value) during administration of PGE$_1$ at infusion rates of 10–30 ng/kg per minute for 15-minute periods.[49] In this same study, PGE$_1$ was also administered continuously for up to 4 months in four patients who responded to PGE$_1$ when given short term. The short-term improvements in LVEF were sustained for the 4-month period with continuous intravenous infusions of PGE$_1$ at a dose of 20 ng/kg per minute.

In another study, PGE$_1$ was administered short term by intravenous administration to five patients following an acute myocardial infarction complicated by left heart failure. Cardiac index was improved; three of the five patients reported complete relief of chest pain during the infusion of PGE$_1$.[50]

PGE$_1$ infusions have been used successfully to treat severe life-threatening right heart failure following cardiac transplantation. In one study, PGE$_1$ (50–100 ng/kg per minute) was administered to three patients for up to 5 days following cardiac transplantation.[51] Pulmonary artery pressure and pulmonary vascular resistance were reduced in all three patients.

Clinical studies with PGI₂

Several uncontrolled studies indicate that synthetic PGI$_2$ (prostacyclin sodium, generic name of epoprostenol) produces beneficial haemodynamic effects when administered for short periods of time to patients with severe, refractory CHF.

In a study by Yui *et al.*, the short-term haemodynamic effects of intravenous prostacyclin, in doses of 22 ± 11 ng/kg per minute, were determined in nine patients with severe symptomatic CHF despite the use of digitalis and diuretics (NYHA class IV CHF).[52] The beneficial *short-term* haemodynamic effects observed following a 1-hour continuous infusion of prostacyclin are shown in Table 13.2. No significant effect on heart rate was observed in this study and no patient experienced chest discomfort or other adverse reactions during or after the prostacyclin infusion. All patients experienced mild facial flushing and warmness of the limbs. Prostacyclin did elevate plasma adrenaline levels; however, there were no significant elevations in plasma aldosterone or noradrenaline concentrations, or plasma renin activity.

In 1986, Nishikawa examined the time course of changes in various haemodynamic parameters in class IV patients who received continuous infusions of prostacyclin for 10 minutes at a rate of 10 ng/kg per minute.[53] The haemodynamic effects observed are shown in Table 13.2. All changes in the haemodynamic parameters peaked within 10 minutes after initiation of the infusion of prostacyclin. No significant effect on heart rate was observed during the infusion. The metabolic responses to prostacyclin were also evaluated in this study. No significant changes were observed in plasma renin activity, angiotension II, aldosterone, adrenaline, blood glucose, insulin, triglycerides or pyruvate. Plasma noradrenaline levels were increased by about twofold by infusions of prostacyclin. Lactate levels were reduced during the infusion, perhaps reflecting the

Table 13.2   Acute haemodynamic effects of epoprostenol and OP-41483 in patients with class IV CHF refractory to digitalis and diuretic therapy: summary of four studies; mean changes (%)

Treatment	Average dose (ng/kg per min)	SAP_m (mmHg)	PCWP (mmHg)	CI (l/m² per min)	SVR (dyn/(s/ cm⁻⁵))	PVR (dyn/(s/ m⁻⁵))	PAP_m (mmHg)	No. of patients studied (ref.)
Epo	22	−23%	−29%	+60%	−47%	−56%	ND	9 (51)
Epo	10	−27%	−41%	+70%	−52%	−44%	−30%	9 (52)
Epo	4	−15%	ND	0%	−14%	ND	−17%	53 (53)
OP-41483	27	−7%	−24%	+33%	−30%	−39%	ND	10 (54)

CI, cardiac index; ND, not done; PAP_m, mean pulmonary artery pressure; PCWP, pulmonary capillary wedge pressure; PVR, pulmonary vascular resistance; SAP_m, mean systemic arterial pressure; SVR, systemic vascular resistance.

haemodynamic improvement produced by prostacyclin. ADP and collagen-induced platelet aggregation were significantly reduced during the infusion.

Kodama *et al.* evaluated the short-term haemodynamic effects of three nitroso-compounds and prostacyclin in 53 patients with CHF following an acute myocardial infarction.[54] The three nitrates (molsidomine, nitroglycerin and isosorbide dinitrate) produced similar haemodynamic effects; mean systemic arterial pressure (SAP_m) and pulmonary artery end-diastolic pressure (PAEDP) decreased by 7–10% and 20–29%, respectively, while systemic vascular resistance (SVR) remained unchanged. In contrast, infusions of prostacyclin (3–4 ng/kg per minute) reduced SAP_m and SVR with a minimal decrease in PAEDP (Table 13.2). None of the agents tested, including these relatively low doses of prostacyclin, produced an increase in cardiac index.

A stable carbacyclin derivative of PGI_2, OP-41483 (Ono Pharmaceuticals, Japan) has also been shown to acutely improve haemodynamics in patients with class IV CHF[55] (see Table 13.2). In this same study, OP-41483 was also shown to significantly inhibit ADP-induced platelet aggregation ($p<0.01$).

Left ventricular ejection fraction (LVEF) in patients with CHF has been shown in two studies to be improved by short-term infusions of prostacyclin. In one study, LVEF was increased in all 10 patients treated with prostacyclin at an infusion rate of 5 ng/kg per minute (mean LVEF of 34.7 ± 14.8% to 43.8 ± 15.8%, $p<0.01$).[56] Slight improvements in LVEF were also noted in 6 of the 10 patients at an infusion rate of 1 ng/kg per minute. Similarly, in another study, LVEF was increased in 8 of 12 patients who received prostacyclin infusion (1–8 ng/kg per minute). Six patients showed improvement in LVEF during administration of 1 ng/kg per minute. Two other patients responded only to prostacyclin at a rate of 5 ng/kg per minute. In all patients, prostacyclin infusions

of 8 ng/kg per minute caused further increases in LVEF.[44]

Infusions of prostacyclin have also been shown to be beneficial in controlling pulmonary hypertension and right ventricular failure that can occur prior to, or following, cardiac transplantation.[57,58]

In all the studies cited above, prostacyclin or the stable analogue, OP-41483, were administered for no longer than a few hours or several days. Recently, a pilot study in 33 patients evaluated the safety and efficacy of chronic administration of prostacyclin sodium (Flolan®, Burroughs Wellcome Co., Research Triangle Park, North Carolina) in patients with severe, refractory CHF.[59] This 12-week study compared the effects of chronic intravenous infusions of prostacyclin plus conventional therapy (digitalis glycoside, diuretic, ACE inhibitor and/or dobutamine) to conventional therapy alone on exercise capacity in patients with class III/IV CHF. Prostacyclin was administered continuously via an indwelling central venous catheter and a small portable infusion pump (Fig. 13.3). At the beginning of the study, all patients received increasing doses of short-term intravenous infusions of prostacyclin prior to randomization into the conventional therapy and prostacyclin groups. This study confirmed the acute beneficial effects of epoprostenol on haemodynamics in patients with severe CHF. At the end of the 12 weeks there was a trend towards improvement in exercise capacity (as measured by distance walked in 6 minutes) in patients who received epoprostenol compared to those patients who received conventional therapy alone (between-group comparison, $p=0.07$) (Table 13.3).

In summary, although only limited clinical data are available, both PGE_1 and PGI_2 show promise for the treatment of right and left heart failure. Clearly, large, well-controlled studies are required to define the usefulness of these agents in this patient population.

Table 13.3 Acute haemodynamic effects of epoprostenol in patients with class III/IV CHF refractory to the triple regimen: digitalis, diuretic and ACE inhibitor (mean changes, $n = 33$)

	CI (l/m² per min)	PCWP (mmHg)	SAP_m (mmHg)	HR (b.p.m.)	SVR (dyn/(s/cm⁻⁵))	PVR (dyn/(s/cm⁻⁵))
Baseline	2.0 ± 0.5	24 ± 10	82 ± 13	86 ± 15	1704 ± 625	217 ± 171
Epoprostenol	2.8 ± 0.6	19 ± 7	73 ± 9	90 ± 14	1040 ± 320	160 ± 104
Change %	$+40$	-21	-11	$+5$	-39	-26

CI, cardiac index; HR, heart rate; PCWP, pulmonary capillary wedge pressure; PVR, pulmonary vascular resistance; SAP_m, mean systemic arterial pressure; SVR, systemic vascular resistance.

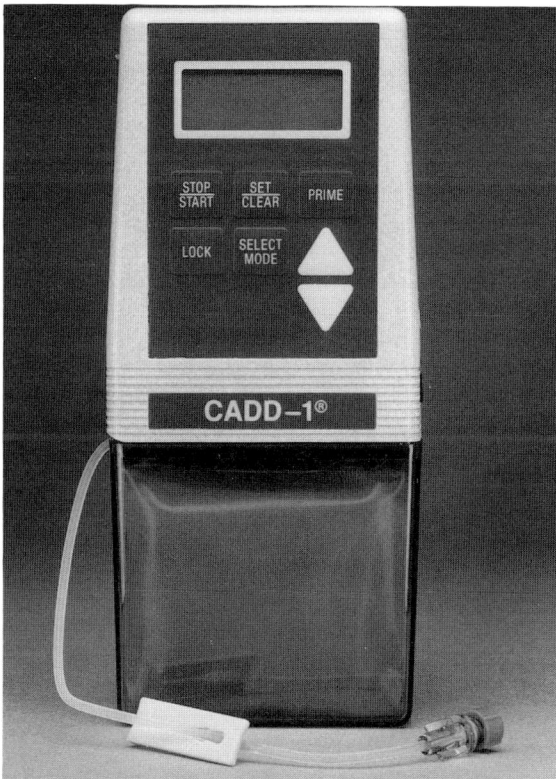

Fig. 13.3 Portable infusion pump (CADD I pump, Pharmacia-Deltec Inc.) used for continuous infusions of epoprostenol in outpatients (reference 58).

Limitations of chronic administration of PGE₁/PGI₂

Although potentially promising in the treatment of CHF, the requirement for continuous intravenous infusions of PGE₁ and PGI₂ (due to chemical/metabolic instability) is a limitation. Development of stable prostaglandin analogues that can be administered via a non-parenteral route will allow for wider use of this therapeutic approach. However, in order to be successful, these analogues must possess a pharmacological profile similar to that of PGE₁ or PGI₂ as well as an acceptable side-effect profile. In addition, because prostaglandins exhibit steep dose–response relationships, safe oral administration may prove difficult due to potential erratic dissolution/absorption. To date, most of the stable analogues have been developed primarily for their antiplatelet rather than their vasodilatory actions. Further studies are needed to determine if these compounds will be useful in the treatment of CHF.

Conclusions

Current treatment modalities do not effectively manage all patients with CHF. Additional therapies are needed that not only can improve haemodynamics but can also translate into improvements in symptoms, exercise capacity, quality of life and survival.

The use of potent prostaglandins that possess pulmonary and vasodilatory actions, such as PGE₁ and PGI₂ or their stable analogues, may offer a new approach to the management of patients with severe CHF that is refractory to current therapies. Large, well-controlled clinical trials are needed to determine the risks and benefits of these compounds. This therapeutic approach may hold great promise, particularly if stable prostaglandin analogues can be developed.

References

1. McKee PA, Castelli WP, McNamara PM, Kannel WB. The natural history of congestive heart failure: the Framingham Study. *N Engl J Med* 1971; **285:** 1441–6.
2. Franciosa JA, Wilen M, Ziesche S, Cohn JN. Survival in men with severe chronic left ventricular failure due

to either coronary heart disease or idiopathic dilated cardiomyopathy. *Am J Cardiol* 1983; **51**: 831–6.

3. Califf RM, Bounous P, Harrell FE, *et al.* The prognosis in the presence of coronary artery disease. In: Braunwald E, Mock MG, Watson JT (eds), *Congestive Heart Failure. Current Research and Clinical Applications.* New York: Grune & Stratton, 1982: 31–50.

4. McLaughlin TJ. Current and emerging therapies for congestive heart failure. *Decision Resources: Spectrum Pharmaceuticals* 1991; **15**: 1–9.

5. Smith WM. Epidemiology of congestive heart failure. *Am J Cardiol* 1985; **55**: 3A–7A.

6. Kannel WB, Belanger AJ. Epidemiology of congestive heart failure. *Am Heart J* 1991; **119**: 951–7.

7. Dzau VJ, Swartz SL, Creager MA. The role of prostaglandins in pathophysiology and therapy of congestive heart failure. *Heart Failure* 1986; **2**: 6–13.

8. Warren S, Dzau VJ. Natriuretic hormones in heart failure. *Heart Failure* 1986; **2**: 33–9.

9. Francis GS, Goldsmith SR, Levine TB, *et al.* The neurohumoral axis in congestive heart failure. *Ann Intern Med* 1984; **101**: 370–7.

10. Curtis C, Cohn JN, Vrobel T, Franciosa JA. Role of the renin–angiotensin system in the systemic vasoconstriction of chronic congestive heart failure. *Circulation* 1978; **58**: 763–70.

11. Kahn JK. Progressive congestive heart failure: ways to approach office management. *Postgrad Med Progressive CHF* 1991; **89**: 102–7.

12. Ferrari A, Gregorini L, Ferrari MC, *et al.* Digitalis and baroreceptor reflexes in man. *Circulation* 1981; **63**: 279–85.

13. Kimmelstiel C, Benotti J. How effective is digitalis in the treatment of congestive heart failure? *Am Heart J* 1988; **116**: 1063–70.

14. Guyatt G, Sullivan M, Fallen E, *et al.* A controlled trial of digoxin in congestive heart failure. *Am J Cardiol* 1988; **61**: 371–5.

15. Jaeschke R, Oxman AD, Guyatt GH. To what extent do congestive heart failure patients in sinus rhythm benefit from digoxin therapy? A systematic overview and meta-analysis. *Am J Med* 1990; **88**: 279–86.

16. Young JB, Uretsky BF, Shahidi FE, *et al.* on behalf of the PROVED Study Investigators. Multicenter, double-blind, placebo-controlled, randomized withdrawal trial of the efficacy and safety of digoxin in patients with mild to moderate chronic heart failure not treated with converting enzyme inhibitors. *J Am Coll Cardiol* 1992; **19**: 259A. [Abstract]

17. Packer M, Gheorghiade M, Young JB, *et al.* on behalf of the RADIANCE Study. Randomized, double-blind, placebo-controlled, withdrawal study of digoxin in patients with chronic heart failure treated with converting enzyme inhibitors. *J Am Coll Cardiol* 1992; **19**: 260A. [Abstract]

18. Feldman AM. Can we alter survival in patients with congestive heart failure? *JAMA* 1992; **26** (14): 1956–61.

19. DiBianco R, Shabetai R, Kostuk W, *et al.* A comparison of oral milrinone, digoxin, and their combination in the treatment of patients with chronic heart failure. *N Engl J Med* 1989; **320**: 677–83.

20. Uretsky BF, Jessup M, Konstam MA, *et al.* Multicenter trial of oral enoximone in patients with moderate to moderately severe congestive heart failure: lack of benefit compared with placebo. *Circulation* 1990; **82**: 774–80.

21. Packer M, Carver JR, Rodenheffer RJ, *et al.* Effect of oral milrinone on mortality in severe chronic heart failure. *N Engl J Med* 1991; **325**: 1468–75.

22. Applefeld MM, Newman KA, Sutton FJ, *et al.* Outpatient dobutamine infusions in the management of chronic heart failure: clinical experience in 21 patients. *Am Heart J* 1987; **114**: 589–95.

23. Dies F, Krell MJ, Whitlow P, *et al.* Intermittent dobutamine in ambulatory outpatients with chronic cardiac failure. *Circulation* 1986; **74** (suppl II): 138. [Abstract]

24. Cohn JN, Archibald D, Johnson G, *et al.* Effects of vasodilator therapy on mortality in chronic heart failure: results of a Veterans Administration Cooperative Study. *N Engl J Med* 1986; **314**: 1547–52.

25. The CONSENSUS Trial Study Group. Effects of enalapril on mortality in severe congestive heart failure: results of the Cooperative North Scandinavian Enalapril Survival Study (CONSENSUS). *N Engl J Med* 1987; **316**: 1429–35.

26. Cohn JN, Johnson G, Ziesche S, *et al.* A comparison of enalapril with hydralazine–isosorbide dinitrate in the treatment of chronic congestive heart failure. *N Engl J Med* 1991; **325**: 303–10.

27. The SOLVD Investigators. Studies of left ventricular dysfunction (SOLVD): rationale, design, and methods: two trials that evaluate the effect of enalapril in patients with reduced ejection fraction. *Am J Cardiol* 1990; **66**: 315–22.

28. Schwartz AB, Chatterjee K. Vasodilator therapy in chronic congestive heart failure (Part 1). *Curr Ther* 1984; **25** (4): 79–92.

29. Pfeffer MA, Lamas GA, Vaugh DE, *et al.* Effects of captopril on progressive ventricular dilatation after anterior myocardial infarction. *N Engl J Med* 1988; **319**: 80–6.

30. Dzau VJ. Vascular and renal prostaglandins as counter-regulatory systems in heart failure. *Eur Heart J* 1988; **9** (suppl H): 15–19.

31. Wennmalm A. Studies of the mechanism controlling the secretion of neurotransmitters in the rabbit heart. *Acta Physiol Scand (Suppl)* 1971; **365**: 1–36.

32. Chazov EI, Pomoinetsky VD, Geiling N, *et al.* Heart adaptation to acute pressure overload: an involvement of endogenous prostaglandins. *Circ Res* 1979; **45**: 205–11.

33. McGiff JC, Wong PYK. Prostaglandins and renal function. *Proceedings, 7th International Congress of Nephrology, Montreal.* Basel: Karger, 1978: 83–91.

34. Dzau VJ, Packer M, Lilly LS, *et al.* Prostaglandins in severe congestive heart failure. Relation to activation of the renin–antiotensin system and hyponatremia. *N Engl J Med* 1984; **310**: 347–52.

35. Punzengruber C, Stanek B, Silberbauer K. Activation of bicycloprostaglandin E_2-metabolite in congestive heart failure. *Am J Cardiol* 1986; **57**: 619–22.

36. Oliver JA, Sciacca RR, Pinto J, Cannon PJ. Participation of the prostaglandins in the control of renal blood flow during acute reduction of cardiac output in the dog. *J Clin Invest* 1981; **67**: 229–37.

37. Holmer SR, Riegger AJG, Notheis WF, *et al.* Hemodynamic changes and renal plasma flow in early heart failure: implications for renin, aldosterone, norepinephrine, atrial natriuretic peptide and prostacyclin. *Basic Res Cardiol* 1987; **82**: 101–8.

38. Silberbauer K, Punzengruber C, Sinzinger H. Endogenous prostaglandin E_2 metabolite levels, renin–angiotensin system and catecholamines versus acute hemodynamic response to captopril in congestive heart failure. *Cardiology* 1983; **60**: 297–301.

39. Swartz SL, Williams GH, Hollenberg NK, *et al.* Captopril-induced changes in prostaglandin production. *J Clin Invest* 1980; **65**: 1257–61.

40. Levin RJ, Jaffe WA, Weksler BB, Tack-Goldman K. Nitroglycerin stimulates production of prostacyclin by cultured human endothelial cells. *J Clin Invest* 1981; **67**: 762–4.

41. Franciosa JA, Park M, Levine TB. Lack of correlation between exercise capacity and indexes of left ventricular performance in heart failure. *Am J Cardiol* 1981; **47**: 33–6.

42. Baker BJ, Wilen MM, Boyd CM, *et al.* Relation of right ventricular ejection fraction to exercise capacity in chronic left ventricular failure. *Am J Cardiol* 1984; **54**: 596–9.

43. Packer M, Lee WH, Medina N, *et al.* Hemodynamic and clinical significance of the pulmonary vascular response to long-term captopril therapy in patients with severe chronic heart failure. *J Am Cardiol* 1985; **6**: 635–9.

44. Kerins DM, Murray R, FitzGerald GA. Prostacyclin and prostaglandin E_1: molecular mechanisms and therapeutic utility. *Prog in Hemost Thromb* 1991; **10**: 307–37.

45. Hall JM, Strange PG. The use of a prostacyclin analogue [^{3}H]iloprost, for studying prostacyclin-binding sites on human platelets and neuronal hybrid cells. *Biosci Rep* 1984; **14**: 941–8.

46. Ashly B. Model of prostaglandin-regulated cyclic AMP metabolism in intact platelets: examination of time-dependent effects on adenylate cyclase and phosphodiesterase activities. *Mol Pharmacol* 1990; **36**: 866–73.

47. Jacobs P, Naeije R, Renard M, *et al.* Effects of prosta-glandin E_1 on hemodynamics and blood gases in severe left heart failure. *J Cardiovasc Pharmacol* 1983; **5**: 170–1.

48. Awan NA, Evenson MK, Needham KE, *et al.* Cardio-circulatory and myocardial energetic effects of prostaglandin E_1 in severe left ventricular failure due to chronic coronary heart disease. *Am Heart J* 1981; **102**: 703–9.

49. Virgolini I, Auinger C, Weissel M, Sinzinger H. Increase in left ventricular ejection fraction induced by PGE_1 and PGI_2. In: Schorr K, Sinzinger H (eds), *Prostaglandins in Clinical Research; Cardiovascular System*, Proceedings of the Fourth International Symposium, Dusseldorf, October 5–7 1988. New York: Liss, 1989; 463–6.

50. Popat KD, Pitt B. Hemodynamic effects of prostaglandin E_1 infusions in patients with acute myocardial infarction and left ventricular failure. *Am Heart J* **103**: 485–9.

51. Armitage JM, Hardesty RL, Griffith BP. Prostaglandin E_1: an effective treatment of right heart failure after orthotopic heart transplantation. *J Heart Transplant* 1987; **6**: 348–51.

52. Yui Y, Nakajima H, Kawai C, Murakami T. Prostacyclin therapy in patients with congestive heart failure. *Am J Cardiol* 1982; **50**: 320–4.

53. Nishikawa H. Intravenous vasodilator therapy in patients with refractory congestive heart failure. *Mie Med J* 1986; **36**: 57–83.

54. Kodama K, Koretsune Y, Nanto S, Taniura K. Hemodynamic and metabolic effects of vasodilator therapy for heart failure in acute myocardial infarction. *Jpn Circ J* 1984; **48**: 380–7.

55. Yui Y, Takatsu Y, Hatti R, *et al.* Vasodilator therapy with a new stable prostacyclin analog, OP41483, for congestive heart failure due to coronary artery disease and comparison of hemodynamic effects and platelet aggregation with nitroprusside. *Am J Cardiol* 1986; **58**: 1042–5.

56. Auinger C, Virgolini I, Weissel M, *et al.* Prostacyclin increases left ventricular ejection fraction. *Prostaglandins, Leukot Essent Fatty Acids* 1989; **36**: 149–51.

57. Esmore D, Keogh A, Spratt P, Chang V. Nitroprusside and prostacyclin in potential cardiac transplant recipients. *Aust NZ J Med* 1989; **19** (5 suppl 1): 564. [Abstract]

58. Esmore D, Spratt PM, Branch JM, *et al.* Right ventricular assist and prostacyclin infusion for allograft failure in the presence of high pulmonary vascular resistance. *J Heart Transplant* 1989; **9**: 136–41.

59. Gheorghiade M, Sueta C, Adams, K, *et al.* Multicenter, randomized trial of epoprostenol in patients with severe heart failure. *J Am Coll Cardiol* 1992; **19**: 216A. [Abstract]

14 Prostaglandins and primary pulmonary hypertension

A Yazdani Butt, TW Higenbottam and J Wallwork

Primary pulmonary hypertension is a fatal disease, which is generally seen in young adults. More women than men develop the disease, but it can also affect children and the elderly.[1] It follows a rapidly downhill course and most patients die within 5 years due to progressive right heart failure[2,3] (Fig. 14.1). Romberg described it for the first time in 1891 from an autopsy examination where sclerosis of pulmonary arteries was noted in the absence of an underlying cardiopulmonary disease.[4] Dresdale *et al.* in 1951 published the first series of patients based on the results of right heart catheterization and introduced the term 'primary pulmonary hypertension'[5] (PPH).

Systolic pulmonary artery pressure at sea level is about 20 mmHg and diastolic pressure is 12 mmHg for a cardiac output of 5–6 litres per minute. For practical purposes, a mean pulmonary artery pressure in excess of 25 mmHg at rest and 30 mmHg on exercise is considered abnormal.[6] Diagnosis of PPH is made on the physiological measurements after ensuring the absence of underlying disease, for example left ventricular failure, mitral valve disease, pulmonary embolism, chronic hypoxic lung disease, hypoventilation or congenital heart disease (Table 14.1).

The World Health Organization classification offers three pathological entities of PPH: plexogenic pulmonary arteriopathy, peripheral thrombotic

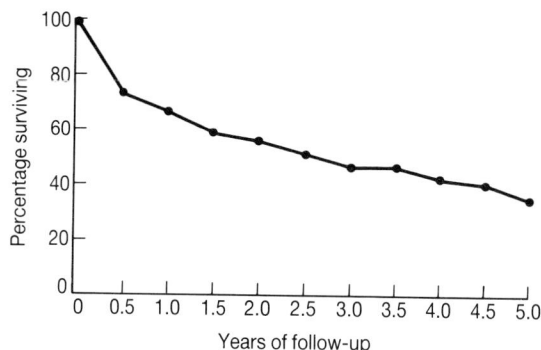

Fig. 14.1 Estimated percentage of patients surviving over time from the baseline catheterization. Number of patients at risk are shown for 0 through 5 years. Median survival is estimated at 2.8 years. Estimated percentages of patients surviving at 1, 3 and 5 years are 68%, 48% and 34%, respectively. (Reproduced, with permission, from D'Alonzo GE *et al.* Survival in patients with primary pulmonary hypertension. *Ann Intern Med* 1991; **115**; 344.)

arterial disease and veno-occlusive disease.[7,8] Plexogenic pulmonary arteriopathy may indicate an underlying pulmonary vasoconstrictor phenomenon as a triggering mechanism along with possible migration of the myofibroblasts[9] towards the intima. It has been suggested to be likely to respond most to vasodilator treatment. This type of PPH is charac-

Table 14.1 Causes of pulmonary hypertension

Secondary pulmonary hypertension
Congenital heart disease with left to right shunt
Mitral valve disease
Primary or secondary myocardial disease
Pulmonary embolism
Intravenous drug abuse
Chronic obstructive lung disease
Interstitial lung disease
Neuromuscular diseases causing hypoventilation
Pickwickian syndrome
Ankylosing spondylitis
Connective tissue disease, e.g. systemic sclerosis
Pulmonary venous obstruction
Chronic liver disease

Primary pulmonary hypertension
Plexogenic arteriopathy
Thrombotic arterial disease
Veno-occlusive disease

(Adapted, with permission, from Rich S. Primary pulmonary hypertention. *Prog Cardiovasc Dis* 1988; **31** (3): 212.)

terized by concentric intimal fibrosis and dilatations in the small pulmonary arteries along with typical plexiform lesions.[10] Peripheral thrombotic arterial disease is characterized by eccentric intimal thickening of the resistant pulmonary arteries associated with recanalized thrombi. In veno-occlusive disease, obstruction occurs in the pulmonary venous system due to intimal proliferation and fibrosis, often resulting in complete obliteration of the venous channels. However, patients with PPH often have both plexogenic and thrombotic changes on histology. As a result, classification is according to the predominant change; i.e. predominantly plexogenic disease or predominantly thrombotic disease.

Certain autoimmune diseases such as systemic lupus erythematosus[11] are associated with PPH.[12] Systemic lupus erythematosus is often associated with a circulating lupus anticoagulant which may contribute to intravascular coagulation. Lupus anticoagulant is an IgG or IgM,[13] which interferes with the formation of prostacyclin and may lead to prostacyclin deficiency.[14-16] It has been postulated that local deficiency of prostacyclin might be a factor in the genesis of PPH, especially as prostacyclin seems experimentally to impede the development of PPH in monocrotaline poisoning.[17,18] Familial PPH occurs which could be associated with deficiency of antithrombin III.[19,20] Susceptible individuals are also more prone to develop pulmonary hypertension

when exposed to dietary treatments such as aminorex fumarate[21] and fenfluramine.[22]

Diagnosis

Clinical features

Diagnosis of PPH is usually delayed for up to 2 years[1] as signs of pulmonary hypertension are missed in the early stages. There should be a high index of suspicion for any young adult presenting with dyspnoea, chest pain and syncope.[1,23,24] There may be a history of Raynaud's phenomenon, which has been recently considered to be associated with a poor prognosis.[25] The patient may have a low volume pulse, prominent a wave, right-sided third and fourth heart sound, loud pulmonary component of the second heart sound, left parasternal heave, a flow murmur from the pulmonary valve, and a murmur of tricuspid regurgitation[1] associated with prominent v waves. Most patients do not present with dependent oedema and this possibly results from elevated levels of atrial natriuretic peptide (ANP) which occur in this condition.[26]

Investigations

The ECG and chest x-ray are abnormal in 90% of the patients and show signs of right ventricular hypertrophy with right axis deviation (Fig. 14.2) and enlarged central pulmonary arteries with peripheral pruning respectively (Fig. 14.3). An autoimmune profile may show raised antinuclear factor (ANF) in many patients.[27] Cross-sectional Doppler echocardiography shows right ventricular hypertrophy with dilatation,[28] distortion of the interventricular septum[29,30] and tricuspid regurgitation (Fig. 14.4). An enlarged pulmonary trunk and some pulmonary regurgitation[28] may also be found, together with an elevated pulmonary artery pressure. Recent developments with colour Doppler enhance the possibility of detecting any intracardiac shunts. Ventilation and perfusion lung scintigraphy (*V*/*Q* scan) is important to exclude proximal pulmonary embolism.[31] Segmental or subsegmental perfusion defects (Fig. 14.5) indicate pulmonary embolism and underline the need to perform pulmonary angiography.[32] A normal *V*/*Q* scan usually represents the plexogenic form of PPH whilst patchy perfusion defects not corresponding to segmental or subsegmental distribution indicate peripheral thrombotic disease.[33] Full pulmonary function tests may show a restrictive pattern with

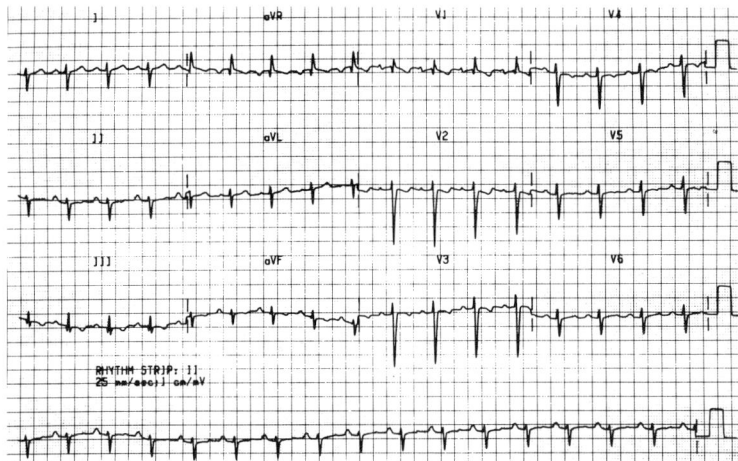

Fig. 14.2 Electrocardiogram of a patient with pulmonary hypertension showing right axis deviation and right ventricular hypertrophy.

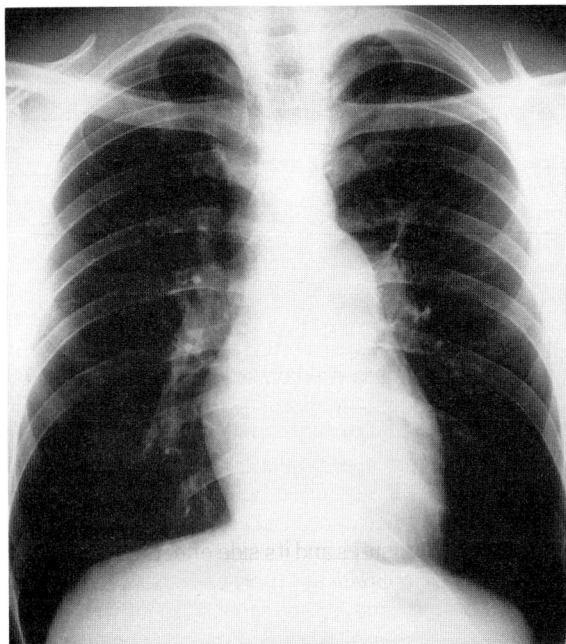

Fig. 14.3 Chest x-ray of patient with primary pulmonary hypertension showing enlargement of the central pulmonary arteries with some peripheral pruning of the vessels.

impairment of gas transfer,[1] and arterial blood gases are usually consistent with hypoxia and hypocapnia.

Right heart catheterization

Right heart catheterization (RHC) is essential, not only to confirm the diagnosis but also to establish the

prognosis for the patient.[1,3,6] Right atrial pressure (RAP), mean pulmonary artery pressure (MPA), cardiac output (CO), pulmonary wedge pressure along with heart rate and systemic arterial pressure are measured during RHC. Systemic and pulmonary arterial blood is taken for gas analysis. Patients with pulmonary artery oxygen saturation ($S\bar{v}o_2$) of less than 63% carry only a 17% chance of survival over 3 years whilst those with $S\bar{v}o_2$ in excess of 63% have a 55% chance of survival over a similar period.[3] Similarly, RAP of more than 20 mmHg, MPA of 85 mmHg or more, and cardiac index of less than 2 litres per minute are associated with a marked reduction in survival.[25]

Treatment

As the aetiology and pathogenetic mechanism in PPH remain unknown, treatment is directed towards alleviating the effects of low cardiac output and pulmonary vasoconstriction.[34,35] Anticoagulants have been shown to be related to improved survival[3] and are useful in preventing thromboembolic episodes, which is a real risk because of the low cardiac output state in PPH. Various parenteral vasodilators such as acetylcholine, tolazoline, phentolamine and isoprenaline have been used, with conflicting results.[9,36] Long-term use of oral vasodilators such as captopril[37] and hydralazine[38] has been disappointing in spite of some early success, and their use has now been largely abandoned. Calcium channel blockers such as nifedipine[39] are currently in use,

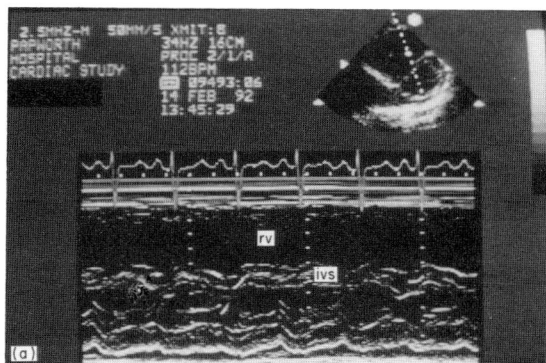

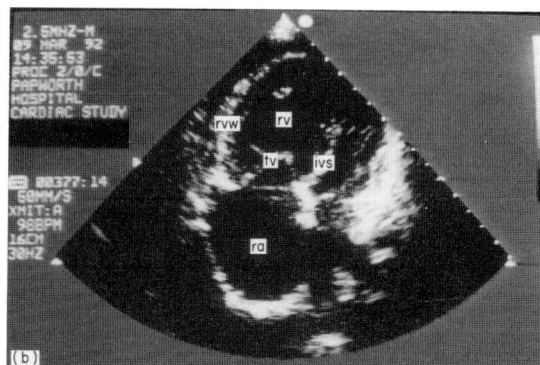

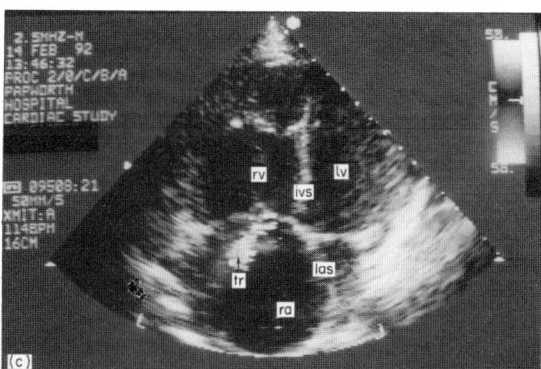

Fig. 14.4 Echocardiographic appearance in pulmonary hypertension. (*a*) M-mode and (*b*) four-chamber view of cross-sectional echocardiogram showing dilated right-sided chambers and right ventricular hypertrophy. (*c*) Colour flow imaging shows a jet due to tricuspid regurgitation, ias, interatrial septum; ivs, intraventricular septum; lv, left ventricle; ra, right atrium; rv, right ventricle; rvw, right ventricular wall; tv, tricuspid valve.

particularly for patients with $S\bar{v}o_2$ of more than 63%. Diltiazem is slightly superior because of its smaller effect on systemic arteries and lower negative inotropic effect on myocardium.[40] In one study high-dose calcium channel-blocking therapy with nifedipine and diltiazem has been shown to cause sustained haemodynamic, symptomatic and electrocardiographic improvement[41] (Table 14.2).

Acute effects of prostaglandin I_2

In recent years interest has grown in using prostaglandin I_2 (prostacyclin or PGI_2), which is derived from arachidonic acid and is a potent vasodilator. This was used in 1980 for the first time as an acute pulmonary vasodilator in a child.[42] Since then, several centres have used this as an investigational agent for its acute effects.[43,44] At this Institute, prostacyclin infusion is given during right heart catherization in order to assess response to its vasodilatory effect.[45] After taking baseline measurements, prostacyclin is commenced at approximately 2 ng/kg per

minute. Haemodynamic measurements are repeated after 5–15 minutes before the dose is increased by 1–2 ng/kg per minute. The prostacyclin infusion is continued until there is a significant drop in pulmonary (PVR) and systemic vascular resistance (SVR) or the patient gets side effects such as headaches, flushing or hypotension. Prostacyclin has a half-life of less than 5 minutes and its side effects can be easily reversed by stopping the infusion. Ideally the aim is for a 30% drop in pulmonary vascular resistance or a 30% increase in cardiac output without a concomitant rise in pulmonary artery pressure. A short-term vasodilator trial with prostacyclin during RHC can be useful in predicting response to long-term vasodilator therapy[40,46,47] (Table 14.3).

Long-term use of prostacyclin infusion in PPH

Because of its short half-life and ability to titrate an optimum pulmonary vasorelaxant dose, the question

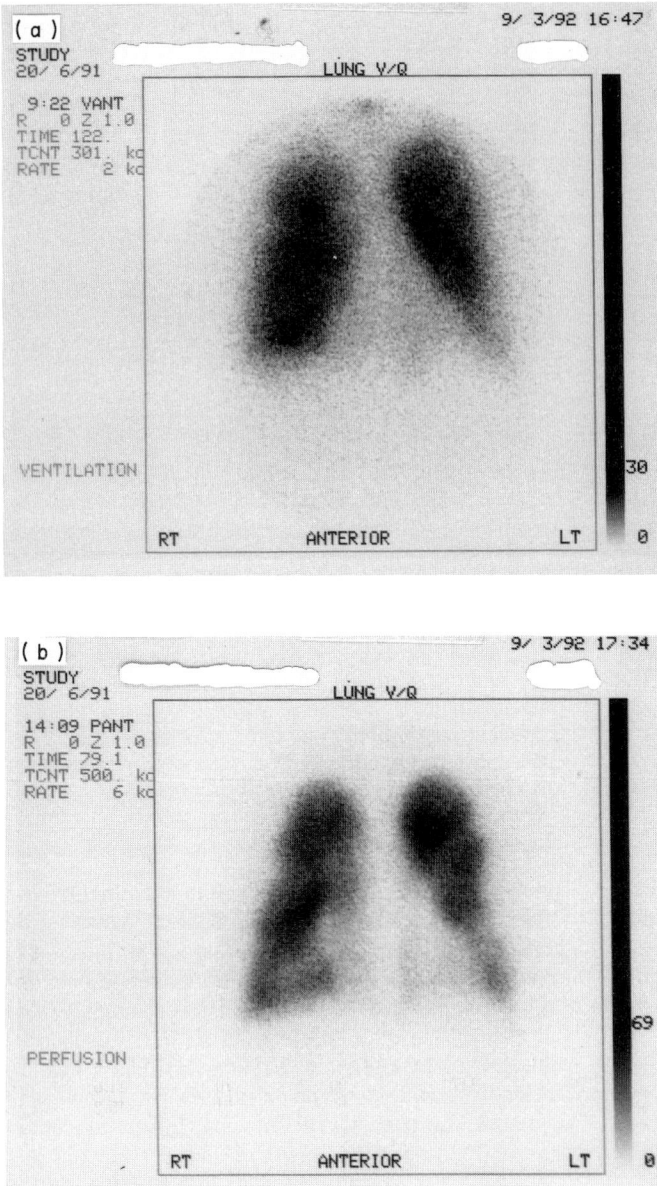

Fig. 14.5   Ventilation and perfusion lung scans of a patient with thromboembolic pulmonary hypertension: (*a*) ventilation scan with normal appearance; (*b*) perfusion scan showing bilateral perfusion defects consistent with thromboembolic disease.

arises about long-term use of prostacyclin as a treatment for pulmonary hypertension. The first study in this regard, preceded by a case report, was carried out at this centre; it showed significant improvement in exercise tolerance and general well-being in the majority of patients with PPH.[45,47] Such improvement is considered to be due to decreased PVR and subsequent increase in cardiac output and oxygen

tissue delivery; however, there was no evidence that prostacyclin reverses the underlying disease process.[45] Since the initial report, Rubin *et al.* have demonstrated that prostacyclin causes substantial and sustained haemodynamic and symptomatic responses in severe primary pulmonary hypertension.[48] At this Institute we consider long-term infusion of prostacyclin for patients who carry a poor

Table 14.2 Results of long-term treatment with high-dose calcium channel blockers

Patient no.	Maintenance (mg/day)	FC	Follow-up (mo)	QRS axis (degrees)	RV_1 (mm)	RVID (mm)
1	720 dil	I	20	95 → 66	2 → 1	31 → 21
2	240 dil*	II	19	115 → 110	4 → 2	32 → 36
3	120 nif	I	17	98 → 76	4 → 1	28 → 16
4	120 nif	I	16	110 → 78	7 → 1	40 → 28
5	120 nif	I	13	125 → 105	5 → 3	34 → 26
6	180 nif	I	6			
7	160 nif	(died)	6			
8	240 nif	I	4			

*Patient reduced dose.
Maintenance, daily dose of drug taken after outpatient readjustments; FC, NYHA functional class at follow-up; Follow-up, current length of follow-up period; QRS axis, initial QRS axis from electrocardiogram and changes after 1 year; RV_1, height of R wave from lead V_1 initially and after 1 year; RVID, right ventricular internal dimension by M-mode echocardiogram initially and after 1 year
dil, diltiazem; nif, nifedipine.
(Reproduced, with permission, from Rich S, Brundage BH. High-dose calcium blocking therapy for primary pulmonary hypertension. *Circulation* 1987; **76** (1): 138.)

Table 14.3 Values for haemodynamic data at baseline and during maximal dose infusion during short-term prostacyclin trial in 10 patients with primary pulmonary hypertension

Patient no.	Max. dose of prostacyclin	SAP (mmHg)	PAP (mmHg)	CI (l/m² per min)	PVR (dyn/(s/cm⁻⁵))	SVR (dyn/(s/cm⁻⁵))	HR (beats/min)	PaO_2 saturation	O_2 delivery (ml/kg per min)
1	Baseline	78	100	1.7	2133	1600	104	45	5.8
	4 ng/kg per min	77	81	2.3	1190	1200	120	50	8.2
2	Baseline	82	71	1.5	1899	1992	70	38	—
	6 ng/kg per min	66	68	1.9	1365	1223	82	45	—
3	Baseline	80	55	1.7	1376	1952	98	52	10.9
	5 ng/kg per min	65	65	1.8	1629	1425	104	53	11.9
4	Baseline	83	80	2.1	1558	1684	87	60	9.5
	4 ng/kg per min	75	80	2.6	1242	1174	90	70	11.6
5	Baseline	73	62	3.0	784	1094	90	51	15.2
	4 ng/kg per min	72	48	3.1	580	1020	90	61	16.8
6	Baseline	93	60	1.5	1583	2187	77	42	8.5
	6 ng/kg per min	80	60	1.8	1358	1457	84	56	9.5
7	Baseline	100	80	1.8	1800	2275	78	51	12.4
	6 ng/kg per min	80	80	2.1	1516	1579	82	57	14.3
8	Baseline	70	50	2.2	869	1440	63	60	11.8
	6 ng/kg per min	61	48	2.8	675	1031	68	68	15.1
9	Baseline	95	105	1.5	2744	2425	84	43	8.3
	8 ng/kg per min	70	105	2.0	2054	1340	96	57	10.9
10	Baseline	76	93	1.3	2523	1723	82	42	7.3
	6 ng/kg per min	62	98	1.45	2400	1048	82	51	8.1
Mean	Baseline	83 (3)	76 (6)	1.83 (0.2)	1727 (202)	1837 (129)	83 (4)	48 (2)	10.0 (1)
(SEM)	5.5 ng/kg per min	71 (2)	73 (6)	2.19 (0.2)	1401 (175)	1250 (61)	90 (4)	57 (2)	11.8 (1)
p value		<0.001	>0.4	<0.005	<0.02	<0.001	<0.005	<0.001	<0.001

CI, cardiac index; HR, heart rate; O_2 delivery, peripheral oxygen delivery; PaO_2 saturation, pulmonary arterial oxygen saturation; PAP, pulmonary artery pressure; PVR, pulmonary vascular resistance; SAP, systemic arterial pressure; SVR, systemic vascular resistance.
(Reproduced, with permission, from Jones *et al.* Treatment of primary pulmonary hypertension with intravenous epoprostenol. *Br Heart J* 1987; **57**: 273.)

prognosis; i.e. those with an S$\bar{v}$o$_2$ of less than 63% and who have evidence of right ventricular dysfunction. These patients are generally accepted for heart/lung transplantation[49] but prostacyclin infusion is used to stabilize their condition during the interim period before suitable donor organs are available.

In order to establish long-term infusion, it is necessary to insert a long intravenous cannula which is tunnelled subcutaneously. Besides, patients need educating on the ward for 2 weeks, during which they are taught how to prepare, store, administer and maintain the infusion. The solution is made by dissolving prostacyclin, available as sodium salt of epoprostenol, with sterile glycine buffer. The 20 ml syringe is mounted on the electrically driven pump (MS 16A, Graseby Dynamics, Bushey, Hertfordshire) with an automatic auditory alarm to indicate pump failure. Long-term intravenous administration of prostacyclin, although expensive and somewhat complicated, provides the means to stabilize these critically ill patients with the option of adjusting the dosage according to response.

However, there are problems with long-term use of prostacyclin. Loose stools, jaw pain and photosensitivity are common side effects and have been seen in 100%, 57% and 36% of the patients, respectively.[48] Headache, cutaneous flushing and abdominal pain are also commonly observed, particularly on increasing the dose, but usually settle within 24 hours.[18] One-third of the patients have experienced dyspnoea during heparin flushing of the catheter, which lasts for 15–30 minutes after commencing prostacyclin.[48] This is probably due to dead space created by heparin flush and can be alleviated by ensuring the removal of dead space with prostacyclin. Pump malfunction occasionally poses difficulty, causing interruption of the infusion which may last up to 12 hours. Pulmonary oedema occasionally occurs with prostacyclin.[48] The exact mechanism is not known but it may be due to increased permeability of pulmonary vascular bed. Septicaemia and ascites are other potential problems.[45] In our study, three patients had ascites that was not due to right heart failure because of the exudate nature of the aspirate and was probably due to leakage from peritoneum. One patient developed chylous ascites before death. Thrombophlebitis and transient neurological ischaemic episodes probably due to paradoxical embolisms have also been reported. Return of symptoms such as syncope have been noticed in a few patients on changing the brand of the syringe, probably causing underdosing of prostacyclin. These complications are related either to prostacyclin or to the delivery system. A syncopal episode on interruption of infusion is a serious indicator of the disease and special attention should be paid to ensuring uninterrupted infusion of prostacyclin in these patients. For patients with severe PPH awaiting transplantation, prostacyclin has improved survival in the first 2 years.[50] It is interesting to see that, with prostacyclin, survival also improved for those patients who failed to respond to prostacyclin during right heart catheterization. Therefore it is conceivable that prostacyclin may not function solely due to its vasorelaxant effects but there may be some additional mechanism responsible for improved survival in severe PPH.

It has been observed that dose requirements for prostacyclin increase during long-term use.[48] This is not necessarily due to progression of the disease because further responsiveness is maintained on increased dosage. Patients intolerant to a certain dose tend to tolerate a higher dose subsequently. This indicates that at least some tachyphylaxis exists with long-term use of prostacyclin. Prostacyclin is generally reserved for more seriously ill patients but there remain a small proportion of patients who do not respond to prostacyclin and their condition remains static or continues to deteriorate. For these selected patients the combination of prostacyclin and a nitrovasodilator such as sodium nitroprusside[51] may produce effective pulmonary vasodilation. Nitrovasodilators cause vascular relaxation by providing nitric oxide (NO) to vascular smooth muscle cells where it stimulates guanylate cyclase enzyme and causes a rise in cyclic 3,5-guanosine monophosphate (cGMP). cGMP mediates vascular relaxation by impairing intracellular calcium. Prostacyclin works through different pathways and instead stimulates adenylate cyclase enzyme and is responsible for increased production of cyclic adenosine monophosphate (cAMP)[52] which also facilitates relaxation. It is quite conceivable that, when used together, these agents may produce a more pronounced pulmonary relaxation. The authors have seen this phenomenon in one patient with pulmonary hypertension who was unresponsive to high-dose prostacyclin but showed a dramatic fall in pulmonary vascular resistance after a combination of prostacyclin and nitroprusside was used. In view of the relatively recent understanding of the molecular mechanisms of prostacyclin and nitrovasodilators, there is scope for investigating new pharmacological applications in the management of primary pulmonary hypertension.

Synthetic analogue of prostacyclin

In recent years a prostacyclin analogue called iloprost has emerged as an alternate agent. Prostacyclin, although an effective pulmonary vasodilator, is expensive, labile at room temperature and has to be protected from light. With these drawbacks and in view of the fact that prostacyclin has shown improvement in symptoms and survival, there has been a need for a synthetic analogue that could be more stable and possibly cheaper. Iloprost has a similar molecular structure to prostacyclin and is provided in an ethanol–TRIS–HCl buffered solution.[53] It seems to exert its vasorelaxant effect through prostacyclin receptors.[54] Iloprost has an oral bioavailability of 13%[55] and might be suitable for oral administration once such a preparation is available. Its favourable action on the kidney leads to increased urinary output as it causes a rise in glomerular filtration rate and reduction in sodium and water resorption.[56] It has a slightly greater half-life of 13 minutes after intravenous administration[57] and it remains stable in isotonic solution, at room temperature and when exposed to light. It has been shown to cause improved exercise tolerance[58] in coronary artery disease, probably by improving coronary blood flow.[59] It has been reported to have an antiarrhythmic[60] effect as well as an antiplatelet effect,[58] and has also been shown to prevent hypoxic pulmonary hypertension[61] and inhibit free radical formation in cardiac ischaemia.[62] In humans, iloprost is comparable to prostacyclin in lowering pulmonary vascular resistance in severe primary pulmonary hypertension.[53] A lower dose of iloprost than of prostacyclin was required in order to obtain similar haemodynamic response. Long-term treatment with iloprost also caused improvement in exercise tolerance of PPH patients, an effect that was comparable to that obtained with prostacyclin[63] (Table 14.4), and the side effect profile of the two has also been similar. Iloprost may be useful in the short-term assessment of patients with PPH and might replace prostacyclin in the long-term treatment of PPH.

Prostaglandins in secondary pulmonary hypertension

Although the role of prostacyclin in the treatment of primary pulmonary hypertension is being established, this agent may also be used at least as an

Table 14.4 Comparable improvement with prostacyclin and with iloprost on exercise tolerance (12 minutes' walk) in patients with PPH

	Inclusion (Baseline)	Prostacyclin	Iloprost
Distance (m)	463 ± 43	640 ± 25**	653 ± 38**
Rest time (s)	197 ± 127	0**	50 ± 41*
▲SaO$_2$ (%)	16 ± 9	5 ± 3*	3 ± 1**
▲HR (min^{-1})	45 ± 6	39 ± 3 NS	31 ± 4 NS

*$p<0.05$; **$p<0.01$.
▲HR (min^{-1}), increase in heart rate per minute; ▲SaO$_2$ (%), arterial oxygen desaturation.
(Reproduced, with permission, from Dinh-Xuan *et al.* Effects of long-term treatment with iloprost, a prostacyclin analogue, on exercise tolerance in patients with primary pulmonary hypertension. *Am Rev Respir Dis* 1990; **141**: A889.)

investigational agent in secondary pulmonary hypertension. The authors have demonstrated pulmonary vasodilatation in response to prostacyclin in chronic obstructive pulmonary disease and pulmonary fibrosis due to sarcoidosis.[44] In these situations, by overcoming hypoxic pulmonary vasoconstriction, ventilation/perfusion imbalance may deteriorate, leading to increased arterial desaturation. However, it has been argued that tissue oxygen delivery may be more important than actual Pao_2,[64] and oxygen delivery is likely to improve in these patients, primarily because of increased cardiac output. Naeije *et al.* have demonstrated improved haemodynamics and pulmonary gas exchange with intravenous prostaglandin E_1 (PGE$_1$) in secondary pulmonary hypertension due to decompensated chronic obstructive pulmonary disease (COPD) (Table 14.5) and have hypothesized that pulmonary vascular tone may be preserved due to adaptation to hypoxia.[65] Therefore, the ventilation/perfusion ratio may not be adversely affected provided an appropriate dose is used in selected patients. Hence there is a potential role for long-term vasodilator therapy in some patients with secondary pulmonary hypertension due to chronic hypoxic lung disease. An oral preparation of a phosphodiesterase inhibitor may provide that role[66] but, before embarking upon such a treatment, it is essential to assess individual response to acute vasodilator challenge.

Prostacyclin can be used effectively in perfusing the combined heart and lung grafts before transplantation to ensure satisfactory graft function postoperatively.[67] It is also conceivable that prostacyclin might play a useful role in improving postoperative

Table 14.5 Mean ± SEM gasometric and haemodynamic measurements before and at 13 minutes of PGE_1 infusion 0.02 µg/kg per minute in 10 patients with secondary pulmonary hypertension due to COPD

	Baseline	PGE_1	p
CI (l/m^2 per min)	3.9 ± 0.3	4.5 ± 0.3	<0.001
HR (beats/min)	110 ± 7	116 ± 7	<0.01
RAM (mmHg)	6 ± 3	5 ± 1	NS
MAP (mmHg)	88 ± 6	82 ± 7	<0.05
SVR (dyn/(s/cm^{-5}))	1082 ± 107	814 ± 131	<0.001
PAM (mmHg)	48 ± 5	38 ± 4	<0.001
PVR (dyn/(s/cm^{-5}))	532 ± 65	368 ± 51	<0.001
Pao$_2$ (mmHg)	38 ± 3	37 ± 2	NS
Pvo$_2$ (mmHg)	26 ± 3	27 ± 2	NS
C(av)o$_2$ (ml/dl)	4.6 ± 0.3	3.9 ± 0.3	<0.01
To$_2$ (ml/m^2 per min)	586 ± 61	657 ± 56	<0.001

C(av)o$_2$, arteriovenous O_2 content difference; CI, cardiac index; HR, heart rate; MAP, mean systemic arterial pressure; NS, not significant; PAM, pulmonary artery mean pressure; Pao$_2$, arterial Po$_2$; Pvo$_2$, mixed venous Po$_2$; PVR, pulmonary vascular resistance; RAM, right atrial mean pressure; SVR, systemic vascular resistance; To$_2$, tissue O_2 delivery.
(Adapted, with permission, from Naeije *et al.* Reduction in pulmonary hypertension by prostaglandin E_1 in decompensated chronic obstructive pulmonary disease. *Am Rev Respir Dis* 1982; **125**: 2.)

morbidity and mortality in recipients of heart transplantation. These patients are likely to have developed pulmonary hypertension due to severe left ventricular failure. Right ventricular function of the donor organ is an important prognostic parameter in the early postoperative period. A vasodilator, such as prostacyclin, which could effectively lower pulmonary vascular resistance should have a beneficial effect on morbidity and mortality in these patients.

Conclusions

PPH is a disease with a fearful prognosis and its exact pathogenesis remains unknown. Patients with pulmonary artery oxygen saturation of more than 63% may be treated with anticoagulants and calcium channel blockers. Those patients with pulmonary artery oxygen saturation of less than 63% and right ventricular dysfunction may be considered for heart/lung or single lung[49,68,69] transplantation but before a suitable donor is available they can be treated with

intravenous prostacyclin, which has improved survival for these severely ill patients.[50] Improved survival in those patients who did not show any pulmonary vasorelaxant response to prostacyclin during RHC indicates that this agent, apart from its vasodilatory effects, may affect some additional mechanism that influences this disease. Further studies are needed to explore that mechanism and also to look for new pharmacological approaches to treat primary pulmonary hypertension. Prostacyclin may be used as an investigational agent in secondary pulmonary hypertension before considering long-term vasodilator therapy.

References

1. Rich S, Dantzker DR, Ayres SM, *et al.* Primary pulmonary hypertension. A national prospective study. *Ann Intern Med* 1987; **107**: 216–23.
2. Voelkel NF, Reeves JT. Primary pulmonary hypertension. In: Mosesr KM (ed), *Pulmonary Vascular Diseases*. New York: Marcel Dekker, 1979: 573–628.
3. Fuster V, Steele PM, Edwards WD, Gersh BJ, McGoon MD, Frye RL. Primary pulmonary hypertension: natural history and the importance of thrombosis. *Circulation* 1984; **70**: 580–7.
4. Romberg E. Uber Sklerose der Lungenarterien. *Dtsch Arch Klin Med* 1891; **48**: 197.
5. Dresdale DT, Schultz M, Michtom RJ. Primary pulmonary hypertension. 1. Clinical and hemodynamic study. *Am J Med* 1951; **11**: 686–705.
6. Weir EK. Diagnosis and management of primary pulmonary hypertension. In: Weir EK, Reeves JT (eds), *Pulmonary Hypertension*. New York: Futura, 1984: 115–68.
7. Hatano S, Strasser T (eds), *Primary Pulmonary Hypertension*. Geneva: World Health Organization 1975: 7–45.
8. Wagenvoort CA, Wagenvoort N. Primary pulmonary hypertension: a pathologic study on the lung vessels in 156 clinically diagnosed cases. *Circulation* 1970; **42**: 1163–84.
9. Heath D, Smith P. Gosney J, *et al.* The pathology of the early and late stages of primary pulmonary hypertension. *Br Heart J* 1987; **58**: 204–13.
10. Giuseppe G, Pietra MD, William D, *et al.* Histopathology of primary pulmonary hypertension. *Circulation* 1989; **80**: 1198–206.
11. Asherson RA, Mockworth-Young CG, Boey RG, *et al.* Pulmonary hypertension in systemic lupus erythematosus. *BMJ* 1983; **287**: 1024–5.
12. Anderson NE, Ali MR. The lupus anticoagulant, pulmonary thromboembolus and fatal pulmonary hypertension. *Ann Rheum Dis* 1984; **43**: 760–3.
13. Harris EN, Gharavi AE, Boey RG. Anti-platelet anti-

bodies: detection by radio-immunoassay and association with thrombosis in lupus erythematosis. *Lancet* 1983; **2**: 1211–14.

14. Cerreras LO, Defreyn G, Machin SJ. Arterial thrombosis, intra-uterine death and 'lupus' anticoagulant: detection of immuno-globulin interfering with prostacyclin formation. *Lancet* 1981; **1**: 244–6.

15. McVerry BA, Machin SJ, Perry H, Goldstone AA. Reduced prostacyclin activity in systemic lupus erythematosus. *Ann Rheum Dis* 1980; **39**: 524–5.

16. Lanham JG, Levin M, Brown M, Gharavi AE, Thomas PA, Hanson GC. Prostacyclin deficiency in a young woman with recurrent thrombosis. *BMJ* 1986; **292**: 435–6.

17. Czer GT, March J, Kanopka R, Moser KM. Low-dose PGI_2 prevents monocrotaline-induced thromboxane production and lung injury. *J Appl Physiol* 1986; **60**: 464–71.

18. Higenbottam T. The place of prostacyclin in the clinical management of primary pulmonary hypertension. *Am Rev Respir Dis* 1987; **136**: 782–5.

19. Loyd JE, Primm RK, Newman JH. Familial primary pulmonary hypertension: clinical patterns. *Am Rev Respir Dis* 1984; **129**: 194–7.

20. Eigeberg O. Inherited antithrombin deficiency causing thrombophilia. *Thromb Diathesis Haemorrhag* 1965; **13**: 516–30.

21. Gurtner HP. Aminorex and pulmonary hypertension. *Cor Vasa* 1985; **27**: 160–71.

22. Douglas JG, Munro JF, Kitchin AH, Muir AL, Proudfoot AT. Pulmonary hypertension and fenfluramine. *BMJ* 1981; **283**: 881–3.

23. Wallcott G, Burchell HB, Brown AL. Primary pulmonary hypertension. *Am J Med* 1970; **49**: 70–9.

24. Hughes JD, Rubin LJ. Primary pulmonary hypertension. An analysis of 28 cases and a review of the literature. *Medicine* 1986; **65**: 65–72.

25. D'Alonzo GE, Barst RJ, Ayres SM, *et al.* Survival in patients with primary pulmonary hypertension. *Ann Intern Med* 1991; **115**: 343–9.

26. Morice AH, Pepke-Zaba J, Brown MJ, Thomas PS, Higenbottam TW. Atrial natriuretic peptide in primary pulmonary hypertension. *Eur Respir J* 1990; **3**: 910–13.

27. Rawson AJ, Woske HM. A study of etiologic factors in so-called primary pulmonary hypertension. *Arch Intern Med* 1960; **105**: 233–43.

28. Goodman J, Harrison DC, Popp RL. Echocardiographic features of primary pulmonary hypertension. *Am J Cardiol* 1974; **33**: 438–43.

29. Visner MS, Arentzen CE, Crumbley AS, *et al.* The effects of pressure-induced right ventricular hypertrophy on left ventricular diastolic properties and dynamic geometry in the conscious dog. *Circulation* 1986; **74**: 410–19.

30. King ME, Braun H, Goldblatt A, *et al.* Interventricular septal configuration as a predictor of right ventricular systolic hypertension in children: a cross-sectional echocardiographic study. *Circulation* 1983; **68**: 68–75.

31. Hull RD, Raskob GE, Heish J. The diagnosis of clinically suspected pulmonary embolism. Practical approaches. *Chest* 1986; **89** (suppl): 417–25.

32. Moser KM, Spragg RG, Utley J, Daily PO. Chronic thrombotic obstruction of major pulmonary arteries. Results of thromboendarterectomy in 15 patients. *Ann Intern Med* 1983; **99**: 299–305.

33. Wilson AG, Harris CN, Lavender JP, Oakley CM. Perfusion lung scanning in obliterative pulmonary hypertension. *Br Heart J* 1973; **35**: 917–30.

34. Reeves JT, Groves BM, Turkevich D. The case for treatment of selected patients with primary pulmonary hypertension. *Am Rev Respir Dis* 1986; **134**: 342–6.

35. Oakley CM. Management of primary pulmonary hypertension. *Br Heart J* 1985; **53**: 1–4.

36. Rich S, Brundage BH. The pharmacologic treatment of primary pulmonary hypertension. In: Bergofsky EH (ed), *Abnormal Pulmonary Circulation*. New York: Churchill Livingstone, 1986: 281–311.

37. Rich S, Martinez J, Lam W, Rosen KM. Captopril as treatment for patients with pulmonary hypertension: problem of variability in assessing chronic drug treatment. *Br Heart J* 1982; **48**: 272–7.

38. Hermiller JB, Bambach D, Thompson MJ, *et al.* Vasodilators and prostaglandin inhibitors in primary pulmonary hypertension. *Ann Intern Med* 1982; **97**: 470–89.

39. Camerini F, Alberti E, Klugmann S, Salvi A. Primary pulmonary hypertension: effects of nifedipine. *Br Heart J* 1980; **44**: 352–6.

40. Roskovec A, Stardling JR, Shepherd G, *et al.* Prediction of favourable response to long term vasodilation of pulmonary hypertension by short term administration of epoprostenol (prostacyclin) or nifedipine. *Br Heart J* 1988; **59**: 696–705.

41. Rich S, Brundage BH. High-dose calcium channel-blocking therapy for primary pulmonary hypertension: evidence for long-term reduction in pulmonary arterial pressure and regression of right ventricular hypertrophy. *Circulation* 1987: **76**: 135–41.

42. Watkins WD, Peterson MB, Crone RK, Shannon DC, Levine L. Prostacyclin and prostaglandin E_1 for severe idiopathic pulmonary artery hypertension. [Letter] *Lancet* 1980; **1**: 1083.

43. Guadagni DN, Ikram H, Maslowski AH. Haemodynamic effects of prostacyclin (PGI_2) in pulmonary hypertension. *Br Heart J* 1981; **45**: 385–8.

44. Jones DK, Higenbottam TW, Wallwork J. Pulmonary vasodilation with prostacyclin in primary and secondary pulmonary hypertension. *Chest* 1989; **96**: 784–9.

45. Jones DK, Higenbottam TW, Wallwork J. Treatment of primary pulmonary hypertension with intravenous epoprostenol (prostacyclin). *Br Heart J* 1987; **57**: 270–8.

46. Reeves JT, Groves BM, Turkevich D. The case for treatment of selected patients with primary pulmonary hypertension. *Am Rev Respir Dis* 1986; **134**: 342–6.

47. Higenbottam TW, Wheeldon D, Wells F, Wallwork J. Long-term treatment of primary pulmonary hypertension with continuous intravenous epoprostenol (prostacyclin). *Lancet* 1984; **1**: 1046–7.

48. Rubin LJ, Mendoza J, Hood M, *et al.* Treatment of primary pulmonary hypertension with continuous intravenous prostacyclin (epoprostenol). *Ann Intern Med* 1990; **112**: 485–91.

49. Reitz BA, Wallwork JL, Hunt SA, *et al.* Heart–lung transplantation: successful therapy for patients with pulmonary vascular disease. *N Engl J Med* 1982; **306**: 557–64.

50. Cremona G, Higenbottam TW, Scott JP. Continuous intravenous infusion of prostacyclin (PGI$_2$) improves survival in primary pulmonary hypertension. [Abstract] *Am Rev Resp Dis* 1991; **143**: A180.

51. Fuleihan DS, Mookherjee S, Potts JL, Obeid AI, Warner RA, Eich RH. Sodium nitroprusside: a new role as a pulmonary vasodilator. [Abstract] *Am J Cardiol* 1979; **43**: 405.

52. Moncada S, Palmer RMJ, Higgs EA. Prostacyclin and endothelium-derived relaxing factor: biological interactions and significance. In: Verstraete M, Vermylen J, Lijnen HR, Arnout J (eds), *Thrombosis and Haemostasis*. Leuven: Leuven University Press, 1987: 597–618.

53. Scott JP, Higenbottam TW, Wallwork J. The acute effect of the synthetic prostacyclin analogue iloprost in primary pulmonary hypertension. *Br J Clin Pharmacol* 1990; **6**: 231–4.

54. Schror K, Darius H, Matzky R, Ohlendorf R. The anti-platelet and cardiovascular actions of a new carbacyclin derivative (ZK36374) – equipotent to PGI$_2$ *in vitro*. *Arch Pharmacol* 1981; **316**: 252–5.

55. Krause W, Humpel M, Hoyer GA. Biotransformation of the stable prostacyclin analogue, iloprost, in the rat. *Drug Metab Dispos* 1984; **12**: 645–51.

56. Yitalo P, Kaukinen S, Nunni A-K, Seppala E, Pessi T, Vapaatala H. Effects of a prostacyclin analog iloprost on kidney function, renin–angiotensin and kallikrein–kinin systems, prostanoids and catecholamines in man. *Prostaglandins* 1985; **29**: 1063–71.

57. Kaukinen S, Ylitalo P, Pessi T, Vapaatalo H. Hemodynamic effects of iloprost, a prostacyclin analog. *Clin Pharmacol Ther* 1984; **36**: 464–9.

58. Bugiardini R, Galvani M, Ferrini D, *et al.* Effects of iloprost, a stable prostacyclin analog, on exercise capacity and platelet aggregation in stable angina pectoris. *Am J Cardiol* 1986; **58**: 453–9.

59. Uchida Y, Murao S. Effects of prostaglandin 12 analogue, ZK 36374, on recurring reduction of coronary blood flow. *Jpn Heart J* 1983; **24** (4): 641–7.

60. Coker SK, Parrat JR. Prostacyclin – antiarrhythmic or arrhythmogenic? Comparison of the effects of intravenous and intracoronary prostacyclin and ZK 36374 during coronary arterial occlusion and reperfusion in anaesthetised greyhounds. *J Cardiovasc Pharmacol* 1983; **5** (5): 557–67.

61. Archer SL, Chesler E, Cohn JN, Weir EK. ZK 36–374. A stable analog of prostacyclin prevents acute hypoxic pulmonary hypertension in the dog. *J Am Cardiol* 1986; **8**: 1189–94.

62. Thiemermann C, Steinhagen-Theissen E, Schor K. Inhibition of oxygen-centred free radical formation by the stable prostacyclin-mimetic iloprost (ZK 36374) in acute myocardial ischaemia. *J Cardiovasc Pharmacol* 1984; **6** (2): 365–6.

63. Dinh Xuan AT, Higenbottam TW, Scott JP, *et al.* Effects of long-term treatment with iloprost, a prostacyclin analogue, on exercise tolerance in patients with primary pulmonary hypertension. *Am Rev Respir Dis* 1990; **141**: A889.

64. Bergofsky EH. Tissue oxygen delivery and corpulmonale in chronic obstructive pulmonary disease. *N Engl J Med* 1983; **308**: 1092–4.

65. Naeije R, Melot C, Mols P, *et al.* Reduction in pulmonary hypertension by prostaglandin E$_1$ in decompensated chronic obstructive pulmonary disease. *Am Rev Respir Dis* 1982; **125**: 1–5.

66. Butt AY, Higenbottam TW, Pepke-Zaba J, *et al.* In vitro pulmonary vasorelaxant effect of the phosphodiesterase inhibitor enoximone. *Angiology* 1993; in press.

67. Hakim M, Higenbottam TW, Bethune D, *et al.* Selection and procurement of combined heart and lung grafts for transplantation. *J Thorac Cardiovasc Surg* 1988; **98**: 474–9.

68. Uren NG, Oakley CM. The treatment of primary pulmonary hypertension. *Br Heart J* 1991; **66**: 119–21.

69. Higenbottam T. Single lung transplantation and pulmonary hypertension. *Br Heart J* 1992; **67**: 121.

15 Prostaglandins in ischaemic peripheral vascular disease

Helmut Sinzinger

Atherosclerosis and its clinical manifestations in the peripheral arteries are a major health problem in industrialized countries. The major risk factors are smoking, hypercholesterolaemia, diabetes and hypertension. Dependent on their prevalence, the incidence of ischaemic peripheral vascular disease (PVD) shows considerable variation. Although no exact epidemiological figures are available as to prevalence and incidence of PVD, the incidence of clinically manifest PVD in people above the age of 50 exceeds 5%, showing a rapid further age-dependent increase.[1] Progressive deterioration that further restricts the arterial blood supply may lead, through the stage of intermittent claudication, to rest pain and trophic lesions such as ulceration and gangrene.[2] The final consequence may be critical limb ischaemia (persistently recurrent ischaemic rest pain requiring regular analgesia for more than 2 weeks) with an ankle systolic pressure ≤ of 50 mmHg and/or a toe systolic pressure of ≤ 30 mmHg, or ulceration or gangrene of the feet or toes with an ankle systolic pressure of ≤ 50 mmHg or a toe systolic pressure of ≤ 30 mmHg[3] with imminent amputation. The prognosis is very poor. Even at specialized centres only about half of such patients were alive and with both legs intact after 1 year,[4] while one-quarter had undergone amputation and another quarter had died. The underlying mechanisms of the disease and the associated impaired interaction between the vascular wall and blood components are heterogeneous in nature and have been outlined in a recent consensus document.[5] The therapeutic management of these patients continues to be a clinical problem.

Stages I–IV (Fontaine) comprise a widely accepted clinical nomenclature in central Europe; four stages are described:

stage I: no palpable pulses, without any other symptoms
stage II: intermittent claudication
stage III: rest pain
stage IV: ischaemic trophic skin changes

Regardless of the stage of PVD, the primary therapeutic aim is to avoid risk factors and attempt to delay the progression of the disease. In intermittent claudication, walking therapy is the treatment of choice together with adjuvant pharmacotherapy if lumen-opening procedures are not indicated. In stage III/IV (critical limb ischaemia), revascularizing procedures (vascular surgery, angioplasty and thrombolysis) may be indicated; there are a number of patients, however, in whom these interventions cannot be performed or have already failed.

Following the discovery and structural identification of prostaglandin E₁ (PGE₁), Carlson and Eriksson reported on ulcer healing and rest pain relief in four patients with PVD who were infused intra-arterially with PGE₁ (1 ng/kg per hour) for 1–3 days.[6] As some improvement was seen after intra-arterial infusion in the contralateral leg as well, a systemic effect of the compound was claimed. A few years later the same authors reported benefit in eight patients receiving a 3-day continuous intravenous infusion of PGE_1. As PGE_1 is metabolized extensively (60–85%) during a single passage through the pulmonary circulation,[7] this finding of benefit in the non-infused leg after intra-arterial therapy and the benefit of intravenous application remained unexplained until recently (see later). In an uncontrolled study, Szczeklik et al.[8] infused 5–10 ng PGI_2/kg per minute continuously intra-arterially for 3 days. They reported disappearance of rest pain as early as on day 2 and on ulcer healing in three patients within 2 months. The other patients exhibited clear improvement, and planned amputation was postponed. The antiaggregatory capacity of PGI_2 and PGE_1 together with the finding of diminished formation of vascular PGI_2 in atherosclerotic[9] vascular segments suggested the hypothesis of prostaglandins as exogenous substitution therapy[8] for an endogenous deficiency.

A great many uncontrolled studies were performed thereafter, mostly because of the ethical difficulty of having a placebo group of patients with critical limb ischaemia. However, clinical trial design, such as the stage of the disease, route of administration, daily and total dose and duration of treatment were selected based on hypothetical concepts only. Choosing different endpoints as a consequence of different disease states further hampered the assessment of the therapeutic potential of this family of compounds. A 3-day regimen of continuous administration was quite common in earlier studies. Extending this to more than 7 days resulted in a rebound phenomenon at cellular (platelet) level, resulting in desensitization, although this was discovered more by accident than by systemic search.[10] This down-regulation at receptor level as a consequence of exogenous substitution has since been proven for both PGI_2[11] and PGE_1[12] as well as for their synthetic analogues.[13] In order to avoid the potential clinical consequences of activated haemostasis, intermittent[14] rather than continuous treatment schemes were introduced and became generally accepted.

It is the aim of this chapter to review only the clinical studies performed on a controlled basis in patients suffering from PVD and thereby to assess the value of therapy with prostaglandins. This is mainly because the high placebo response rate (up to 50%) in this condition makes it very difficult to assess the results of uncontrolled treatment.[15] The data available are grouped according to the substance used and the route of administration. Some controlled studies concerned primarily with pharmacological measurements are discussed, but not listed in the tables.

Table 15.1   Controlled studies with intra-arterial PGE_1 in PVD stages II–IV

Author	Design	n	Dose	Duration	Fontaine stage	Endpoint	Results (S/NS)
Sakaguchi, 1984[16]	C* DB	65	0.05 ng/kg per min 0.15 ng/kg per min	24 d	III/IV	UH	UH (S) PR (S) with higher dose
Blume, 1987[55]	PC DB	50	10–20 µg/90 min	21 d	IIb	Walking	PW (S)
Creutzig et al., 1987[56]	C†	30	2 × 5 µg/50 min	17 d	IIb	Walking	(S)
Creutzig et al., 1988[57]	C† DB	40	2 × 5 µg/50 min	21 d	IIb	Walking	PW (NS)
Rudofsky et al, 1987[58]	PC DB	50	20 µg/120 min	21 d	IIb	Walking	PW (S)
Trübestein et al., 1987[59]	C‡	57	20 µg/60 min	21 d	III/IV	Analgesics UH Amputation	(S) (S) (S)
Böhme et al., 1989[17]	C‡	34	10–20 µg/60 min	23 d	III/IV	Stage UH LR	(NS) (NS) (S)

*vs niacinate; †vs nucleotide-nucleoside mixture; ‡vs ATP.
NS, not significant; S, significant.
C, controlled; DB, double-blind; LR, long-term results; PC, placebo-controlled; PR, pain reduction; PW, pain-free walking; UH, ulcer healing.

Table 15.2   Controlled studies with intravenous PGE$_1$ in PVD stages II–IV

Author	Design	n	Dose	Duration	Follow-up	Fontaine stage	Endpoint	Results (S/NS)
Short studies								
Telles *et al*, 1984[40]	PC DB	30	10 ng/kg per min continuous	3 d		IV		RP (NS) UH (NS)
Jogestrand & Olsson, 1985[41]	C cross-over	16	ca.3 ng/kg per min continuous	3 d		IV		RP (NS) UH (NS)
Schuler *et al.*, 1984[19]	PC DB	123	20 ng/kg per min continuous	3 d		IV		RP (NS) UH (NS)
Eklund *et al.*, 1982[39]	PC DB	22	7 × 20 µg/d	3 d		IV		UH (NS) Negative late results
Long-term studies								
Diehm *et al.*, 1988[60]	PC DB	46	1 × 60 µg/d	21 d		III	Analgesics. PR stage	(S) (S) (S)
Rudofsky, 1988[61]	PC DB	50	1 × 60 µg/d	28 d		IIb	Walking	PW (S)
Trübestein *et al.*, 1989[62]	C*	70	2 × 40 µg/d	28 d	(S)	IV	UH	PR (NS) Analg. (S) UH (S)
Diehm *et al.*, 1989[63]	C†	48	1 × 60 µg/d	21 d		IIb	Walking	PW (NS) Positive LR (S)
Hepp *et al.*, 1991[64]	C*	195	2 × 40 µg/d	28 d		IIb	Walking	(S)

*vs pentoxifylline; †vs naftidrofuryl.
NS, not significant; S, significant.
C, controlled; DB, double-blind; LR, long-term results; PC, placebo-controlled; PR, pain reduction; PW, pain-free walking; RP, rest pain; UH, ulcer healing.

Results of trials with PGE$_1$ and PGI$_2$

PGE$_1$ (Tables 15.1 and 15.2)

The initial choice of continuous intra-arterial treatment[16] was technically difficult and associated with frequent local complications. However, in this multicentre, randomized, controlled, double-blind study, the patients treated for an average of 24 days showed ulcer healing in 27% and pain relief in 82%. The other studies (Tables 15.1 and 15.2), in contrast, used discontinuous administration in a dose of 5–20 µg over 1 or 2 hours for 3–4 weeks.

PGE$_1$ was compared with placebo in two studies that included patients with less severe disease. Other studies compared PGE$_1$ with intra-arterial adenosine triphosphate or a nucleotide–nucleoside mixture. These studies revealed significant benefits, as compared to controls, on rest pain, consumption of analgesic, ulcer healing, amputation rate and walking distance, the benefits lasting up to 12 months or more. Böhme *et al.*[17] observed that 39% of patients improved from stage III/IV to II and a 78% improvement in ulceration. These changes were not significantly different from the control group, though long-term improvement was significantly better in PGE$_1$-treated patients.

Intravenous administration of PGE$_1$ was initially studied over a relatively short period of 3 days (upper part of Table 15.2). These studies did not result in a significant benefit for the patient. In contrast, however, use of intermittent PGE$_1$ therapy over a longer period of 3–4 weeks (lower part of Table 15.2) resulted in significant benefits in all four studies. Of these, two were in comparison with placebo and the others in comparison with naftidrofuryl and pentoxifylline (oxpentifylline). The majority of the studies resulted in reduced analgesic consumption and in pain relief. The paper by Rhodes and Heard[18] is not listed in Table 15.2 because the data

($n=8$) are part of the results ($n=123$) described by Schuler *et al.*[19] The former reported that in eight patients treated for 3 days only, no pain relief was obtained and even an increase in ulcer size occurred. The uncontrolled studies performed especially with PGE_1 are so numerous, and the infusion scheme (route, dose, titration, duration, endpoints, follow-up, etc.) varies to such an extent, that the large amount of information produced does not allow any concise conclusion.

Prostacyclin (PGI_2)

Controlled studies with prostacyclin have been few. As they were performed between 1980 and 1987, the substance was continuously administered intra-arterially for a relatively short time, except in the studies by Cronenwett,[20] Karnik *et al.*[21] and Virgolini *et al.*,[22] and the last two used intermittent intravenous administration (Table 15.3). The findings for two of the five studies were positive, data being available for stage II and critical limb ischaemia as well. The largest double-blind trial published so far[22] randomly allocated 108 patients to receive either prostacyclin (6 ng/kg per minute over 8 hours daily for 5 consecutive days) or placebo. After 1 month, 44% (24 out of 54) of the prostacyclin-treated and 15% (8 out of 54) of the placebo-treated patients responded positively to treatment. Patients receiving prostacyclin showed significant ($p<0.01$)

prolongation of absolute and relative walking times, as compared to placebo-treated patients up to the second follow-up month. In the open-label study[23] which followed the double-blind trial, 44% of the patients receiving prostacyclin responded favourably (>20% improvement in walking); of the non-responders in the controlled segment of the trial, 31% showed improvement. Interestingly, when improvement occurred, it was generally sustained for at least 2 months. Two other placebo-controlled studies[24,25] were designed primarily to examine aspects of clinical pharmacology. Although treatment and follow-up were short (7 days), the authors achieved positive ($p<0.05$) findings in terms of pain relief and ulcer healing.

The early studies with PGI_2 were criticized because they were performed in an open fashion.[8,26–28] The basic dose regimen, moreover, was in sharp contrast to the one that is favoured today – i.e. intermittent rather than continuous, long-term rather than short-term, intravenous instead of intra-arterial and low-dose instead of high-dose. This may explain the poor clinical outcome of those early trials as compared to those with the stable analogue iloprost or with PGE_1.

In all the studies (Table 15.3) the dose of prostacyclin was above 5 ng/kg per minute, and facial flushing was encountered in more than 25% of patients, so limiting the extent to which they were truly double-blind.

Table 15.3 Controlled studies with prostacyclin in patients with PVD stages II–IV

Author	Design	n	Dose	Duration	Follow-up	Fontaine stage	Endpoint	Results (S/NS)
Belch *et al.*, 1983[65]	DB	28	2.5–10 ng/kg per min	96 h i.a.	6 m	III	PR	PR (S)
Nizankowski *et al.*, 1985[66]	DB	30	5 ng/kg per min	72 h	6 w	III/IV	UH PR	NM PR
Negus *et al.*, 1985[67]	C*	33	6–8 ng/kg per min	72 h i.a.	4 y	III/IV	UH PR	UH (NS) PR
Cronenwett, 1986[20]	DB, PC	26	6 ng/kg per min	72 h i.v.	6 m	III/IV	UH PR	UH (NS) PR (NS)
Karnik *et al*, 1987[21]	C†	20	5 ng/kg per min × 10 h	5 d i.v.	4 w	III/IV	UH PR	UH (NS) PR (NS)
Virgolini *et al.*, 1990[22]	DB, PC	108	6 ng/kg per min × 8 h	5 d i.v.	4–11 m	II	PW	(S)

*no difference from Praxilene (naftidrofuryl).
†vs naftidrofuryl.
NS, not significant; S, significant.
C, controlled; DB, double-blind; i.a., intra-arterial; i.v., intravenous; NM, not mentioned; PC, placebo-controlled; PR, pain reduction; PW, pain-free walking; UH, ulcer healing.

Stable prostaglandin analogues

Chiesa *et al.*[29] first reported clinical benefit with ilo-prost in a diabetic patient in whom amputation was avoided.

Iloprost

Six controlled studies with iloprost given over 2–4 weeks in a total of 728 patients are available (Table 15.4). Significant improvement was reported for pain relief, ulcer healing and amputation rate.

In a randomized multicentre study in 133 patients suffering from Buerger's disease (thromboangiitis obliterans) iloprost and aspirin (100 mg) were compared.[30] Iloprost was administered at 0.5–2 ng/kg per minute (maximum tolerable dose) for 6 hours a day for 28 days. At the end of treatment the findings were significantly in favour of iloprost (pain relief 63% vs 28%, complete ulcer healing 35% vs 13%). After 6 months the response rate was 88% vs 21%. In a randomized, placebo-controlled cross-over study, aimed essentially to examine clinical pharmacology, 10 patients with stage III/IV, receiving 0.8–2.5 ng/kg per minute over 12 hours for 1 week, showed a significant reduction in rest pain. In contrast to the improvement normally seen in such patients in response to placebo, a deterioration in the placebo group of patients was observed.[25]

Taprostene (CG-4203)

In a randomized double-blind study in 30 patients with stage II disease,[31] taprostene 25 ng/kg per minute was given for 6 hours a day for 5 days. Two months after the end of therapy the absolute walking distance, as determined by treadmill testing, was increased by 12% over placebo ($p<0.01$) and the pain-free walking distance by 7% over placebo ($p<0.01$).

In general, side effects were significantly higher in patients treated with the intra-arterial as compared to the intravenous route of administration. Intra-arterial application may be associated with local complications at the puncture site (haematoma, bleeding, swelling, redness, pain, aneurysm) and, rarely, embolism. General symptoms after PGE_1 include gastrointestinal symptoms (5%) and headache (2%). Changes in blood pressure and heart rate occur in less than 1%. The usual dose of 40 µg PGE_1 over 2 hours (i.e. about 5 ng/kg per minute) does not significantly change blood pressure and heart rate. Whilst such low doses do improve the microcirculation, myocardial contractility and blood pressure are affected only at doses higher than 20 ng/kg per minute. Both PGE_1 and PGI_2 increase left ventricular ejection fraction, and this effect may start at therapeutic doses.[17] Intravenous infusion may cause a phlebitis-like redness at the infusion site (7%). This redness disappears immediately after therapy and does not reflect a true phlebitis.[55] Due to differences in dosing, a comparison of incidence and severity of

Table 15.4   Controlled studies with iloprost administered intravenously in PVD stages III–IV

Author	Design	n	Dose	Duration	Follow-up	Fontaine stage	Endpoint	Results (S/NS)
Brock *et al.*, 1990[68]	PC, MC DB	109	0.5–2 ng/kg per min* × 6 h	28 d	—	IV	UH Pain	UH (S) PR (NS)
Balzer *et al.*, 1987[69]	PC, MC DB	112	0.5–2 ng/kg per min* × 6 h	14 d	—	III	Pain	PR (S) Doppler (NS)
Diehm *et al.*, 1989[63]	PC, MC DB	99	0.5–2 ng/kg per min* × 6 h	28 d	6 m	IV	UH	UH (S)
Bliss *et al*, 1991[70]	PC, MC DB	151	0.5–2 ng/kg per min* × 6 h	14 d 28 d	6 m	III/IV	UH	UH (S) Amputation (S)
Norgren *et al*, 1990[71]	PC, MC DB	103	0.5–2 ng/kg per min* × 6 h	14 d	6 m	IV	UH	UH (NS)
Guilmot *et al.*, 1991[72]	PC	128	0.5–2 ng/kg per min* × 6 h	21 d	4 m	III/IV	UH Pain	PR (S) UH (NS)

*dose titration, highest individually tolerated dose was administered (0.5 ng/kg per minute incremental dose).
NS, not significant; S, significant.
DB, double-blind; MC, multicentre; PC, placebo-controlled; PR, pain reduction; UH, ulcer healing.

side effects is impossible. Whilst prostacyclin at a rate of 3 ng/kg per minute i.v. causes almost no side effects, further increase results in typical vasodilation-related effects such as facial flushing and headache. The unique 'jaw pains', especially during gum chewing, have been reported so far only for PGI_2 and not for PGE_1 or iloprost. The side effects of iloprost, a stable analogue, are very similar, the dose 1 ng/kg per minute being comparable (concerning side effects) to 3 ng/kg per minute of prostacyclin.

Local therapy with prostaglandins

The local treatment of arterial ulcers with PGI_2 (dissolved in albumin), PGE_1 (in albumin and ointment) as well as with OP-1206 and iloprost (in ointment) has been attempted in uncontrolled studies, with equivocal results. No data on controlled studies, however, are available so far, although one multicentre trial (using iloprost) is in progress.

Comment

Endogenous prostaglandins affect haemostasis. The antiplatelet and vasodilator actions[32] and the concept of exogenously substituting an endogenous deficiency[9] served as an early rationale[8,28] for clinical trials. It is well accepted now that either PGE_1 or PGI_2 (as well as their synthetic analogues) has a wide spectrum of anti-atherosclerotic actions.[33-36] These include beneficial effects (for review, see 33, 37) on thromboresistance, endothelial stabilization, neutrophils, monocytes, fibrinolysis, haemorrheology, vascular lipid metabolism, smooth muscle cell proliferation and extracellular matrix generation including inhibition of mitogen release[36,38] among others. One beneficial action of E-compounds on white blood cell function seems not to be shared by the I-compounds.[35] Nevertheless, the relevant actions underlying the proven clinical efficacy have not been identified. The continuous infusion scheme which was favoured in early trials has been abandoned after the finding that these compounds cause a 'rebound phenomenon'[10] as a result of desensitization at receptor level.[13] Furthermore, a treatment lasting for only a few days has been identified as being too short. For example, comparison of the negative results obtained by Eklund *et al.*,[39] Schuler,[19] Telles *et al.*[40] and Jogestrand and Olsson[41] with PGE_1 and early results with PGI_2 explain the more recent 2- to 4-week therapy. The longer the

treatment, the better have been the results.[30,42,55,56] Daily infusions lasting 2–8 hours are the most common. This daily duration of treatment has also been shown to be most effective in inducing vascular thromboresistance and in improving systemic haemostatic balance.[14,43] Interestingly, nitric oxide derived from exogenous nitrate (isosorbide dinitrate) potentiated the increase in thromboresistance caused by PGE_1.[44]

PGI_2 is not significantly metabolized during lung passage. Importantly, during infusions of PGE_1, an active metabolite, 13,14-dihydro PGE_1, which shares the biological activities of its parent compound, is formed[45] via enzymatic oxidation and subsequent reduction of the 13,14 double bond.[46] This may take place in the pulmonary circulation, which would explain the efficacy of intravenous infusions of PGE_1. Further confirmation of this result is required to substantiate the hypothesis. The discovery of this metabolic route could explain the early findings by Carlson's group of an improvement in the contralateral leg after intra-arterial PGE_1 therapy.[6]

Insufficient information is available as to whether repeated treatment with prostaglandins results in continued improvement. The only study that examined this question found no significant difference.[22,23] Data on a controlled comparison between prostaglandins as well as of different doses or routes of one compound are not yet available. The selection of endpoints, such as amputation, walking distance, pain and analgesic consumption, is not without problems and is thus under debate. Although the Fontaine classification of PVD is useful as a clinical tool, a change of the Fontaine stage should not be used as a measure of efficacy in clinical trials.[4] As walking has been shown not to be predictive of the development of clinical limb ischaemia, this variable is also under criticism as an endpoint. Clearly, there are 'responders' and 'non-responders' to prostaglandin therapy, but an intensive search for a possible mechanism of action or a powerful predictive test for clinical efficacy has so far failed. There are still some contradictions concerning dosing. Whilst there is generally a trend towards lower doses in order to prevent subjective side effects as well as steal phenomena (especially with PGE_1 and PGI_2), some groups still prefer individual (once or even daily) titration up to the maximum tolerated dose, and this has been the general practice in the clinical trials with iloprost. Although some clinical pharmacological studies have shown something like a minimal effective dose, no clear dose–response relationship has been demonstrated except by Scheffler, regarding blood flow and tissue oxygen concentration using PGE_1. Thromboresistance induced by prostaglandins has been demonstrated in arteries[47] as well as in prosthetic grafts.[48] Clinical pharmacological studies measuring thromboresistance of atherosclerotic lesions did not reveal any difference between two doses for PGE_1 (5 vs 20 ng/kg per minute i.v.[49]) between the intra-arterial and the intravenous route,[50] or between PGI_2 (3 vs 5 ng/kg per minute i.v.[43]) and iloprost (1 vs 2 ng/kg per minute i.v.[51]). The interpretation of results is further complicated by the different dose calculations being given either on the basis of ng substance per kg per minute or as total amount per hour, the latter not taking into consideration the body weight of the patient when given over a period of 1 hour.

Prostaglandins improve utilization of oxygen and glucose and decrease lactate and pyruvate concentrations.[52] PGE_1 increased glucose utilization five-fold, paralleled by increased protein synthesis and inhibition of protein degradation.[54]

To summarize, there is clear evidence from controlled studies that PGE_1 and iloprost are of benefit at least in a subpopulation of PVD patients. Positive data are available also for prostacyclin, although to a more limited extent. Treatment for only 3 days mostly did not result in benefit, whilst almost all the long-term studies treating for more than 2 weeks did. This was seen in terms of pain relief and an increase in the number of patients achieving preservation of a viable limb. Discovery of the mechanism of action and optimizing the therapeutic applications of these compounds could further improve the rate, extent and duration of therapeutic benefit. Considering, furthermore, the many proven antiatherosclerotic actions, the development of stable orally active analogues of prostaglandins offers the most promising pharmacotherapy for PVD and, in particular, critical limb ischaemia. Two such compounds are already on the market in Japan.

Acknowledgements

I am grateful to L Heeck, RA Henry (Schering, Berlin, Germany) and Waltraud Rogatti (Schwarz Pharma, Monheim, Germany) for providing me with the detailed study data. The valuable help of Susanne Granegger and Eva Unger in preparing and typing the manuscript is gratefully acknowledged.

References

1. Dormandy JA and the European Working Group on Critical Leg Ischemia. Clinical experience with iloprost in the treatment of critical leg ischemia. In: Rubanyi GM (ed), *Cardiovascular Significance of Endothelium-derived Vasoactive Factors*. Mount Kisco NY: Future Publ. 1991: 335–47.
2. Editorial. European consensus on critical limb ischaemia. *Lancet* 1989; **1**: 737–8.
3. European Working Group on Critical Leg Ischemia. Second European consensus document on chronic critical leg ischemia. *Circulation* 1991; **84**/IV: 1–26.
4. Wolfe JHN. The definition of critical ischaemia: is this a concept of value? In: Greenholgh RM, Jamieson CW, Nicolaides AN (eds), *Limb Salvage and Amputation for Vascular Disease*. Philadelphia: WB Saunders, 1988.
5. Dormandy JA. *European Consensus Document of Critical Limb Ischaemia*. New York: Springer, 1989.
6. Carlson LA, Eriksson I. Femoral-artery infusion of prostaglandin E_1 in severe peripheral vascular disease. *Lancet* 1973; **1**: 155–6.
7. Vane JR. The release and fate of vasoactive hormones in the circulation. *Br J Pharmacol* 1968; **35**: 209–14.
8. Szczeklik A, Nizankowski R, Skawinski S, Szczeklik J, Gluszko P, Gryglewski RJ. Successful therapy of advanced arteriosclerosis obliterans with prostacyclin. *Lancet* 1979; **1**: 1111–14.
9. Sinzinger H, Feigl W, Silberbauer K. Prostacyclin generation in atherosclerotic arteries. *Lancet* 1979; **2**: 442–4.
10. Sinzinger H, Silberbauer K, Horsch AK, Gall A. Decreased sensitivity of human platelets to PGI_2 during long term intraarterial prostacyclin infusion in patients with peripheral vascular disease. A rebound phenomenon? *Prostaglandins* 1981; **21**: 49–51.
11. Sinzinger H, Leithner C, Silberbauer K. Rebound platelet activation during continuous epoprostenol infusion. *Lancet* 1984; **1**: 759.
12. Sinzinger H, Reiter S. The intrainfusion platelet rebound following PGE_1-infusion is faster and more intensive than that with PGI_2. *Prostaglandins Leukot Med* 1984; **13**: 281–7.
13. Modesti PA, Fortini A, Poggesi L, Boddi M, Abbate R, Gensini GF. Acute reversible reduction of PGI_2 platelet receptors after iloprost infusion in man. *Thromb Res* 1987; **48**: 663–9.
14. Sinzinger H, Fitscha P, Kaliman J. The optimal PGI_2 infusion time as judged by autologous platelet-labeling in patients with active atherosclerosis. In: Schrör K (ed), *Prostaglandins and Other Eicosanoids in the Cardiovascular System*. Basel: Karger, 1985: 358–64.
15. Sinzinger H, Virgolini I, O'Grady J. Clinical trials of PGE_1, PGI_2 and mimetics in patients with peripheral vascular disease. *Prog Clin Biol Res* 1989; **301**: 85–96.

16. Sakaguchi S. Prostaglandin E_1 intraarterial therapy in patients with ischemic ulcer of the extremities. *Int Angiol* 1984; **3:** 39–42.

17. Böhme H, Brülisauer M, Härtel U, Bollinger A. Periphere arterielle Verschlusskrankheit im Stadium III und IV-kontrollierte Zweizentren-Studie zur Wirksamkeit von intraarteriellen Prostaglandin E_1-Infusionen. *Med Welt* 1989; **40:** 1501–3.

18. Rhodes RS, Heard SE. Detrimental effect of high-dose prostaglandin E_1 in the treatment of ischemic ulcers. *Surgery* 1983; **93:** 839–42.

19. Schuler JJ, Flanigan DP, Holcroft JW, Ursprung KK, Mohrland JS, Pyke E. Efficacy of prostaglandin E_1 in the treatment of lower extremity ischemic ulcers secondary to peripheral vascular occlusive disease. *J Vasc Surg* 1984; **1:** 160–70.

20. Cronenwett JL. The use of prostaglandins PGE_1 and PGI_2 in peripheral arterial ischemia. *J Vasc Surg* 1986; **3:** 370–4.

21. Karnik R, Valentin A, Slany I. Prostacyclin versus naftidrofuryl. *Herz/Kreislauf* 1987; **1:** 23–6.

22. Virgolini I, Fitscha P, Linet OI, O'Grady J, Sinzinger H. A double blind placebo controlled trial of intravenous prostacyclin (PGI_2) in 108 patients with ischaemic peripheral vascular disease. *Prostaglandins* 1990; **39:** 657–64.

23. Virgolini I, Fitscha P, Weiss K, Linet OI, O'Grady J, Sinzinger H. Intravenous prostacyclin (PGI_2) infusion to 108 patients with ischaemic peripheral vascular disease: phase II – open study. *Prostaglandins* 1991; **42:** 9–14.

24. Hossmann V, Auel H, Rücker W, Schrör K. Prolonged infusion of prostacyclin in patients with advanced stages of peripheral vascular disease: a placebo-controlled cross-over study. *Klin Wochenschr* 1984; **62:** 1108–12.

25. Hossmann V, Auel H, Schrör K. Plazebo-kontrollierte Cross-over-Studie über die Wirkung von Iloprost (ZK 36374) auf fortgeschrittene Stadien der arteriellen Verschlusskrankheit. In: Trübestein G (ed), *Konservative Therapie arterieller Durchblutungsstörungen.* Stuttgart: Georg Thieme, 1986: 186–91.

26. Olsson AG. Intravenous infusion of prostacyclin for ischaemic ulcers in peripheral vascular disease. *Lancet* 1980; **2:** 1076.

27. Pardy BC, Lewis JD, Eastcott HHG. Preliminary experience with prostaglandins E_1 and I_2 in peripheral vascular disease. *Surgery* 1980; **88:** 826–31.

28. Szczeklik A, Gryglewski RJ, Nizankowski R, Skawinski S, Gluszko P, Korbut R. Prostacyclin therapy in peripheral arterial disease. *Thromb Res* 1980; **19:** 191–6.

29. Chiesa R, Vicavi A, Mari G, Golineberti M, DiCarlo V, Pozza G. Use of stable prostacyclin analogue ZK 36374 to treat severe lower limb ischaemia. *Lancet* 1985; **2:** 95–6.

30. Fiessinger JN, Schäfer M for the TAO study. Trial of iloprost versus aspirin treatment for the critical limb ischaemia of thromboangiitis obliterans. *Lancet* 1990; **335:** 555–7.

31. Fitscha P. Prostaglandine in Pathogenese und Therapie der peripheren arteriellen Verschlusskrankheit (PVK). In: Kraupp O, Sinzinger H, Widhalm K (eds), *Atherogenesis 7.* Wien, München, Bern: Wilhelm Maudrich, 1986.

32. Moncada S, Gryglewski RJ, Bunting S, Vane JR. An enzyme isolated from arteries transforms prostaglandin endoperoxides to an unstable substance that inhibits platelet aggregation. *Nature* 1976; **263:** 663–5.

33. De Gaetano G, Bertele V, Cerletti C. Mechanism of action and clinical use of prostaglandins. In: Dormandy JA, Stock G (eds), *Critical Leg Ischaemia: its pathophysiology and management.* Berlin: Springer, 1989: 117–43.

34. Sinzinger H, Virgolini I, Fitscha P. Pathomechanisms of atherosclerosis beneficially affected by prostaglandin E_1 (PGE_1) – an update. *VASA Suppl* 1989; **28:** 6–13.

35. Sinzinger H. Prostaglandins and -analogs in the treatment of platelet vessel wall interaction. In: Herman AG (ed), *Antithrombotics.* Antwerp: Kluwer, 1991: 205–20.

36. Willis AL, Smith DL, Vigo C. Suppression of principal atherosclerotic mechanisms by prostacyclin and other eicosanoids. *Prog Lipid Res* 1986; **48:** 1–22.

37. Sinzinger H, Rogatti W. Prostaglandin E_1 in der Therapie der peripheren arteriellen Durchblutungsstörung. *Wr klin Wochenschr* 1991; **103:** 558–65.

38. Sinzinger H, Kefalides A, Hoche C. Is the platelet derived growth factor (PDGF) a main regulator in atherosclerosis? *Circulation* 1982; **66:** 192.

39. Eklund AE, Eriksson G, Olsson AG. A controlled study showing significant short term effect of PGE_1 in healing of ischaemic ulcers of the lower limb in man. *Prostaglandins Leukot Med* 1982; **8:** 265–71.

40. Telles GS, Campbell WB, Wood RF, Collin J, Baird RN, Morris PJ. Prostaglandin E_1 in severe lower limb ischaemia: a double-blind controlled trial. *Br J Surg* 1984; **71:** 506–8.

41. Jogestrand T, Olsson AG. The effect of intravenous prostaglandin E_1 on ischemic pain and on leg blood-flow in subjects with peripheral artery disease: a double-blind controlled study. *Clin Physiol* 1985; **5:** 495–502.

42. Diehm C, Abri O, Baitsch G, *et al.* Iloprost, ein stabiles Prostacyclinderivat, bei arterieller Verschlusskrankheit im Stadium IV. *Dtsch med Wochenschr* 1989; **114:** 783–8.

43. Sinzinger H, Fitscha P, Kaliman J, O'Grady J. Search for the optimal PGI_2-infusion protocol – advantages of a 6-hour intermittent infusion. *Thromb Haemost* 1985; **54:** 85–6.

44. Sinzinger H, Fitscha P, O'Grady J, Rauscha F, Rogatti W, Vane JR. Synergistic effect of prostaglandin E_1

and isosorbide dinitrate in peripheral vascular diease. *Lancet* 1989; **1**: 627–8.

45. Peskar BA, Hesse WH, Rogatti W, *et al.* Formation of 13,14-dihydro-prostaglandin E_1 during intravenous infusions of prostaglandin E_1 in patients with peripheral arterial occlusive disease. *Prostaglandins* 1991; **41**: 225–8.

46. Änggard E, Larsson C. The sequence of the early steps in the metabolism of prostaglandin E_1. *Eur J Pharmacol* 1971; **14**: 66–70.

47. Sinzinger H, Fitscha P. Epoprostenol and platelet deposition in atherosclerosis. *Lancet* 1984; **1**: 905–6.

48. Sinzinger H, O'Grady J, Cromwell M, Höfer R. Epoprostenol (prostacyclin) decreases platelet deposition on vascular prosthetic grafts. *Lancet* 1983; **2**: 1275–6.

49. Sinzinger H, O'Grady J, Fitscha P. Effect of prostaglandin E_1 on deposition of autologous labelled platelets onto human atherosclerotic lesions in vivo. *Postgrad Med J* 1987; **63**: 245–7.

50. Sinzinger H, O'Grady J, Fitscha P, Rauscha F, Kaliman J. Comparable effect of prostaglandin E_1 in decreasing *in vivo* platelet deposition on human lesion sites after intravenous and intraarterial application. *Thromb Res* 1988; **50**: 749–55.

51. Fitscha P, Tiso B, Krais T, Sinzinger H. Effect of iloprost on *in vivo* and *in vitro* platelet function in patients with peripheral vascular disease. *Adv Prostaglandin Thromboxane Leukotriene Res* 1987; **17**: 450–4.

52. Bergström S, Carlson LA, Weeks JR. The prostaglandins: a family of biologically active lipids. *Pharmacol Rev* 1968; **20**: 1–48.

53. Rexroth W, Amendt K, Römmele U, Stein U, Wagner E, Hild R. Effekte von Prostaglandin E_1 auf Hämodynamik und Extremitätenstoffwechsel bei Gesunden und Patienten mit arterieller Verschlusskrankheit Stadium III und IV. *VASA* 1985; **14**: 220–4.

54. Stiegler H, Relt K, Wicklmayr M, Mehnert H. Metabolic effects of prostaglandin E_1 on human skeletal muscle with special regard to the amino acid metabolism. *VASA* 1989; **28**: 14–18.

55. Blume J. Klinische Wirksamkeit der intraarteriellen Infusionstherapie mit Prostaglandin E_1 im Stadium IIb der arteriellen Verschlusskrankheit. *Therapiewoche* 1987; **37**: 4819–23.

56. Creutzig A, Caspary L, Alexander K. Intermittent intraarterial prostaglandin E_1 therapy of severe claudication. *VASA Suppl* 1987; **17**: 44–6.

57. Creutzig A, Caspary L, Radeke U, Specht S, Ranke C, Alexander K. Prospektive randomisierte Doppelblindstudie zur Wirksamkeit von i.a. Prostaglandin E_1 bei der schweren Claudicatio intermittens. In: Heidrich H, Böhme H, Rogatti W (eds), *Prostaglandin E1-Wirkung und therapeutische Wirksamkeit.* Heidelberg: Springer, 1988: 95–102.

58. Rudofsky G, Altenhoff B, Meyer P, Lohman A. Intraarterial perfusion with prostaglandin E_1 in patients with intermittent claudication. *VASA* 1987; **17** (suppl): 47–51.

59. Trübestein G, Ludwig M, Diehm C, Gruss JD, Horsch S. Prostaglandin E_1 bei arterieller Verschlusskrankheit im Stadium III und IV. Ergebnisse einer multizentrischen Studie. *Dtsch Med Wochenschr* 1987; **112**: 955–9.

60. Diehm C, Hübsch-Müller C, Stammler F. Intravenöse Prostaglandin E_1-Therapie bei Patienten mit peripherer arterieller Verschlusskrankheit (AVK) im Stadium III – eine doppelblinde, plazebokontrollierte Studie. In: Heidrich H, Böhme H, Rogatti W (eds), *Prostaglandin E1-Wirkung und therapeutische Wirksamkeit.* Heidelberg: Springer, 1988: 133–43.

61. Rudofsky G. Intravenöse PGE_1-Infusionsbehandlung bei Patienten mit arterieller Verschlusskrankheit im Stadium IIb. In: Heidrich H, Böhme H, Rogatti W (eds), *Prostaglandin E1-Wirkung und therapeutische Wirksamkeit.* Heidelberg: Springer, 1988: 103–11.

62. Trübestein G, von Bary S, Breddin K, *et al.* Intravenous prostaglandin E_1 versus pentoxifylline therapy in chronic arterial occlusive disease – a controlled randomized multicenter study. *VASA* 1989; **28**: 44–9.

63. Diehm C, Kühn A, Strauss R, Hübsch-Müller C, Kübler W. Effects of regular physical training in a supervised class and additional intravenous prostaglandin E_1 and naftidrofuryl infusion therapy in patients with intermittent claudication. *VASA* 1989; **28**: 26–30.

64. Hepp W, von Bary S, Corovic D, *et al.* Therapeutic efficacy of intravenous prostaglandin E_1 versus pentoxifylline in patients with intermittent claudication. In: Diehm C, Sinzinger H, Rogatti W (eds), *Prostaglandin E1. New Aspects of Pharmacology, Metabolism and Clinical Efficacy.* Heidelberg: Springer, 1991: 101–8.

65. Belch JJF, McKay A, McArdle B, *et al.* Epoprostenol (prostacyclin) and severe arterial disease. A double blind trial. *Lancet* 1983; **1**: 315–17.

66. Nizankowski R, Krolikowski W, Bielatowicz J, Schaller J, Szczeklik A. Prostacyclin for ischemic ulcers in peripheral arterial disease: a random assignment, placebo-controlled study. In: Gryglewski R, Szczeklik A, McGiff JC (eds), *Prostacyclin. Clinical Trials.* New York: Raven Press, 1985: 15–27.

67. Negus D, Irving JD, Friedgood A. Intraarterial prostacyclin compared to praxilene in the management of advanced atherosclerotic lower limb ischemia. In: Gryglewski R, Szczeklik A, McGiff JC (eds), *Prostacyclin. Clinical Trials.* New York: Raven Press, 1985: 107–19.

68. Brock FE, Abri O, Baitsch G, *et al.* Iloprost in der Behandlung ischämischer Gewebsläsionen bei Diabetikern. *Schweiz Med Wochenschr* 1990; **120**: 1477–82.

69. Balzer K, Bechara G, Bisler H, *et al.* Placebokontrollierte, doppel-blinde Multizenterstudie zur

Wirksamkeit von Iloprost bei der Behandlung ischämischer Ruheschmerzen von Patienten mit peripheren
arteriellen Durchblutungsstörungen. *VASA Suppl*
1987; **20:** 379–81.

70. Bliss BP, Wilkins DC, Campbell WB, and the UK
Severe Limb Ischaemia Study Group. Treatment of
limb-threatening ischaemia with intravenous iloprost:
a randomised double-blind placebo controlled study.
Eur J Vasc Surg 1991; **5:** 511–16.

71. Norgren L, Alwmark A, Ängqvist KA, *et al*. A stable
prostacyclin analogue (iloprost) in the treatment of
ischaemic ulcers of the lower limb. *Eur J Vasc Surg*
1990; **4:** 463–7.

72. Guilmot JL, Diot E, for the French Iloprost Study
Group. Treatment of lower limb ischaemia due to
atherosclerosis in diabetic and nondiabetic patients
with iloprost, a stable analogue of prostacyclin. Results of a French Multicentre Trial. *Drug Invest* 1991;
3: 351–9.

16 Prostaglandins in Raynaud's phenomenon

JJF Belch

Man has evolved as a tropical animal, better suited to losing heat than to retaining it. His neutral environmental temperature when naked and at rest is 28°C. After a fall of only 8°C in environmental temperature metabolic rate must double or body temperature will fall. Man's response to cold, the use of clothes, has enabled him to survive in temperate areas. However, some people respond abnormally to cold and suffer from conditions such as chilblains, cold urticaria, cryoglobulinaemia, prurigo heimalis and Raynaud's phenomenon. Of these cold-related disorders the best recognized is Raynaud's phenomenon (RP). The clinical manifestations and laboratory abnormalities detected in RP make it a disorder theoretically likely to benefit from treatment with the antiplatelet vasodilator prostaglandins (PG). These abnormalities, the potential beneficial effects of prostaglandins and the clinical studies are reviewed below.

The clinical problem

In 1862 Maurice Raynaud first defined Raynaud's phenomenon as episodic digital ischaemia provoked by cold and emotion.[1] It is classically manifest by pallor of the digits followed by cyanosis and rubor. The pallor reflects vasospasm in the digital vessels (Fig. 16.1); the cyanosis deoxygenation of the static venous blood; and the rubor-reactive hyperaemia following the return of blood flow. RP is nine times more common in women than men[2] and has an overall prevalence in the population of approximately 10%, although it may affect as many as 20–30% of women in the younger age groups.[3] RP can be a benign condition, however – if severe, it can cause digital ulceration and gangrene (Fig. 16.2). Until recently little was known about the true aetiology and extent of this disorder. This lack of knowledge has led to difficulties in the treatment and prediction of prognosis in RP. It is now known that Raynaud's

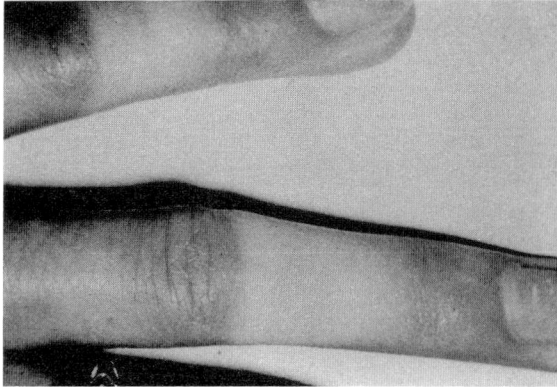

Fig. 16.1 The vasospasm of Raynaud's phenomenon.

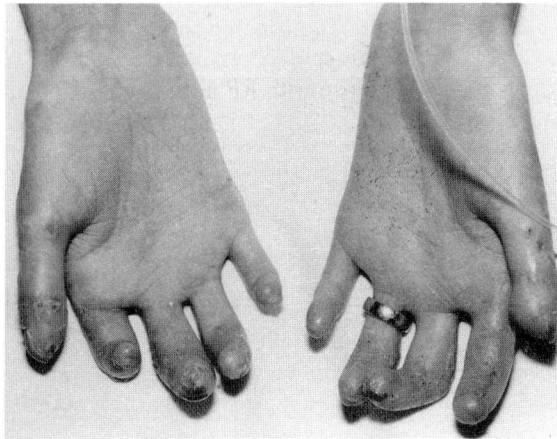

Fig. 16.2 Digit loss in Raynaud's syndrome.

original definition requires modification. For example, the full triphasic colour change is not now thought to be essential for the diagnosis.[4] A history of cold-induced blanching with subsequent reactive hyperaemia can still reflect significant vasospasm/ RP; moreover, stimuli other than cold and emotion can provoke an attack, for example, trauma, hormones and chemicals including those in tobacco smoke.[5] Raynaud's limitation of symptoms to the digits also needs expansion as the tip of the nose, tongue and earlobes may be involved. The hypothesis which suggests that more widespread vasospasm occurs in this disorder has been supported by the findings of decreased oesophageal[6] and myocardial[7] perfusion after cold challenge. Some workers have speculated that the lesions of the kidney and lung seen in severe cases of RP associated with connective tissue disorders (CTDs) may be ac-

counted for in the same way.[8] This concept of 'systemic vasospasm' may have important therapeutic implications.

Phenomenon, syndrome or disease?

One of the major problems for workers in this area of medicine has been the inconsistent terminology used to describe Raynaud's attacks. In Europe RP is the blanket term used to describe anyone suffering from cold-related digital vasospasm. RP is subdivided into secondary Raynaud's syndrome (RS) where there is an associated disorder and primary Raynaud's disease (RD) where there is not. Unfortunately, this European classification is not accepted globally and researchers in America and Australasia tend to use syndrome and phenomenon interchangeably.[9] Furthermore, the definition of RS, often not specified in published work, varies from investigator to investigator; consequently, assessment of the literature may be difficult. The situation is further complicated by the fact that long-term studies have shown that RP may be the precursor of systemic illness by over 20 years[10] and recently developed sensitive laboratory procedures have shown that more than one-half of patients referred to hospital have an associated systemic disease (RS). There is a wide spectrum of diseases associated with RS, the best recognized being the CTDs and RS of occupational origin.

RS is found in the majority of patients with systemic sclerosis (SSc) and mixed connective tissue disease,[11] and also in patients with systemic lupus erythematosus (SLE), polymyositis and dermatomyositis, and Sjögren's syndrome.[12] RS occurs in rheumatoid arthritis and hyperviscosity syndromes in a percentage similar to that seen in the normal population (10%). However, the symptomatology tends to be more severe (Fig. 16.3).

RP of occupational origin can also occur. Vinyl chloride disease occurring in workers exposed to this chemical has been well described with the incidence of RS estimated to be approximately 3% in exposed workers.[13] A more common form of occupational RS is vibration white finger disease (VWF). As its name suggests, VWF occurs in workers exposed to vibrating machines such as chain-saws, pneumatic drills and buffs. It is estimated that between 40 and 90% of all workers using vibratory equipment will have RS although the symptoms may

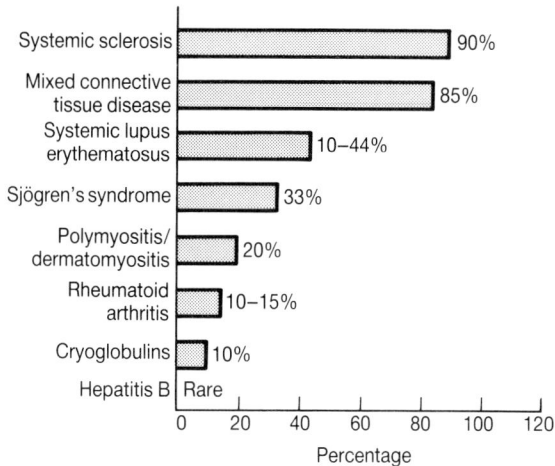

Fig. 16.3 Raynaud's syndrome and the rheumatic diseases.

Table 16.1 Other conditions associated with Raynaud's disease

Obstructive arterial disease
Atherosclerosis (especially thrombangiitis obliterans)
Thoracic outlet syndromes (including cervical rib)
Emboli

Drugs
β-Blockers
Ergot and other antimigraine drugs
Cytotoxics
Bromocriptine

Miscellaneous
Cryoglobulinaemia
Hypothyroidism
? Neoplasm

resolve in 25% of cases if a job change is effected early in the course of the disease.[14] Clinicians previously thought that the symptoms of this form of RP affected only the hands; however, vibration-induced RP affecting both hands and feet has recently been described.[15] The troublesome nature of the symptomatology of VWF and the severity of the symptoms in RS associated with immunological disorders has particular relevance to the use of PGs as a treatment for such RPs. Nevertheless, it should be remembered that other conditions and situations are also associated with the development of RS and include obstructive vascular disease and some drug therapies (Table 16.1).

At present the frequency with which such secondary conditions are recognized varies widely with reported studies and may depend, in part, on the duration of the RP symptoms at the time seen, the thoroughness with which a search for an associated disorder is undertaken and physician referral patterns. This fact is clearly illustrated in a review by Edwards and Porter.[16] In 1976 the authors reported an 81% incidence of secondary RS in their population of 100 RP patients. By 1988 the study population had grown to 615 patients but the percentage of those with secondary RS had fallen to 46%. The authors commented that in the early years of their study the patients were only referred if severely symptomatic. As the authors' interest in RP became more widely known, more patients with mild symptoms were referred. In general patients with RP attending hospitals are far more likely to have a sec-

ondary RS than those with RP in the general population.[16] However, both from a treatment and prognostic point of view it is important to be able to detect as soon as possible those patients with RP who will develop a CTD. Such early detection can be difficult but some clearly defined abnormalities have been linked with disease progression to secondary RS. These abnormalities are (1) certain clinical features, (2) abnormal nailfold vessels and (3) abnormal immunological tests.[17]

Suspicious clinical symptoms include the findings of any features of CTD such as sclerodactyly and in particular digital ulceration which does not occur in primary RD.[18] Also predictive is the finding of an abnormal capillary pattern seen at the nailfold which is strongly associated with the subsequent development of SSc.[19] These vessels can be clearly seen using only a hand-held ophthalmoscope at the highest magnification. The presence of anticentromere antibody or scleroderma 70 (anti-topoisomerase) antibodies in patients otherwise presenting as RD is also predictive of the development of limited SSc (calcinosis, Raynaud's phenomenon, oesophageal involvement, sclerodactyly, telangiectasia – CREST) and diffuse SSc respectively.[20] Antinuclear antibody positivity in the serum is also associated with future development of CTD.[12] LeRoy and Lomea[21] suggest that nailfold capillary microscopy and serum antinuclear antibody detection can together predict more than 95% of patients destined to have a CTD.

Treatment strategies must, of course, be based on patient diagnosis and the detection of an associated disorder in the patient with RP is an important step in the management of these patients. Of equal importance in the design of treatment protocols is a clear understanding of the underlying pathology, particularly aspects which may be modified by such treatment regimens.

Pathophysiology of Raynaud's phenomenon

Several factors are considered to have an aetiological importance in RP. They fall into three broad categories: neurogenic mechanisms, blood and blood vessel wall interactions, and abnormal inflammatory and immunological responses. The latter two categories are the most relevant with regard to PG treatment. However, the importance of the former should not be ignored.

Neurogenic mechanisms

Two major theories have been presented to explain the vasospasm seen in RP. Maurice Raynaud believed that hyperactivity of the sympathetic nervous system caused an increased vasoconstrictor response to cold[1] whereas Lewis[22] hypothesized a 'local fault' in which precapillary resistance vessels were hypersensitive to local cooling. Supporting evidence for the theory of Maurice Raynaud is the demonstration that normal blood flow is attained in the hands and fingers by warming or sympathetic blockade,[23] that there is exaggerated digital vasoconstriction in response to postural changes,[24] and that emotional stress produces attacks in patients with RP. However, normal microelectrode recordings of skin sympathetic nerve activity at rest and with various stimuli,[25] normal vasoconstriction of the contralateral hand during cooling[26] and normal catecholamine levels[27] in patients with RP do not substantiate this theory. Lewis,[22] credited with the theory of a 'local fault', produced vasospastic attacks in single fingers by direct cooling and induced attacks in sympathetically denervated fingers as have others subsequently[28] who suggest that there is a peripheral abnormality in the vascular response to temperature change in RP independent of central sympathetic control. Further support for the 'local fault' theory comes from Bunker *et al.*[29] who suggest, however, that the fault may lie in a dysfunction of a calcitonin gene-related peptide (CGRP) dependent neurovascular axis. They examined the distribution and quantity of CGRP-containing neurons in the digital skin of RD and RS patients and normal subjects. In

both RP groups there were significant reductions in the numbers of these CGRP immunoreactive neurons and the authors suggest this may be of aetiological importance in RP. It is possible that such findings are a consequence of ischaemia and not a cause as the authors did not study ischaemia of non-RP origin. However, a deficiency of CGRP remains an aetiological hypothesis. In the same way, abnormalities of vasodilator prostaglandins and their precursors have been described in RP[30,31] which may be relevant to blood flow in the vessel. The conflicting results of some of the above studies are not easily explained either in terms of the methodology or the patient study groups and they serve to remind us that the exact pathophysiology of vasospasm is still uncertain and probably multifactorial.

Other putative abnormalities of the RP nervous system have also been described. Klimiuk *et al.*[32] suggested an autonomic dysfunction in RS secondary to SSc as detected by the alteration in blood pressure response to standing. However, Suarez-Almazor *et al.*,[33] using six standard tests of autonomic function, reported normal results in all but the blood pressure response. It is possible that in normal subjects systolic blood pressure and heart rate increase rapidly after standing mainly owing to an increase in sympathetic activity caused by the initial fall in peripheral resistance. The difference seen in patients could be due to the extensive perivascular fibrosis seen in RS complicated by SSc which could cause an alteration in the normal variation in pulse rate because of the loss of elasticity of the vessels. The other cardiac reflexes are normal. This suggests that autonomic control in RP is probably intact.

Blood and blood vessel wall interactions

Abnormal blood vessel tone does not, however, explain all the features of RP. For example, the digits of patients with RP can appear cyanotic between blood vessel spasm attacks. In addition, patients with RS and SSc who die of myocardial infarction may have normal coronary arteries, and decreased renal cortical blood flow has been described with body cooling or a cold pressor stimulus in these patients.[34] As the neurogenic control of the digital, coronary and renal circulation is different in each case it is possible that a blood-borne or blood vessel factor(s) is involved. The flow in the microcirculation is critically dependent on the intactness of the endothelium and on the properties of the cellular and liquid elements of blood. Abnormalities in these parameters are likely to contribute to poor blood flow and aggravate RP symptoms. Conversely a therapy such as the prostaglandins, designed to resolve these abnormalities, might be expected to improve blood flow in RP.

The endothelium and Raynaud's phenomenon

The endothelium has an important role in maintaining haemostasis but preventing inappropriate thrombosis. It is a functioning organ, releasing important chemicals, one of which is prostacyclin (PGI_2). Endothelial damage is probably an important feature of RP. Factor VIII von Willebrand factor antigen (FVIIIvWFAg) is a blood clotting factor made and released by the endothelium. Damage to the vasculature will elevate plasma levels and such an elevation has been well documented in RP.[35,36] Those who have an associated CTD have a higher FVIIIvWFAg level than those who do not[37] and it has been suggested that FVIIIvWFAg may have a role as a predictor of the progression of RD to RS, and as a measure of the severity of the RP attacks.[38] Greaves et al.[39] extended this work by demonstrating high levels of FVIIIvWFAg in patients with CTD visceral involvement when compared to those without and James et al.[37] published an intriguing study showing that 20% of first degree relatives of patients with RS also had high levels of FVIIIvWFAg, suggesting a genetic predisposition towards microvascular injury.

Although the FVIIIvWFAg itself could propagate the vascular damage by participating in the coagulation cascade and by promoting platelet activation, the actual mechanism by which vascular damage originates is not fully understood. Kahaleh and LeRoy[40] have shown the presence of endothelial cell cytotoxic activity in RP serum which is removed by plasmapheresis. If such a factor exists then it could be responsible for other manifestations of endothelial dysfunction such as abnormal fibrinolysis. Plasma fibrinolysis is largely controlled by the endothelium through its ability to produce tissue plasminogen activator (t-PA) and tissue plasminogen activator inhibitor (PAI). t-PA, as its name suggests, promotes the activation of plasminogen to plasmin. Plasmin then lyses fibrin. The balance between fibrinolysis and fibrin deposition is controlled to a great extent by the balance between t-PA and PAI. Hyperviscosity and hyperfibrinogenaemia have been reported in RP.[41] These abnormalities have been related to a deficiency in the fibrinolytic system[42,43]

as measured by these endothelial cell products. Both the increase in fibrinogen and the abnormalities of fibrinolysis are limited to RS patients with normal levels being found in RD[44] and they are likely, therefore, to be a consequence of the vasospasm. Such abnormalities, however, may further augment the ischaemia.

Endothelin, another endothelial product, is a vasoactive peptide with potent and prolonged *in vitro* and *in vivo* vasoconstrictor activity. Elevated baseline plasma levels of endothelin have been reported in RP which are further increased by digital cold challenge.[45] As with PAI and t-PA, it seems likely that this abnormality is once again consequent upon the vasospasm, yet with the potential to profoundly augment the resultant ischaemic process.

Prostacyclin is another endothelial product. Work investigating endothelial production of prostacyclin in RP was hindered initially by the difficulty in measuring its stable metabolite 6-keto-$PGF_{1\alpha}$ in plasma. Initial reports of increased levels of 6-keto-$PGF_{1\alpha}$ in RS[46,47] as a response to vessel injury were balanced by work suggesting that serum from patients with RP inhibited prostacyclin production by the endothelial cell as measured by a platelet aggregation bioassay.[48] As more superior assay techniques have been developed and a better understanding of endothelial cell culture obtained, it has become apparent that RS serum does not directly decrease prostacyclin production[49] though any sustained and widespread endothelial cell damage will ultimately impair its function. Of interest is the concept of cellular resistance to prostaglandin effects in RS. This may effect the RS platelet,[50] phagocyte or macrophage. Whicher et al.[51] demonstrated a diminished acute phase response after prostaglandin infusion in RS, reflecting either macrophage or liver resistance and Kirby et al.[52] postulated a prostaglandin resistance of the cyclic nucleotide response of RS lymphocytes. It is also of interest that cooling decreases endothelial synthesis of prostacyclin[53] and although cooling also decreases the synthesis of platelet thromboxane A_2 (TXA_2) the inhibition of the latter is proportionately greater than the former and this may be related to the finding of increased platelet aggregation in RP described below.

Cellular elements of blood and Raynaud's phenomenon

If platelets are activated in the circulation they release vasoconstrictor substances such as TXA_2 and serotonin and form aggregates which may be expected to aggravate the disease by further decreasing digital blood flow. Reilly *et al.*[54] demonstrated increased synthesis of TXA_2 in RP as measured by analysis of urine metabolites by gas chromatography, and Klimiuk *et al.*[55] showed decreased platelet serotonin levels in RS which they suggest reflect widespread platelet activation. Other platelet release products such as β-thromboglobulin are also elevated in RP[56] and this parallels the well documented increase in the rate of platelet aggregation itself.[44,57,58]

The part played by the red blood cell (RBC) has also been studied. Its diameter of approximately 5 μm is greater than that of some of the capillaries so flow in the microcirculation may be critically dependent on RBC deformability. RBC deformability measured by a filtration technique is diminished in patients with RS.[47,59] Cold temperatures also reduce RBC deformability as does the acidosis present in cold ulcerated fingers, so hard red cells may contribute to a further decrease in flow.[44] RBCs from patients with RS were also found to be more adherent to cultured endothelial cells and to have a lower electrophoretic velocity,[59] these latter results suggesting slower passage of the cells in the microcirculation. These abnormalities may be brought about by a serum/plasma factor capable of altering RBC behaviour and later studies support this concept by showing RS serum enhances calcium influx into the RBC induced by the calcium ionophore A23817.[60] Alternatively the decreased deformability could be the result of the increased activity of lysosomal glycosidase, an enzyme which can split off carbohydrate chains of membrane glycoprotein.[61] No matter what the cause, as with other changes these RBC abnormalities are likely to be due to the associated condition but may contribute to decreased digital flow.

An important role for the white blood cell (WBC) in maintaining flow in small blood vessels has also been suggested.[62] Polymorphonuclear leucocytes (PMNs) are almost 2000 times less deformable than the erythrocyte[63] and when they become activated they project pseudopods and their cytoplasmic stiffness increases further. Another property of the neutrophil that has important implications with respect to its effect in the microcirculation is adhesion to the endothelium and other cells including other WBCs, forming cellular microemboli. Once the PMN has become fixed in the microvasculature it can deliver a variety of further insults to the vessel lining including the release of active oxygen species (ROS, free radicals).[64] Increased WBC activity as measured by PMN release of leukotriene B_4 (LTB_4) is increased in RS, as are markers for pathological ROS activity.[65] The migration of leucocytes[66] and immune complex deposition[67] are also increased in RS of immunological origin and may provide a mechanism for the vascular damage seen in these diseases. These changes may be further augmented by the vasospasm itself when the flowing blood is halted by the constriction of the blood vessel. After resolution of the spasm, blood re-enters the digits, setting the scene for the classic reperfusion injury where reoxygenation of ischaemic tissue leads to a burst of free radical production. This has been seen to occur following other reperfusion situations such as balloon angioplasty.[68]

Inflammatory and immune response in Raynaud's phenomenon

More conventionally the white blood cell has been considered to be important as the producer and modifier of the inflammatory and immune response. The endothelium is also involved in these processes by the production of its vasoactive agents, growth factors and growth inhibitors. It is recognized that disordered immunity/inflammation occurs in the majority of severe cases of RS via its association with the CTDs.[12] Interestingly, however, abnormal PMN behaviour also occurs in VWF, a RS which has no clear immune/inflammatory basis.[65] Tumour necrosis factor (TNF) and lymphotoxin are monocyte/macrophage and T-cell-derived proteins whose major functions are believed to be the mediation of cytotoxicity to tumour cells.[69] TNF and lymphotoxin also inhibit endothelial cell growth and stimulate fibroblast growth and collagen synthesis. Furthermore, they promote the release of FVIIIvWFAg from endothelial cells and have thus been linked in theory to its abnormal release in RS. Leroy *et al.*[70] suggest a possible role of TNF in vascular injury in RS and it is likely that the importance of this factor and other growth factors such as growth factor β and platelet-derived growth factor[69] will be more fully realized in the future.

Prostaglandin treatment for Raynaud's phenomenon: theoretical considerations

It is of interest that of all the above vessel and blood cell abnormalities detected in RP only FVIIIvWFAg, a marker of blood vessel damage, has been reported to be elevated in primary RD.[36] All other abnormalities occur only in secondary RS. It is likely, therefore, that the majority of these are a consequence of the vasospasm/vessel damage rather than a direct cause, or indeed occur partly as a result of the underlying disorder. Nevertheless, impaired endothelial cell function, adherent WBCs and platelets, and hard red cells will contribute to impaired blood flow and their correction by such therapies as prostaglandins may produce clinical improvement. Furthermore, for the secondary RS associated with CTDs certain prostaglandins may be expected to exert a beneficial effect on the abnormal immune/inflammatory response.

Prostacyclin and also PGE_1 are potent antiplatelet vasodilators and as such might be expected to be useful in a disease characterized by vasospasm and platelet aggregation. It is likely that there is a relationship between platelet behaviour and control of vascular tone. Cowley *et al.*[71] have shown a close correlation between the maximum vasoconstrictor response to cold and the threshold concentration of sodium arachidonate required to induce platelet aggregation in normal volunteers. Prostacyclin favourably altered both this maximum vasoconstrictor response and the threshold dose of sodium arachidonate required in a parallel way, suggesting a link between platelet behaviour and vascular tone which is modified by prostacyclin. Additionally, prostacyclin has been shown to increase fibrinolysis,[72] probably in a passive fashion as a result of the intense vasodilatation. Early reports suggested that both PGI_2 and PGE_1 may increase red cell deformability.[73–75] Others have found no effect[76] or even decreased filterability.[77] This variation may reflect either differences in the prostaglandin concentrations used or the effect of the prostaglandins on platelets and leucocytes which may have contaminated the test erythrocyte suspensions. This latter suggestion is thought to be the most likely as both

prostaglandins have profound antiplatelet effects and also modify WBC behaviour. Such an effect on the WBC is likely to modify both the thrombotic and the inflammatory aspects of these cells' behaviour. Prostacyclin decreases WBC adhesion to the endothelium[78] and PGE_1 can scavenge free radicals, thus promoting further blood flow in the microcirculation.[79] These antithrombotic effects of PGI_2 and PGE_1 are well known and fully documented in other chapters. They are probably relevant in the treatment of RP.

Less well understood but probably equally important in RP are the prostaglandin effects in inflammation. Prostaglandins are released from all the major immuno-inflammatory cell types[80] and whilst they are initially responsible for the development of the five cardinal signs of inflammation, a later anti-inflammatory role for some of the prostaglandins has been described. PGI_2, PGE_1 and PGE_2 increase intracellular cyclic AMP and this increase in PMN cyclic AMP results in a decrease in lysosomal enzyme release, decreased PMN chemotaxis and diminished margination and adhesion of the leucocytes in the blood vessel.[81] Similarly, the effect of the PGEs and PGI_2 on the lymphocyte is thought to be mainly inhibitory as exogenous addition of these prostaglandins inhibited *in vitro* function of lymphocytes and *in vivo* responses mediated by lymphocytes.[82] It has been suggested that some of the endogenous prostaglandins have a negative feedback role in chronic inflammation, initially aiding the development of the cardinal signs of inflammation followed by a later suppressant effect. The cellular resistance to the effects of the prostaglandins in RP as documented earlier[50–52] could be relevant here. It may be that excess prostaglandin production during the initial phase of inflammation in patients with secondary RS allows the development of cellular resistance to the later suppressant effects of these prostaglandins. The introduction of even higher doses of PGs such as those infused pharmacologically would then suppress cellular function and this could explain the apparent paradox which occurs in other inflammatory diseases such as adjuvant arthritis, where despite high levels of PGEs being found in the joint, an infusion of PGE_1 appears to prevent and suppress the arthritis.[83]

Thus it can be seen that the abnormalities of coagulation and thrombosis, and of the inflammatory and immune systems seen in RP appear also to be those which might potentially be modified by PGI_2 and PGE therapy.

Prostaglandin treatment for Raynaud's phenomenon: the clinical trials

Although much work has been carried out in the area of prostaglandin treatment for Raynaud's phenomenon it should be remembered that not all patients require drug therapy. Much can be done for patients with mild disease without the need for drugs. Stopping smoking can be useful,[5] as can changing occupation and withdrawing drugs known to be associated with RP. Many patients are apprehensive about their disease, fearing that the white dead appearance of the fingers immediately precedes gangrene and amputation; information regarding self-help groups and advice on how to protect the digits from cold can be helpful. Electrically heated gloves and socks are the perfect solution for some patients[84] and padded soles in shoes keep the feet warm and relieve pressure on the toes which can augment the vasospasm.

The majority of patients, however, requiring referral to a hospital specialist because of the severe nature of their vasospasm, will require some form of drug therapy. The calcium channel antagonist nifedipine is probably the treatment of first choice with many studies showing benefit using 20–60 mg nifedipine per day,[75] the retard preparation being used to attenuate the vasodilatory side effects.[85] This drug, however, is not universally effective and many of the patients whose RP is complicated by the presence of digital ulceration and/or a CTD find nifedipine at best only partially successful and more often obtain no benefit. It is within this particular group of patients that the prostaglandins have found their niche as a treatment for RP. Early work evaluates PGE_1 and PGI_2; more recently the stable prostaglandin analogues have been assessed as have some alternative drug delivery concepts and other ways of increasing a prostaglandin effect within the digits. These will be examined in turn.

Prostaglandin E₁

The first published work using PGE_1 as a treatment for RP was carried out by Clifford *et al.* in 1980[86] (Table 16.2) who administered up to 10 ng/kg per minute PGE_1 using an incremental dosage schedule. It was given through a central line into 26 patients for 72 hours at a time. A subjective response was reported in all but one patient during the treatment phase; 21/26 maintained this improvement at 2

weeks and 17/26 at 6 weeks. Hand and finger temperatures were elevated by the infusion and this was also maintained at 2 and 6 weeks following the infusion. Side effects were reported as minimal but included flushing, headache and postural hypotension. The same group also published the first controlled study in 1980[87] using a cross-over design to treat 12 patients with RS secondary to SSc. A saline/dextrose mix was used as control and the study documented a definite patient preference for the PGE_1 study leg (10/12). Two of the five patients with ulcers experienced healing and skin temperature measured by thermography rose an average of 2°C after PGE_1 which was maintained until the 2 weeks follow-up. This objective evidence of increased blood flow secondary to PGE_1 treatment was supported by their 1982 study[88] where the authors reported increased capillary pressure, digital blood flow and skin temperature following PGE_1.

Thereafter, isolated case reports continued to suggest a benefit from this form of treatment[89-92] and Pardy and Eastcott[93] retrospectively reviewed the outcome of 21 of their patients so treated. This uncontrolled, almost anecdotal, work is of interest as, although the same PGE_1 regimen was employed, for the first time patients who had a definite diagnosis of primary RD (*n*=8) were separated from those who had RS. Pardy and Eastcott found that none of the primary group experienced any benefit from the infusion whereas 12/13 RS patients had a favourable subjective response and the authors witnessed 10/23 healed digits. Objective measures such as digital skin temperature supported this concept of ineffectivity in primary disease by showing only a transient increase in temperature during the infusion versus 9/13 RS patients who demonstrated a sustained elevation in temperature for up to 11 weeks.

This persistence of drug effect after the infusion time period has been a feature of all the above studies and has been emphasized by later ones. Kyle *et al.*[94] in 1985 studied 11 RS patients in which 9/11 patients showed an immediate symptomatic response which was maintained in 6 at 6 weeks. A normalized thermographic response to cold challenge was seen immediately after the infusion in 10/11 and this was also maintained in 6 of these patients for 8 weeks.

After such encouraging reports, therefore, it was with some disappointment that Mohrland *et al.*[95] published their negative multicentre double-blind controlled study. Fifty-five patients were enrolled and received either the usual PGE_1 infusion regimen or saline placebo. For the first time subjective re-

Table 16.2 PGE_1 and Raynaud's phenomenon

Authors	Infusion regimen	Patients	Study design	Outcome: symptomatic	Outcome: objective
Clifford et al., 1980[86]	6–10 ng/kg per min 72 h	11 SSc 1 SLE	Uncontrolled	Less severe attacks (subjective) 5/8 ulcers healed	Finger pulse volume and hand temperature increased up to 6 w
Martin et al., 1981[87]	6–10 ng/kg per min 72 h	12 SSc	Single-blind Cross-over	83% improved during PGE_1 25% placebo Maintained at 2 w 2/5 ulcers healed	Hand and digit temperature (thermography) increased with PGE_1 Maintained at 2 w
Allen & O'Reilly, 1981[89]	10 ng/kg per min 72 h	1 CTD	Uncontrolled	Immediate improvement No long-term benefit	Immediate increase in cold tolerance Maintained at 4 w
Baron et al., 1982[90]	50 ng/kg per min for 10 min every 1 h for 2–3 days	2 SSc	Uncontrolled	2/2 ulcers healed	Immediate increase in finger temperature
Cohen et al., 1989[91]	5.5 ng/kg per min 76 h	1 MCTD	Uncontrolled	Much improved (subjective) Maintained at 6 w	None measured
Yoshikawa et al., 1990[92]	10 ng/kg per min 72 h	1 SSc 1 SLE 1 Polyarteritis 1 RA	Uncontrolled	4/4 ulcers healed	4/4 decreased circulating immune complexes
Pardy & Eastcott, 1983[93]	8–10 ng/kg per min 72 h	8 RD 13 RS	Uncontrolled	RD no benefit 12/13 RS improved (subjective) 10/23 ulcers healed	RD 7/8 transient increase digit temperature RS 9/13 increased digit temperature maintained at 11 w
Kyle et al., 1985[94]	10 ng/kg per min 72 h	6 SSc 1 SLE 1 Dermatomyositis 2 uCTD	Uncontrolled	8/10 improved at 1 w 6/10 at 6 w (subjective) 5/6 ulcers healed	9/10 immediate improvement in cold challenge response 6/10 at 6 w
Mohrland et al., 1985[95]	10 ng/kg per min 72 h	24 RD 31 SSc	Double-blind Placebo-controlled	63% improved during PGE_1 48% placebo (diary cards)	Immediate mild increase in skin temperature and finger systolic pressure at 15°C after PGE_1
Langevitz et al., 1989[97]	6–10 ng/kg per min 72 h	10 SSc 1 SLE 1 uCTD	Uncontrolled	17/20 infusions produced improvement (subjective) 35/65 ulcers healed Maintained for 4–72 w	None measured
Mizushima et al., 1987[98]	Lipo-PGE_1 bolus dose i.v. daily for 4 w	135 CTD	Double-blind Placebo-controlled	No difference attacks (diary cards) Significant ulcer healing	None measured

MCTD mixed CTD, uCTD undifferentiated CTD.

sponses were formally assessed using a diary card assessment of frequency and duration of vasospastic attacks. No difference between active and placebo groups could be detected; indeed, both groups appreciably improved. Objectively although a few of the temperature measures appeared better in the active group no definite overall improvement was seen in the PGE_1 patients when compared to the controls. This large study therefore raises salient doubts about the effectiveness of such a treatment for RP although a number of questions still need to be addressed regarding the study design. As noted by Pardy and Eastcott and also supported by work with prostacyclin,[96] primary RD patients do not appear to benefit from prostaglandin treatment. Twenty-four of the 55 patients enrolled into the controlled study had RD and this may partially explain the results. Nevertheless, both groups improved and this stresses the need for such studies to be double blind and controlled. It appears that 3 days of 'relaxing' in a warm hospital bed is an effective way to reduce attacks. However, whilst this might explain the immediate effects, the persistence of symptomatic improvement in both groups is suspicious of a climatic change and it may be that with a November to June study some improvement was due to the weather alone. Interestingly, despite the negative nature of this study, uncontrolled reports of successful treatment still appear in the literature although the treatment is clearly being reserved for intractable digital ulceration.[97] It appears, therefore, that the large percentage of RD patients, now known to be unlikely to benefit from treatment, included in the analysis of the double-blind study considered with the possibility of a climatic effect has obviously left workers unconvinced as to the validity of this study. One has to conclude that no clear consensus exists regarding the efficacy of PGE_1 in RS. A further large double-blind placebo-controlled study enrolling only RS patients is still required to adequately assess this treatment. Unfortunately, such a study is unlikely to be undertaken. PGE_1 is an inflammatory mediator and produces the five cardinal signs of inflammation round the site of the peripheral venous access.[86,95] This necessitates its infusion through a central line which is an invasive procedure involving the risk of pneumothorax,[94,97] a complication best avoided in patients at risk of developing pulmonary fibrosis secondary to their SSc. Of interest, therefore, is a novel approach to this concern. PGE_1 has been incorporated into lipid microspheres and has been given as a bolus intravenous dose through a peripheral vein daily for 4 weeks.

In this multicentre, double-blind, placebo-controlled study by Mizushima et al.[98] no objective measures of improvement were assessed. However, in the 135 patients with RS secondary to CTD the ulcer healing was reported to be significantly better after lipo-PGE_1 treatment than with placebo. As both lipo-PGE_1 and PGI_2 and the newer prostaglandin analogues do not require central line infusion, these, therefore, appear to be a more attractive approach.

Prostacyclin

A similar assessment of the vasodilator antiplatelet prostaglandin, prostacyclin, was being carried out over the same decade (Table 16.3). In 1981 we completed the first pilot study of five RS patients who received four 5-hour infusions at weekly intervals.[99] The first infusion was placebo and the three later infusions were prostacyclin, given by an incremental increase in dose up to a maximum peak dose of 10 ng/kg per minute. Symptomatic improvement measured by diary card recording of decreased frequency and duration of attacks was found in four out of five of the patients. As with PGE_1 this benefit persisted to the 6-week assessment time point. Objective measures of finger and hand temperature showed an increase after prostacyclin treatment. These findings were supported by a later larger open study of 24 patients with SSc.[100] Similar long-term clinical and laboratory improvements were detected although a different infusion regimen was employed. Prostacyclin was given by continuous intravenous infusion for 72 hours. Both groups reported a high incidence of vasodilatory side effects using this dose of 10 ng/kg per minute and the majority of subsequent work reports on lower dose regimens. In our double-blind placebo-controlled study[101] we infused 7.5 ng/kg per minute prostacyclin on three occasions for 5 hours at weekly intervals. Diary card recording showed a decrease in the frequency and duration of vasospastic attacks over the 6 weeks following the infusions in six of seven prostacyclin-treated patients. This compares to only one of seven placebo patients improving. Hand and finger temperatures remained elevated for between 1 and 6 weeks after the treatment.

The intermittent infusion regimen rather than a continuous one was chosen to allow the outpatient management of patients. The fortuitous nature of such a choice became apparent when Sinzinger et al.[102] published data showing a decreased sensitivity of human platelets to prostacyclin between 24

Table 16.3 PGI$_2$ and Raynaud's phenomenon

Authors	Infusion regimen	Patients	Study design	Outcome: symptomatic	Outcome: objective
Belch *et al.*, 1981[99]	10 ng/kg per min 5 h × 4 Weekly intervals	2 SSc 1 SLE 2 uCTD	Run in placebo infusion	4/5 improved after PGI$_2$ (diary cards) Maintained at 6 w 2/2 ulcers healed	Immediate increase in hand and finger temperature Maintained at 6 w
Dowd *et al.*, 1982[100]	7.5–10 ng/kg per min 72 h	24 SSc	Uncontrolled	21/24 improved warmth, pain and cold tolerance (diary cards) Maintained for 4–28 w	Significant immediate increase in hand temperature (thermography only) 63% maintained at 6 w
Belch *et al.*, 1983[101]	7.5 ng/kg per min 5 h × 3 Weekly intervals	8 SSc 6 uCTD	Double-blind Placebo-controlled	6/7 improved after PGI$_2$ (diary cards) 1/7 placebo (diary cards) Maintained at 6 w 3/3 ulcers healed PGI$_2$ 1/3 placebo	Significant increase in hand and finger temperature after PGI$_2$ at 1 w Finger warmth maintained at 6 w
Bellucci *et al.*, 1986[104]	7.5 ng/kg per min 5 h × 3 Weekly intervals	4 SSc	Uncontrolled	7/8 improved (diary cards) Maintained between 2 and 12 w	5/8 improved capillary microscopy Maintained 2–12 w No change digital pulse volume
Fitscha *et al*, 1988[96]	5 ng/kg per min 6 h × 5 Daily	13 RD	Uncontrolled	No benefit (diary cards)	No improvement in hand temperatures
San Lazaro *et al.*, 1985[105]	10 ng/kg per min 72 h Further course 2 days later for 10 days	1 RS	Uncontrolled	Improved (subjective) Maintained at 3 w	None measured
Ruthlein *et al.*, 1991[107]	5–6 ng/kg per min 120 h	9 SSc 2 Atherosclerosis	Uncontrolled	11/11 immediate benefit (subjective) 7/11 maintained at 6 w 3/5 ulcers healed	Plasma PGF$_{1\alpha}$ levels normal 30 min after infusion

uCTD undifferentiated CTD.

and 42 hours after starting a continuous infusion treatment. This, combined with a post-infusion rebound in platelet aggregation,[103] made an intermittent regimen a management necessity rather than a patient convenience. Later studies, therefore, all selected our intermittent regimen.[104]

Prostacyclin has been evaluated mainly in patients with RS usually secondary to SSc. Fitscha *et al.*[96] provided scientific support to the growing opinion that prostacyclin was ineffective in primary RD in their study of 13 patients. No symptomatic or objective response was detected after prostacyclin treatment, these results being in agreement with those being obtained with PGE$_1$ at the same time.[93] In a similar fashion to PGE$_1$ a prolonged beneficial effect

occurred lasting weeks after the end of the infusion period. This time the data were supported by a small though controlled study.[101] The antiplatelet effects of prostacyclin do not persist past the termination of the infusion by more than 2 hours in normal volunteers[106] and in two[101,104] out of the three[100] studies involving RS patients in which platelet aggregation was measured no alteration in platelet aggregation could be detected immediately after the termination of the infusion. In the third study[100] the 50% of patients who did show a decrease in aggregation immediately after termination of the infusion lost this effect by 2 hours. Similarly, the clinical effects of vasodilatation such as headache and flushing pass off quickly after the end of the infusion.[107] At the time of the first recording of this prolonged benefit it was common to read, therefore, of an unexplained 'cyto-protective effect' of prostacyclin. This term has been poorly defined but has been used by many authors to explain the long-term beneficial effects of the vasodilatory prostaglandins. In a stomach pretreated with prostacyclin, acid or alcohol can be added without ulceration developing.[108] We now know that this is due to the rapidity of tissue repair rather than the prevention of damage and this may be relevant in RP. Sinzinger *et al.*[103] went some way to providing an explanation in their study of labelled platelets in patients with active atherosclerosis. Prior to treatment the labelled platelets became adherent to atherosclerotic plaques. A platelet uptake ratio could be assessed by comparing the platelet deposition over the lesion to the plaque-free contralateral side. Prostacyclin decreased the platelet uptake ratio and this was maintained long after the infusion had been terminated. It is possible, therefore, to speculate that the drug may facilitate endothelial repair, thereby breaking the vicious cycle of endothelial cell damage and altered blood flow. Alternatively, the majority of patients studied have RS secondary to SSc or other rheumatological conditions. Abnormalities of WBC behaviour occur in these conditions as part of the inflammatory process.[65] We now know that the WBC also has a powerful role in modulating blood flow in the microcirculation[62] and an alteration in neutrophil and lymphocyte function by prostacyclin might well be important in the provision of this therapeutic response seen with prostacyclin.

Synthetic prostaglandin analogues

Both PGE_1 and PGI_2 require careful storage, handling and preparation. They are both unstable and of short duration of action. They therefore have to be freshly made up and given by continuous intravenous infusion. Prolonged treatment usually means hospitalization of the patients. Other problems associated with the intravenous administration of any drug can also occur, for example, infection at the site of the cannula insertion. This is in addition to the local side effects occurring if there is leakage of the prostaglandin from the cannula into the tissue. The prostaglandin's narrow therapeutic window also means that patients have to be carefully monitored with slow incremental increases in dosage to a maximum tolerated dose which can vary from patient to patient. Although serious side effects are uncommon using the above dosage regimens, most patients will experience facial flushing and headache. A few will re-

quire a decrease in drug dosage usually because of nausea, some may vomit and occasionally hypotension occurs. These problems would be tolerable if the treatment were curative. Unfortunately, repetition of the regimen is required at varying intervals with all the above attendant problems. In our own patient population repetition of the treatment is required between 6 weeks and 6 months for most patients.

One of the newer prostaglandin analogues, iloprost (Schering Chemicals AG), addresses one of these problems. Iloprost, a carbacyclin derivative of prostacyclin, is chemically stable and it appears equipotent to prostacyclin in its antiplatelet effects in most studies.[109] Like prostacyclin, it also has anti-WBC effects.[110] Its chemical stability means it retains more than 95% of its antiplatelet activity after 7 days at room temperature[111] and though still currently being given by intravenous infusion its stability makes its use much more convenient.

The first published study investigated the effects of 2 ng/kg per minute iloprost given intravenously for 8 hours a day for 3 days to 13 patients with SSc in an open study[112] (Table 16.4). Disappointingly, analysis of the diary cards was not possible due to poor compliance; however, in 19/26, ulcers healed over 10 weeks and 9/13 'felt improved'. The peripheral vascular resistance also fell after treatment and this was maintained for up to 6 weeks.

Yardumian *et al.*[113] and McHugh *et al.*[114] carried out double-blind placebo-controlled studies, both using the possibly inappropriate cross-over design. With a drug capable of producing a variable long-term effect some 'hangover' effect into the next treatment phase could occur and indeed was seen here.[113] Nevertheless, both studies investigating 12 and 29 RS patients respectively showed a significant decrease in duration and severity of vasospastic attacks over the study period of 6 weeks.

In these studies and in another[115] the dose of 2 ng/kg per minute iloprost appeared effective but vasodilatory side effects did occur. As we believe that the mechanism by which these prostaglandins provide benefit is not fully known, neither therefore, is the optimum dose. The above regimen involves titrating the dose to the maximum tolerated dose, often less than 2 ng/kg per minute due to the side effects induced. The subsequent study by Torley *et al.*[116] was therefore designed to establish whether the long-term benefits of iloprost were independent of the acute vasomotor effects. Dosage regimens of 2 ng/kg per minute and of 0.5 ng/kg per minute were equally effective in decreasing the frequency, dur-

Table 16.4 Iloprost and Raynaud's phenomenon

Authors	Infusion regimen	Patients	Study design	Outcome: symptomatic	Outcome: objective
Rademaker et al., 1987[112]	2 ng/kg per min 8 h × 3 daily	13 SSc	Uncontrolled	9/13 improved (subjective) Maintained at 10 w 19/26 ulcers healed	Digital peripheral vascular resistance fell Maintained at 6 w
Yardumian et al., 1988[113]	1–3 ng/kg per min 5 h × 3 daily	10 SSc 1 MCTD 1 uCTD	Single-blind placebo-controlled cross-over 6 w wash out	Significantly decreased attacks (diary cards) Maintained at 6 w	Significantly increased digital flow (laser doppler) Maintained at 6 w
McHugh et al., 1988[114]	2 ng/kg per min 6 h × 3 daily	26 SSc 3 RD	Double-blind placebo-controlled cross-over 6 w wash out	30% reduction attacks after iloprost 2% placebo (diary cards) Maintained at 6 w	Significant immediate decrease in thermal gradient Not maintained
Keller et al., 1993[115]	2–4 ng/kg per min 5 h × 6 daily	18 SSc 4 MCTD 3 RD	Run in placebo infusion	75% improved after iloprost 11/11 ulcers healing	13/15 immediate increase hand, digit temperature Not maintained
Torley et al., 1991[116]	0.5 ng/kg per min versus 2 ng/kg per min 6 h × 3 daily	43 SSc 5 MCTD 4 uCTD 1 RA 1 Sjögren's 1 Dermato-myositis	Double-blind comparison of 2 doses	Both doses gave significant decrease in attacks (diary cards) Maintained at 8 w	None measured
Rademaker et al., 1989[117]	2 ng/kg per min 8 h × 3 daily 1 further 8 h at 8 w versus nifedipine 30–60 mg/day	23 SSc	Double-blind double dummy	50% improved after iloprost or nifedipine	Significant increase in digital blood flow iloprost
Watson & Belcher, 1991[118]	2 ng/kg per min 6–8 h × 3 daily	84 CTD	Retrospective case sheet analysis	58% improved after iloprost 43% other treatments 50% previous non-responders improved after iloprost	

MCTD mixed CTD, uCTD undifferentiated CTD.

ation and severity of vasospastic attacks in 55 patients. Ulcer healing occurred to a similar degree in both treatment groups, that is in 44% of patients receiving the standard dose and 39% of patients receiving the lower dose. The low dose was associated with fewer side effects and was better tolerated by the patients.

Another study which has clinical relevance is that carried out by Rademaker *et al.* in 1989.[117] This study compared iloprost to the current 'gold standard' treatment, nifedipine. Twenty-three patients were enrolled and given iloprost or nifedipine 30–60 mg/day. Both treatments effectively reduced attacks; however, nifedipine was less effective at healing digital ulcers and produced more side effects. The beneficial effect of iloprost treatment was also emphasized by a retrospective study of iloprost against other treatments for RP.[118] Eighty-four patients who had received other treatments for their RP prior to receiving iloprost were investigated. Fifty-eight per cent were improved by the iloprost compared to 43% who had had a previous response to another treatment. Furthermore, of the 48 patients who had not responded at all to any treatment for RP 50% found iloprost to be beneficial. The authors suggest that even patients resistant to other treatments may benefit from iloprost infusion.

Despite its efficacy as a treatment and its equipotency with nifedipine, it still remains a second choice treatment because of its mode of administration. Studies of the orally active prostacyclin analogue, cicaprost, proved disappointing.[119] In contrast, a pilot study of oral limaprost, a PGE_1 analogue, was encouraging.[120] Forty-seven patients with RP were given 30 µg of limaprost a day by mouth over 4 months. Fifteen similar patients received no treatment and acted as control. Seventy-four per cent of treated patients improved and seven of eight patients with ulcers experienced healing. Recovery time after cold challenge was measured by thermography and was also improved in the majority of patients receiving limaprost. Further controlled studies with this compound are underway. Delivery through the skin has also been studied.[121] This transdermal approach has become popular generally with patients and, indeed, studies of the transdermally absorbed PGE_2 analogue were popular with the RS patient as well as providing both subjective and objective improvements in the disorder.[122,123] Unfortunately, development of this particular compound was not undertaken; however, the acceptability of such a mode of administration was established. Other orally and transdermally active prostaglandins are under development and will be evaluated in RP in the future. The need for a double-blind controlled not cross-over design for these studies is stressed.

Achieving a prostaglandin-like effect through manipulation of the arachidonic pathway

If the aim of treatment is to provide a vasodilatory antiplatelet effect then there are a number of ways of achieving this (Fig. 16.3) without the need for direct prostaglandin infusion.

Inhibition of the cyclo-oxygenase enzyme

Inhibition of this enzyme by non-steroidal anti-inflammatory agents (NSAIs) produces a significant antiplatelet effect. Van der Meer *et al.*[124] studied the effect of acetylsalicylic acid together with dipyridamole in 25 patients with RP over 1 week. No significant changes in the symptoms of RP or in the fingertip pulse response to cooling were found compared to placebo despite the demonstration of an inhibitory effect of the drugs on platelet function. As aspirin inhibits the cyclo-oxygenase enzyme it can prevent not only the production of TXA_2 but also prostacyclin. Although some thrombotic situations have been improved by NSAI treatment such a treatment has not proven effective in RP.

Inhibition of thromboxane synthetase

A TX synthetase inhibitor should selectively block the transformation of the cyclic endoperoxides into TXA_2 without loss of prostacyclin formation. Dazoxiben is an orally active imidazole derivative which has been shown to significantly inhibit TX synthetase activity and it has been studied in RP in the hope that it would block the vasoconstrictor effects of TXA_2 and perhaps increase prostacyclin formation via substrate diversion to prostacyclin synthetase. Disappointingly, none of the double-blind and placebo-controlled studies could show benefit in patients with either primary or secondary RP.[125,126] In only one study was there any suggestion of improvement where flow recovery time was faster after a challenge of cold air in the treated group; however, the finger blood flow itself as measured by plethysmography was unchanged.[127] Thus, dazoxiben cannot be recommended as a treatment for RP. The subsequent discovery that the endoperoxides themselves cause vasoconstriction probably accounts for some of the lack of effect. Attenuation of the TX effect through receptor blockade might be more successful as it does not lead to a build-up of the endoperoxides which may have a direct vasoconstrictor effect or act as substrate for other vasoconstrictor compounds such as $PGF_{2\alpha}$. A single-dose placebo-controlled study of a thromboxane receptor blocker in RP confirmed the potent antiplatelet effect of the drug, though only a minimal change in blood flow response occurred.[128] Other compounds which combine thromboxane synthetase inhibition with thromboxane receptor blockade have also been shown to have potent antiplatelet effects in patients with vascular disease[129] and should be evaluated in RP.

Dietary manipulation of essential fatty acids

Prostaglandins of the 2 series are derived from arachidonic acid (AA). Other essential fatty acids (EFAs) are metabolized to different prostaglandin series. The ingestion of a diet rich in evening primrose oil (EPO) will elevate levels of dihomo-γ-linolenic acid (DGLA) which will result in monoenoic or 1-series prostaglandins. One of these is the potent vasodilator antiplatelet agent PGE_1 discussed earlier.[86] Theoretically the desired antiplatelet vasodilator effect should be maintained by the PGE_1 without the opposing effects of TXA_2. Leukotrienes (LTs) are also produced through EFA metabolism. LTB_4 is one of the LTs resulting from 5-lipoxygenase action on AA. This is a potent WBC activator. In contrast to AA, metabolism of DGLA to LT does not occur, merely the production of an inert 15-hydroxyl derivative which blocks further transformation of AA to the LTs.[130] With the evidence that WBC activity may be relevant to vascular disease in general,[62,65] attenuation of LTB_4 effects may be useful. Twelve capsules of EPO a day contain a total dose of 540 mg γ-linolenic acid, the precursor of DGLA. After a 2-week placebo run-in phase, 11 patients with RP were given this dose of EPO[131] and their response compared to 12 patients given 12 capsules per day of placebo. Despite the detection of an antiplatelet effect in the blood and a clinical worsening of diary card attacks recorded only in the placebo group as the winter weather set in, no objective improvement in blood flow could be detected. Interpretation of this study, however, is hindered by the mixing of primary and secondary RP patients; although divided equally between the two treatment groups, 50% of the patients had RD and we now know that these might not have been expected to respond to such a treatment.

High dietary levels of another EFA, eicosapentanoic acid (EPA), provides the substrate for production of the prostaglandins of the 3 series. PGI_3 has been shown to be equipotent to PGI_2 whereas TXA_3 is a much less effective platelet aggregant than TXA_2,[132] the net effect again being a gain in vasodilatation and a decrease in platelet aggregation. EPA forms the 5-series LTs. The potency of LTB_5 in inducing leucocyte aggregation is 10% of the potency of LTB_4.[133] Thus an additional anti-white-cell effect

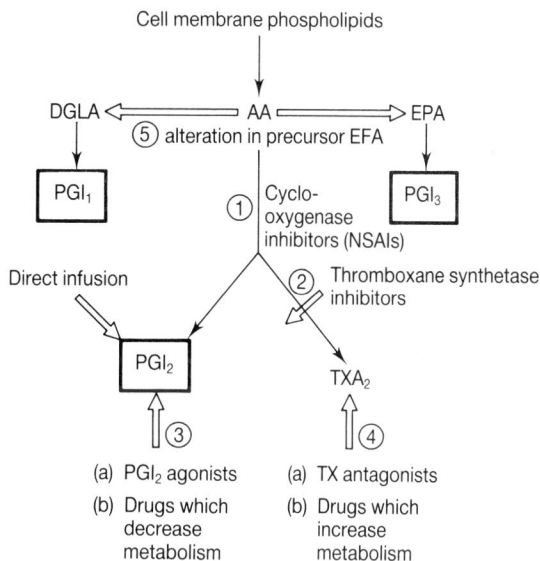

Fig. 16.4 Therapeutic approaches to the arachidonic acid cascade.

might be expected during administration of this therapy.

Fish oil supplements containing both EPA and docosahexaenoic acid (DHA) have been given to patients with RP in an olive oil placebo-controlled study.[134] Both placebo and fish oil supplementation increased the time interval before induction of Raynaud's attacks after cold challenge in 32 patients with RP. This reached statistical significance in the fish oil supplemented group at 6 weeks but the effect was not maintained at 12 weeks. Attenuation of documented benefit in the fish oil group may have occurred due to the use of an active placebo as olive oil contains various EFAs including a proportion of EPA.

Two other features of this study are of interest. The first is that the beneficial effect seen at 6 weeks was lost by 12 weeks. This agrees with the earlier work in EPO when a significant antiplatelet effect detected between 2 and 6 weeks was lost at 8 weeks. Could the tachyphylaxis seen with continuous prostaglandin infusion[102] occur with oral dosing of prostaglandin precursors? This may be relevant to the development of orally active prostaglandin analogues. The second unusual feature of the above study is that the RD patients (11/16) benefited, not those with RS secondary to SSc. This is in contrast to other prostaglandin work[93] and suggests an alternative, possibly direct mechanism of action for the EFAs such as a beneficial change in membrane fluidity following incorporation of the EFA itself into the cell. Currently only the above two studies have investigated EFA supplementation in RP. From the results it has to be concluded that such treatments have at best only a modest effect. However, now that genetic engineering has allowed the development of EFA-producing yeasts, studies with larger, possibly more effective, doses are now possible.

Conclusion

Theoretically the documented abnormalities of blood flow and blood constituents in RP should benefit from treatment by the vasodilator antiplatelet prostaglandins. Their additional anti-WBC and possible fibrinolytic effects may also be relevant. Prostaglandin E_1 treatment is beneficial in the majority of studies. However, the largest placebo-controlled study could not confirm this beneficial effect. It is possible, however, that the proportion of primary RD patients in this study influenced the results as these patients do not have the coagulation and haemorrheological abnormalities which may be modified by PGE_1. A similar lack of effect with prostacyclin treatment in primary RD has also been documented; however, it does appear to be effective in RS as does the synthetic analogue, iloprost. This prostaglandin effect lasts for a variable amount of time after infusion documented at usually between 2 and 6 weeks. Other methods of achieving the vasodilator antiplatelet effect of these prostaglandins by interfering with AA metabolism have been evaluated. However, at present no convincing evidence exists as to their benefit. Further work involving the above and orally and transdermally active prostaglandin compounds is being undertaken. These studies should be double blind and placebo controlled. A cross-over design should be avoided and an intermittent regimen considered. Long-term studies evaluating rate of disease progression during treatment, particularly in SSc, should be of interest.

Acknowledgements

JJFB receives support from the Sir Jules Thorn Trust and the Oliver Bird Foundation.

References

1. Raynaud M. De l'asphyxre et de la gangrene symétriques des extrémités. Paris 1862. (Translated by Thomas Barlow, London: New Sydenham Society, 1988).
2. Porter JM, Bardona EJ, Baur GM, Wesche DH, Andrasch RH, Rosch J. The clinical significance of Raynaud's syndrome. *Surgery* 1976; **80**: 756–64.
3. Olsen N, Neilsen SL. Prevalence of primary Raynaud phenomena in young females. *Scand J Clin Lab Invest* 1978; **37**: 761–4.
4. Belch JJF. Management of Raynaud's phenomenon. *Ther Update* 1990; **41**: 253–60.
5. Goodfield MJD, Hume A, Rowell NR. The acute effects of cigarette smoking on cutaneous blood flow in smoking and non-smoking subjects with and without Raynaud's phenomenon. *Br J Rheumatol* 1990; **29**: 89–91.
6. Belch JJF, Land D, Park RHR, McKillop JH, McKenzie JF. Decreased oesophageal blood flow in patients with Raynaud's phenomenon. *Br J Rheumatol* 1988; **27**: 426–30.
7. Kahan A, Devaux JY, Amor B, *et al.* Nifedipine and thallium-201 myocardial perfusion in progressive systemic sclerosis. *N Engl J Med* 1986; **314** (22): 1397–402.
8. Baron M, Feiglin D, Hyland R, Urowitz MB, Shiff B. Gallium lung scans in progressive systemic sclerosis. *Arthritis Rheum* 1983; **26**: 967–74.
9. Porter JM, Rivers SP, Anderson CJ, Baum GM. Evaluation and management of patients with Raynaud's syndrome. *Am J Surg* 1987; **142**: 183–9.
10. Allen EV, Brown GE. Raynaud's disease: a critical review of minimal requisites for diagnosis. *Am J Med Sci* 1932; **183**: 187–200.
11. Gifford RW, Hines EA. Raynaud's disease among young women and girls. *Circulation* 1957; **16**: 1012–21.
12. Kallenberg CGM, Wouda AA, Hoet MA, van Venrooij WJ. Development of connective tissue disease in patients presenting with Raynaud's phenomenon: a six year follow up with emphasis on the predictive value of antinuclear antibodies as detected by immunoblotting. *Ann Rheum Dis* 1988; **47**: 634–41.
13. Maricq HR, Johnson MN, Whetstone CC. Capillary abnormalities in polyvinyl chloride production workers in examinations by *in vivo* microscopy. *JAMA* 1976; **236**: 1368–71.
14. Taylor W. The hand–arm vibration syndrome, secondary Raynaud's phenomenon of occupational origin. *Proc R Coll Phys, Edinb* 1989; **19**: 7–14.
15. Hedlund U. Raynaud's phenomenon of fingers and toes of miners exposed to local and whole-body vibration and cold. *Int Arch Occup Environ Health* 1989; **61**: 457–61.
16. Edwards JM, Porter JM. Associated disease in

patient with Raynaud's syndrome. *Vasc Med Rev* 1990; **1**: 51–8.

17. Fitzgerald O, Hess EV, O'Connor GT, Spencer-Green G. Prospective study of the evolution of Raynaud's phenomenon. *Am J Med* 1988; **84**: 718–26.

18. Gerbracht DD, Steen VD, Ziegler GL, Medsger ThA, Rodnan GP. Evolution of primary Raynaud's phenomenon (Raynaud's disease) to connective tissue disease. *Arthritis Rheum* 1985; **28**: 87–92.

19. Maricq HR. Raynaud's phenomenon and microvascular abnormalities in scleroderma (systemic sclerosis). In: Jayson MIV, Black CM (eds), *Systemic Sclerosis: Scleroderma*. Chichester: John Wiley, 1988: 151–66.

20. Kallenberg CGM, Wouda AA, The TH. Systemic involvement and immunological findings in patients presenting with Raynaud's phenomenon. *Am J Med* 1980; **69**: 675–80.

21. LeRoy EC, Lomea R. The spectrum of scleroderma. *Hosp Pract* 1989; **10**: 33–42.

22. Lewis T. The pathological changes in the arteries supplying the fingers in warm-handed people and in cases of so-called Raynaud's disease. *Clin Sci* 1938; **3**: 288–311.

23. Peacock JH. Vasodilatation in the human hand: observations on primary Raynaud's disease and acrocyanosis of the upper extremities. *Clin Sci* 1957; **17**: 575–86.

24. Olsen N, Petring OU, Rossing N. Exaggerated postural vasoconstrictor reflex in Raynaud's phenomenon. *BMJ* 1987; **294**: 1186–8.

25. Fagius J, Blumberg H. Sympathetic outflow to the hand in patient with Raynaud's phenomenon. *Cardiovasc Res* 1985; **19**: 249–53.

26. Downey JA, Frewin DB. The effect of cold on blood flow in the hand of patients with Raynaud's phenomenon. *Clin Sci* 1973; **44**: 279–89.

27. Kontos HA, Wasserman AJ. Effect of reserpine in Raynaud's phenomenon. *Circulation* 1969; **34**: 259–65.

28. Freedman RR, Mayes MD, Sabharwal SC. Induction of vasospastic attacks despite digital nerve block in Raynaud's disease and phenomenon. *Circulation* 1989; **80**: 859–62.

29. Bunker CB, Terenghi G, Springall DR, Polak JM, Dowd PM. Deficiency of calcitonin gene-related peptide in Raynaud's phenomenon. *Lancet* 1990; **336**: 1530–3.

30. Belch JJF. Eicosanoids and rheumatology: inflammatory and vascular aspects. *Prostaglandins Leukot Essent Fatty Acids* 1989; **36**: 219–34.

31. Manku MS, Morse N, Belch JJF. Effects of gamma-linoleic acid supplementation on plasma essential fatty acids. *Prog Lipid Res* 1986; **25**: 469–73.

32. Klimiuk PS, Taulor L, Baker RD, Jayson MIV. Autonomic neuropathy in systemic sclerosis. *Ann Rheum Dis* 1988; **47**: 542–5.

33. Suarez-Almazor ME, Bruera E, Russell AS. Normal cardiovascular autonomic function in patients with systemic sclerosis (CREST variant). *Ann Rheum Dis* 1988; **47**: 672–4.

34. Belch JJF. Raynaud's phenomenon: its relevance to scleroderma. *Ann Rheum Dis* 1991; **50**: 839–45.

35. Kahaleh MB, Osborn I, LeRoy EC. Increased factor VIII von Willebrand factor antigen and von Willebrand factor activity in scleroderma and in Raynaud's phenomenon. *Ann Rheum Dis* 1981; **94**: 482–4.

36. Belch JJF, Zoma A, Richards I, Forbes CD, Sturrock RD. Vascular damage and factor VIII related antigen in the rheumatic diseases. *Rheumatol Int* 1987; **7**: 107–11.

37. James JP, Stevens TRJ, Hall ND, *et al*. Factor VIII related antigen in connective tissue disease patients and relatives. *Br J Rheumatol* 1990; **29**: 6–9.

38. Lau CS, McLaren M, Belch JJF. Factor VIII/von Willebrand factor antigen levels correlate with symptom severity in patients with Raynaud's phenomenon. *Br J Rheumatol* 1991; **30**: 433–6.

39. Greaves M, Malia RG, Milford Ward A, *et al*. Elevated von Willebrand factor antigen in systemic sclerosis: relationship to visceral disease. *Br J Rheumatol* 1988; **27**: 281–5.

40. Kahaleh MB, LeRoy EC. Vascular factors in the pathogenesis of systemic sclerosis. In: Jayson MIV, Black CM (eds), *Systemic Sclerosis: Scleroderma*. Chichester: John Wiley, 1988: 107–18.

41. Pringle R, Walder DN, Weaver JP. Blood viscosity and Raynaud's disease. *Lancet* 1965; **1**: 1086–8.

42. Jarrett PEM, Browse M, Browse NL. Treatment of Raynaud's phenomenon by fibrinolytic enhancement. *BMJ* 1978; **2**: 523–5.

43. Belch JJF, Zoma A, McLaughlin K, *et al*. Fibrinolysis in SLE: effect of desamino D arginine vasopressin infusion. *Br J Rheumatol* 1987; **25**: 262–6.

44. Belch JJF, Drury J, Flannigan P, *et al*. Abnormal biochemical and cellular parameters in the blood of patients with Raynaud's phenomenon. *Scott Med J* 1987; **32**: 12–14.

45. Zamora MR, O'Brien RF, Rutherford RB, Weill JV. Serum endothelium-1 concentrations and cold provocation in primary Raynaud's phenomenon. *Lancet* 1990; **336**: 1144–7.

46. Kinney EL, Demers LM. Plasma 6-keto PGF_1 concentration in Raynaud's phenomenon. *Prostaglandins Med* 1981; **7**: 389–93.

47. Belch JJF, McLaren M, Anderson J, *et al*. Increased prostacyclin metabolites and decreased red cell deformability in patients with systemic sclerosis and Raynaud's syndrome. *Prostaglandins Leukot Med* 1985; **17**: 1–9.

48. Rustin MHA, Bull HA, Machin SJ, Koro O, Dowd PM. Serum from patient with Raynaud's phenomenon inhibits prostacyclin production. *J Invest Dermatol* 1987; **89**: 555–9.

49. Holt CM, Moult J, Lindsey N, Hughes P, Greaves

M, Rowell NR. Prostacyclin production by human umbilical vein endothelium in response to serum from patients with systemic sclerosis. *Br J Rheumatol* 1989; **28**: 216–20.

50. Belch JJF, O'Dowd A, Forbes CF, Sturrock RD. Platelet sensitivity to a prostacyclin analogue in systemic sclerosis. *Br J Rheumatol* 1986; **24**: 346–50.

51. Whicher JT, Bell AM, Martin FR, Marshall LA, Dieppe PA. Prostaglandins cause an increase in serum acute-phase proteins in man, which is diminished in systemic sclerosis. *Clin Sci* 1984; **66**: 165–71.

52. Kirby JDT, Dowd PM, Lima DRA, Kilfeather S, Turner P. Prostacyclin increases cyclic-nucleotide responsiveness of lymphocytes from patient with systemic sclerosis. *Lancet* 1980; **2**: 453–4.

53. Jeremy JY, Mikhailidis DP, Hutton RA, Dandona P. The effect of cooling on *in vitro* vascular prostacyclin and platelet thromboxane A$_2$ synthesis: relevance to cold-induced pathology. *Microcirc Endothelium Lymphatics* 1988; **4** (1): 3–20.

54. Reilly IAG, Roy L, Fitzgerald GA. Biosynthesis of thromboxane in patients with systemic sclerosis and Raynaud's phenomenon. *BMJ* 1986; **292**: 1037–9.

55. Klimiuk PS, Grennan A, Weinkove C, Jayson MIV. Platelet serotonin in systemic sclerosis. *Ann Rheum Dis* 1989; **48**: 586–9.

56. Kahaleh MB, Osborn I, Leroy EC. Elevated levels of circulating platelet aggregates and beta-thromboglobulin in scleroderma. *Ann Intern Med* 1982; **96**: 610–13.

57. Zahavi J, Hamilton WAP, O'Reilly MJG, Leyton J, Cotton LT, Kakkar VV. Plasma exchange and platelet function in Raynaud's phenomenon. *Thromb Res* 1980; **19**: 85–93.

58. Hutton RA, Mikhailidis DP, Bernstein RM, Jeremy JY, Hughes GRV, Dandona P. Assessment of platelet function in patient with Raynaud's syndrome. *J Clin Pathol* 1984; **37**: 182–7.

59. Kovacs IB, Sowemimo-Coker SO, Kirby JDT, Turner P. Altered behaviour of erythrocytes in scleroderma. *Clin Sci* 1983; **65**: 515–19.

60. Rademaker M, Thomas RH, Kirby JD, *et al.* Calcium influx into red cells: the effects of sera from patients with systemic sclerosis. *Clin Exp Rheumatol* 1991; **9** (3): 247–51.

61. Herrmann K, Haustein UF, Bohme HJ, *et al.* Acid lysosomal hydrolases in systemic sclerosis and other connective tissue diseases. *Br J Dermatol* 1982; **106**: 523–8.

62. Belch JJF. The role of the white blood cell in arterial disease. *Blood Coag Fibrinol* 1990; **1**: 183–92.

63. Schmid-Schonbein GW, Engler RC. Granulocytes as active participants in acute myocardial ischemia and infarction. *Am J Cardiovasc Pathol* 1986; **1**: 15–30.

64. Belch JJF, Chopra M, Hutchinson S, *et al.* Free rad-ical pathology in chronic arterial disease. *Free Radic Biol Med* 1989; **6** (4): 375–8.

65. Lau CS, O'Dowd A, Belch JJF. White blood cell activation in Raynaud's phenomenon of systemic sclerosis and vibration induced white finger syndrome. *Ann Rheum Dis* 1992; **51**: 249–52.

66. Spisani S, Dovigo L, Colamussi V. Leukocyte migration and phagocytosis in progressive systemic sclerosis. *Scand J Rheumatol* 1981; **10**: 299–300.

67. van der Meulen J, Wouda AA, Mandema E, The TH. Immune complexes in peripheral blood polymorphonuclear leucocytes of patients with Raynaud's phenomenon. *Clin Exp Immunol* 1979; **35**: 62–6.

68. Lau CS, Scott N, Shaw JW, Belch JJF. Increased activity of oxygen free radical during reperfusion in patients with peripheral arterial disease undergoing percutaneous peripheral artery balloon angioplasty. *Int Angiol* 1991; **10** (4): 244–6.

69. Kahaleh MB, Smith EA, Soma Y, Leroy EC. Effect of lymphotoxin and tumour necrosis factor on endothelial and connective tissue cell growth and function. *Clin Immunol Immunopathol* 1988; **49**: 261–72.

70. Leroy EC, Smith EA, Kahaleh MB, Trojanowska M, Silver RM. A strategy for determining the pathogenesis of systemic sclerosis: is transforming growth factor-beta the answer? *Arthritis Rheum* 1989; **32**: 817–25.

71. Cowley AJ, Stainer K, Cockbill S, Heptinstall S. Correlation between platelet behaviour and cold-induced vasoconstriction in man, and the effects of epoprostenol infusion. *Clin Sci* 1984; **67**: 511–14.

72. Utsunomiya T, Kransz MM, Valeri CR, Shepro D, Hechtman HB. Treatment of pulmonary embolism with prostacyclin. *Surgery* 1980; **88**: 25–30.

73. Dowd PM, Kovacs IB, Bland CJH, Kirby JDT. Effect of prostaglandins I$_2$ and E$_1$ on red cell deformability in patients with Raynaud's phenomenon and systemic sclerosis. *BMJ* 1981; **283**: 350.

74. Kury PG, Ramwell PW, Connell HM. The effect of prostaglandins E$_1$ and E$_2$ on the human erythrocyte as monitored by spin labels. *Biochem Biophys Res Commun* 1974; **56**: 478–88.

75. Rodeheffer RJ, Rommer JA, Wigley F, Smith CR. Controlled double-blind trial of nifedipine in the treatment of Raynaud's phenomenon. *N Engl J Med* 1983; **308**: 880–3.

76. Lucas GS, Sims MH, Caldwell NM, Alexander SJC, Stuart J. Haemorrheological effects of prostaglandin E$_1$ infusion in Raynaud's syndrome. *J Clin Pathol* 1984; **37**: 870–3.

77. Belch JJF, Lowe GDO, Drummond MM, Forbes CD, Prentice CRM. Prostacyclin reduces red cell deformability. *Thromb Haemost* 1981; **45**: 189.

78. Higgs GA. Prostaglandins and the microcirculation. In: Herman AG, van Houtte PM, Denolin H, Goossens A (eds), *Cardiovascular Pharmacology of the Prostaglandins*. New York: Raven Press, 1982: 315–25.

79. Zimmerman JJ. Pharmacologic modulation by prostaglandin E₁ of superoxide anion production by human polymorphonuclear leukocytes. *Crit Care Med* 1986; **14:** 761–4.

80. Winkelstein A, Kelley VE. The effects of PGE₁ on lymphocytes in NZB/NZW mice. *Clin Immunol Immunopathol* 1980; **17:** 212.

81. Korchak HM, Abramson SB. The role of arachidonic acid metabolites in the regulation of neutrophil function. In: Goodwin JS (ed), *Prostaglandins and Immunity*. Boston: Martinus Nijhoff, 1985: 179.

82. Rogers TJ. The role of arachidonic acid metabolites in the function of murine suppressor cells. In: Goodwin JS (ed), *Prostaglandins and Immunity*. Boston: Martinus Nijhoff, 1985: 80.

83. Editorial. Prostaglandins and immunity. *Lancet* 1981; **2:** 24.

84. Kempson GE, Coggon D, Acheson ED. Electrically heated gloves for intermittent digital ischaemia. *BMJ* 1983; **286:** 268.

85. Finch MB, Copeland S, Passmore AP, Johnston GD. A double-blind cross-over study of nifedipine retard in patients with Raynaud's phenomenon. *Clin Rheumatol* 1988; **7** (3): 359–65.

86. Clifford PC, Martin MFR, Sheddon EJ, Kirby JD, Baird RN, Dieppe PA. Treatment of vasospastic disease with prostaglandin E₁. *BMJ* 1980; **281:** 1031–4.

87. Martin MFR, Dowd PM, Ring EFJ, Cooke ED, Dieppe PA, Kirby JDT. Prostaglandin E₁ infusions for vascular insufficiency in progressive systemic sclerosis. *Ann Rheum Dis* 1981; **40:** 350–4.

88. Martin MFR, Tooke JE, Wright V. Microvascular changes produced by prostaglandin E₁. *Ann Rheum Dis* 1982; **41:** 309–10.

89. Allen JA, O'Reilly MJG. Treatment of severe Raynaud's phenomenon with prostaglandin E₁. *Ir J Med Sci* 1981; **150:** 190.

90. Baron M, Skrinskas G, Urowitz MB, Madras PN. Prostaglandin E₁ therapy for digital ulcers in scleroderma. *Can Med Assoc J* 1982; **126:** 42–5.

91. Cohen LE, Faske I, Fenske NA, Greist MA. Prostaglandin infusion therapy for intermittent digital ischaemia in a patient with mixed connective tissue disease. *J Am Acad Dermatol* 1989; **20:** 893–7.

92. Yoshikawa T, Suzuki H, Kato H, Yano S. Effects of prostaglandin E₁ on collagen diseases with high levels of circulating immune complexes. *J Rheumatol* 1990; **17** (11): 1513–14.

93. Pardy BJ, Eastcott HHG. Prostaglandin therapy in severe limb ischaemia. *World J Surg* 1983; **7:** 353–62.

94. Kyle V, Parr G, Salisbury R, Thomas PP, Hazelmann B. Prostaglandin E₁ vasospastic disease and thermography. *Ann Rheum Dis* 1985; **44:** 73–8.

95. Mohrland JS, Porter JM, Smith EA, Belch JJF, Simms MH. A multiclinic, placebo-controlled, double-blind study of prostaglandin E₁ in Raynaud's syndrome. *Ann Rheum Dis* 1985; **44:** 754–60.

96. Fitscha P, Kaliman J, Weidinger F, Sinzinger H, O'Grady J. Epoprostenol in patients with Raynaud's disease. *Prostaglandins Leukot Essent Fatty Acids* 1988; **33** (1): 23–7.

97. Langevitz P, Buskila D, Lee P, Urowitz MB. Treatment of refractory ischemic skin ulcers in patients with Raynaud's phenomenon with PGE₁ infusions. *J Rheumatol* 1989; **16** (11): 1433–5.

98. Mizushima Y, Shiokawa Y, Homma M, *et al.* A multicenter double-blind controlled study of lipo-PGE₁, PGE₁ incorporated in lipid microspheres in peripheral vascular disease secondary to connective tissue disorders. *J Rheumatol* 1987; **14:** 97–103.

99. Belch JJF, Newman P, Drury JK, *et al.* Successful treatment of Raynaud's syndrome with prostacyclin. *Thromb Haemost* 1981; **45** (3): 255–6.

100. Dowd PM, Martin MFR, Cooke ED, *et al.* Therapy of Raynaud's phenomenon by intravenous infusion of prostacyclin (PGI₂). *Br J Dermatol* 1982; **81:** 106–10.

101. Belch JJF, Drury JK, Capell H, *et al.* Intermittent epoprostenol (prostacyclin) infusion in patients with Raynaud's syndrome – a double-blind controlled trial. *Lancet* 1983; **1:** 313–15.

102. Sinzinger H, Silberbauer K, Horsch AK, Gall A. Decreased sensitivity of human platelets to PGI₂ during long-term intra-arterial prostacyclin infusion in patients with peripheral vascular disease – a rebound phenomenon? *Prostaglandins* 1981; **21:** 49–51.

103. Sinzinger H, Fitscha P, Kaliman J. The optimal PGI₂ infusion time as judged by autologous platelet-labelling in patients with active atherosclerosis. In: Schror K (ed), *Prostaglandins and Other Eicosanoids in the Cardiovascular System*. Basel: Karger, 1985: 358–64.

104. Bellucci S, Kedra AW, Courmelle JM, *et al.* Prolonged remission in Raynaud's phenomenon after prostacyclin infusion. *Scand J Rheumatol* 1986; **15:** 392–8.

105. San Lazaro C de, Colver AF, Parkin JM. Prostacyclin in severe peripheral vascular disease. *Arch Dis Child* 1985; **60:** 370–84.

106. O'Grady J, Warrington S, Mote MJ, *et al.* Effects of intravenous infusion of prostacyclin (PGI₂) in man. *Prostaglandins* 1980; **19:** 319–32.

107. Ruthlein HJ, Reigger G, Auer IO. Treatment of severe Raynaud syndrome in scleroderma or thromboangiitis obliterans with prostacyclin (PGI₂). *Z Rheumatol* 1991; **50:** 16–20.

108. Soll AH, Whittle BJR. Prostacyclin inhibits canine parietal cell activity and cyclic AMP formation. *Prostaglandins* 1981; **21:** 353–65.

109. Belch JJF, Greer I, McLaren M, *et al.* The effects of intravenous ZK36–374, a stable prostacyclin analogue, on normal volunteers. *Prostaglandins* 1984; **28:** 67–77.

110. Belch JJF, Saniabadi A, Dickson R, Sturrock RD, Forbes CD. Efefct of Iloprost (ZK 36 374) on white cell behaviour. In: Gryglewski RJ, Stock G (eds), *Prostacyclin and Its Stable Analogue Iloprost.* Berlin: Springer-Verlag, 1987: 97–102.

111. Skubulla W, Raduchel B, Vorgruggen H. Chemistry of stable prostacyclin analogues: synthesis of iloprost. In: Gryglewski RJ, Stock G (eds), *Prostacyclin and Its Stable Analogue Iloprost.* Berlin: Springer-Verlag, 1987: 17–24.

112. Rademaker M, Thomas RHM, Provost G, Beacham JA, Cooke ED, Kirby JD. Prolonged increase in digital blood flow following iloprost infusion in patients with systemic sclerosis. *Postgrad Med J* 1987; **63:** 617–20.

113. Yardumian DA, Isenberg DA, Rustin M, *et al.* Successful treatment of Raynaud's syndrome with iloprost, a chemically stable prostacyclin analogue. *Br J Rheumatol* 1988; **27:** 220–6.

114. McHugh NJ, Csuka M, Watson H, *et al.* Infusion of iloprost, a prostacyclin analogue, for treatment of Raynaud's phenomenon in systemic sclerosis. *Ann Rheum Dis* 1988; **47:** 43–7.

115. Keller J, Kaltenecker A, Schricker Th, Krais Th, Lindner R, Hornstein OP. Vascular and antiplatelet actions of intermittent infusion with a new stable prostacyclin derivative in patients with Raynaud's phenomenon and scleroderma. *J Dermatol* 1993; (in press).

116. Torley HI, Madhok R, Capell HA, *et al.* A double blind, randomised, multicentre comparison of two doses of intravenous iloprost in the treatment of Raynaud's phenomenon secondary to connective tissue diseases. *Ann Rheum Dis* 1991; **50:** 800–4.

117. Rademaker M, Cooke ED, Almond NE, *et al.* Comparison of intravenous infusions of iloprost and oral nifedipine in treatment of Raynaud's phenomenon in patient with systemic sclerosis: a double blind randomised study. *BMJ* 1989; **298:** 561–4.

118. Watson HR, Belcher G. Retrospective comparison of iloprost with other treatments for secondary Raynaud's phenomenon. *Ann Rheum Dis* 1991; **50:** 359–61.

119. Lau CS, McLaren M, Saniabadi A, Scott N, Belch JJF. The pharmacological effects of cicaprost, an oral prostacyclin analogue, in patients with Raynaud's syndrome secondary to systemic sclerosis – a preliminary study. *Clin Exp Rheumatol* 1991; **9:** 271–3.

120. Murai C, Sasaki T, Osaki H, Hatakeyama A, Shibata S, Yoshinaga K. Oral limaprost for Raynaud's phenomenon. *Lancet* 1989; **1:** 1218.

121. Belch JJF, Ansell D, Saniabadi A, Forbes CD, Sturrock RD. Transdermally applied iloprost (ZK 36–374) decreases whole blood platelet aggregation. In: Sinzinger H, Schror K (eds), *Prostaglandins in Clinical and Biological Research*, vol 242. New York: Liss, 1987: 413–17.

122. Belch JJF, Shaw B, Sturrock RD, Madhok R, Leiberman P, Forbes CD. Double-blind trial of CL 115,347, a transdermally absorbed prostaglandin E2 analogue, in treatment of Raynaud's phenomenon. *Lancet* 1985; **1:** 1180–3.

123. Besson JAO, Glen AIM. Treatment of childhood Raynaud's disease by transdermal prostaglandin E2 analogue. *Lancet* 1985; **1:** 50.

124. van der Meer J, Wouda AA, Kallenberg CGM, Wesseling H. A double-blind controlled trial of low dose acetylsalicylic acid and dipyridamole in the treatment of Raynaud's phenomenon. *VASA* 1987; **18:** 71–4.

125. Belch JJF, Cormie J, Newman P, *et al.* Dazoxiben, a thromboxane synthetase inhibitor, in the treatment of Raynaud's syndrome: a double-blind trial. *Br J Clin Pharmacol* 1983; **15:** 1135–6.

126. Jones EW, Hawkey CJ. A thromboxane synthetase inhibitor in Raynaud's phenomenon. *Prostaglandins Leukot Med* 1983; **12:** 67–71.

127. Tindall H, Tooke JE, Menys VC, Martin MFR, Davies JA. Effect of dazoxiben, a thromboxane synthetase inhibitor of skin-blood flow following cold challenge in patients with Raynaud's phenomenon. *Eur J Clin Invest* 1985; **15:** 20–3.

128. Lau CS, Khan F, McLaren M, Bancroft A, Walker M, Belch JJF. The effects of thromboxane receptor blockade on platelet aggregation and digital skin blood flow in patient with secondary Raynaud's syndrome. *Rheumatol Int* 1991; **11:** 163–8.

129. Hoet B, Arnout J, Van Geet C, Deckmyn H, Verhaeghe R, Vermylen J. Ridogrel, a combined thromboxane synthetase inhibitor and receptor blocker, decreases elevated plasma – thromboglobulin levels in patients with documented peripheral arterial disease. *Thromb Haemost* 1990; **64** (1): 87–90.

130. Voorlees JJ. Leukotrienes and other lipoxygenase products in the pathogenesis and therapy of psoriasis and other dermatoses. *Arch Dermatol* 1983; **119:** 541–7.

131. Belch JJF, Shaw B, O'Dowd A, *et al.* Evening primrose oil (Efamol) in the treatment of Raynaud's phenomenon: a double blind study. *Thromb Haemost* 1985; **54** (2): 490–4.

132. Dyerberg J, Bang HO, Stoffersen E, Moncada S, Vane JR. Eicosapentanoic acid and prevention of thrombosis and atherosclerosis. *Lancet* 1978; **2:** 117–19.

133. Prescott SM. The effect of eicosapentanoic acid on

leukotriene β_4 production by human neutrophils. *J Biol Chem* 1984; **259**: 7615–17.

134. DiGiacomo RA, Kremer JM, Shah DM. Fish-oil dietary supplementation in patients with Raynaud's phenomenon: a double-blind, controlled, prospective study. *Am J Med* 1989; **86**: 158–64.

17 Prostanoids in cerebral ischaemia and stroke

Richard J Gryglewski

Endogenous prostanoids in experimental cerebral ischaemia

The levels of free arachidonic acid and of prostanoids in brain tissue or in cerebrospinal fluid are very low.[1-5] For instance, the basal levels of prostacyclin (PGI_2) or thromboxane A_2 (TXA_2) are of the order of a few picograms per milligram of protein in the brain cortex of rats sacrificed by microwave radiation.[5] However, insults to neural tissue such as death by decapitation, trauma, ischaemia, hypoxia, reperfusion or subarachnoid haemorrhage cause a considerable increase in amounts of free arachidonic acid and the products of its oxidation in brain[5-7] and in cerebrospinal fluid.[2,8,9] Paradoxically, an increased turnover of arachidonic acid in ischaemic piglet brain is associated with the suppressed production of prostanoids in response to hypercapnia and hypotension.[10] This complex prostanoid reaction to the brain ischaemia seems to depend on changes in activities of phospholipases A_2 or C and lipoxygenation of arachidonic acid, rather than on activation of prostaglandin H synthase.[8-10] Of the various biochemical events that characterize cerebral ischaemia, enhanced generation of eicosanoids mostly exacerbates and only rarely improves the outcome of ischaemic or reperfusion injury.

Marked species differences exist in the composition of products of PGH synthase (i.e. prostanoids) in cerebral tissue. For instance, in the brain of the rat, gerbil or rabbit the predominant prostanoid is prostaglandin D_2, and the concentrations of other prostanoids decrease in the order: PGD_2, $PGF_{2\alpha}$, $PGE_2 > 6$-keto-$PGF_{1\alpha}$, TXB_2.[6,11] This profile of prostanoids is in contrast with that in the canine brain in which PGD_2 levels are negligible and 6-keto-$PGF_{1\alpha}$ levels are relatively high. In the human brain $PGF_{2\alpha}$ is represented most abundantly, followed by PGE_2, while prostacyclin (i.e. 6-keto-$PGF_{1\alpha}$) levels are low.[3] On the contrary, prostacyclin metabolites are the principal prostanoids in human cerebrospinal fluid;[7,12] most likely this particular prostacyclin derives from choroid plexus or pial vessels and not from neural tissue.

Ischaemic/reperfusion insult is followed by marked increases in PGD_2, $PGF_{2\alpha}$, PGE_2 and TXB_2 in the rat and gerbil brain,[4,6,13,14] $PGF_{2\alpha}$, PGE_2 and 6-keto-$PGF_{1\alpha}$ in the canine brain,[3] TXB_2, 6-keto-$PGF_{1\alpha}$ and PGE_2 in the fetal rabbit brain,[15,16] and 6-keto-$PGF_{1\alpha}$, TXB_2, PGE_2, $PGF_{2\alpha}$, but not peptidoleukotrienes, in the newborn piglet brain.[9] The postischaemic production of prostanoids was extensively studied in gerbil brain because of its total dependence on blood supply from carotid arteries.[17-19] Distinct differences have been found in gerbils in the pattern of prostanoid levels depending on the time course and brain region. For instance, the greatest rise was found for PGD_2 in cortex and in the hypothalamus immediately after reperfusion, and for PGE_2 in hippocampus and in striatum 4 hours after reperfusion. Interestingly, the production of PGD_2 decreased below the control levels in all brain areas tested 4 hours after reperfusion. Changes in TXB_2 levels were small, whilst changes in 6-keto-$PGF_{1\alpha}$ were pronounced only in hippocampus. Because the hippocampus is the most sensitive to ischaemia, the enhanced production of PGI_2 could represent an attempt by the injured tissue to protect itself.[19] In gerbils a massive synthesis of $PGF_{2\alpha}$ during cerebral ischaemia/reperfusion was associated with a rapid progression of cytotoxic brain oedema, whereas late accumulation of PGE_2 in cerebral tissues was coupled with development of vasogenic brain oedema.[18]

In patients with stroke[2,20] or with aneurysmal subarachnoid haemorrhage[21] the dominant prostanoid found in cerebrospinal fluid was $PGF_{2\alpha}$, which might have been involved in delayed clinical vasospasm in these patients. An imbalance between vasoconstrictor PGD_2 and vasodilator PGI_2 as measured in cerebrospinal fluid was also implicated as promoting vasospasm in patients with subarachnoid haemorrhage.[22-24] An increase in the TXB_2/6-keto-$PGF_{1\alpha}$ ratio (i.e. TXA_2/PGI_2 ratio) was proposed as another indicator of the risk of developing cerebral vasospasm in humans,[25-27] cynomolgus monkeys[28] and dogs[29] following an insult to the brain.

In monkeys an imbalance in constrictor prostanoids and prostacyclin is likely to arise from a relative deficiency of PGI_2 rather than from a surplus of TXA_2.[28] On the other hand, in dogs with subarachnoid haemorrhage a deficiency in PGI_2 was not observed. Despite high levels of PGI_2 in cerebrospinal fluid, marked angiographic constriction of the basilar artery occurred. This might be associated with increased levels of TXA_2 and PGE_2.[29] In patients with acute stroke the prostanoid pattern was different. A rise in the TXB_2/6-keto-$PGF_{1\alpha}$ ratio in their cerebrospinal fluid occurred owing to increased production of TXA_2 while no change in the generation of PGI_2 was observed.[25]

The physiological role of prostanoids in the regulation of cerebral blood flow is debatable,[30,31] although prostanoids contribute to determination of the range of autoregulation of cerebral blood flow, at least in newborn animals.[32] Nevertheless, as discussed above, enhanced generation of vasoconstrictor prostanoids or suppressed production of prostacyclin might contribute to cerebral vasospasm following an insult. It is important to realize that, among dienoic prostanoids, prostacyclin is the only one that relaxes cerebral arteries in humans, baboons[33] and dogs,[34] whereas prostaglandins A_2, B_2, D_2, E_2, $F_{2\alpha}$ and TXA_2 contract or have little effect on cerebral arteries,[31,33,35,36] although PGE_2 and even $PGF_{2\alpha}$ increase cerebral blood flow in newborn piglets.[32] Among monoenoic prostanoids, PGE_1 resembles PGI_2 in its vasodilatory action on cerebral blood vessels.[37] For eicosanoids in general, the products of enzymatic lipoxygenation of arachidonic acid such as leukotrienes are thought to cause vasoconstriction and increase vascular permeability in cerebral ischaemia.[12,38] Leukotriene C_4 (LTC_4) was found to be generated by slices of rat brain following stimulation with calcium ionophore A23187.[39] In newborn piglets the brain levels of peptidoleukotrienes (LTC_4–LTF_4) are lower than those of prostanoids and they are not changed by cerebral ischaemia.[9] In the cerebral circulation the vasodilator action of PGI_2 is augmented by complementary 'endothelium-derived relaxing factors', one of which seems to be a free radical generated in association with the activation of PGH synthase by bradykinin, and the other a nitrosothiol released by acetylcholine.[40]

Cerebral prostanoids generated in abundance during the ischaemia/reperfusion injury not only affect local vascular tone but also influence coagulation and fibrinolytic activity of blood. For instance, PGI_2 and PGD_2 inhibit while TXA_2 stimulates platelet aggregation and their release reaction. Therefore, prostacyclin and PGD_2 inhibit thrombus formation whilst TXA_2 is thrombogenic. Indeed, metabolic and functional protection of the ischaemic brain of the spontaneously hypertensive rats was provided by antiplatelet pretreatment with a PGI_2 analogue or a TXA_2 synthase inhibitor or an antiplatelet serum.[41] Moreover, prostacyclin has fibrinolytic action, perhaps because it releases tissue plasminogen activator (t-PA) from endothelial cells.[42] During the cerebral ischaemia/reperfusion insult, liberation of unsaturated fatty acid from phospholipids is followed by their lipoxygenation to lipid peroxides[43] while some of lysophospholipids may be used as substrates for the formation of platelet-activating factor (PAF). PAF along with lipid peroxides are strongly neurotoxic and promote cerebral vasospasm.[44] Ginsenosides, which are PAF antagonists, protect rats against cerebral ischaemia/reperfusion injury, inhibit lipid peroxidation and stimulate PGI_2 release.[45] Cerebral ischaemia is also associated with the generation of oxygen free radicals during the reperfusion phase. Oxygen free radicals (superoxide anion, hydroxyl radical, singlet oxygen or peroxynitrite) exert direct detrimental effects on neurons. Alternatively, through inhibition of glutamine synthetase, they lead to accumulation of an excitatory neurotoxin, glutamate.[46] Superoxide anions inactivate an 'endothelium-derived relaxing factor' (EDRF)[47] which in aortic endothelial cells is nitric oxide[48] or in cerebral circulation it may be a nitrosothiol.[40] Superoxide anions when dismuted to hydroxyl radicals such as lipid peroxides inhibit the activity of PGI_2 synthase[49] and, at much higher concentrations, they inactivate PGH synthase. Superoxide anions may also interact with nitric oxide to form peroxynitrite, a free radical that inactivates a number of enzymes that contain sulphydryl groups.

In summary, experimental cerebral ischaemia/reperfusion models are associated with the local generation of oxygen free radicals and with the release of free unsaturated fatty acids from cerebral phospholipids. Oxygen free radicals promote direct damage to neurons, accumulation of neurotoxic glutamate, inactivation of EDRF and generation of peroxynitrites or lipid peroxides. These cause further damage to cell membranes and inhibit PGI_2 synthase. Thus, subsequent cyclo-oxygenation of free arachidonic acid yields only vasoconstrictor or cytotoxic eicosanoids which also contribute to postischaemic hypoperfusion,[38,50] brain oedema[51] and neuronal hypermetabolism,[52] especially in the presence of PAF.[44] In addition, prostacyclin deficiency may promote formation of cerebral microthrombi and suppress plasma fibrinolytic activity. In patients with ischaemic stroke a reduction of serum prostacyclin stability[53] and a defective platelet responsiveness to prostacyclin have been reported.[54]

Prostacyclin and related therapy in experimental cerebral ischaemia

The reports on this subject are inconsistent and therapeutic effects depend on animal species, type of ischaemia (global or regional), the presence of reperfusion phase and experimental protocols. In one of the early studies on 95 anaesthetized beagle dogs[38] the recurring reduction of carotid artery and cerebral blood flow was induced by a partial constriction of carotid artery. It was eliminated by prostacyclin (0.25–0.5 µg/kg) or TXA_2 synthase inhibitors OKY-046 and OKY-1580, and induced by the PGI_2 synthase inhibitor tranylcypromine.[49] The recurring reduction was also eliminated by aspirin and ketoprofen but not by indomethacin, whilst it was induced

by $PGF_{2\alpha}$ and LTC_4. The authors concluded that TXA_2 had acted as an inducer and PGI_2 as an inhibitor of the recurring reduction of cerebral blood flow in dogs. However, in 12 mongrel dogs with global brain ischaemia followed by reperfusion a TXA_2 synthetase inhibitor UK-38485 (dazmegrel) failed to improve postischaemic brain hypoperfusion,[55] as it failed in cats with acute focal cerebral ischaemia[56] and in rabbits with global cerebral ischaemia.[57] Because dazmegrel produced almost complete inhibition of the postischaemic increase in the TXB_2 production and only a modest increase in blood levels of 6-keto-$PGF_{1\alpha}$,[55] it could be that subsequent to inhibition of TXA_2 synthase a shift from PGH_2 to PGI_2 was less pronounced than a shift from PGH_2 to other (vasoconstrictor) prostanoids. On the other hand, in cats TXA_2 synthetase inhibition with imidazole increased local blood flow in the ischaemic penumbra.[58]

In patients with ischaemic cerebrovascular disease OKY-046 increased the urinary excretion of 6-keto-$PGF_{1\alpha}$ in parallel with a decrease in urinary TXB_2.[59] It is not known if the intensity of this shift towards the generation of PGI_2 would be sufficient to justify the therapeutic use of TXA_2 synthetase inhibitors for the treatment or prevention of stroke. It may well be that the PGI_2/TXA_2 balance is not a causative factor in postischaemic cerebral hypoperfusion. On the other hand, in spontaneously hypertensive rats with cerebral ischaemia the inhibition of TXA_2 synthesis by OKY-046 or trapidil did not produce a further increase in 6-keto-$PGF_{1\alpha}$ plasma levels, but it did prevent a reduction in cortical blood flow,[60] development of cerebral oedema and appearance of deleterious metabolic events in brain.[61] In gerbils, eicosapentaenoic acid protected against postischaemic cerebral oedema without affecting the levels of dienoic prostanoids, including PGI_2 and TXA_2.[62] So far, a selective pharmacological inhibition of TXA_2 synthase has been shown to be beneficial in only a few experimental models of cerebral ischaemia. This may be due to an unpredictable fate of PGH_2 which accumulates in consequence of inhibition of TXA_2 synthase or because insufficient amounts of endogenous PGI_2 are generated. Studies with TXA_2/PGH_2 receptor antagonists may help in resolving this dilemma.

The pharmacological inhibition of cyclo-oxygenase removes not only TXA_2 but also other prostanoids; however, there is no shift of metabolism of arachidonic acid towards leukotrienes. Of non-steroidal anti-inflammatory drugs (NSAIDs) that are cyclo-oxygenase inhibitors, aspirin halted the recurring reduction of cerebral blood flow in a canine model of cerebral ischaemia.[38] In patients with stroke, aspirin at a low dose of 40–75 mg daily inhibited the generation of TXA_2[63] and it did not reduce the generation of PGI_2.[64] In dogs with subarachnoid haemorrhage, ibuprofen prevented cerebral vasospasm,[65] and it widened a range of autoregulation of cerebral blood flow in newborn pigs, whilst indomethacin was paradoxically decreasing basal cerebral blood flow.[32]

Hallenbeck and his colleagues[50,66–68] developed a most interesting approach to the treatment of canine brain ischaemia. They established that a concomitant administration of PGI_2 and indomethacin,[50] or, even more so, PGI_2, indomethacin and heparin,[52,68] prevented the impairment of postischaemic brain reperfusion and promoted postischaemic neuronal recovery.

The mechanism of action of this protective cocktail is not clear; antiplatelet[68] and leucocyte-suppressive[67] mechanisms were excluded. The data with NSAIDs in experimental cerebral ischaemia encouraged clinical trials with aspirin alone or combined with dipyridamole, sulphinpyrazone, warfarin, heparin, streptokinase or ticlopidine in secondary stroke prevention.[69] These trials are not the subject of this review; however, out of a plethora of retrospective and prospective studies the latest meta-analysis of seven randomized controlled trials tested the effectiveness of aspirin in the treatment of 6409 patients with transient ischaemic attacks and minor strokes. Significant risk reductions were observed for total death, total strokes, and total strokes and cardiovascular death, odds ratios ranging from 0.59 to 0.78. Although the dosage of aspirin, concurrent medication and selection of patients are proposed as possible factors influencing the efficacy of treatment, in large-scale trials aspirin has proved itself to be useful as a preventive measure in cerebroprotection in patients with transient ischaemic attacks and minor strokes.[70]

The studies carried out by Hallenbeck and co-workers[50,67,68,71] posed a question concerning the mechanism of the cerebroprotective action of PGI_2 during experimental brain ischaemia and reperfusion. Three mechanisms are most commonly proposed:

1. Vasodilation resulting in an increase in regional cerebral blood flow.
2. Antiplatelet and fibrinolytic actions which lead to improvement in the microcirculation in infarcted areas.
3. Ill-defined 'cytoprotection' of cerebral regions exposed to ischaemia.

In cats with acute cerebral infarction PGI_2 reduced upstream resistance but global and regional cerebral blood flow did not improve because systemic blood pressure also fell, although no intracerebral steal phenomenon was observed.[72] In dogs with focal cerebral ischaemia the protective effect of PGI_2 does not seem to depend on its effects on platelets and granulocytes.[67,69] However, a direct protective action of PGI_2 against anoxic damage to cultured cerebral tissue *in vitro* was reported.[73]

In rabbits with transient complete brain ischaemia, PGI_2 (2 µg/kg per minute, i.v.) prevented early morphological changes, especially in bulbar motorneurons and hippocampal neurons. Prostacyclin also diminished perivascular swelling, although it did not affect ultrastructural damage in motor cortex neuron nuclei and glial cell nuclei.[74,75] Rabbits treated with PGI_2 recovered their cortical and hippocampal bioelectrical activity in a shorter time than control animals.[76] It seems that in this model PGI_2 protects against early morphological and functional changes induced by brain ischaemia, although it fails to provide similar protection in the late stage of postischaemic injury, possibly because prostacyclin is unable to prevent nuclear injury in glial and neuronal cells induced by protracted ischaemia.[77,78] Hence increased efficacy of PGI_2 in experimental cerebral ischaemia was sought by combining PGI_2 with other drugs such as indomethacin,[50] indomethacin and heparin,[52] α-adrenolytics,[79] dimethyl sulphoxide,[80] various NSAIDs and calcium channel blockers.[81]

In a feline model of transorbital occlusion of the middle cerebral artery, PGI_2 (100 ng/kg per minute i.a.) diminished regional blood flow to ischaemic focus (a steal phenomenon) and produced no decrease in infarct size.[82] In a similar feline model of cerebral ischaemia a stable prostacyclin analogue TRK-100 prevented microcirculatory aberrations in the acute phase of ischaemic stroke.[83] This discrepancy in effects of PGI_2 or its stable analogue in focal cerebral ischaemia led to a discussion between the authors,[84,85] in which a superiority of stable PGI_2 analogues over native PGI_2 was raised.[85] Apart from the PGI_2-induced 'cerebral steal phenomenon' which was found by Awad *et al.*[82] but not by Tanaka *et al.*[83] or by Date and Hossman,[72] there is not as much difference between the findings of both groups of researchers[82–85] as it might seem at first glance. In the early stage of ischaemia, PGI_2 protected the blood–brain barrier against ischaemic damage[82] and at the same time TRK-100 prevented the microcirculatory derangements.[83] The fact that PGI_2 had no effect on infarct size[82] is in keeping with ultrastructural findings which failed to reveal a beneficial effect of PGI_2 in the delayed phase of ischaemia.[77]

Beneficial effects of stable PGI_2 analogues in the early phase of cerebral ischaemia were confirmed in a number of studies. In cats with occlusion of the middle cerebral artery, PGI_2 (50 ng/kg per minute, i.v.) and its stable analogue OP-2507 (10–50 ng/kg per minute, i.v.) did not affect systemic blood pressure, heart rate or regional cerebral blood flow, but they prevented the postischaemic cerebral oedema, most likely due to their cytoprotective effects.[86] In gerbils with unilateral ligation of the common carotid artery OP-2507 (1–30 μg s.c.) in a dose-dependent manner decreased the occurrence of neurological symptoms of cerebral ischaemia such as circling behaviour and rolling fits, in parallel with the attenuation of neuropathological severity of cerebral infarction.[87] In dogs with cerebral ischaemia induced by ligation of the intercostal, left subclavian and brachiocephalic arteries a stable PGI_2 analogue beraprost (1 μg/kg per minute, i.v.) abolished the decrease in baroreceptor reflex sensitivity, which was an indicator of the extent of the residual blood flow in the medulla oblongata during ischaemia. As beraprost did not influence this blood flow, the authors concluded that the beneficial action of beraprost in brain ischaemia had been exerted through cytoprotection.[88]

In contrast with the above-presented models of acute complete cerebral ischaemia, transient incomplete cerebral ischaemia in rats was produced by association of mild systemic hypotension with bilateral carotid artery occlusion for 1 hour. These oligaemic animals were later infused for 3 days with a stable analogue of PGI_2, iloprost (167 ng/kg per minute) using Alzet osmotic minipumps. This long-term treatment with iloprost (and with its more potent derivative ZK-96480) reduced postoligaemic cerebral oedema, diminished accumulation of calcium in the brain and improved the learning capacity of the injured animals.[89] Iloprost is a potent relaxant of isolated cerebral arteries[90] but in this case a direct cytoprotective action is a more likely explanation for the beneficial effects of iloprost. Another long-term experiment was performed in male, stroke-prone, spontaneously hypertensive rats with focal ischaemia which was produced by occlusion of the middle cerebral artery. The postischaemic treatment with a stable PGI_2 analogue TTC 909 incorporated into lipid microspheres (100 ng/kg per day, i.v., for 7 days) prevented the development of brain oedema and improved secondary metabolic derangement coupled to flow in the postischaemic area.[91] These cerebroprotective effects were also seen with postischaemic administration of an oligomeric PGE_1 (6 mg/kg, i.p.) to rats with focal brain ischaemia[51] or oligomeric PGB (10 mg/kg i.p) to gerbils with global brain ischaemia.[92] Both types of prostaglandin oligomers improved the neurological status of the animals and protected against neuropathological damage. These last series of experiments suggest that PGI_2 and PGE_1 may be not only protective at an early stage of experimental brain ischaemia but they may also reverse the neurological deficit after the insult has occurred.

Clinical trials with prostacyclin in stroke

Therapy of ischaemic cerebral vascular disease has been reviewed by Kistler *et al.*[93,94] As the brain cannot repair itself by forming new neurons, the treatment of ischaemic cerebral vascular disease is primarily preventive. Transient ischaemic attacks or minor strokes are signals to start preventive therapy. Surgical therapy with carotid endarterectomy is the main treatment for carotid stenosis. A pharmacological approach with anticoagulant or antiplatelet treatment has been frequently criticized for the small number of patients studied in trials, lack of controlled trials and the lack of proper diagnostic entry rules into a trial. More recent prospective multicentre randomized studies[95,96] and the results of the meta-analysis of several smaller trials[70] point to benefits of antiplatelet therapy in the prevention of stroke. There is little evidence to support the use of heparin once a completed fixed major stroke deficit exists; however, if a spontaneous improvement occurs or the deficit is small, anticoagulant therapy may prevent further damage.[94]

Only a few trials of the treatment of ischaemic stroke with prostacyclin have been reported. In 1983 we published[97] the results of an open trial in ten patients with fresh completed stroke who were treated with prostacyclin at a dose of 2.5–5.0 ng/kg per minute, i.v., in 6-hour courses four to ten times over 1–2.5 days. In all patients a dramatic regression of hemiplegia or hemiparesis or aphasia occurred in the first few hours of the prostacyclin infusion. At the end of 8 weeks one patient had died because of a sudden occlusion of carotid artery, six patients left the clinic without any sign of neurological deficit and three patients showed residual hemiparesis. In a preliminary report on the effectiveness of prostacyclin in stroke, Hakim *et al.*[98] observed that 1 month after the treatment of five patients with prostacyclin (2–10 ng/kg per minute, i.v. for 8 hours daily for 5 consecutive days) two patients had complete resolution and three patients moderate improvement of their deficit. In another open trial, Miller *et al.*[99] administered prostacyclin (5–8 ng/kg per minute, i.v. for 25–49 hours) to seven patients with acute cerebral infarction. Four patients without computed axial tomographic (CT scan) evidence of cerebral infarction improved on prostacyclin therapy, whereas the remaining three patients who had evidence of infarction on CT scan did not benefit.

The above findings encouraged us to carry out a controlled trial on the efficacy of prostacyclin in the treatment of patients with stroke. Our group[100] accomplished a controlled randomized trial in 27 patients with completed ischaemic stroke who received either prostacyclin (2.5–5 ng/kg per minute, i.v. for 6 hours repeated to a total of five such periods separated by 6-hour intervals without drug) or placebo. A significant alleviation of neurological deficit occurred at 6 and 54 hours after treatment in patients receiving prostacyclin; however, this improvement lost its statistical significance at the end of a 2-week follow-up period. Thus, we were not able to demonstrate that prostacyclin was effective in the treatment of ischaemic stroke. Our patients in the open trial[97] were significantly younger (53 ± 1.8 years old) than in our controlled randomized trial[100] (65 ± 3.1 years old, mean ± SE). This may partially explain an apparent benefit of the prostacyclin therapy observed by us in the open trial, since, according to Martin *et al.*,[101] age is related to the neurological score at 14 days after stroke with a 6.8% decrease in improvement for each additional 10 years of age.

Martin *et al.*[101,102] reported a double-blind controlled trial of prostacyclin in cerebral infarction. Thirty-two patients with sudden onset of aphasia, cranial nerve palsies or hemiparesis and no sign of cerebral haemorrhage on CT scan entered the trial. Prostacyclin (5 ng/kg per minute, i.v.) or placebo was infused intermittently for 65 hours. In the short term (2 weeks after the treatment) there was a comparative improvement in speech, but minimal changes in neurological score or disability status in the prostacyclin-treated group, accompanied by lack of change in pulse, systemic blood pressure, cerebral blood transit time and the CT scan-determined infarct volume. The assessment of the long-term (10–18 months after stroke) efficacy of prostacyclin showed no significant differences between the control and the treatment groups. No evidence was produced that prostacyclin had improved mortality or morbidity in patients after cerebral infarction.

Pokrupa *et al.*[103] treated 28 patients suffering from acute ischaemic stroke either with prostacyclin (up to 10 ng/kg per minute, i.v., 8 hours daily for 5 days, 16 patients) or with placebo (12 patients). Six control and five treated patients also underwent positron emission tomography (PET) to determine cerebral blood flow and cerebral oxygen metabolism. Patients in the prostacyclin group showed PET changes comparable to those of patients in the placebo group. There was no significant difference in neurological scores between the placebo and the prostacyclin-treated groups at any time during the trial.

The biggest multicentre placebo-controlled double-blind trial of prostacyclin for the treatment of acute non-haemorrhagic stroke was presented by the Prostacyclin Study Group in 1987.[104] Five neurological centres were involved in that trial. A total of 80 patients with stroke onset within 24 hours were randomized into placebo (37 patients) and prostacyclin (43 patients) groups. Patients in the prostacyclin group received a continuous infusion of prostacyclin at a dose of 8.5 ng/kg per minute, i.v., for 64 hours. The placebo group received only vehicle. Prostacyclin at that dose resulted in reduction in systemic blood pressure, flushing and tachycardia. Neurological deficit scores were determined on admission, on day 3 and after 1, 2 and 4 weeks. A significant improvement in the score for neurological deficit was noted in both groups; however, the placebo group tended to fare better throughout the study. Two patients in the placebo group and one in the prostacyclin group died. The results of this multicentre trial suggest a lack of therapeutic efficacy of prostacyclin in patients with non-haemorrhagic cerebral infarction.

Recently, Hoshi and Mizushima[105] published the results of a preliminary double-blind cross-over trial on the effectiveness of Lipo-PGI$_2$, a prostacyclin analogue (isocarbacyclin methylester) incorporated in lipid microspheres for the treatement of 17 patients with cerebral infarction. Although the authors suggest that Lipo-PGI$_2$ at a low dose of 2 µg daily relieves the clinical symptoms of chronic cerebral infarction, final conclusions will await the completion of the multicentre randomized controlled studies now in progress.

In conclusion, the experimental data on metabolism of eicosanoids in the ischaemic brain, the cerebroprotection by prostacyclin in experimental brain ischaemia as well as vasodilator, antiplatelet, fibrinolytic and cytoprotective properties of prostacyclin all provide a rationale for clinical trials with prostacyclin in stroke.

The clear outcome of three major placebo-controlled, randomized trials[100,101,104] is that between 2 weeks and 18 months there is no evidence for therapeutic benefit from prostacyclin given at a dose of 2.5–8.5 ng/kg per minute, i.v., either intermittently or continuously for 30–64 hours to patients with acute completed stroke. In the short term, in two[100,101] out of three studies a comparative improvement in speech in the prostacyclin-treated group was recorded, though it disappeared in longer term observation. The failure to demonstrate long-term beneficial actions of prostacyclin in patients with stroke seems to depend neither on dosage of prostacyclin nor on 'rebound phenomenon'.[106] In one trial[104] prostacyclin was given in a continuous intravenous infusion at the highest tolerated dose, and in two trials[100,101] an intermmittent pattern of treatment should have prevented the desensitization of platelets to prostacylin.

The failure to demonstrate therapeutic actions of prostacyclin sodium salt in patients with completed stroke should not discourage further randomized, controlled trials of new stable prostacyclin analogues with an improved profile of pharmacological actions; for example with less hypotensive effects or greater cytoprotective potency,[83,86–89,105] especially for the prevention of threatened stroke. A failure of controlled trials to demonstrate efficacy of prostacyclin might result from cerebral accumulation of vasoconstrictor and cytotoxic eicosanoids, lipid peroxides, nitric oxide, peroxynitrites, oxygen free radicals, excitatory amino acids and calcium. Their detrimental effects may not be offset by endogenous prostacyclin or even by pharmacological concentrations of exogenous prostacyclin.

If this is the case, the treatment of stroke patients with prostacyclin may benefit from the addition of heparin and indomethacin,[66–68] aspirin and other NSAID,[38,63,65,70] ticlopidine,[107] TXA_2 synthase inhibitors or TXA_2/PGH_2 receptor antagonists,[38,41,60] calcium channel blockers[81] or dimethyl sulphoxide.[80]

The present state of the art of pharmacological treatment of cerebral ischaemia gives rise to a somewhat nihilistic attitude among many clinicians dealing with stroke. Prostacyclin alone with its vasodilator, thrombolytic and cytoprotective actions appeared to be too weak to prevent the development of signs of ischaemic insult in completed stroke. Nevertheless, a transient improvement in speech in prostacyclin-treated patients and beneficial effects of prostacyclin and its analogues in the treatment of experimental brain ischaemia support such an approach. Stable, orally active prostacyclin analogues may in future be tested in secondary prevention (perhaps along with aspirin) in patients with transient ischaemic attacks.

References

1. Pace-Asciak CJ, Nashat M. Catabolism of prostaglandin endoperoxides into prostaglandin E_2 and $F_{2\alpha}$ by the rat brain. *J Neurochem* 1976; **27**: 551–6.
2. Egg D, Herold M, Rumpl E. Prostaglandin $F_{2\alpha}$ in cerebrospinal fluid after stroke. *Lancet* 1978; **1**: 990.
3. Abdel-Halim MS, Lunden J, Cseh G, Anggard E. Prostaglandin profiles in nervous tissue and blood vessels of the brain of various animals. *Prostaglandins* 1980; **19**: 249–58.
4. Wolfe LS, Pappius HM. Arachidonic acid metabolism in cerebral ischemia and brain injury. *Cereb Ischemia* 1984; **10**: 223–31.
5. Petroni A, Socini A, Blasevich M, Borghi A, Galli C. Differential effects of various vasoactive drugs on basal and stimulated levels of TXB_2 and 6-keto-$PGF_{1\alpha}$ in rat brain. *Prostaglandins* 1985; **29**: 579–87.
6. Gaudet RJ, Alan I, Levine L. Accumulation of cyclooxygenase products of arachidonic acid metabolism in the gerbil brain during reperfusion after bilateral common carotid artery occlusion. *J Neurochem* 1980; **35**: 653–8.
7. Wolfe LS, Pappius HM, Pokrupa R, Hakim A. Involvement of arachidonic acid metabolites in experimental brain injury. Identification of lipoxygenase products in brain. Clinical studies on prostacyclin infusion in acute cerebral ischemia. *Adv Prostaglandin Thromboxane Leukotriene Res* 1985; **15**: 585–8.
8. Katz B, Sofonio M, Lyden PD, Mitchell MD. Prostaglandin concentrations in cerebrospinal fluid of rabbits under normal and ischemic conditions. *Stroke* 1988; **19**: 349–51.
9. Hsu P, Zuckerman S, Mirro R, Armstead WM, Leffer CW. Effects of ischemia/reperfusion on brain tissue prostanoids and leukotrienes in newborn pigs. *Prostaglandins* 1991; **42**: 557–69.
10. Leffler CW, Mirro R, Armstead WM, Busija DW, Thelin O. Prostanoid synthesis and vascular responses to exogenous arachidonic acid following cerebral ischemia in piglets. *Prostaglandins* 1990; **40**: 241–8.
11. Abdel-Halim MS, Anggard E. Regional and species differences in endogenous prostaglandin biosynthesis by brain homogenates. *Prostaglandins* 1979; **17**: 411–18.
12. Chen ST, Hsu CY, Hogan EL, Halushka PV, Linet OI, Yatsu FM. Thromboxane, prostacyclin and leukotrienes in cerebral ischemia. *Neurology* 1986; **36**: 466–70.

13. Shohami E, Rosenthal J, Lavy S. The effect of incomplete cerebral ischemia on prostaglandin levels in rat brain. *Stroke* 1982; **13**: 494–9.

14. Dorman RV. Effects of cerebral ischemia and reperfusion on prostanoid accumulation in unanesthetized and pentobarbital-treated gerbils. *J Cereb Blood Flow Metab* 1988; **8**: 609–12.

15. Goldin E, Harel S, Tomer A, Yavin E. Thromboxane and prostacyclin levels in fetal rabbit brain and placenta after intrauterine partial ischemic episodes. *J Neurochem* 1990; **54**: 587–91.

16. Yavin E, Goldin E, Magal E, Tomer A, Harel S. Ischemia stress and arachidonic acid metabolites in the fetal brain. *Ann NY Acad Sci* 1989; **559**: 248–58.

17. Gaudet RJ, Levine L. Effect of unilateral common carotid artery occlusion on levels of prostaglandins D_2, $F_{2\alpha}$ and 6-keto-prostaglandin $F_{1\alpha}$ in gerbil brain. *Stroke* 1980; **11**: 648–52.

18. Bhakoo KK, Crockard HA, Lascelles PC, Avery SF. Prostaglandin synthesis and oedema formation during reperfusion following experimental brain ischaemia in the gerbil. *Stroke* 1984; **15**: 891–5.

19. Kempski O, Shohami E, von Lubitz D, Hallenbeck JM, Feuerstein G. Postischemic production of eicosanoids in gerbil brain. *Stroke* 1987; **18**: 111–19.

20. Egg D, Herold M, Rumpl E, Gunther K. Prostaglandin $F_{1\alpha}$ levels in human cerebrospinal fluid in normal and pathological conditions. *J Neurol* 1980; **222**: 239–48.

21. Chehrazi BB, Giri S, Joy RM. Prostaglandins and vasoactive amines in cerebral vasospasm after aneurysmal subarachnoid hemorrhage. *Stroke* 1989; **20**: 217–24.

22. Rodriguez-y-Baena R, Gaetani P, Folco G, Branzoli U, Paoletti P. Cisternal and lumbar CSF concentration of arachidonate metabolites in vasospasm following subarachnoid hemorrhage from ruptured aneurysm: biochemical and clinical considerations. *Surg Neurol* 1985; **24**: 428–32.

23. Rodriguez-y-Baena R, Gaetani P, Folco G, Vigano T, Paoletti P. Arachidonate metabolites and vasospasm after subarachnoid haemorrhage. *Neurol Res* 1986; **8**: 25–32.

24. Rodriguez-y-Baena R, Gaetani P, Silvani V, Vigano T, Crivellari MT, Paoletti P. Cisternal and lumbar CSF levels of arachidonate metabolites after subarachnoid haemorrhage: an assessment of the biochemical hypothesis of vasospasm. *Acta Neurochir (Wien)* 1987; **84**: 129–35.

25. Fagan SC, Castellani D, Gengo FM. Prostanoid concentrations in human CSF following acute ischaemic brain infarction. *Clin Exp Pharmacol Physiol* 1986; **13**: 629–32.

26. Seifert V, Stolke D, Kaever V, Dietz H. Arachidonic acid metabolism following aneurysm rupture. *Eur Arch Psychiatry Neurol Sci* 1986; **236**: 94–101.

27. Seifert V, Stolke D, Kaever D, Dietz H. Arachidonic acid metabolism following aneurysm rupture. *Surg Neurol* 1987; **3**: 243–52.

28. Nosko M, Schulz R, Weir B, Cook DA, Grace M. Effects of vasospasm on levels of prostacyclin and thromboxane A_2 in cerebral arteries of the monkey. *Neurosurgery* 1988; **22**: 45–50.

29. Seifert V, Stolke D, Kunz U, Resch K. Influence of blood volume on cerebrospinal fluid levels of arachidonic acid metabolites after subarachnoid hemorrhage. *Neurosurgery* 1988; **23**: 313–21.

30. Wahl M. Local chemical, neural and humoral regulation of cerebrovascular resistance vessels. *J Cardiovasc Pharmacol* 1985; **7** (suppl 3): S36–46.

31. Murphy S, Pearce B. Eicosanoids in the CNS: sources and effects. *Prostaglandins Leukot Essent Fatty Acids* 1988; **31**: 165–70.

32. Chemtob S, Beharry K, Rex J, Varma DR, Aranda JV. Prostanoids determine the range of cerebral blood flow autoregulation of newborn piglets. *Stroke* 1990; **21**: 777–84.

33. Boullin DJ, Bunting S, Blaso WP, Hunt TM, Moncada S. Response of human and baboon arteries to prostaglandin endoperoxides and biologically generated and synthetic prostacyclin; their relevance to arterial cerebral spasm in man. *Br J Clin Pharmacol* 1979; **7**: 139.

34. Chapleau CE, White RP. Effects of prostacyclin on the canine isolated basilar artery. *Prostaglandins* 1979; **17**: 573–80.

35. Ellis EF, Nies AS, Oates JA. Cerebral arterial smooth muscle contraction by thromboxane A_2. *Stroke* 1977; **8**: 480–3.

36. Toda N. Different responsiveness of a variety of isolated dog arteries to prostaglandin D_2. *Prostaglandins* 1982; **23**: 99–112.

37. Toda N, Miyazaki M. Responses of isolated dog cerebral and peripheral arteries to prostaglandins after application of aspirin and polyphloretin phosphate. *Stroke* 1978; **9**: 490–8.

38. Uchida Y, Murao S. Role of prostaglandin I_2 and thromboxane A_2 in recurring reduction of carotid and cerebral blood flow in dogs. *Stroke* 1981; **12**: 786–92.

39. Dembińska-Kieć A, Simmet T, Peskar BA. Formation of leukotriene C_4-like material by rat brain tissue. *Eur J Pharmacol* 1984; **99**: 57–62.

40. Marshall JJ, Kontos HA. Endothelium-derived relaxing factors. A perspective from *in vivo* data. *Hypertension* 1990; **16**: 371–86.

41. Katayama Y, Shimizu J, Suzuki S, *et al.* Role of arachidonic acid metabolism on ischemic brain edema and metabolism. *Adv Neurol* 1990; **52**: 105–8.

42. Gryglewski RJ, Botting RM, Vane JR. Prostacyclin: from discovery to clinical applications. In: Rubanyi GM (ed), *Cardiovascular Significance of Endothelium-derived Vasoactive Factors*. New York: Futura, 1991: 3–37.

43. Yoshida S, Inoh S, Asano T, *et al.* Lipid peroxidation

as a cause of postischemia brain injury. In: Betz E, *et al.* (eds), *Pathophysiology and Pharmacotherapy of Cerebrovascular Disorders*. Baden Baden, Köln, New York: Verlag Gerhard Witzstrock, 1980: 85–9.

44. Lindsberg PJ, Hallenbeck JM, Feuerstein G. Platelet-activating factor in stroke and brain injury. *Ann Neurol* 1991; **30**: 117–29.

45. Chu GX, Chen X. Anti-lipid peroxidation and protection of ginsenosides against cerebral ischemia reperfusion injuries in rats. *Chung Kuo Yao Li Hsueh Pao* 1990; **11**: 119–23.

46. Floyd RA. Role of oxygen free radicals in carcinogenesis and brain ischemia. *FASEB J* 1990; **4**: 2587–97.

47. Gryglewski RJ, Palmer RMJ, Moncada S. Superoxide anion is involved in the breakdown of endothelium-derived vascular relaxing factor. *Nature* 1986; **320**: 454–6.

48. Palmer RMJ, Ashton DS, Moncada S. Vascular endothelial cells synthetize nitric oxide from L-arginine. *Nature* 1988; **333**: 664–6.

49. Gryglewski RJ, Bunting S, Moncada S, Flower RJ, Vane JR. Arterial walls are protected against deposition of platelet thrombi by a substance (prostaglandin X) which they make from prostaglandin endoperoxides. *Prostaglandins* 1976; **12**: 685–713.

50. Hallenbeck JM, Furlow TW Jr. Prostaglandin I_2 and indomethacin prevent impairment of postischemic brain reperfusion in the dog. *Stroke* 1979; **10**: 629–37.

51. Tsuyoshi-Ohnishi S, Tominaga T, Katsuoka M. Inhibition of ischemic brain edema formation by postischemic administration of a prostaglandin oligomer. *Prostaglandins Leukot Essent Fatty Acids* 1989; **37**: 107–11.

52. Hallenbeck JM, Leitch DR, Dutka AJ, Greenbaum LJ, McKee AE. Prostaglandin I_2, indomethacin and heparin promote postischemic neuronal recovery in dogs. *Ann Neurol* 1982; **12**: 145–56.

53. Stein RW, Papp AC, Weiner WJ, Wu KK. Reduction of serum prostacyclin stability in ischemic stroke. *Stroke* 1985; **16**: 16–18.

54. Pettigrew C, Papp A, Wu KK. Dose-related stimulation of platelet cyclic adenosine monophosphate by prostacyclin in thrombotic stroke. *Thromb Res* 1987; **45**: 669–74.

55. Prough DS, Kong D, Watkins WD, Stout R, Stump DA, Beamer WC. Inhibition of thromboxane A_2 production does not improve post-ischemic brain hypoperfusion in the dog. *Stroke* 1986; **17**: 1272–6.

56. Moufarrij NA, Little JR, Skrinska V. Thromboxane synthase inhibition in acute focal cerebral ischemia in cats. *J Neurol* 1984; **61**: 1107–12.

57. Sofeir M, Deshayes S, Plotkine M, Boulu RG. Influence of imidazole in rabbits submitted to global cerebral ischemia. *J Cereb Blood Flow Metab* 1983; **3** (suppl 1): S295–6.

58. Roy MW, Dempsey RJ, Cowen DE, Donaldson DL,

Young AB. Thromboxane synthetase inhibition with imidazole increases blood flow in ischemic penumbra. *Neurosurgery* 1988; **22**: 317–23.

59. Uyama O, Nagatsuka K, Nakabayashi S, *et al.* The effect of a thromboxane synthetase inhibitor OKY-046, 6-keto-prostaglandin $F_{1\alpha}$ in patients with ischemic cerebrovascular disease. *Stroke* 1985; **16**: 241–4.

60. Sadoshima S, Ooboshi H, Okada Y, Yao H, Ishitsuoka T, Fudjishima M. Effect of thromboxane synthetase inhibitor on cerebral circulation and metabolism during experimental cerebral ischemia in spontaneously hypertensive rats. *Eur J Pharmacol* 1989; **169**: 75–83.

61. Katayama Y, Terashi A, Shimizu J, *et al.* Role of platelets as a factor aggravating cerebral ischemia. *Jpn Circ J* 1990; **54**: 1511–16.

62. Black KL, Hoff JT, Radin NS, Desmukh GD. Eicosapentaenoic acid: effect on brain prostaglandins, cerebral blood flow and edema in ischemic gerbils. *Stroke* 1984; **15**: 65–9.

63. Weksler BB, Kent JL, Rudolph D, Scherer PB, Levy DE. Effects of low dose aspirin on platelet function in patients with recent cerebral ischemia. *Stroke* 1985; **16**: 5–9.

64. Poungvarin N, Ketsa-Ard K. Low-dose aspirin and its antithrombotic effect in ischaemic stroke patient. *J Med Assoc Thai* 1989; **72**: 421–6.

65. Chyatte D. Prevention of chronic cerebral vasospasm in dogs with ibuprofen and high-dose methylprednisolone. *Stroke* 1989; **20**: 1021–6.

66. Hallenbeck JM, Leitch DR, Dutka AJ, Greenbaum LJ Jr. PGI₂, indomethacin and heparin promote postischemic neuronal recovery in dogs when administered therapeutically. In: Wu KK, Rossi EC (eds), *Prostaglandins in Clinical Medicine – Cardiovascular and Thrombotic Disorders*. Chicago, London: Year Book Medical, 1982: 335–41.

67. Kochanek PM, Dutka AJ, Hallenbeck JM. Indomethacin, prostacyclin and heparin improve postischemic cerebral blood flow without affecting early postischemic granulocyte accumulation. *Stroke* 1987; **18**: 634–7.

68. Kochanek PM, Dutka AJ, Kumaroo KK, Hallenbeck JM. Effects of prostacyclin, indomethacin and heparin on cerebral blood flow and platelet adhesion after multifocal ischemia of canine brain. *Stroke* 1988; **19**: 693–9.

69. Barnett HJ. Aspirin in stroke prevention. An overview. *Stroke* 1990; **21**: IV40–3.

70. Stachenko SJ, Bravo G, Cote R, Boucher J, Battista RN. Aspirin in transient ischemic attacks and minor stroke: a meta-analysis. *Fam Pract Res J* 1991; **11**: 179–91.

71. Hallenbeck JM. Prostaglandin I_2 and indomethacin prevent impairment of post-ischemic brain reperfusion in the dog. *Stroke* 1979; **10**: 629–37.

72. Date H, Hossmann KA. Effect of vasodilating drugs

on intracortical and extracortical vascular resistance following middle cerebral artery occlusion in cats. *Ann Neurol* 1984; **16**: 330–6.

73. Renkawek K, Herbaczynska-Cedro K, Mossakowski MJ. The effect of prostacyclin on the morphological and enzymatic properties of CNS cultures exposed to anoxia. *Acta Neurol Scand* 1986; **73**: 111–18.

74. Pluta R. Influence of prostacyclin on early morphological changes in the rabbit brain after complete 20-min ischemia. *J Neurol Sci* 1985; **70**: 305–16.

75. Pluta R. The effects of prostacyclin on early ultrastructural changes in the neuron nuclei of the motor cortex in rabbits after complete 20 min cerebral ischemia. *Exp Mol Pathol* 1988; **48**: 161–73.

76. Pluta R, Salinska E, Lazarewicz JW. Prostacyclin attenuates in the rabbit hippocampus early consequences of transient complete cerebral ischemia. *Acta Neurol Scand* 1991; **83**: 370–7.

77. Pluta R. Experimental treatment with prostacyclin of global cerebral ischemia in rabbit – new data. *Neuropatol Pol* 1990; **28**: 205–15.

78. Mossakowski MJ, Gadamski R. Effect of prostacyclin (PGI$_2$) and indomethacin on ischemic damage of sector CA1 of Ammon's horn in the Mongolian gerbil (Pol). *Neuropatol Pol* 1987; **25**: 21–34.

79. Nikolov R, Dikova M, Nikolova M, Voronina T, Nerebkova L, Garibova T. Cerebroprotective effect of nicergoline and interference with the antihypoxic effect of prostacyclin. *Methods Find Exp Clin Pharmacol* 1987; **9**: 479–84.

80. de la Torre JC. Synergic activity of combined prostacyclin: dimethyl sulfoxide in experimental brain ischemia. *Can J Physiol Pharmacol* 1991; **69**: 191–8.

81. Nikolov R. Prostacyclin as a cerebroprotective agent against brain hypoxia. *Biomed Biochim Acta* 1989; **48**: S183–7.

82. Awad I, Little JR, Lucas F, Skrinska V, Slugg R, Lesser RP. Treatment of acute focal cerebral ischemia with prostacyclin. *Stroke* 1983; **14**: 203–9.

83. Tanaka K, Gotoh F, Fukuuchi Y, *et al.* Stable prostacyclin analogue preventing microcirculatory derangement in experimental cerebral ischemia in cats. *Stroke* 1988; **19**: 1267–74.

84. Awad IA. Prostacyclin in experimental ischemic models. [letter] *Stroke* 1989; **20**: 698.

85. Tanaka K, Gotoh F, Fukuuchi Y, Amano T. Prostacyclin in experimental ischemic methods. [reply] *Stroke* 1989; **20**: 698.

86. Terawaki T, Takakuwa T, Iguchi S, *et al.* Effect of a prostacyclin analog OP-2507 on acute ischemic cerebral edema in cats. *Eur J Pharmacol* 1988; **152**: 63–70.

87. Masuda Y, Yasuba M, Zushi K, Ochi Y, Kadokawa T, Okegawa T. Effect of OP-2507, a stable prostacyclin analogue on cerebral ischaemia induced by unilateral ligation of common carotid artery in gerbils. *Arch Int Pharmacodyn Ther* 1988; **294**: 125–36.

88. Kurihara J, Sahara T, Kato H. Protective effect of beraprost sodium, a new chemically stable prostacyclin analogue, against the deterioration of baroreceptor reflex following transient global cerebral ischaemia in dogs. *Br J Pharmacol* 1990; **99**: 91–6.

89. Borzeix MG, Cahn R, Cahn J. Effects of new chemically and metabolically stable prostacyclin analogues (iloprost and ZK 96480) on early consequences of a transient cerebral oligaemia in the rat. *Prostaglandins* 1988; **35**: 653–64.

90. Egemen N, Birler K, Avman N, Turker RK. Experimental cerebral vasospasm: resolution by iloprost. *Acta Neurochir (Wien)* 1988; **95**: 131–5.

91. Shima K, Ohashi K, Umezawa H, *et al.* Postischaemic treatment with the prostacyclin analogue TTC-909 reduces ischaemic brain injury. *Acta Neurochir* 1990; **51** (suppl): 242–4.

92. von Lubitz DKJE, Redmond DJ. Cerebral ischemia in gerbils: improvement of survival after postischemic treatment with oligoprostaglandin B$_1$. *Eur J Pharmacol* 1989; **164**: 405–14.

93. Kistler JP, Ropper AH, Heros RC. Therapy of ischemic cerebral vascular disease due to atherothrombosis. *N Engl J Med* 1984; **311**: 27–34.

94. Kistler JP, Ropper AH, Heros RC. Therapy of ischemic cerebral vascular disease due to atherothrombosis. II. *N Engl J Med* 1984; **311**: 100–5.

95. Goyan JE. The 'trials' of a long-term clinical trial: the Ticlopidine Aspirin Stroke Study and the Canadian–American Ticlopidine Study. *Controlled Clin Trials* 1989; **10**: 236S–44S.

96. ESPS Group. European Stroke Prevention Study. *Stroke* 1990; **21**: 1122–30.

97. Gryglewski RJ, Nowak S, Kostka-Trąbka E, *et al.* Treatment of ischaemic stroke with prostacyclin. *Stroke* 1983; **14**: 197–202.

98. Hakim AM, Pokrupa RP, Wolfe LS. Preliminary report on the effectiveness of prostacyclin in stroke. *J Can Sci Neurologiques* 1984; **11**: 409.

99. Miller VT, Coull BM, Yatsu FM, Shah AB, Beamer NB. Prostacyclin infusion. *Neurology* 1984; **34**: 1431–5.

100. Huczyński J, Kostka-Trąbka E, Sotowska W, *et al.* Double-blind controlled trial of the therapeutic effects of prostacyclin in patients with completed ischaemic stroke. *Stroke* 1985; **16**: 810–14.

101. Martin JF, Hamdy N, Nicholl J, *et al.* Double-blind controlled trial of prostacyclin in cerebral infarction. *Stroke* 1985; **16**: 386–90.

102. Martin JF, Hamdy N, Nicholl J, *et al.* Prostacyclin in cerebral infarction. *N Engl J Med* 1985; **312**: 1652.

103. Pokrupa R, Hakim AM, Villaneuva J. Clinical study of prostacyclin infusion after acute ischemic stroke. Cerebrovascular disease. *Can J Neurol Sci* 1986; **13**: 165.

104. Hsu CY, Faught RE Jr, Furlan AJ, *et al.* Intravenous prostacyclin in acute nonhemorrhagic stroke: a

placebo controlled double-blind trial. *Stroke* 1987; **18:** 352–8.

105. Hoshi K, Mizushima Y. A preliminary double-blind cross-over trial of lipo-PGI$_2$, a prostacyclin derivative incorporated in lipid microspheres in cerebral infarction. *Prostaglandins* 1990; **40:** 155–64.

106. Sinzinger H, Silberbauer K, Harsch AK, Gall A. De-creased sensitivity of human platelets to PGI$_2$ during long-term intraarterial prostacyclin infusion in patients with peripheral vascular disease – a rebound phenomenon. *Prostaglandins* 1981; **21:** 49–51.

107. Barnett HJ. Clinical trials in stroke prevention. *Arzneimittelforschung* 1991; **41:** 340–4.

18 Prostaglandins in liver disease, organ transplantation and extracorporeal circulation

AES Gimson, JF Martin and M Greaves

In recent years much evidence has accumulated demonstrating the importance of eicosanoids in hepatic pathophysiology.[1] The products of arachidonic acid metabolism, via both cyclo-oxygenase and 5-lipoxygenase pathways, are mediators of these processes and many therapeutic applications are being derived.

The importance of eicosanoids in these pathological states is a reflection of the role of the liver as a major source of eicosanoid production,[2,3] a target for their action whether produced from within the liver or from extrahepatic sources,[4-6] and an important site of their metabolic inactivation.[7] Within the liver hepatocytes are targets for prostanoid actions[8] and in man may effectively clear eicosanoids from the circulation,[9] whilst non-parenchymal cells including Kupffer cells, hepatic mast cells and inflammatory cells infiltrating the liver, are sources of leukotriene B_4 (LTB$_4$)[10] and the cysteinyl leukotrienes (LTC$_4$, LTD$_4$, LTE$_4$).[11,12] Numerous stimuli may affect production and release of leukotrienes from these cellular sites including complement

components C5a, bacterial endotoxin, platelet activating factor, phospholipase A_2 or calcium ionophores.[1]

In addition to widely recognized effects of prostanoids, specific actions within the liver have also been found. Thus PGD$_2$ enhances glycogenolysis in the isolated perfused liver[6] and PGE$_2$ may suppress the release of cytokines from endotoxin stimulated hepatic Kupffer cells.[13] Thromboxane A$_2$ (TXA$_2$) stimulates glycogenolysis and can elevate portal pressure by increasing portal venous resistance.[14] The cysteinyl leukotrienes are potent mediators of inflammatory responses, contracting smooth muscle, causing plasma extravasation.[15]

Eicosanoids and liver injury

Mechanisms of liver cell injury have been considerably clarified in recent years.[16] A final common pathway of liver membrane damage associated with an increase in intracellular calcium and activation of

251

phospholipase, which in turn liberates arachidonic acid, has been proposed.[17]

Prior to these events an important role for non-parenchymal cells in mediating the hepatotoxicity of compounds as diverse as bacterial endotoxin, paracetamol, galactosamine and carbon tetrachloride[18,19] has recently been demonstrated. Hepatotoxicity due to paracetamol is associated at an early stage by significant increase in the number of macrophages and endothelial cells in the liver,[20] and activators of both these cell lines have been shown to enhance the hepatotoxicity of these agents.[18] Such cell lines may release numerous mediators including reactive oxygen and nitrogen intermediates (superoxide, nitric oxide), platelet activating factor, cytokines (tumour necrosis factor, IL-1, IL-6) as well as LTB$_4$ and the cysteinyl leukotrienes[10] that could contribute further to liver injury.[21] Leukotriene levels are found to increase early after carbon tetrachloride- and galactosamine-induced liver injury,[22] with rises in PGE$_2$ and 6-keto-PGF$_{1\alpha}$ occurring later.[23]

The role of leukotrienes as mediators of liver injury is also demonstrated by abolition of the hepatotoxicity from the coadministration of hepatic RNA synthesis inhibitors (galactosamine or α-amanitin) and lipopolysaccharide, by the use of diethylcarbamazine which inhibits LTA$_4$ synthesis and FPL-55712, a receptor antagonist of cysteinyl leukotrienes.[21] D-Galactosamine-induced hepatitis in rats is also prevented by a dual arachidonate lipoxygenase and cyclo-oxygenase inhibitor BW-755C[21], and a specific 5-lipoxygenase inhibitor (AA-861) also protects against carbon tetrachloride toxicity.[22]

Prostaglandins and hepatic cytoprotection

Whilst lipoxygenase products may be involved in mediating some models of liver injury, the role of cyclo-oxygenase products in the prevention of hepatotoxicity has also been investigated. In some animal models cyclo-oxygenase inhibition during the initial stages of the liver injury may exacerbate hepatotoxicity,[24] but Stachura *et al.*, using pretreatment with 16,16-dimethyl PGE$_2$, was able to protect against galactosamine-induced liver damage.[25]

These findings have also been confirmed in models of carbon tetrachloride and bromobenzene hepatotoxicity.[26,27] Both prostacyclin (PGI$_2$) and PGE$_1$ have similar protective effects[24,28,29] but the synthetic prostaglandin analogue BW-245C which acts through the PGD$_2$ receptor is inactive.[28] The synthetic PGI$_2$ derivatives iloprost and 9β-methylcarbacyclin are also protective in other animal models.[30,31]

The mechanism of prostanoid protection from liver injury is controversial. Changes in blood flow or distribution are unlikely as compounds with potent vasodilatory action such as BW-245C are ineffective[28] and cytoprotection is also observed in isolated hepatocytes.[24,31,32] An effect upon hepatic non-parenchymal cells with prevention of release of mediators including cytokines and leukotrienes, by lipopolysaccharide, has been demonstrated.[13] Prostacyclin has been shown to increase intracellular cAMP and cGMP within liver cells.[33] Intracellular cAMP plays a major role in the control of calcium ion transport,[34] which is important in the preterminal rise in intracellular calcium after liver injury. Lysosomal membrane stabilization associated with changes in intracellular cAMP[35] represents a further mechanism whereby prostanoids may prevent toxic liver injury. Prostaglandins including prostacyclin, 16,16,-dimethyl PGE$_2$, misoprostol and thromboxane synthetase inhibitors are also protective against ischaemia and hypoxia–induced liver damage.[33,36–38] As hepatic sinusoidal disruption by activated leucocytes, platelets and fibrin is observed during toxic liver injury and may impair microcirculatory blood flow and oxygen delivery,[39] prostanoids may protect such hypoxic hepatocytes.

Eicosanoids and viral hepatitis

Viral hepatitis is associated with a marked portal, and to lesser extent lobular infiltration by proinflammatory cells with subsequent hepatocellular necrosis. Frog-virus-3-induced liver damage in rats has close histological and biochemical similarity to human viral hepatitis.[40]

In this model a marked increase in biliary excretion of cysteinyl leukotrienes is observed within 4 hours of virus inoculation[41] and both a selective lipoxygenase inhibitor (AA-861) and a dual lipoxygenase and cyclo-oxgenase inhibitor (BW-755C) prevent rises in hepatic enzyme by up to 80%.[41]

Prostaglandins exhibit significant immunosuppressive effects[42] including a reduction in the expression of class II histocompatibility antigens on murine macrophages.[43] Certain prostaglandins are potent inhibitors of viral replication.[44] Abecassis *et al.* used the murine hepatitis virus type 3 (MHV-3) in genetically susceptible BALB/cJ mice ↄ develop a model of fulminant hepatic failure.[45] ⸱⸱⸱ this virus is directly cytopathic *in vitro*, genetic susceptibility is also dependent on T-lymphocyte controlled expression of procoagulant activity,[46] with the deposition of sinusoidal microthrombi and focal avascular necrosis, similar to that seen in fulminant viral hepatitis in man.[39] In this virus model 16,16-dimethyl PGE_2 was fully protective in both the intact animal and isolated cultured hepatocytes.[45] The enhanced procoagulant activity was also inhibited, whereas viral replication was unchanged, suggesting that the mechanism of protection may be due to an inhibition of immune stimulated coagulation rather than any direct effect on the virus.

In man the mortality of fulminant viral hepatitis with grade 3 or 4 encephalopathy has often been 80%, with little change in these figures despite significant improvements in many aspects of intensive care.[47] In these circumstances the Toronto group have studied the use of intravenous PGE_1 (0.2 µg/kg per hour – 0.6 µg/kg per hour) in patients with fulminant viral hepatitis.[48] Seventeen patients were treated in the initial study (three HAV, six HBV, and eight presumed non-A–non-B cases), with 14 having grade 3 or 4 encephalopathy. Twelve of the cases responded rapidly to the PGE_1 infusion with dramatic falls in transaminase levels (1540 ± 833 to 188 ± 324 iu/l) and a decrease in prothrombin time (27 ± 7 to 12 ± 1 seconds), and five patients with non-A–non-B hepatitis who relapsed when the infusion was stopped, improved again on retreatment.

Although this report was met with considerable interest, no control group was included. Furthermore, recent evidence suggests that patients with fulminant viral hepatitis do not represent a homogeneous group with respect to prognosis, with hepatitis type A and B cases having a survival of up to 50%, whereas those with non-A–non-B hepatitis have only a 10–15% survival.[49] A retrospective analysis from the Institute of Liver Studies at King's College Hospital demonstrated specific criteria of independent prognostic significance which, if applied to the Toronto patients, would indicate that the majority of such patients would have been expected to survive with intensive care procedures alone and irrespective of any use of PGE_1. A blinded controlled trial will therefore be required to clarify the real efficacy of prostaglandins in this clinical situation.

Eicosanoids and haemodynamics in liver disease

Chronic liver disease

Patients with cirrhosis have a high cardiac output and low systemic vascular resistance with a high arterial oxygen delivery and a low oxygen extraction ratio.[50] The cause of this profound systemic vasodilation remains unclear but systemic release of prostanoids has been implicated. Guarner *et al.* and others have demonstrated that systemic production of PGI_2, as assessed by urinary excretion of the 2,3-dinor-6-oxo-$PGF_{1\alpha}$ is increased in decompensated liver disease, with increased urinary excretion of the TXA_2 metabolite 2,3-dinor-TXB_2,[51,52] although the levels observed are not high enough to produce such profound peripheral vasodilation.

Systemic vasodilation is also associated with a low pulmonary vascular resistance, when severe, hepatogenic pulmonary angiodysplasia may develop with an increased alveolar–arterial oxygen gradient and severe hypoxaemia. Shijo *et al.* reported a case in whom indomethacin combined with intravenous $PGF_{2\alpha}$ caused an increase in pulmonary vascular resistance and arterial oxygen saturation, raising the possibility that vasodilator eicosanoids may modulate the pulmonary circulation in such patients.[53]

The hepatorenal syndrome (HRS) is typically characterized by vasoconstriction of the renal arterioles, reduced glomerular filtration rate, low urinary sodium with preserved renal water retention and normal renal histology. There has been considerable interest in the role of prostanoids in mediating these changes. Vasodilatory prostanoids may be of importance in the maintenance of renal function in patients with chronic liver disease as non-steroidal anti-inflammatory drugs induce a predictable fall in glomerular filtration rate.[54] Initial studies found urinary excretion of TXA_2 metabolites to be increased and prostacyclin metabolites to be decreased.[55] In more recent studies where the cases have been controlled for severity of liver disease, urinary excretion rates of both vasodilator and vasoconstrictor prostanoids (renal and extrarenal) have been increased, even during the early phase of HRS, and subsequently fell with the reduction in creatinine clearance as the condition deteriorated.[52] As hepatic decompensation with severe jaundice and ascites but in the absence of HRS was also associated with a progressive increase in production and excretion of both prostacyclin and TXA_2, an imbalance in their production/ release is unlikely to mediate the renal haemodynamic changes of HRS. Thromboxane synthetase inhibitors have also not improved renal function in these patients.[56] Fevery *et al.* reported that oral misoprostol (PGE_1 analogue) was able to reverse the HRS in four patients, producing a marked diuresis and increase in creatinine clearance.[57] Unfortunately these patients had also received a colloid infusion to produce volume expansion and this manoeuvre alone may have accounted for the observed effect.

Cysteinyl leukotrienes in hepatorenal syndrome

The cysteinyl leukotrienes C_4 and D_4 are potent vasoconstrictors which may modulate glomerular filtration.

Urinary excretion of the metabolite leukotriene E_4 increases with severity of liver disease, but following correction for creatinine clearance (cr.cl) levels were considerably higher only in patients with HRS (54.1 pg/ml cr.cl) compared to normal controls (1.0 pg/ml cr.cl), compensated liver disease (1.9 pg/ml cr.cl) and those with severe hepatocellular dysfunction (11.0 pg/ml cr.cl).[58] Whether cysteinyl leukotrienes are an important factor in the pathogenesis of HRS will await the development of specific 5-lipoxygenase inhibitors or leukotriene antagonists for clinical use.

Fulminant hepatic failure (FHF)

A high cardiac output with systemic vasodilatation are also a feature of FHF and may be accompanied by marked hyperlactataemia. These features, and an abnormal relationship between oxygen extraction ratio and the position of the oxygen–haemoglobin dissociation curve, may be evidence of a covert tissue hypoxia due to functional shunting around actively respiring tissues.[59] Similar changes in the relationship between oxygen supply and demand have also been observed in critically ill patients, in whom changes in cardiac output and oxygen extraction move in parallel over a greater range than normal, and in whom an elevated arterial oxygen delivery may still be inadequate for tissue requirements. The diagnosis of tissue hypoxia in such cases is difficult and cannot rely on single measurements of oxygen consumption or extraction ratio, but require an oxygen flux test whereby the response to manoeuvres which increase oxygen delivery to tissues is observed. Oxygen extraction rising when oxygen supply is increased implies that the tissues are hypoxic.

Harrison *et al.* used prostacyclin, with potent vasodilatory actions within the microcirculation, in a group of patients with grade 4 encephalopathy due to fulminant hepatic failure in order to increase oxygen delivery to tissues, in an attempt to detect a covert tissue oxygen debt.[60] Prostacyclin 5 ng/kg per minute increased cardiac output and oxygen delivery and was associated with a dramatic increase in total body oxygen consumption of more than 25%.

Significant falls in mixed venous lactate and an increase in oxygen extraction ratio were also observed. The exact site of this increased oxygen extraction remains unclear but the results suggest that a covert tissue oxygen debt is common in these patients despite apparently adequate arterial pressure and oxygen content and emphasizes the importance of optimizing oxygen delivery in preventing the development of organ dysfunction.

Eicosanoids and organ transplantation

Organ preservation and cold ischaemia

Graft viability following cold ischaemia is of prime importance in organ transplantation. Whilst ischaemia/reperfusion-induced liver injury may affect hepatocyte and biliary epithelial function, sinusoidal endothelial cells are the predominant target of warm ischaemia and are critical to graft survival after transpantation.[61] Extensive endothelial damage results in platelet and fibrin deposition with loss of graft perfusion and function. Prostacyclin has many properties that are potentially beneficial in organ preservation including vasodilation, inhibition of platelet aggregation/adherence and leucocyte adherence as well as cellular cytoprotection. Araki demonstrated that prostacyclin was cytoprotective during hypoxia in isolated perfused livers[62] and this has been confirmed by others showing preservation of mitochondrial function, ATP and cyclic nucleotide levels[63] and prevention of ischaemic damage.[33,37] Prostacyclin also attenuates lung ischaemic injury on reperfusion, resulting in lower pulmonary vascular resistance and improved arterial oxygenation.[64] Thromboxane synthetase inhibitors may also reduce ischaemic liver injury.[37] Nevertheless, the metabolic and chemical stability of prostacyclin has limited its therapeutic application as a useful addition to preservation fluids. Stable prostacyclin analogues (iloprost, OP-41483) improve pulmonary function after lung transplantation[65] and reduce alanine transferase release and lipid peroxidation after liver transplantation.[66,67] A reduction in lipid peroxidation may result from reduced adherence of activated polymorphonuclear leucocytes which generate toxic oxygen species.

Primary graft non-function after orthotopic liver transplantation is associated with minimal bile production, rapidly rising transaminases, hypoglycaemia, coagulopathy and progression to encephalopathy and may develop in some degree in between 2 and 8%. Many factors are implicated in the pathogenesis but a reperfusion injury with sinusoidal cell disruption has been considered important. Because of the previously discussed effects of prostaglandins during hepatic hypoxia and preservation[35,37,62–64] Greig *et al.* treated 10 patients with primary graft non-function 4–34 hours after liver transplantation with a PGE$_1$ infusion (up to 0.6 µg/kg per hour).[68] Within 12 hours of treatment eight patients responded with a significant fall in transaminases, prothrombin time and improvement in bile production.[68] These promising results require further confirmation in controlled studies.

Prostaglandin analogues have also been investigated in the prevention of graft rejection in renal transplant recipients.[69] The rationale for their use includes their immunosuppressive effects,[42] reduction in ischaemic renal injury and reversal of cyclosporin nephrotoxicity in animal models.[70] In this group of patients treatment with misoprostol was associated with a significant improvement in graft function as judged by mean serum creatinine concentration (128 ± 7 vs 158 ± 11 µmol/l at 12 weeks, $p=0.03$), and a reduction in the incidence of acute rejection episodes. Cyclosporin blood levels and the frequency of nephrotoxicity were similar in both groups.

Prostaglandins in extracorporeal circulation

Extracorporeal circuits are now frequently used in clinical medicine, often for the treatment of life-threatening disorders. Haemodialysis (HD) for chronic renal failure is widely practised and the equipment and techniques are constantly under development and have reached a high degree of sophistication.

More recently high-flux postdilutional haemofiltration (HF) has been applied as an alternative for the treatment of uraemic subjects as well as in the management of some other disorders. The use of highly permeable membranes permits the removal of medium range solutes. Haemoperfusion (HP) through charcoal columns has been successful in the management of severe liver failure. Finally, extracorporeal membrane oxygenation is now a routine procedure for the maintenance of gas exchange during cardiac surgery.

All of these procedures require the prolonged and repeated contact of blood components with a substantial surface area of foreign material. Whilst there have been considerable advances in the biocompatibility of the components used in all parts of these extracorporeal circuits, blood platelet activation and fibrin formation remain major concerns and their occurrence can cause life-threatening complications in this mode of treatment.

When blood is exposed to a synthetic surface there is the potential for complex interactions between the foreign material and all the cellular and plasma components. Proteins are rapidly adsorbed onto the surface and many subsequently undergo structural or chemical change. Fibrinogen is present in plasma in high concentration and is selectively adsorbed to a foreign surface;[71] however, other components, including fibronectin, coagulation factors, globulins and albumin, may contribute to the surface layer depending upon the individual characteristics of the biomaterial in use, in particular its hydrophobic properties. The composition of this protein layer, which accumulates extremely rapidly, influences the subsequent interactions with cellular components of the blood.[72]

Platelets can adhere to a foreign surface within seconds of exposure and, depending upon the flow characteristics operating and the degree of stimulation, may progress to aggregation to form a platelet mass.[73,74] Involved platelets may not re-enter the circulation, resulting in a thrombocytopenic, and hence potentially haemorrhagic, state.

Alternatively, some partially activated platelets and platelet aggregates may re-enter the blood flow and give the potential for significant systemic embolization and consequent tissue hypoxia and even infarction. Furthermore, platelet activation may result in the acceleration of fibrin deposition, through the contribution of essential phospholipid components which act as cofactors in the reactions in the intrinsic and final common pathways of blood coagulation. Also the release of platelet cytoplasmic granules may make available components which can further augment the thrombotic process, including platelet agonists and cofactors (ADP, von Willebrand factor and fibrinogen), and others which can act as inflammatory mediators (prostaglandins and products of the lipoxygenase pathway).

Activation due to exposure of blood to an artificial surface is not confined to the coagulation and haemostatic mechanism. Activation of granulocytes and of the complement systems during extracorporeal blood passage have been demonstrated[75,76] and other interactions may also be of clinical importance.

Clinical consequences of coagulation activation in extracorporeal circuits

Gross thrombus formation in extracorporeal circuits is clearly undesirable. However, more subtle activation may also be important. It has long been recognized that the level of coagulation and platelet activation which occurs during haemodialysis (HD)[77–79] can result in the consumption of coagulation factors and platelets and thus contribute to the post-dialysis haemorrhagic state.[80] Although the development of modern dialysis apparatus has probably reduced the incidence and severity of these phenomena, anticoagulation is generally required for safe dialysis.[81] There is also concern that, conversely, coagulation activation during dialysis could lead to a prethrombotic state[82] and this could theoretically contribute to the premature atherosclerosis which develops in a large proportion of subjects on long-term dialysis programmes. Furthermore, passage of microemboli, formed in the dialyser circuit, into the circulation could result in tissue hypoxia during dialysis.

When clotting occurs in extracorporeal HD circuits erythrocytes become trapped and are not available for reinfusion. This tends to exacerbate the often clinically important anaemia of chronic renal failure.

During cardiopulmonary bypass (CPB) platelet activation and consumption make a major contribution to postoperative haemorrhage.[83–85] Furthermore, microembolic phenomena may well have a role in the post-CPB syndrome of cerebral dysfunction[86–88] and products of platelet activation could have an adverse effect on myocardial function.[89] Similar considerations apply to procedures involving haemofiltration and haemoperfusion and it is accepted that pharmacological anticoagulation is required for the safe performance of procedures which involve the exposure of blood to an extracorporeal circuit.

Anticoagulation in extracorporeal circuits

Heparin has most commonly been utilized to prevent thrombosis in extracorporeal circuits. Systemic anticoagulation can be easily achieved. By making use of the efficient heparin-neutralizing capacity of protamine, 'regional' anticoagulation within the extracorporeal circuit is an alternative possibility. Heparin is a highly sulphated glycosaminoglycan extracted from mast cell-rich mammalian tissues. Unfractionated heparins consist of a mixture of fragments with a mean molecular weight of 12 000 (range 5 000–30 000). Fractionated heparins (molecular weight <7 000) are becoming increasingly available for clinical use and offer certain advantages.

Heparin binds to the plasma protein antithrombin thus facilitating inhibition of the proteases of the intrinsic and common coagulation pathways resulting in a profound anticoagulant effect. This is reflected in prolongation of the clotting times, particularly the KCCT and thrombin time, but also the prothrombin time.

The major anticoagulant effect of unfractionated heparin is through the inhibition of thrombin but other proteases, including factor Xa, are also inhibited. In contrast, low molecular weight (fractionated) heparins accelerate factor Xa inhibition at doses similar to those of unfractionated heparin but the antithrombin activity is greatly reduced.

Heparin, used therapeutically, is an extremely effective and efficient anticoagulant. However, its use in extracorporeal circuits is associated with several disadvantages. As discribed above, an early and important event in extracorporeal circuits is platelet activation and aggregation with formation of platelet microemboli and the development of thrombocytopenia. Heparin has no inhibitory effect on these events, indeed platelets possess heparin-binding sites and, *in vitro*, heparin can induce a degree of platelet aggregation. A modest degree of thrombocytopenia is common during full-dose heparin therapy, due to platelet activation.[90] Furthermore, an idiosyncratic response is less often seen; this involves the formation of a heparin-dependent platelet antibody after several days of exposure to heparin.[91] The antibody results in more severe thrombocytopenia, commonly associated with arterial and venous thromboembolic events, which may be life-threatening: this syndrome of 'heparin-induced thrombocytopenia' is fortunately uncommon in clinical practice.

Although the half-life of administered heparin is short, excessive dosage or incomplete neutralization by protamine can result in a severe, persisting coagulopathy. This is disadvantageous, especially in those subjects who already suffer from disturbed haemostatic mechanisms due to their underlying disorder or therapy. Thus, many subjects with severe renal impairment manifest a bleeding tendency which is due mainly to disturbed platelet–subendothelial interactions, with a defect of platelet release.[92]

Disseminated intravascular coagulation, with a potentially severe coagulopathy due to consumption of labile clotting factors, fibrinogen and platelets, is commonly present in acutely ill subjects, such as those with septicaemia or shock, who may require life-saving haemofiltration or haemodialysis treatment. Here, the haemorrhagic risk from heparin anticoagulation may be of great importance. Where haemoperfusion is performed against a background of liver disease, the potentially severe coagulopathy and thrombocytopenia of liver failure may render anticoagulation with heparin hazardous.

Subjects who are exposed to heparin for prolonged periods appear to be at increased risk of developing osteoporosis.[93] Fortunately, this is not commonly clinically important and has been described mainly after prolonged continuous heparin exposure during thrombosis prophylaxis. However, any increased tendency to bone loss, additional to that already present, in subjects with chronic renal failure would be undesirable.

Other theoretical disadvantages of heparin as anticoagulant in extracorporeal circuits include its variable neutralization by platelet factor 4 released from the α-granules of platelets stimulated by exposure to the components of the extracorporeal circuit, and the theoretical possibility that heparin–protamine macromolecules could contribute to microembolic complications. Clearly, an alternative antithrombotic drug is desirable in order to overcome some of these problems.

Use of prostacyclin in extracorporeal circuits

Prostacyclin in haemodialysis

Prostacyclin possesses properties which could be predicted to be useful in the prevention of activation of haemostatic mechanisms on exposure of blood to an artificial surface. From the comments above it is apparent that uncontrolled adhesion and aggregation of platelets is a major factor in the early stages of thrombus formation within extracorporeal circuits. Although heparin is highly efficient in the prevention of subsequent thrombin generation and fibrin deposition, it has no, or even an adverse effect on platelet activation.

The potent inhibitory activity of prostacyclin on both adhesion and aggregation offers attractive possibilities.

Early experiments were performed using PGE$_1$[94] which also possesses potent antiplatelet activity. However, side effects of the use of this prostanoid were unacceptable. Subsequently Woods *et al.*[95] were able to demonstrate the apparently safe substitution of prostacyclin for heparin during HD in dogs. Encouragingly, this could be achieved without any evidence for clotting in the dialysis circuit despite the absence of any prolongation of clotting times. Furthermore, microembolization from the dialyser, as assessed by change in screen filtration pressure, and thrombocytopenia were abolished when prostacylin was used. In these experiments a high dose of prostacyclin (30–50 ng/kg per minute) was administered.

Subsequently smaller doses of prostacyclin (5 ng/kg per minute) were successfully administered to human subjects undergoing dialysis with heparin anticoagulation.[96] Two potentially beneficial effects were observed. The early fall in platelet count (by around 10%) seen with heparin alone was abolished, and ongoing platelet activation with release of β-thromboglobulin also was inhibited. More surprisingly, the prolongation of thrombin time was enhanced, confirming earlier observations of an apparent 'heparin-sparing effect' in animal studies.[96] This may be through the inhibition of platelet release of platelet factor 4, a heparin inhibitor, and offers the possibility of use of lower heparin doses during dialysis, with a reduction in the potential adverse effects of the anticoagulant. This heparin-sparing activity of prostacyclin has not been found in all studies[97] and may be dependent upon the degree of heparin anticoagulation achieved and on the type of dialyser.

The studies of Woods *et al.*[95] and Turney *et al.*[96] raised the possibility of the substitution of prostacyclin, as the sole antithrombotic agent, for heparin during HD in man. A potential risk would be the unopposed generation of thrombin with fibrin deposition within the extracorporeal circuit.

Zusman *et al.*[98] successfully used prostacyclin as the sole antithrombotic agent during HD in 10 subjects with chronic renal failure. A dosage of 4 ng/kg per minute was administered by intravenous infusion for 10 minutes prior to dialysis, then prostacyclin was given into the arterial line during the procedure, the dose being limited by tolerance (hypotension, headache, nausea or abdominal pain). Platelet responsiveness to ADP *ex vivo* was reduced but no change in coagulation was noted. No haemorrhage or clot formation in the dialyser circuit was found. Subsequently Smith *et al.*[99] reported similar success in 12 subjects using prostacyclin at a dose of 3–12 ng/kg per minute, adjusted according to blood pressure and given into the arterial line. However, significant hypotension complicated the procedure in four cases and was prolonged and severe in two. In the latter an acetate bath was used as opposed to the standard bicarbonate dialysate, and the authors postulated that the cardiosuppressant effect of acetate may augment the hypotensive effect of prostacyclin. *Ex vivo* platelet responsiveness was diminished when compared to that during subsequent dialysis with conventional heparin anticoagulation, but neither heparin nor prostacyclin resulted in prolongation of the bleeding time.

Prostacyclin did not prevent dialysis-associated leucopenia. Interestingly, there was an apparent minor increase in dialysis efficiency, in three of four subjects studied, when prostacyclin was compared to heparin. Similar findings had previously been noted in normal dogs,[100] but not by Zusman *et al.*[98] who used a lower total dose of prostacyclin and a different type of dialyser.

It is noteworthy that major clotting in the dialyser occurred in one subject studied by Smith *et al.* and in one further subject a less severe episode was noted. Others have found unacceptable clotting within the dialyser to be a major problem when prostacyclin is used alone during HD, even when the more biocompatible hollow fibre dialysers are used and the safety of this approach was subsequently questioned.[101]

Furthermore, the hypotensive effect can be hazardous, and particular problems have been noted in critically ill patients with combined renal and respiratory failure, where prostacyclin administered intravenously at a dose of 5 ng/kg per minute prior to dialysis caused a reduction in mean arterial pressure, pulmonary and systemic vascular resistance and cardiac filling pressure without increase in cardiac output. Tissue oxygen delivery was substantially reduced.[102]

The principal role for prostacyclin in HD is perhaps to allow reduced heparin dosage in those subjects at high risk of bleeding.[103] Also, the demonstrable reduction in platelet microaggregate formation[104] could be an advantage where microembolization is perceived to be a deleterious phenomenon. In most units in the UK, however, prostacyclin is not considered to be necessary for uncomplicated dialysis.

Prostacyclin in cardiopulmonary bypass

Postoperative haemorrhage and cerebral dysfunction are major complications of bypass surgery. Bleeding is predominantly due to thrombocytopenia and platelet dysfunction secondary to platelet activation and release in the extracorporeal circuit.

Early experiments utilizing the antiplatelet effects of PGE_1 suggested a significant preservation of platelet numbers and function.[105] A similar effect of prostacyclin was noted by Longmore *et al.*[106] during CPB experiments in greyhounds. Although prostacyclin alone did not prevent fibrin deposition, the consumption of platelets was abolished and heparin and prostacyclin in combination allowed the preservation of platelet numbers and fibrinogen concentration.

In an early study in man, platelet numbers were preserved during CPB using prostacyclin, but the dose required was unclear.[107]

The benefits of prostacyclin infusion during CPB have been confirmed in two placebo-controlled trials.[108,109] A dose of 10 ng/kg per minute from induction of anaesthesia, increasing to 20 ng/kg per minute at start of bypass, together with heparin infusion resulted in a marked reduction in the degree of the thrombocytopenia resulting from the use of heparin alone. Some evidence for a 'heparin-sparing' effect on the activated clotting time was noted and fewer subjects on prostacyclin required extra heparin doses. Total blood loss was lower in the prostacyclin group, presumably due to preservation of platelet numbers. Although blood pressure was lowered by prostacyclin, this did not result in clinical problems.[108]

Similar results were obtained by Walker *et al.*[109] who also demonstrated a reduction in platelet release (as plasma β-thromboglobulin and platelet factor 4) in the presence of prostacyclin. More recently Malpass *et al.*[110] successfully administered prostacyclin during CPB.

A major advance would be the prevention of the post-CPB cerebral syndrome. Only in one study were psychometric and neurological tests performed on groups who had received prostacyclin and heparin or heparin alone. Demonstrable impairment in cerebral function was present at 3 days after CPB, but no difference between the groups could be demonstrated.[108]

Prostacyclin in haemofiltration

Haemofiltration (HF) utilizes highly permeable membranes which allow passage of medium-range solutes. Although the membranes used may be more biocompatible than those used in dialysis, high shear stresses are generated, with the potential for cell damage and platelet activation with coagulation. Heparin is therefore routinely used during HF. In a small study, prostacyclin 4 ng/kg per minute given in addition to heparin reduced platelet loss and inhibited release. However, hypotensive episodes were common.[111]

A possible indication for prostacyclin in HF is the management of subjects at high risk of bleeding.

Prostacyclin alone has been compared with prostacyclin and heparin during HF in subjects with acute renal failure after liver transplantation. However, no important difference in bleeding time or blood loss was noted.[112]

Prostacyclin in charcoal haemoperfusion

During HP for fulminant hepatic failure, thrombocytopenia and the development of cellular aggregates are major problems.[113] Hypotension frequently develops and may lead to abandonment of the procedure. It has been proposed that release of vasoactive substances from damaged blood cells, including platelets, may be pathogenic in these hypotensive complications.[114] Prostacyclin apparently prevented platelet activation during HP in dogs.[115]

In man prostacyclin 16 ng/kg per minute was given, in addition to heparin, during a 4-hour HP through a column of polymer-coated activated charcoal.[116] Six subjects with hepatic encephalopathy were compared with six others treated identically with heparin alone. Although platelet counts remained higher in the prostacyclin-treated group, differences were not significant and severe thrombocytopenia developed in no subject in this study. However, β-thromboglobulin release was greater in the subjects given heparin alone.

Hypotension developed in two subjects in the heparin group and none in the prostacyclin and heparin group. Thus, prostacyclin can be given safely during

HP, but this small study did not provide strong evidence for its routine use.

Prostacyclin analogues

Used therapeutically, prostacyclin suffers from the disadvantage of a somewhat low therapeutic ratio: hypotension and colic occur in some subjects at doses around 5 ng/kg per minute. Also, once reconstituted in aqueous solution, it degrades *in vitro* with a half-life of around 12 hours, which can be inconvenient.

Analogues have been developed and studied as alternatives to prostacyclin for use in extracorporeal circuits. Iloprost (ZK-36374, Schering) is a carbacyclin derivative which is stable in aqueous solution at pH 7.4, is at least equipotent to prostacyclin in antiplatelet effect, but has considerably weaker vasodilatory activity.[117]

Treatment with iloprost (50 ng/kg per minute) during cardiopulmonary bypass with 30 minutes of global ischaemia in mongrel dogs resulted in less platelet consumption and myocardial platelet deposition than that which occurred in similar experiments with a saline control. Furthermore, given at a dose of 150 ng/kg per minute for the initial 30 minutes of an extracorporeal membrane oxygenation procedure in dogs, the platelet protective effect appeared to persist for the full 3 hours of the procedure.[118] In these experiments, in comparison to dogs given heparin alone, the platelet count remained stable, and the persisting defect of platelet aggregation to ADP which occurs in CPB was not seen after termination of the iloprost infusion, suggesting an ongoing protective effect against procedure-induced platelet activation and subsequent dysfunction.

Iloprost has been compared to prostacyclin in human subjects during HD on heparin for chronic renal failure.[97] Iloprost 2 ng/kg per minute and prostacyclin 5 ng/kg per minute seemed indistinguishable in terms of the changes in platelet numbers and release which occurred during the procedure.

CG-4203 (taprostene; Grunenthal GmbH) is an alternative, stable prostacyclin analogue which has approximately one-fifth of the platelet inhibitory potency of prostacyclin *ex vivo*. When administered at a dosage of 25–35 ng/kg per minute, with heparin, to chronic renal failure patients undergoing HD for 5 hours, inhibition of ADP-induced platelet responsiveness *ex vivo* was noted.[119] Although marked heparin-sparing was achieved, dialysis with CG-4203 alone resulted in clot formation and premature termination of the procedure. Also, the therapeutic ratio of this analogue appears to be small, as the 35 ng/kg per minute infusion resulted in nausea and headache in all subjects.

Clearly prostacyclin analogues offer some advantages over prostacyclin itself but, as with prostacyclin, the precise place for these agents in procedures involving extracorporeal circulation remains unclear. One indication, albeit an uncommon one, is the prevention of the potentially lethal platelet activation by heparin which could occur during cardiopulmonary bypass in a subject with a heparin-dependent platelet antibody due to previous heparin exposure. Iloprost has been successfully utilized in this particular situation.[120]

The future

There have been major advances in the development of anticoagulant and antiplatelet drugs over recent years. It is not yet known whether the fractionated (low molecular weight) heparins or the heparinoids will be superior to unfractionated heparins as anticoagulants in extracorporeal circuits. Used in combination with prostacyclin or an analogue, further improvement in safety can perhaps be achieved.

Hirudin is the anticoagulant agent from the medicinal leech. Recombinant hirudin has been used for anticoagulation during HD in nephrectomized dogs. Platelet count and fibrinogen level remained unchanged and no haemorrhagic problem was observed.[121,122] If these results are reproduced in human subjects the requirement for an additional antiplatelet agent may be abolished.

New antiplatelet agents are also under development. A thromboxane synthetase inhibitor has been compared with iloprost during cardiopulmonary bypass in dogs; iloprost was possibly more efficacious in the prevention of platelet activation in the doses used, however.[89] Ticlopidine, a potent inhibitor of ADP-induced platelet aggregation, has been used in HD and during CPB.[123-125] Other drugs may eventually prove to be superior to prostacyclin in this area, but at the present time only prostacyclin, among antiplatelet agents, has been thoroughly studied as an anticoagulant for use in extracorporeal circuits in man.

References

1. Huber M, Keppler D. Eicosanoids and the liver. In: Popper H, Schaffner F (eds), *Progress in Liver Disease.* Vol IX. Philadelphia: WB Saunders, 1990: 117–42.
2. Decker K. Eicosanoids. Signal molecules of liver cells. *Semin Liver Dis* 1985; **5**: 175–90.
3. Spolarics Z, Tanacs B, Garzo B, *et al.* Prostaglandin and thromboxane synthesizing activity in isolated murine hepatocytes and nonparenchymal liver cells. *Prostaglandins Leukot Med* 1984; **16**: 379–88.
4. Birmelin M, Decker K. Synthesis of prostanoids and cyclic nucleotides by phagocytosing rat kupffer cels. *Eur J Biochem* 1984; **142**: 219–25.
5. Ouwendijk R, Zijlstra F, van den Broeck A, Wilsons S, Vincent J. Comparison of the production of eicosanoids by human and rat peritoneal macrophages and rat Kupffer cells. *Prostaglandins* 1988; **35**: 437–46.
6. Casteleijn E, Kuiper J, Van Rooij H, Koster J, Van Berkel T. Prostaglandin D$_2$ mediates the stimulation of glycogenolysis in the liver by phorbol ester. *Biochem J* 1988; **250**: 77–80.
7. Okumura T, Nakayama R, Sago T, Saito K. Identification of prostaglandin E metabolites from primary cultures of rat hepatocytes. *Biochim Biophys Acta* 1985; **837**: 197–207.
8. Casteleijn E, Kuiper J, Van Rooij H, Kamps S, Van Berket T. Endotoxin stimulates glycogenolysis in the liver by means of intercellular communication. *J Biochem Chem* 1988; **263**: 6953–5.
9. Wernze H, Titor W, Goerig M. Release of prostanoids into the portal and hepatic vein in patients with chronic liver disease. *Hepatology* 1986; **6**: 911–16.
10. Hagman W, Denzlinger C, Keppler D. Role of peptide leukotrienes and their hepatobiliary elimination in endotoxin action. *Circ Shock* 1984; **14**: 223–35.
11. Keppler D, Hagmann W, Rapp S, Denzlinger C, Koch H. The relation of leukotrienes to liver injury. *Hepatology* 1985; **5**: 883–91.
12. Sakagami Y, Mizoguchi Y, Seki S, Kobayashi K, Morishawa S, Yamamoto S. Release of peptide leukotrienes from rat Kupffer cells. *Biochem Biophys Res Commun* 1988; **156**: 217–21.
13. Kart U, Peters T, Decker K. The release of tumor necrosis factor from endotoxin-stimulated rat Kupffer cells is regulated by prostaglandin E$_2$ and dexamethasone. *J Hepatol* 1988; **7**: 352–61.
14. Iwai M, Gardemann A, Puschel G, Jungermann K. Potential role for prostaglandin F$_{2\alpha}$, D$_2$, E$_2$ and thromboxane A$_2$ in mediating the metabolic and haemodynamic actions of sympathetic nerves in perfused rat liver. *Eur J Biochem* 1988; **175**: 45–50.
15. Piper P, Samhoun M. Leukotrienes. *Br Med Bull* 1987; **43**: 297–311.
16. Reed D. Status of calcium and thiols in hepatocellular

injury by oxidative stress. *Semin Liver Dis* 1990; **10** (4): 285–92.

17. Acosta D, Sorenson E. Role of calcium in cytotoxic injury of cultured hepatocytes. *Ann NY Acad Sci* 1983; **407**: 78–92.

18. Laskin D. Nonparenchymal cells and hepatotoxicity. *Semin Liver Dis* 1990; **10** (4): 293–304.

19. Nolan J. Endotoxin, reticuloendothelial function and liver injury. *Hepatology* 1981; **1**: 458–65.

20. Laskin D, Pilaro A. Potential role of activated macrophages in acetaminophen hepatotoxicity. 1. Isolation and characterisation of activated macrophages from rat liver. *Toxicol Appl Pharmacol* 1986; **86**: 204–15.

21. Keppler D, Forsthove C, Hagmann W. Leukotrienes and liver injury. In: Bianchi L, Gerok W, Popper H (eds), *Trends in Hepatology*. Lancaster: MTP Press Ltd, 1985: 137–45.

22. Kawada N, Mizoguchi Y, Kobayashi K, Yamamoto S, Morisawa S. Arachidonic acid metabolites in carbon tetrachloride-induced liver injury. *Gastroenterol Jpn* 1990; **25**: 363–8.

23. Koyama Y, Imoto M, Tanaka M, Fukuda Y, Satake T, Ozawa T. Changes in endogenous prostaglandin levels during D-galactosamine-induced liver injury. *Biochem Int* 1989; **19**: 421–8.

24. Guarner F, Fremont-Smith M, Prieto J. Cytoprotective effect of prostaglandins on isolated rat liver cells. *Liver* 1985; **5**: 35–9.

25. Stachura J, Tarnawski A, Ivey K, *et al.* Prostaglandin protection of carbon tetrachloride-induced liver cell necrosis in the rat. *Gastroenterology* 1981; **81**: 211–17.

26. Ruwart M, Rush B, Friedle N, Piper R, Kolaja G. Protective effect of 16,16-dimethyl PGE$_2$ on the liver and kidney. *Prostaglandins* 1982; **21** (suppl): 97–102.

27. Funck-Brentano C, Tinel M, Degott C, Letteron P, Babany G, Pessayre D. Protective effect of 16,16-dimethyl prostaglandin E$_2$ on the hepatotoxicity of bromobenzene in mice. *Biochem Pharmacol* 1984; **33**: 89–96.

28. Noda Y, Hughes R, Williams R. Effect of prostacyclin and a prostaglandin analogue BW 245C on galactosamine-induced hepatic necrosis. *J Hepatol* 1986; **2**: 53–64.

29. Mizoguchi Y, Tsutsui H, Miyajima K, *et al.* The protective effects of prostaglandin E$_1$ in an experimental massive hepatic cell necrosis model. *Hepatology* 1987; **7**: 1184–8.

30. Bursch W, Taper H, Somer M, Meyer S, Putz B, Schulte-Hermann R. Histochemical and biochemical studies on the effect of the prostacyclin derivative iloprost on CCl$_4$-induced lipid peroxidation in rat liver and its significance for hepatoprotection. *Hepatology* 1989; **9**: 830–8.

31. Gove C, Hughes R, Zmiec Y, Williams R. *In vivo* and *in vitro* studies on the protection effects of 9β-methylcarbacyclin, a stable prostacyclin analogue,

in galactosamine-induced hepatocellular damage. *Prostaglandins Leukot Essent Fatty Acids* 1990; **40**: 73–7.

32. Bursch W, Schulte-Hermann R. Cytoprotective effects of iloprost against liver cell death induced by carbon tetrachloride or bromobenzene. In: Gryglewski R, Stock G (eds), *Prostacyclin and its Stable Analogue Iloprost*. Berlin: Springer Verlag, 1987: 258–68.

33. Sikujara O, Monden M, Toyoshima K, Okamura J, Kosaki G. Cytoprotective effect of prostaglandin I$_2$ on ischaemia-induced hepatic cell injury. *Transplantation* 1983; **36**: 238–43.

34. Levine R. The role of cyclic AMP in hepatic and gastrointestinal function. *Gastroenterology* 1970; **59**: 280–300.

35. Goldfarb R, Glenn T. Regulation of lysosomal membrane stabilisation via cyclic nucleotides and prostaglandins – the effect of steroids and indomethacin. In: Lefer A, Schumer W (eds), *Molecular and Cellular Aspects of Shock and Trauma*. New York: Alan R Liss Inc., 1983: 146–66.

36. Meren M, Varin F, Ruwart M, Thurman R. Effect of 16,16-dimethyl prostaglandin E$_2$ on oxygen uptake and microcirculation in the perfused rat liver. *Hepatology* 1986; **6**: 917–21.

37. Besse T, Gustin T, Claeys N, Schroeyers P, Lambotte L. Effect of PGI$_2$ and thromboxane antagonist of liver ischaemic injury. *Eur Surg Res* 1989; **21**: 213–17.

38. Kurokawa T, Nonami T, Harada A, *et al.* Effects of prostaglandin E$_1$ on the recovery of ischaemia-induced liver mitochondrial dysfunction in rats with cirrhosis. *Scand J Gastroenterol* 1991; **26**: 269–74.

39. Horney J, Galambos J. The liver during and after hepatic necrosis. *Gastroenterology* 1979; **73**: 639–45.

40. Kirn A, Gut J, Bingen A. Murine hepatitis induced by frog virus 3; a model for studying the effect of sinusoidal cell damage. *Hepatology* 1983; **3**: 105–11.

41. Hagman W, Steffan A-M, Kirn A, Keppler D. Leukotrienes as mediators in frog virus 3-induced hepatitis in rats. *Hepatology* 1987; **7**: 732–6.

42. Rappaport R, Dodge G. Prostaglandin E inhibits the production of human interleukin 2. *J Exp Med* 1982; **155**: 943–8.

43. Tripp C, Wyche A, Unanue E, Needleman P. The functional significance of the regulation of macrophage Ia expression by endogenous arachidonate metabolites *in vitro*. *J Immunol* 1986; **137**: 3915–20.

44. Santoro M, Benedetto A, Zaniratti E, Garaci E, Jaffe G. The relationship between prostaglandins and virus replication: endogenous prostaglandin synthesis during infection and the effect of exogenous PGA on virus production in different cell lines and in persistently infected cell lines. *Prostaglandins* 1983; **25**: 353–63.

45. Abecassis M, Falk J, Makowka L, Didzans V, Falk R, Levy G. 16,16-Dimethyl prostaglandin E_2 prevents the development of fulminant hepatitis and blocks the induction of monocyte/macrophage procoagulant activity after murine hepatitis virus strain 3 infection. *J Clin Invest* 1987; **80:** 881–9.

46. Bourne H, Lichtenstein L, Melmon K, Henney C, Weinstein Y, Shearer G. Modulation of inflammation and immunity of cyclic AMP. *Science* 1974; **184:** 19–28.

47. Williams R, Gimson A. Intensive liver care and management of acute hepatic fever failure. *Dig Dis Sci* 1991; **36:** 820–6.

48. Sinclair S, Levy G. Treatment of fulminant viral hepatic failure with prostaglandin E. A preliminary report. *Dig Dis Sci* 1991; **36:** 791–800.

49. O'Grady J, Gimson A, O'Brien C, Pucknell A, Hughes R, Williams R. Controlled trials of charcoal haemoperfusion and prognostic factors in fulminant hepatic failure. *Gastroenterology* 1988; **94:** 1186–92.

50. Sherlock S. Vasodilatation associated with hepatocellular disease: relation to functional organ failure. *Gut* 1990; **31:** 365–7.

51. Guarner F, Guarner C, Prieto J, *et al.* Increased synthesis of systemic prostacyclin in cirrhotic patients. *Gastroenterology* 1986; **90:** 687–94.

52. Moore K, Ward P, Taylor G, Williams R. Systemic and renal production of thromboxane A_2 and prostacyclin in decompensated liver disease and hepatorenal syndrome. *Gastroenterology* 1991; **100:** 1069–77.

53. Shijo H, Sasaki H, Miyajima Y, Okumura M. Prostaglandin $F_{2\alpha}$ and indomethacin in hepatogenic pulmonary angiodysplasia. Effects on pulmonary haemodynamics and gas exchange. *Chest* 1991; **100:** 873–5.

54. Boyer T, Zia P, Reynolds T. Effects of indomethacin and prostaglandin A on renal function and plasma renin activity in alcoholic liver disease. *Gastroenterology* 1979; **77:** 215–22.

55. Zipser R, Radvan G, Kronberg I, Duke R, Little T. Urinary thromboxane B_2 and prostaglandin E_2 in the hepatorenal syndrome: evidence for increased vasoconstrictor and decreased vasodilator factors. *Gastroenterology* 1983; **84:** 697–703.

56. Zipser R, Kronberg I, Rector W, Daskalopoulos G. Therapeutic trial of thromboxane synthesis inhibition in the hepatorenal syndrome. *Gastroenterology* 1984; **87:** 1228–32.

57. Fevery J, Van Cutsem E, Nevens F, Van Steenbergen W, Verberckmoes R, De Groote J. Reversal of hepatorenal syndrome in four patients by peroral misoprostol (prostaglandin E_2 analogue) and albumin administration. *J Hepatol* 1990; **11:** 153–8.

58. Moore K, Taylor G, Maltby N, *et al.* Increased production of cysteinyl leukotrienes in hepatorenal syndrome. *J Hepatol* 1990; **11:** 263–71.

59. Bihari D, Gimson A, Watson A, Williams R. Tissue hypoxia in fulminant hepatic failure. *Crit Care Med* 1985; **13:** 1034–9.

60. Harrison P, Wendon J, Gimson A, Alexander G, Williams R. Improvement by *N*-acetyl cysteine of haemodynamics and oxygen transport in fulminant hepatic failure. *N Engl J Med* 1991; **324:** 1853–7.

61. Caldwell-Kenkel J, Currin R, Tanaka Y, Thurman R, Lemasters J. Reperfusion injury to isolated endothelial cells following cold ischaemic storage to rat liver. *Hepatology* 1989; **10:** 282–6.

62. Araki H, Lefer A. Cytoprotective action of prostacyclin during hypoxia in the isolated perfused liver. *Am J Physiol* 1980; **238:** H176–81.

63. Okabe K, Malchesky P, Nose Y. Protective effect of prostaglandin I_2 on hepatic mitochondrial function of the preserved rat liver. *Tohoku J Exp Med* 1986; **150:** 373–9.

64. Hooper T, Thomson D, Jones M, *et al.* Amelioration of lung ischaemic injury with prostacyclin. *Transplantation* 1990; **49:** 1031–5.

65. Klepetko W, Muller M, Khurl-Brady G. Beneficial effect of iloprost on early pulmonary function after lung preservation with modified Euro-Collins solution. *Thorac Cardiovasc Surg* 1989; **37:** 174–8.

66. Sanchez-Urdazpal L, Gores G, Ferguson D, Krom R. Improved liver preservation with addition of iloprost to Euro-Collins and University of Wisconsin storage solutions. *Transplantation* 1991; **52:** 1105–7.

67. Goto S, Kim Y, Kodama Y, *et al.* Beneficial effect of a stable prostacyclin analogue (OP-41483) on rat liver preserved for twenty-four hours with lactobionate solution. *Transplantation* 1991; **52:** 926–8.

68. Greig P, Woolf G, Sinclair S, *et al.* Treatment of primary graft nonfunction with prostaglandin E_1. *Transplantation* 1989; **48:** 447–53.

69. Moran M, Mozes M, Maddux M, *et al.* Prevention of acute graft rejection by the prostaglandin E_1 analogue misoprostol in renal-transplant recipients treated with cyclosporin and prednisolone. *N Engl J Med* 1990; **322:** 1183–8.

70. Paller M. Effects of the prostaglandin E_1 analogue misoprostol on cyclosporin nephrotoxicity. *Transplantation* 1988; **45:** 1126–31.

71. Lee RG, Adamson C, Kim SW. Competitive adsorption of plasma protein onto polymer surfaces. *Thromb Res* 1974; **4:** 485–8.

72. George JN. Direct assessment of platelet adhesion to glass: a study of the forces of interaction and the effects of plasma and serum factors, platelet function and modification of the glass surface. *Blood* 1972; **40:** 862–4.

73. Bruck SD. *Properties of Biomaterials in the Physiological Environment.* Boca Raton, FL: CRC Press, 1980.

74. Baumgartner HR, Muggli R, Tschopp TB, Turitto VT. Platelet adhesion, release and aggregation in flowing blood: effects of surface properties and

platelet function. *Thromb Haemost* 1976; **35:** 124–38.

75. Ivanovich P, Chenoweth DE, Schmidt R, *et al.* Symptoms and activation of granulocytes and complement with two dialysis membranes. *Kidney Int* 1983; **24:** 758–63.

76. Wegmuller E, Montandon A, Nydegger U, Descoeudres C. Biocompatibility of different haemodialysis membranes. Activation of complement and leukopenia. *Int J Artif Organs* 1986; **9:** 85–92.

77. Lindsay RM, Prentice CRM, Davidson JG, Burton JA, McNichol GP. Haemostatic changes during dialysis associated with thrombus formation of dialysis membranes. *BMJ* 1972; **4:** 454–8.

78. Zucker WH, Shinoda BA, Mason RG. Experimental interactions of components of haemodialysis units with human blood. *Am J Pathol* 1974; **75:** 139–56.

79. Marshall JW, Ahearn DJ, Nothum RJ, Esterly J, Nolph KD, Maher JF. Adherence of blood components to dialyzer membranes: morphological studies. *Nephron* 1974; **12:** 157–70.

80. Lazarus JM. Complications of hemodialysis. *Kidney Int* 1981; **18:** 783–96.

81. Hathiwala S. Dialysis without anticoagulation. *Int J Artif Organs* 1983; **6:** 64–6.

82. Turney JH, Woods HF, Weston MJ. Regular haemodialysis therapy induces a prethrombotic state. *Thromb Haemost* 1979; **42:** 67–71.

83. McKenna R, Bachmann F, Whittaker B, Gilson JR, Weinberg M. The hemostatic mechanism after open-heart surgery. *J Thorac Cardiovasc Surg* 1975; **70:** 298–308.

84. Friedenberg WR, Myers WO. Plotke ED, *et al.* Platelet dysfunction associated with cardiopulmonary bypass. *Ann Thorac Surg* 1978; **25:** 298–305.

85. Harker LA, Malpass TW, Branson HE, Hessel EA, Slichter SJ. Mechanism of abnormal bleeding in patients undergoing cardiopulmonary bypass. Acquired transient platelet dysfunction associated with selective alpha-granule release. *Blood* 1980; **56:** 824–34.

86. Bass RM, Longmore DB. Cerebral damage during open heart surgery. *Nature* 1969; **222:** 30–3.

87. Lee WH, Brady MP, Rowe JM, Miller WC. Effects of extracorporeal circulation upon behaviour, personality and brain function. Part II. Haemodynamic, metabolic and psychometric correlations. *Ann Surg* 1971; **173:** 1013–23.

88. Branthwaite MA. Neurological damage related to open-heart surgery. *Thorax* 1972; **27:** 748–53.

89. Huddleston CB, Hammon JW, Wareing TH, *et al.* Amelioration of the deleterious effects of platelets activated during cardiopulmonary bypass. *J Thorac Cardiovasc Surg* 1985; **89:** 190–5.

90. Salzman EW, Rosenberg RD, Smith MH, Lindon JN, Favreau L. Effect of heparin and heparin fractions on platelet aggregation. *J Clin Invest* 1980; **65:** 64–7.

91. Chong BH, Ismail F, Cade J, Gallus AS, Gordon S, Chesterman CN. Heparin-induced thrombocytopenia: studies with a new low molecular weight heparinoid, Org 10172. *Blood* 1989; **73:** 1592–5.

92. Moosa A, Ford I, Brown CB, Greaves M. Fibrinopeptide A, thromboxane B_2 and beta-thromboglobulin levels in bleeding time blood in uraemia. *Platelets* 1991; **2:** 157–60.

93. Squires JW, Pinch LW. Heparin induced spinal fractures. *JAMA* 1979; **241:** 2417–19.

94. Addonizio VP, Macarak EJ, Niewiarowski S, Colman RW, Edmunds JH. Preservation of platelets during extracorporeal circulation with prostaglandin E_1. *Trans Am Soc Artif Intern Organs* 1977; **23:** 639–41.

95. Woods HF, Ash G, Weston MJ, Bunting S, Moncada S, Vane JR. Prostacyclin can replace heparin in haemodialysis in dogs. *Lancet* 1978; **2:** 1075–7.

96. Turney JH, Williams LC, Fewell MR, Parsons V, Weston MJ. Platelet protection and heparin sparing with prostacyclin during regular dialysis therapy. *Lancet* 1980; **2:** 219–22.

97. Dibble JB, Kalra PA, Orchard MA, Turney JH, Davies JA. Prostacyclin and iloprost do not affect action of standard dose heparin on haemostatic function during haemodialysis. *Thromb Res* 1988; **29:** 385–92.

98. Zusman RM, Rubin RH, Cato AE, Cocchetto DM, Crow JW, Tolkoff-Rubin N. Hemodialysis using prostacyclin instead of heparin as the sole antithrombotic agent. *N Engl J Med* 1981; **304:** 934–9.

99. Smith MC, Danviriyasup K, Crow JW, *et al.* Prostacyclin substitution for heparin in long-term hemodialysis. *Am J Med* 1982; **73:** 669–78.

100. Patak RV, Wiegmann TB, Diederich DA. Effect of prostacyclin (PGI_2) on urea clearance (U_{cl}) in conscious dog. *Kidney Int* 1981; **19:** 155A.

101. Knudsen F, Nielsen AH, Kornerup HJ, Pedersen JC, Dyerberg J. Epoprostenol as sole antithrombotic treatment during haemodialysis. *Lancet* 1984; **1:** 235–6.

102. Davenport A, Will EJ, Davison AM. Adverse effects of prostacyclin administered directly into patients with combined renal and respiratory failure prior to dialysis. *Intensive Care Med* 1990; **16:** 431–5.

103. Turney JH, Dodd NJ, Weston MJ. Prostacyclin in extracorporeal circulations. *Lancet* 1981; **1:** 1101.

104. Kuzniewski M, Sulowicz W, Hanicki Z, *et al.* Effect of heparin and prostacyclin/heparin infusion on platelet aggregation in hemodialyzed patients. *Nephron* 1990; **56:** 174–8.

105. Addonizi VP, Strauss JF, Colman RW, Edmunds LH. Effects of prostaglandin E_1 on platelet loss during *in vivo* and *in vitro* extracorporeal circulation with a bubble oxygenator. *J Thorac Cardiovasc Surg* 1979; **77:** 119–26.

106. Longmore DB, Bennet G, Guierrara D, *et al.* Prosta-

cyclin: a solution to some problems of extracorporeal circulation. Experiments in greyhounds. *Lancet* 1979; **1**: 1002–5.

107. Radegran K, Papaconstantinou C. Prostacyclin infusion during cardiopulmonary bypass in man. *Thromb Res* 1980; **19**: 267–70.

108. Longmore DB, Bennet JG, Hoyle PM, *et al*. Prostacyclin administration during cardiopulmonary bypass in man. *Lancet* 1981; **1**: 800–4.

109. Walker ID, Davidson JF, Faichney A, Wheatley DJ, Davidson KG. A double blind study of prostacyclin in cardiopulmonary bypass surgery. *Br J Haematol* 1981; **49**: 415–23.

110. Malpass TW, Amory DW, Harker LA, Ivey TD, Williams BD. The effect of prostacyclin infusion on platelet haemostatic function in patients undergoing cardiopulmonary bypass. *J Thorac Cardiovasc Surg* 1984; **87**: 550–5.

111. Canaud B, Mion C, Arujo A, *et al*. Prostacyclin (epoprostanol) as the sole antithrombotic agent in postdilutional haemofiltration. *Nephron* 1988; **48**: 206–12.

112. Legat K, Zimpfer M, Steltzer H, Gabriel A, Muller C, Tuchy GL. Heparin and prostacyclin in hemofiltration after orthotopic liver transplantation. *Transplant Proc* 1984; **3**: 1984.

113. Silk DBA, Williams R. Experiences in the treatment of fulminant hepatic failure by conservative therapy, charcoal haemoperfusion and polyacrylonitrile haemodialysis. *Int J Artif Organs* 1978; **1**: 29–33.

114. Weston MJ, Langley PG, Rubin MH, Hanid MA, Mellon PJ, Williams R. Platelet function in fulminant hepatic failure and effect of charcoal haemoperfusion. *Gut* 1977; **18**: 897–902.

115. Bunting S, Moncada S, Vane JR, Woods HF, Weston MJ. Prostacyclin improves hemocompatibility during charcoal hemoperfusion. In: Vane JR, Bergstrom S (eds), *Prostacyclin*. New York: Raven Press, 1979.

116. Gimson AES, Langley PG, Hughes RD, *et al*. Prosta-

cyclin to prevent platelet activation during charcoal haemoperfusion in fulminant hepatic failure. *Lancet* 1980; **1**: 173–5.

117. Bergman G, Kiff PS, Atkinson L, Kerkey S, Jewitt DE. Dissociation of platelet aggregation and vasodilation with iloprost, a stable, orally active prostacyclin derivative. *Circulation* 1983; **68** (suppl III): 398.

118. Cottrell ED, Kappa JR, Stenach N, *et al*. Temporary inhibition of platelet function with iloprost (ZK36374) preserves canine platelets during extracorporeal membrane oxygenation. *J Thorac Cardiovasc Surg* 1988; **96**: 535–41.

119. Maurin N, Ballmann M. Prevention of coagulation during hemodialysis by a combination of the stable prostacyclin analogue CG4203 and low-dose heparin. *Clin Nephrol* 1988; **30**: 35–41.

120. Kappa JR, Horn MK, Fisher CA, Cottrell ED, Ellison N, Addonizio VP. Efficacy of iloprost (ZK36374) versus aspirin in preventing heparin-induced platelet activation during cardiac operations. *J Thorac Cardiovasc Surg* 1987; **94**: 405–13.

121. Bucha E, Markwardt F, Nowak G. Hirudin in haemodialysis. *Thromb Res* 1985; **40**: 563–70.

122. Markwardt F, Nowak G, Bucha E. Hirudin as anticoagulant in experimental haemodialysis. *Haemostasis* 1991; **21** (suppl 1): 149–55.

123. Renner C, Guilmet D, Curtet JM. Ticlopidine in cardiac surgery with extracorporeal circulation. *Nouv Presse Med* 1980; **9**: 3249–51.

124. Installe E, Gonzalez M, Schoevaerdts JC, Tremouroux J. Prevention by ticlopidine of platelet consumption during extracorporeal circulation for heart surgery and lack of effect on operative and postoperative bleeding. *J Cardiovasc Pharmacol* 1981; **3**: 1174–83.

125. Traietti P, Chippini MG, Belfiglio A, Bartoli R, Bologna E. Effect of ticlopidine treatment in haemodialysis patients. *Clin Ter* 1988; **127**: 27–35.

19 Future therapeutic opportunities

H Graf, GM Rubanyi and G Stock

The pharmacological properties and the clinical use of prostaglandins has been discussed in great detail in the previous chapters. Many efforts have been undertaken to increase chemical and metabolic stability of prostaglandins by chemical modification in order to obtain more suitable compounds for effective therapeutic use.

Prostaglandins and their analogues have been utilized successfully in the termination of pregnancy, for the induction of labour, as 'cytoprotective' agents in gastroduodenal ulceration, in ischaemic peripheral vascular disease, thrombangiitis obliterans and Raynaud's syndrome.

Preliminary studies using prostacyclin,[1-3] PGE$_2$[4-6] and its stable analogues[7,8] demonstrated beneficial effects in patients with congestive heart failure. Clinical efficacy of iloprost, the most intensively investigated prostacyclin analogue, was used in the treatment of diabetic neuropathy[9] and this compound proved to be superior to prostacyclin.[10,11] Novel therapeutic opportunities arise from ongoing preclinical studies in tumour metastasis[12-14] and atherosclerosis[15-17] using stable prostacyclin analogues. Additionally, these compounds were found to reduce the size of myocardial infarction in experimental animals and to enhance functional and anatomical recovery of the ischaemic heart and to prevent coronary thrombosis.[18] Unfortunately, prostacyclin and its analogues failed to reveal beneficial therapeutic effects in patients with myocardial ischaemia.[19] It was speculated that this lack of efficacy might be due to the impaired generation of endothelium-derived relaxing factor (EDRF) in the coronary arteries of these patients.[20] Nitric oxide donors (nitrovasodilators) were found to show synergistic effects with iloprost on platelet aggregation[21] and leucocyte activation and migration,[22] but do not synergize as vasodilators.[23]

Prostacyclin analogues and metastasis

Antimetastatic properties of the stable prostacyclin analogues iloprost, cicaprost and eptaloprost (for structural details see Chapter 4) were demonstrated in tumour metastasis models using rats and mice. Intravenous administration of prostacyclin has been found to reduce the formation of lung nodules after intravenous injection of B16 melanoma cells.[24-26] Treatment of mice bearing a Lewis lung carcinoma cell line (3LL) with iloprost reduced the formation of metastases. The effect was comparable in magnitude with that obtained using natural prostacyclin, but this effect was seen with much smaller dosages and had a significantly longer duration. Similar results were obtained using iloprost in the treatment of spontaneous metastasis with increased survival time of the hosts when combined with tumour removal by surgery.[27] Preoperative treatment with the prostacyclin analogue followed by surgical removal of the primary tumour was found to be synergistic with postoperative treatment with cyclophosphamide.[28]

Cicaprost, a metabolically stable and orally available prostacyclin analogue, was recently investigated in various animal tumour models. The compound dose dependently inhibited the formation of metastases of a prostate carcinoma in the rat[29] and reticulum sarcoma[29] and mammary carcinoma in mice.[30]

The number of metastases in the lung of C57 B16 mice bearing B16BL6 myeloma cells injected intravenously was found to depend on the duration of pretreatment using iloprost, cicaprost or eptaloprost.[13] Results indicated that the analogues should be administered close to the day of injection of the tumour cells to achieve a maximal beneficial effect. The mechanism by which prostacyclin mimetics interfere in the complex sequential events leading to tumour metastases remains to be elucidated. Up to now, no striking effects of prostacyclin analogues were found on the growth of the primary tumour. Therefore, the decreased number of metastases due to cicaprost therapy cannot be correlated with a decrease in the cell number disseminated from the primary tumour.

Much evidence suggests that prostacyclin mimetics inhibit tumour cell-induced platelet aggregation which is said to be required for tumour dissemination.[26,31] However, there are also results questioning an important role of platelets in the course of tumour metastasis. Significant inhibition of metastases is still evident 24 hours after treatment whereas tumour cell-associated platelet aggregation is not reduced at this time point. This clearly indicates a dissociation of the effect of iloprost on platelet aggregation and metastasis.

It has also been proposed, that prostacyclin analogues might inhibit the adhesion of tumour cells to the vascular endothelium by down-regulation of the expression of receptors on the surface of tumour cells.[32] Additionally, modification of the host immunocompetence by prostacyclin mimetics was discussed as a possible mechanism of its antimetastatic activity.[33] Iloprost significantly increased macrophage-mediated tumour cell growth inhibition, increased the *in vivo* clearence of tumour cells from the lungs, enhanced natural killer cell activity and effectively improved T-cell-mediated immune response.

In this respect, the beneficial therapeutic effect of prostacyclin mimetics seems to be due to the combined action of these compounds on different target cells: endothelial cells, tumour cells, platelets and immune competent cells such as macrophages and T cells.

Prostacyclin in the treatment of atherosclerosis

A diminished capacity of the vascular wall to generate prostacyclin has been demonstrated in the coronary arteries, the aortae and mesenteric arteries of patients suffering from atherosclerosis and in experimental animal models.[34–38] These results could be verified in cell culture.[39] Furthermore, lipid hydroperoxides were able to inhibit prostacyclin formation[40] as a result of irreversible inhibition of prostacyclin synthase. This enzyme was demonstrated to show many characteristics of a cytochrome P450 enzyme[41] and hydrophobic peroxides serve as suicide substrates. The elevated urinary metabolites of prostacyclin in patients suffering from severe atherosclerosis[42] may be explained by an increased production of prostacyclin in parts of the vasculature not affected by the atheromatous process. The mechanism of this compensatory pathway seems to be at least in part due to the 'steal' of PGH_2 from activated platelets by intact vascular endothelium.[34]

In spite of these findings, replacement therapy using orally availble prostacyclin mimetics should be promising. As outlined before, the potential of prostacyclin mimetics seems to be to act on different target cells involved in the crucial steps of atherogenesis. Endothelial cell activation appears to be a key step in atherogenesis. In contrast to the 'normal' endothelium, activation causes thrombogenicity, release of cytokines and growth factors, increase in endothelial permeability and transendothelial migration of immunocompetent cells and lipid peroxidation. Aggregating platelets and invading monocytes release growth factors and cytokines[43,44] and lead to the inflammatory and proliferative responses characteristic of sclerotic plaques. Oxidized LDL produces injury to cultured endothelial cells[45] and in this way, uncontrolled oxidation of LDL by the activated endothelium not only gives rise to the formation of foam cells and cell necrosis within the surrounding tissue but also may cause further damage to the endothelium. The risk of high serum levels of LDL in the development of atherosclerosis might be explained in this way as might the beneficial effect of HDL which increases prostacyclin formation by the intact endothelium. Prostacyclin is able to counteract several mechanisms of endothelial cell activation as mentioned above. It additionally inhibits accumulation of cholesterol in macrophages[43] and vascular smooth muscle cells[46] presumably by stimulating ACEH (acid cholesterol ester hydrolase).

Pathophysiological events ultimately leading to atherosclerosis unfortunately appear to be too complex and therefore sclerotic diseases need to be treated with more than one drug. It would be of advantage to use the synergistic action of a prostacyclin mimetic and a drug or drugs selected in order to minimize side effects unavoidable with single drug therapy.

As far as lipid accumulation is concerned, PGE_2 in inhibiting ACAT (acetyl-CoA:cholesterol acetyltransferase) could synergistically lower cholesterol accumulation in the tissues affected. Radical scavenger and lipid lowering drugs used in combination with prostacyclin mimetics could help to avoid endothelial activation by oxidized lipoproteins.

PGD_2 was shown to be a potent leucocyte inhibitor and its stable analogues thus would be candidates for use together with prostacyclin mimetics in a combined antiatherosclerotic therapy. Unfortunately, PGD_2 also acts as a pulmonary vasoconstrictor. Therefore, it may be a challenge to develop more selective analogues with minimal vascular activity.

As NO donors synergize with prostacyclins in inhibiting activation of platelets and leucocytes but not as vasorelexants[22] this combination could be of help in interrupting the vicious cycle of intercellular activation of the cells involved in atherogenesis.

Prostaglandins and cytoprotection

Cytoprotective effects were originally described for the gastroprotective activity of prostaglandins and its analogues. Stable analogues or prostaglandins E_1 and E_2 analogues such as rioprostil, enprostil and nocloprost[47,48] were developed as anti-ulcer drugs differing in their effects on gastric acid secretion, gastroprotection and ulcer healing. Although prostaglandin E_2 and its analogues are the most widely used drugs in investigating gastroduodenal ulceration, prostacyclin plays an important role as an endogenous, locally formed cytoprotective agent within the gastric mucosa. Exogenous prostacyclin was effective in inhibiting the development of gastric ulcers in the rat[49] and significantly accelerated healing of gastric peptic ulcers.[50,51] Further preclinical investigation and clinical trials are necessary to identify prostaglandin analogues which besides their protective effect enhance healing of acute gastric ulceration in a dose range which does not affect normal gastrointestinal and cardiovascular function.

Protection of cell integrity independent of selective cell function has additionally been described in hepatocytes,[52,53] brain cells,[54] adrenal nerve terminals[55] and cardiac myocytes.[56]

Protection of cardiac myocytes by prostacyclin from postischaemic injury was demonstrated in a variety of animal models.[57-60] To analyse the potential role of endogenous prostacyclin experiments were designed to study coronary effluent for eicosanoids after myocardial ischaemia.[61] Compared to the massive enhancement of compounds deleterious to the myocardium – leukotrienes, hydroperoxides, thromboxane A_2 and HETEs – only a minor increase in prostacyclin formation was observed.[62,63]

Animal studies suggest that this increase in prostacyclin biosynthesis is insufficient to protect the injured myocardium against ischaemic injury. Consistently, stimulation of endogenous prostacyclin production by defibrotide revealed beneficial effects in myocardial ischaemia[64] and compounds inhibiting endogenous prostacyclin biosynthesis like indomethacin and aspirin aggravate ischaemic myocardial injury.[65,66] However, clinical studies in acute myocardial infarction showed only mild improvement or failed to demonstrate any beneficial therapeutic effects of prostacyclin administered systemically.[19,67,68] It was concluded that prostacyclin and its analogues are of limited therapeutic benefit for patients with ischaemic heart disease.[19]

As prostaglandins are locally acting mediators of intercellular signalling pathways, beneficial effects may be enhanced by the interaction with other endogenous mediators and lack of therapeutic benefit may also be caused by the attenuation of one or more endogenous intercellular signalling compounds acting in concert with prostaglandins. As EDRF production is reduced dramatically under conditions of experimental ischaemia[69,70] and inhibition of endogenous prostacyclin biosynthesis appears to simultaneously reduce EDRF formation,[71] exogenous NO donors may be likely candidates for a combined therapy with prostacyclin mimetics. NO donors are much more potent inhibitors of leucocyte release reaction[22] compared to prostacyclin. The release of proteases and cytotoxic radicals from activated leucocytes is deleterious to the ischaemic myocardium[72] and EDRF (NO) and prostacyclin inhibits this process in a synergistic manner similar to their effect on platelet aggregation.[21] This synergism of EDRF and prostacyclin as activators of the cGMP and cAMP signalling pathways does not occur with respect to their vasodilating properties.[23] Therefore, the combination of NO donors and stable prostacyclin analogues in the treatment of myocardial ischaemia should be of clinical advantage in avoiding or minimizing cardiovascular side effects. It would certainly be worthwhile to test this concept in clinical trials and analogous preliminary studies have been conducted in peripheral vascular disease.[73]

Prostaglandins and bone remodelling

In bone fracture repair and osteomyelitis a simultaneous increase of bone resorption and new bone formation is observed in order to achieve bone remodelling. PGE_2 is the most potent prostanoid in resorbing bone in tissue culture.[74] Increase in invading leucocytes, vasodilatation and the initial production of osteogenic cells was suggested to be the mechanism of prostaglandin action *in vivo*, where PGE_2 stimulates bone formation in the fetal rat and in chick embryo. Clinical relevance of the influence of prostaglandins in bone formation was found in infants with cyanotic congenital heart disease and cortical hyperostosis after treatment with PGE_1[75,76]

PGD_2 stimulates calcification of human osteoblastic cells cultured from explants of human periosteum.[77] PGD_2 and its non-enzymatic metabolite Δ^{12}-PGJ_2 both enhance calcification with an efficacy similar to that found for $1,25$-$(OH)_2$-vitamin D_3. The mechanism of action was supposed to be due to an induction of collagen, osteocalcin and alkaline phosphatase and this increase led to the accumulation of hydroxyapatite within the matrix of osteoblasts. It remains unclear whether PGD_2 itself or its more stable metabolite is responsible for the biological effect.

Stable PGD_2 agonists (ZK-110841 and ZK-118182; for structural details see Chapter 4) are now available[78] to test the therapeutic potential of PGD_2 in bone remodelling including osteoporosis.

Conclusion

Over the past two decades numerous important functions of prostaglandins have been discovered, excellently summarized in the previous chapters. Every effort has been made to optimize their therapeutic potential by synthesizing stable analogues and also selective antagonists. Nonetheless, there is still the challenge to elucidate the precise mechanism of action, not only in the control of vascular tone and platelet aggregation but also in the more complex

field of immunomodulation and those biological activities summarized by the term 'apoprotection'. There is still the challenge to use more selective prostaglandin mimetics and analogues in order to get a close insight into the signal transduction pathways and a better understanding of the target cells involved. These new insights will hopefully lead to a more precise utilization in pharmacotherapy and novel therapeutic opportunities.

References

1. Yui Y, Nakajama H, Kawai C. Prostacyclin therapy in patients with congestive heart failure. *Am J Cardiol* 1982; **50**: 320–4.
2. Auinger G, Virgolini I, Weissel M, Bergmann H, Sinzinger H. Prostacyclin I_2 (PGI_2) increases left ventricular ejection fraction (LVEF). *Prostaglandins Leukot Essent Fatty Acids* 1989; **36**: 149–54.
3. Yui Y, Sakurai T, Nakajina H, Kawai C. Effect of prostacyclin and prazocin in the treatment of congestive heart failure, with special reference in the sympathetic nervous system. *Jpn Circ J* 1984; **1**: 365–72.
4. Awan NA, Evenson MK, Needham KE, Beattie JM, Armsterdam EA, Mason OT. Cardiocirculatory and myocardial energic effects of prostaglandin E_1 in patients with acute myocardial infarction and left ventricular failure. *Am Heart J* 1981; **102**: 703–9.
5. Popat KD, Pitt BP. Hemodynamic effects of prostaglandin E_1 in patients with acute myocardial infarction and left ventricular failure. *Am Heart J* 1982; **103**: 485–9.
6. Jacobs P, Naeije R, Renard M, Melot C, Mols P, Hallemans R. Effects of prostaglandin E_1 on hemodynamic and blood gases in severe left heart failure. *J Cardiovasc Pharmacol* 1983; **5**: 170–1.
7. Yui Y, Takatsu Y, Hattori R, *et al.* Vasodilator therapy with a new stable prostacyclin analog, OP-41483, for congestive heart failure due to coronary artery disease and comparison of hemodynamic effects and platelet aggregation with nitroprusside. *Am J Cardiol* 1986; **58**: 1042–5.
8. Elsner D, Kramer EP, Riegger AJG. Hemodynamic, humoral, and renal effects of the prostacyclin analogue iloprost in conscious dogs with and without heart failure. *J Cardiovasc Pharmacol* 1990; **16**: 601–8.
9. Shindo H, Tawata M, Aida K, Onaya T. Clinical efficacy of a stable prostacyclin analog, Iloprost in diabetic neuropathy. *Prostaglandins* 1991; **41**: 85–96.
10. Tohijma T, Sawada K, Funayama H, Shiokawa Y. Treatment of diabetic neuropathies with prostaglandin E_1. In: Goto Y, Horiuchi A, Kogure K (eds), *Diabetic Neuropathy*. Amsterdam–Oxford–Princeton: Excerpta Medica, 1982: 358.
11. Goto Y, Toyoda T, Suzuki H, *et al.* Evaluation of the therapeutic effect of prostaglandin E_1 on diabetic

peripheral neuropathy. A multi-center clinical study. *J Jpn Diabet Soc* 1984; **27** (1): 3.

12. Giraldi T, Rapozzi V, Perissin L, Zorzet S. Antimetastatic action of stable prostacyclin analogs in mice. *Adv Prostaglandin Thromboxane Leukotriene Res* 1991; **21**: 913–16.

13. Costantini V, Giampietri A, Allegrucci M, Agnelli G, Nenci GG, Fioretti MC. Mechanisms of the antimetastatic activity of stable prostacyclin analogues: modulation of host immunocompetence. *Adv Prostaglandin Thromboxane Leukotriene Res* 1991; **21**: 917–20.

14. Schneider MR, Schillinger E, Schirner M, Skuballa W, Stürzebecher S, Witt W. Effects of prostacyclin analogues in *in vivo* tumor models. *Adv Prostaglandin Thromboxane Leukotriene Res* 1991; **21**: 901–8.

15. Gryglewski RJ. Prostaglandins, platelets and atherosclerosis. In: Fasman JD (ed), *CRC Critical Reviews on Biochemistry*. New York: CRC Press Inc, 1980; **7**: 291–338.

16. Szczeklik A, Gryglewski RJ, Nizankowski R, Musial J, Pieton R, Mruk J. Circulatory and anti-platelet effects of intravenous prostacyclin in healthy men. *Pharmacol Res Commun* 1987; **10**: 545–56.

17. Szczeklik A, Nizankowski R, Skawinski S, Gluszko P, Gryglewski RJ. Successful therapy of advanced arteriosclerosis obliterans with prostacyclin. *Lancet* 1979; **1**: 1111–14.

18. Müller B, Witt W, McDonald FM. Iloprost: stable prostacyclin analogue. In: Rubanyi GM (ed), *Cardiovascular Significance of Endothelium-derived Vasoactive Factors*. Mount Kisco, New York: Futura Publ Co, 1991: 309–33.

19. Gryglewski RJ, Botting RM, Vane JR. Prostacyclin: from discovery to clinical application. In: Rubanyi GM (ed), *Cardiovascular Significance of Endothelium-derived Vasoactive Factors*. Mount Kisco, New York: Futura Publ Co, 1991: 3–38.

20. Ganz P, Vekshtein VI, Yeung AC, *et al.* Impaired endothelial vasodilator function in human coronary arteries. In: Rubanyi GM (ed), *Cardiovascular Significance of Endothelium-derived Vasoactive Factors*. Mount Kisco, New York: Futura Publ Co, 1991: 113–24.

21. Radomski MW, Palmer RMJ, Moncada S. The antiaggregating properties of vascular endothelium: interaction between prostacyclin and nitric oxide. *Br J Pharmacol* 1987; **92**: 639–46.

22. Korbut R, Trabka-Janik E, Gryglewski RJ. Cytoprotection of human polymorphonuclear leukocytes by stimulators of adenylate and guanylate cyclases. *Eur J Pharmacol* 1989; **165**: 171–2.

23. Gryglewski RJ, Korbut R, Trabka-Janik E, Zembowicz A, Trybulec M. Interaction between NO-donors and iloprost in human vascular smooth muscle, platelets and leukocytes. *J Cardiovasc Pharmacol* 1989; **14**: 124–8.

24. Honn KV, Cicone B, Skoff A. A potent antimetastatic agent. *Science* 1981; **212**: 1270–2.

25. Honn KV, Canavaugh P, Evans C, Taylor JD, Sloane BF. Tumor cell-platelet aggregation: induced by cathepsin-B-like proteinase and inhibited by prostacyclin. *Science* 1982; **217**: 540–2.

26. Costantini V, Fuschiotti P, Allegrucci M, Agnelli G, Nenci GG, Fioretti MC. Platelet–tumor cell interaction: effect of prostacyclin and a synthetic analog on metastasis formation. *Cancer Chemother Pharmacol* 1988; **22** (4): 289–93.

27. Sava G, Perissin L, Zorzet S, Piccini P, Giraldi T. Antimetastatic action of the prostacyclin analog iloprost in the mouse. *Clin Exp Metastasis* 1989; **7**: 671–8.

28. Giraldi T, Rapozzi V, Perissin L, Zorzet S. Antimetastatic action in mice of PGI₂ analog iloprost. In: *Eicosanoids and Bioactive Lipids in Cancer and Radiation Injury*. Proceedings of the 1st International Conference. Dordrecht: Kluwer, 1990: 415–18.

29. Schirner M, Schneider MR. Cicaprost inhibits metastases of animal tumors. *Prostaglandins* 1991; **42**: 451–61.

30. Welch DR, Neri A, Nicolson GL. Comparison of 'spontaneous' and 'experimental' metastases using rat 13762 mammary adenocarcinoma metastatic cell clones. *Invasion Metastasis* 1982; **3**: 65–80.

31. Gasic GJ. Role of plasma, platelets, and endothelial cells in tumor metastasis. *Cancer Metastasis Rev* 1984; **3**: 99–116.

32. Grossi IM, Taylor JD, Honn KV. Prostacyclin and prostacyclin analogs inhibit tumor cell adhesion to substrata, through inhibition of membrane expression of the integrin receptor IRGpIIb/IIIa. *Proc Am Assoc Cancer Res* 1989; **30**: 324 (Abs).

33. Constantini V, Fuschiotti P, Giampietri A, *et al.* Effects of a stable prostacyclin analogue on platelet activity and on host immunocompetence in mice. *Prostaglandins* 1990; **39** (6): 581–99.

34. D'Angelo V, Mysliwiec M, Donati MB, De Gaetano G. Defective fibrinolytic and prostacyclin-like activity in human atheromatous plaque. *Thromb Haemost* 1978; **39**: 535–6.

35. Sinzinger H, Silberbauer K, Feigl W. Diminished PGI₂ function by human atherosclerotic arteries. *Lancet* 1979; **1**: 469–70.

36. Sinzinger H, Silberbauer K, Feigl W. Prostacyclin activity is diminished in differential types of morphologically controlled human atherosclerotic lesions. *Thromb Haemost* 1979; **42**: 803–5.

37. Dembinska-Kiec A, Gryglewska T, Zmuda A, Gryglewski RJ. The generation of prostacyclin by arteries and by coronary vascular bed is reduced in experimental atherosclerosis in rabbits. *Prostaglandins* 1977; **14**: 1025–35.

38. Dembinska-Kiec A, Gryglewski RJ, Zmuda A, Gryglewska T. Prostacyclin and thromboxane A₂ biosynthesis capacities of heart, arteries and platelets at various stages of experiential atherosclerosis in rabbits. *Atherosclerosis* 1987; **31**: 385–94.

39. Larrue J, Leroux C, Daret D, Bricaud H. Decreased prostacyclin production in cultured smooth muscle cells from atherosclerotic rabbit aorta. *Biochim Biophys Acta* 1982; **710**: 257–63.

40. Terashita Z, Nishikawa K, Terao S, Nakagawa M, Hino T. A specific prostaglandins I_2 synthetase inhibitor 3-hydroperoxy-3-methyl-Z-phenyl- ^{3}H-indole. *Biochem Biophys Res Commun* 1979; **91**: 72–8.

41. Ullrich V, Graf H. Prostacyclin and thromboxane synthase as P-450 enzymes. *TIPS* 1984; **5**: 352–5.

42. Fitzgerald GA, Smith B, Pedersen AK, Brash AR. Increased prostacyclin biosynthesis in patients with severe atherosclerosis and platelet activation. *N Engl J Med* 1984; **310**: 1060–5.

43. Willis AL, Smith DL, Vigo C. Suppression of principal atherosclerotic mechanisms by prostacyclins and other eicosanoids. *Prog Lipid Res* 1986; **25**: 645–66.

44. Willis AL, Smith DL, Vigo C, Kluge AF. Effects of prostacyclin and orally stable mimetic agent RS-93427–007. *Lancet* 1987; **2**: 682–3.

45. Henriksen T, Evensen SA, Carlander B. Injury to cultured endothelial cells induced by low density lipoproteins. *Scand J Clin Lab Invest* 1979; **39**: 369–75.

46. Hajjar DP. Prostaglandins and cyclic nucleotides: modulators of arterial cholesterol metabolism. *Biochem Pharmacol* 1985; **34**: 295–300.

47. Konturek SJ, Brzozowski T, Drozdowicz D, *et al.* Nocloprost, a unique PGE_2 analog, with local gastroprotective and ulcer healing activity. *Adv Prostaglandin Thromboxane Leukotriene Res* 1991; **21**: 793–7.

48. Hawkey CJ. Prostaglandins and mucosal protection: laboratory evidence versus clinical performance. In: Garner A, Whittle BJR (eds), *Advances in Drug Therapy of Gastrointestinal Ulcerations*. Chichester: John Wiley, 1989: 89–94.

49. Whittle B Jr. Temporal relationship between cyclooxygenase inhibition as measured by prostacyclin biosynthesis and the gastrointestinal damage induced by indomethacin in the rat. *Gastroenterology* 1981; **80**: 94–8.

50. Dembinska-Kiec A, Kostka-Trabka E, Kosiniak-Kamysz A, *et al.* Prostacyclin in patients with peptic gastric ulcers. *Hepatogastroenterology* 1985; **33**: 262–6.

51. Uchida M, Kawano O, Misaki N, Saitoh K, Irino O. Healing of acetic acid-induced gastric ulcer and gastric mucosal PGI_2 level in rats. *Dig Dis Sci* 1990; **35**: 80–5.

52. Araki H, Lefer AM. Cytoprotective actions of prostacyclin during hypoxia in the isolated perfused cat liver. *Am J Physiol* 1980; **238**: H176–81.

53. Bursch W, Schulte-Hermann R. Cytoprotective effect of iloprost against liver cell death induced by carbon tetrachloride or bromobenzene. In: Gryglewski RJ, Stock G (eds), *Prostacyclin and its Stable Analogue Iloprost*. First International Workshop on Iloprost. Berlin: Springer-Verlag, 1987: 257–68.

54. Renkawek K, Herbaczynska-Cedro K, Mossakowski MJ. The effect of prostacyclin on the morphological and enzymatic properties of CNS cultures exposed to anoxia. *Acta Neurol Scand* 1986; **73** (2): 111–18.

55. Schrör K, Darius H, Addicks K, Köster R, Smith EF. PGI_2 prevents ischemia-induced alterations in cardiac catecholamines without influencing nerve-stimulation-induced catecholamine release in nonischemic conditions. *J Cardiovasc Pharmacol* 1982; **4**: 741–8.

56. Araki H, Lefer AM. Role of prostacyclin in the preservation of ischemic myocardial tissue in the perfused cat heart. *Circ Res* 1980; **47**: 757–63.

57. Jouve R, Puddu E. Prostacyclin and protection of the ischaemic myocardium. *Cardiologia* 1988; **33**: 339–41.

58. Jugdutt BJ, Hutchins GM, Bulkley BH, Becker LC. Dissimilar effects of prostacyclin, prostaglandin E_1 and prostaglandin E_2 on myocardial infarct size after coronary occlusion in conscious dogs. *Circ Res* 1981; **49**: 685–700.

59. Lefer AM, Ogletree ML, Smith JB, Silver MJ, Nicolau KC, Barnette WE, Gasic GP. Prostacyclin: a potentially valuable agent for preserving myocardial tissue in acute myocardial ischaemia. *Science* 1978; **200**: 52–4.

60. Melin JA, Becker LC. Salvage of ischaemic myocardium by prostacyclin during experimental myocardial infarction. *J Am Coll Cardiol* 1983; **2**: 279–86.

61. Schrör K. Eicosanoids and myocardial ischaemia. *Basic Res Cardiol* 1987; **82** (1): 235–43.

62. Coker SJ, Parratt JR, Ledingham JMCA. Thromboxane and prostacyclin release from ischaemic myocardium in relation to arrhythmias. *Nature* 1981; **291**: 323–4.

63. Engels W, Van Bilsen M, De Groot MJM, *et al.* Ischemia and reperfusion induced formation of eicosanoids in isolated rat hearts. *Am J Physiol* 1990; **258**: H1865–71.

64. Hohlfeld Th, Strobach H, Schrör K. Stimulation of prostacyclin synthesis by defibrotide: improved contractile recovery from myocardial 'stunning'. *J Cardiovasc Pharmacol* 1991; **17** (1): 108–15.

65. Forman MB, Uderman H, Jackson EK, *et al.* Effects of indomethacin on systemic and coronary hemodynamics in patients with coronary artery disease. *Am Heart J* 1985; **110**: 311–18.

66. Husted SE, Kraemmer-Nielsen H, Krusell LR, Faergeman O. Acetylsalicylic acid 100 mg and 1000 mg daily in acute myocardial infarction suspects: a placebo-controlled trial. *J Intern Med* 1989; **226**: 303–10.

67. Henriksson P, Edhag O, Wennmalm A. Prostacyclin infusion in patients with myocardial infarction. *Br Heart J* 1985; **53**: 173–9.

68. Kiernan FJ, Kluger J, Regnier JC, Rutkowski M, Fieldman A. Epoprostenol sodium (prostacyclin) infusion in acute myocardial infarction. *Br Heart J* 1986; **56**: 428–32.

69. Tsao PS, Lefer AM. Time course and mechanism of endothelial dysfunction in isolated ischemic- and hypoxic-perfused rat hearts. *Am J Physiol* 1990; **259**: H1660–6.
70. Siegfried MR, Ma X-L, Rider T, Lefer AM. Cardioprotective effects of C-87, 3786, an organic NO donor in feline myocardial ischemia–reperfusion injury. *Circulation* 1991; **84** (II): II-620.
71. Woditsch I, Strobach H, Schrör K. Nitric oxide and prostacyclin formation in isolated rabbit hearts during ischemia and reperfusion. *Circulation* 1991; **84** (II): II-276.
72. Simpson PJ, Mitsos SE, Ventura A. Prostacyclin protects ischemic reperfused myocardium in the dog by inhibition of neutrophil activation. *Am Heart J* 1987; **113**: 129–37.
73. Gryglewski RJ, Bieron K, Demdinska-Kiec AM, Kostaka-Trabka E, Zembowicz A. Interaction between prostacyclin and molsidomine in blood cells and plasma. *Adv Prostaglandin Thromboxane Leukotriene Res* 1990; **21**: 655–8.
74. Dietrich JW, Goodson JM, Raisz LG. Stimulation of bone resorption by various prostaglandins in organ culture. *Prostaglandins* 1975; **10**: 231–40.
75. Ueda K, Saito A, Nakano H, et al. Cortical hyperostosis following long-term administration of prostaglandin E_1 in infants with cyanotic congenital heart disease. *J Pediatr* 1980; **97**: 843–6.
76. Jorgenson HR, Svanholm H, Host A. Bone formation induced in an infant by systemic prostaglandin-E_2 administration. *Acta Orthop Scand* 1988; **59**: 464–6.
77. Koshihara Y, Toshikazu A, Riko T. Prostaglandin D_2 stimulated calcification by human osteoblastic cells. *Adv Prostaglandin Thromboxane Leukotriene Res* 1990; **21B**: 847–50.
78. Schulz BG, Beckmann R, Müller B, et al. Cardio- and hemodynamic profile of selective PGD_2-analogues. *Adv Prostaglandin Thromboxane Leukotriene Res* 1990; **21B**: 591–4.

Index